# Problem-Oriented
# Medical Diagnosis

D1072327

# Problem-Oriented Medical Diagnosis

## Fifth Edition

Edited by

**H. Harold Friedman, M.D.**
Clinical Professor of Medicine,
University of Colorado School of
Medicine; Director, Electrocardio-
graphic Laboratory, and Attending
Physician, Rose Medical Center;
Attending Physician, Saint Joseph
Hospital, Denver

Little, Brown and Company
Boston/Toronto/London

Library of Congress Catalog Card No.
91-60593

ISBN 0-316-29387-3

Printed in the United States of America

SEM

To my granddaughter,
Stefanie Anne

# Contents

# Preface

The objective of this fifth edition of *Problem-Oriented Medical Diagnosis* is unchanged from that of the first edition. Briefly, it is to provide a concise but comprehensive, logical, stepwise approach to the diagnosis of medical problems encountered in the everyday practice of adult medicine.

Problem identification begins with a complete history and physical examination. From the information thus obtained, it is possible to select appropriate laboratory procedures that may assist in establishing a diagnosis. Many physicians also order routinely a battery of laboratory tests for screening purposes. The findings of the history, physical examination, and laboratory investigations provide the essential data on which the diagnosis, prognosis, and management of the patient are based.

The problem-oriented medical record devised by Weed has largely supplanted the traditional methods for medical record-keeping. Although the merits of the problem-oriented system may be debated by some, it is hardly disputable that, regardless of the method of record-keeping employed, one of the physician's major responsibilities is to discover all the patient's problems. Such problems may present themselves as symptoms, physical signs, laboratory or radiologic abnormalities, symptom complexes or syndromes, and clinical diagnoses. The subjects selected for discussion in this manual were chosen because they occur frequently or because they are clinically important. In a field as vast as internal medicine, a great deal of selectivity must be exercised to keep the book within reasonable limits.

The problems chosen for consideration are listed as sections within the chapters. To deal with these problems, I have chosen academically oriented physicians who are engaged primarily in the care of patients. It is hoped that their work will give this manual the imprimatur of both authenticity and practicality.

This book is intended for the medical student, the intern, the family practice or internal medicine resident, and the private practitioner, whether a family physician or an internist. It should also be useful to the nurse practitioner and the physician's assistant.

Most textbooks of medicine are organized in terms of diseases rather than patients, and properly so. Such books, however, do not provide the methodology for proceeding from symptoms, signs, or abnormal laboratory findings to the diagnosis of disease. This text, which gives the diagnostic approach to the problems presented, should help to bridge the gap. It is intended to supplement, not to replace, conventional textbooks of medicine.

The book is written primarily in outline form for clarity and conciseness while maintaining a reasonable degree of comprehensiveness. Because individual contributors were permitted some latitude in dealing with the topics assigned to them, the presentations of the various problems are not uniform throughout the book. Most of the authors, however, have used the following format: definition of the entity, consideration of its etiology and significant clinical features, and presentation of a practical diagnostic approach to the problem. Brief interpretations of the relevant laboratory tests also are given. Discussions of pathophysiology, prognosis, and treatment have been omitted, however, not only because they are outside the scope of the book but also because this information is readily available from other sources. For similar reasons, a bibliography is not included.

In this edition, the entire text has been updated and much of it has been revised.

New sections on Sleep Disorders, Chronic Fatigue Syndrome, and Acquired Immunodeficiency Syndrome have been added. Drs. George E. Bokinsky, Henry G. Fieger, Jr., and Kenneth P. Glassman have joined the group of contributing authors.

H. H. F.

# Contributing Authors

**George E. Bokinsky, M.D.**

Associate Professor of Medicine, University of Vermont College of Medicine, Burlington, Vermont; Attending Physician, Maine Medical Center, Portland, Maine

**Walter G. Briney, M.D.**

Clinical Professor of Medicine, University of Colorado School of Medicine; Attending Rheumatologist, Rose Medical Center, Denver

**Robert G. Chapman, M.D.**

Associate Professor of Medicine, University of Colorado School of Medicine; Staff Physician, University Hospital and Veterans Administration Medical Center, Denver

**S. Robert Contiguglia, M.D.**

Associate Clinical Professor of Medicine, University of Colorado School of Medicine; Chairman, Renal Division, Rose Medical Center, Denver

**Paul M. Cox, Jr., M.D.**

Professor of Medicine, University of Vermont College of Medicine, Burlington, Vermont; Chief of Critical Care Medicine, Maine Medical Center, Portland, Maine

**Lane D. Craddock, M.D.**

Clinical Professor of Medicine, University of Colorado School of Medicine; Attending Physician, Rose Medical Center, Denver

**Sidney Duman, M.D.**

Clinical Professor of Medicine, and Associate Clinical Professor of Neurology, University of Colorado School of Medicine; Attending Neurologist, Rose Medical Center, Denver

**William C. Earley, M.D.**

Formerly Associate Clinical Professor of Radiology, University of Colorado School of Medicine; Staff Radiologist, Rose Medical Center, Denver

| | |
|---|---|
| **James H. Ellis, Jr., M.D.** | Clinical Professor of Medicine, University of Colorado School of Medicine; Chief, Division of Pulmonary Medicine, Rose Medical Center, Denver |
| **Henry G. Fieger, Jr., M.D.** | Assistant Clinical Professor of Neurological Surgery, University of Colorado School of Medicine; Attending Neurosurgeon, Saint Joseph Hospital, Denver |
| **Barry W. Frank, M.D.** | Clinical Professor of Medicine, University of Colorado School of Medicine; Chief, Gastrointestinal Laboratory, Saint Joseph Hospital; Attending Physician, Rose Medical Center, Denver |
| **H. Harold Friedman, M.D.** | Clinical Professor of Medicine, University of Colorado School of Medicine; Director, Electrocardiographic Laboratory, and Attending Physician, Rose Medical Center; Attending Physician, Saint Joseph Hospital, Denver |
| **Stanley H. Ginsburg, M.D.** | Associate Clinical Professor of Neurology, University of Colorado School of Medicine; Attending Neurologist, Rose Medical Center, Denver |
| **Kenneth P. Glassman, M.D.** | Assistant Clinical Professor of Medicine, University of Colorado School of Medicine; Attending Rheumatologist, Rose Medical Center, Denver |
| **Arnold Heller, M.D.** | Assistant Clinical Professor of Orthopedic Surgery, University of Colorado School of Medicine; Attending Orthopedic Surgeon, Rose Medical Center, Denver |
| **Gilbert Hermann, M.D.** | Clinical Professor of Surgery, University of Colorado School of Medicine; Attending Surgeon, Rose Medical Center, Denver |
| **Walter A. Huttner, M.D.** | Clinical Professor of Medicine, University of Colorado School of Medicine; Director of Diabetes Treatment Center, and Attending Physician, Rose Medical Center, Denver |
| **Robert C. Jacobs, M.D.** | Associate Clinical Professor of Medicine, University of Colordao School of Medicine; Attending Rheumatologist, Rose Medical Center, Denver |

**Herbert Kaplan, M.D.**

Clinical Professor of Medicine, University of Colorado School of Medicine; Attending Rheumatologist, Rose Medical Center, Denver

**Harvey B. Karsh, M.D.**

Associate Clinical Professor of Medicine, University of Colorado School of Medicine; Attending Physician, Rose Medical Center, Denver

**Fred H. Katz, M.D.**

Clinical Professor of Medicine, University of Colorado School of Medicine; Attending Physician, Rose Medical Center, Denver

**Melvyn H. Klein, M.D.**

Associate Clinical Professor of Medicine, University of Colorado School of Medicine; Attending Physician, Rose Medical Center, Denver

**Andrew Mallory, M.D.**

Clinical Professor of Medicine, University of Colorado School of Medicine; Attending Physician, Rose Medical Center, Denver

**Sunder J. Mehta, M.D.**

Associate Clinical Professor of Medicine, University of Colorado School of Medicine; Attending Physician, Rose Medical Center, Denver

**Jeffrey L. Mishell, M.D.**

Associate Clinical Professor of Medicine, University of Colorado School of Medicine; Attending Physician, Rose Medical Center, Denver

**Kenneth H. Neldner, M.D.**

Professor and Chairman, Department of Dermatology, Texas Tech University Health Sciences Center School of Medicine, Lubbock, Texas

**Jerome S. Nosanchuk, M.D.**

Adjunct Professor of Clinical Pathology and Pathology, New York State School of Veterinary Medicine, Ithaca, and Cornell University Medical College, New York; Director of Laboratories, Tompkins Community Hospital, Ithaca, New York

**Stanley B. Reich, M.D.**

Vice Chairman and Professor, Department of Radiology, University of California, Davis, School of Medicine, Davis; Chairman of Radiology, Veterans Administration Medical Center, Martinez, California

**John C. Riley, M.D.**

Radiologist, Porter Hospital and Swedish Hospital, Englewood, Colorado

**David H. Rubinstein, M.D.**

Assistant Clinical Professor of Psychiatry, University of Colorado School of Medicine, Denver; Medical Director, Columbine Psychiatric Center, Littleton, Colorado

**John H. Saiki, M.D.**

Professor of Medicine, University of New Mexico School of Medicine, Albuquerque

**Janet E. Schemmel, M.D.**

Clinical Professor of Medicine, University of Colorado School of Medicine; Attending Physician, Saint Joseph Hospital and Rose Medical Center, Denver

**Marvin I. Schwarz, M.D.**

Professor of Medicine, and Head, Division of Pulmonary Sciences, University of Colorado School of Medicine, Denver

**David Shander, M.D.**

Associate Clinical Professor of Medicine, University of Colorado School of Medicine; Attending Physician, Rose Medical Center, Denver

**N. Balfour Slonim, M.D., Ph.D.**

Director, Cardiopulmonary Laboratory, and Staff Physician, Department of Medicine, Rose Medical Center, Denver

**Charley J. Smyth, M.D., M.S.D.**

Clinical Professor of Medicine, University of Colorado School of Medicine, Denver

**Joseph C. Tyor, M.D.**

Associate Clinical Professor of Medicine, University of Colorado School of Medicine; Attending Physician, Rose Medical Center, Denver

**Alan A. Wanderer, M.D.**

Clinical Professor of Pediatrics, University of Colorado School of Medicine; Clinical Staff Physician, Department of Allergy and Immunology, National Jewish Hospital, Denver

**Phillip S. Wolf, M.D.**

Professor of Medicine, University of Colorado School of Medicine; Chief of Cardiology, University Hospital, Denver

# Problem-Oriented
# Medical Diagnosis

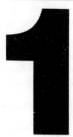

# General Problems

## EDEMA
H. Harold Friedman

### Definition

Edema is an increase in the volume of interstitial fluid (i.e., the extravascular portion of the extracellular compartment). The plasma volume may or may not be increased.

### Diagnosis

There may be a considerable increase in the interstitial fluid volume before it is clinically appreciated. The symptoms and signs of edema are unexplained weight gain, tightness of a ring or shoe, puffiness of the face, swollen extremities, enlarged abdominal girth, and persistence of indentation of the skin following pressure.

### Etiology

#### Localized Edema

This term usually refers to edema produced by regional obstruction to venous or lymphatic flow, or both. It is usually limited to one or two limbs. Examples include unilateral lower extremity edema due to deep venous thrombosis or thrombophlebitis, venous insufficiency, popliteal (Baker's) cyst, cellulitis, and trauma. The term is sometimes used to refer to patches of "vascular" edema seen in allergic states.

Hydrothorax and ascites may be localized phenomena or may occur in any generalized edematous state. When such an association is not evident, or if the effusions do not respond to treatment, the involved serous cavity should be tapped and the fluid examined by appropriate means (see Differential Diagnosis of Pleural Effusion, Chapter 4, and Abdominal Distention and Ascites, Chapter 5). Unilateral leg edema may be produced by increased hydrostatic pressure due to deep vein thrombophlebitis, venous insufficiency, or popliteal (Baker's) cysts. It can also be the result of increased capillary permeability from cellulitis or trauma. Local lymphatic obstruction or pelvic neoplasm is sometimes causative.

Bilateral leg edema is usually a manifestation of generalized edema. In some instances, however, it is the result of bilateral venous insufficiency.

### Generalized Edema

The more common causes of generalized edema are listed below.
1. Congestive heart failure.
   a. *Symptoms.* A history of heart disease can usually be obtained. Exertional dyspnea, orthopnea, paroxysmal nocturnal dyspnea, fatigue, weakness, and swelling of the lower extremities are common.
   b. *Signs.* Physical examination usually reveals distended jugular veins, cardiomegaly, bibasilar rales, hepatomegaly, and dependent edema.
   c. *Laboratory findings.* The hemogram is usually normal. Urinalysis may disclose proteinuria (trace to 2 + ). Mild azotemia due to renal hypoperfusion is not unusual.
2. Pericardial disease.
   a. Chronic constrictive pericarditis.
      (1) *Symptoms.* The major symptoms are dyspnea, fatigue, weakness, abdominal distention, and edema.
      (2) *Signs.* The classic findings are markedly elevated venous pressure, often with a deep Y trough and Kussmaul's sign; pulsus paradoxus; a quiet precordium; slight to moderate cardiac enlargement; and absence of significant murmurs.
   b. Pericarditis with effusion.
      (1) *Symptoms.* Chest pain is common but may not be present. Dyspnea, orthopnea, and cough are frequent complaints.
      (2) *Signs.* The area of cardiac dullness is increased. The apical impulse may be impalpable or if present may be located well within the lateral border of cardiac dullness. A pericardial friction rub is often but not always present. When cardiac tamponade occurs, there may be elevated venous pressure, decreased blood pressure with a narrow pulse pressure, pulsus paradoxus, ascites, and edema.
   c. *Laboratory findings.* Chest films and an electrocardiogram are helpful in the diagnosis of pericardial disease. Echocardiography and other procedures may be useful in the diagnosis of pericardial effusion. Hemodynamic studies are important in the evaluation of chronic constrictive pericarditis (see Table 3-15).
3. Liver disease.
   a. *Symptoms.* A history of alcoholism and jaundice may be obtained. Weakness, fatigability, anorexia, and weight loss are common.
   b. *Signs.* Physical examination usually reveals evidence of liver disease: jaundice, spider nevi, palmar erythema, hepatomegaly, sometimes splenomegaly, parotid swelling, gynecomastia, testicular atrophy, and clubbing. Although lower extremity edema is not uncommon, the edema may be limited to the peritoneal cavity (ascites).
   c. *Laboratory findings.* An elevated serum bilirubin level, abnormal liver function tests, and reduced serum albumin level are typical. Urinalysis may reveal proteinuria (0 to 1 + ).
4. Hypoalbuminemic states.
   a. Nephrotic syndrome.
      (1) *Symptoms.* The history may or may not reveal evidence of renal disease or a systemic illness that can produce the nephrotic syndrome (e.g., diabetes mellitus, systemic lupus erythematosus). Constitutional symptoms may be present but are nonspecific.
      (2) *Laboratory findings.* Urinalysis shows marked proteinuria (> 3.5 g in 24 h) and lipiduria. Hypoalbuminemia, hyperlipemia, and hypercholesterolemia are typically present.
   b. Protein-losing enteropathy.
      (1) *Symptoms.* This is a rare disorder that may occur in association with disorders such as chronic inflammatory enterocolonopathies, Ménétrier's disease, and gastric carcinoma. The symptoms are those of the underlying disease.

(2) *Signs.* There are no specific signs.

(3) *Laboratory findings.* Decreased serum albumin level and a normal urinalysis are typical.

c. Malnutrition associated with severe protein deficiency may result in edema.

5. Miscellaneous causes.

   a. Acute nephritic syndrome. This disorder is characterized by oliguria, proteinuria, hematuria, red blood cell casts, hypertension, and edema. Acute poststreptococcal glomerulonephritis is the most common cause of the acute nephritic syndrome.

   b. Idiopathic edema. This condition occurs almost exclusively in premenopausal women. Its etiology is unknown. The characteristic feature of the disorder is excessive weight gain (usually from 4 to 12 lb) from morning to evening when the patient is up and about. Purely cyclic edema is rare, but is sometimes superimposed on the aforementioned pattern.

   c. Myxedema. Patients with hypothyroidism often have puffiness below the eyes and in the pretibial region. At the latter site it may be firm and nonpitting.

   d. Trichinosis. This disease, commonly associated with the ingestion of raw or improperly cooked pork, has as symptoms and signs muscle aches, fever, periorbital edema, and eosinophilia.

   e. Hemiplegia. Unilateral edema in the paralyzed extremity or extremities is a common finding in stroke victims.

   f. Lymphedema.

   g. Filariasis.

---

## Diagnostic Approach

1. As a first step it is essential to determine whether the edema is localized or generalized. This can usually be accomplished by careful attention to the history and physical examination. Once localized edema and its causes have been excluded, it can be assumed that the edema is generalized.

2. The three most common causes of generalized edema are congestive heart failure, liver disease, and the nephrotic syndrome. The diagnosis is usually apparent on clinical grounds in the first two conditions, whereas heavy proteinuria suggests the third.

   a. Congestive heart failure and cardiac tamponade sometimes present a problem in differential diagnosis. The presence of an apical impulse that is displaced downward and to the left and a gallop rhythm are strong evidence in favor of congestive heart failure rather than cardiac tamponade. It is also worth noting that congestive heart failure is so frequently associated with cardiomegaly that a normal cardiac silhouette almost excludes the diagnosis.

   b. Liver disease as the cause of edema is usually evident from the physical examination. Abnormal liver function tests support the diagnosis.

3. When generalized edema is found not to be due to cardiovascular or hepatic disease or to the nephrotic syndrome, consideration must be given to other, less frequent causes.

4. Routine studies in patients with edema should include the following:

   a. CBC.

   b. Urinalysis.

   c. Biochemical screening, including $T_4$ and $T_3$ resin uptake, serum albumin and total protein, serum cholesterol, and liver function tests.

   d. Chest films.

   e. Electrocardiogram.

5. Urinary findings of heavy proteinuria, hematuria, cylindruria, and formed elements in the sediment are generally indicative of renal parenchymal disease (see Renal and Urinary Tract Disorders, Chapter 7).

6. Moderate to heavy proteinuria, with or without hypoalbuminemia, suggests the nephrotic syndrome. Additional studies are necessary to determine its etiology.

7. Hypoalbuminemia without proteinuria requires investigation for malnutrition or protein-losing enteropathy, provided liver disease is excluded.
8. The diagnosis of idiopathic cyclic edema is based on an appropriate clinical setting, the exclusion of other causes, and a positive water-loading test.

## FATIGUE
### H. Harold Friedman

Fatigue is one of the most common symptoms for which patients seek medical attention.

## Definition

Fatigue is a sense of weariness, described by patients variously as exhaustion, tiredness, lack of pep and energy, loss of ambition or interest, low vitality, or a feeling of being "all in." It is often accompanied by a subjective sensation of weakness and a strong desire to rest or sleep.

## Etiology

Fatigue is normal when it is the result of a full day's work or sustained physical activity. It may also be a consequence of a period of prolonged emotional stress or mental strain. In these circumstances, the cause of the fatigue is usually evident to the patient, and he rarely seeks advice because of it. Chronic fatigue, however, is not a normal state. Although chronic fatigue may be due to a physical ailment, it is most often psychogenic in origin. Table 1-1 lists the more common causes of chronic fatigue.

## Diagnostic Approach

### History

1. Much can be learned from the history of a patient with fatigue. Because fatigue is most commonly psychic in origin and the result of anxiety, anger, or chronic conflict, a careful inquiry into the emotional state of the patient and his life situation is warranted. Depressive reactions, also a common cause of fatigue, are often associated with weakness, anorexia, weight loss, apathy, insomnia, withdrawal, lack of a desire to go on, and self-depreciation. The presence of such symptoms should alert the physician to the possibility of serious depression with its attendant risk of suicide. Therapy should be instituted promptly, even before diagnostic studies are completed.
2. Clues to the etiology of fatigue may be found in the analysis of the symptom itself.
   a. Patients with fatigue due to anxiety are typically tired when they go to bed and just as tired when they wake up in the morning. As a general rule the fatigue appears to lessen during the day. Many patients complain that they are "always tired" and that no amount of rest or sleep seems to improve their weariness or give them strength. Inquiry will often disclose that there is considerable variation in the patient's fatigue: at one time he feels exhausted, and at another time—sometimes only a few minutes later—he is full of energy and capable of any task confronting him. Motivation appears to be a large factor in the patient's ability to cope with the situations of everyday life. Headaches and other pains, as well as subjective weakness, commonly accom-

**Table 1-1.** Causes of chronic fatigue

A. Fatigue of psychogenic origin (80% of cases)
   1. Anxiety states
   2. Depression
B. Fatigue of physical origin (20% of cases)
   1. Infectious disease
     a. Febrile states
     b. Tuberculosis
     c. AIDS or AIDS-related complex
   2. Metabolic disorders
     a. Diabetes mellitus
     b. Hypothyroidism
     c. Hyperparathyroidism
     d. Hypopituitarism
     e. Addison's disease
   3. Blood dyscrasias
     a. Anemia
     b. Lymphoma and leukemia
   4. Renal diseases
     a. Acute renal failure
     b. Chronic renal failure
   5. Liver diseases
     a. Acute hepatitis
     b. Chronic hepatitis and cirrhosis
   6. Inflammatory diseases
     a. Connective tissue disease
     b. Inflammatory bowel disease
     c. Sarcoid
   7. Chronic pulmonary disease
   8. Chronic cardiovascular disease
   9. Neoplastic diseases
  10. Chronic fatigue syndrome
  11. Neuromuscular diseases (see Weakness of Neuromuscular Origin, Chapter 10)
  12. Miscellaneous causes
     a. Medications
     b. Alcoholism
     c. Drug abuse

pany the fatigue. The problem of anxiety is considered in detail later in this chapter.

  **b.** Fatigue due to depression follows no set pattern, but is almost invariably accompanied by other stigmata of the depressed state (namely, a persistent mood of sadness coupled with pessimism, cognitive changes, and physiologic disturbances). The problem of depression is discussed in detail later in this chapter.

  **c.** Fatigue due to physical illness, on the other hand, is relieved by decreased activity and by rest and sleep. The patient probably awakens refreshed in the morning, but less than ordinary activity causes fatigue.

  **d.** Denial or minimization of fatigue in a patient who looks tired or is described as being weak or tired by his family usually implies organic disease rather than a psychological disturbance.

### Physical Examination

  **1.** Fatigue per se is not associated with any specific physical findings.
  **2.** The patient who is pale, wan, and sickly in appearance, who looks tired and worn,

and whose face sags and body slumps should be suspected of having organic illness.
3. The facial expression of the depressed patient, once seen, is rarely forgotten.
4. Most physical ailments that cause fatigue can be diagnosed by clinical observation alone.
5. A careful neurologic examination is indicated in all cases.

### Diagnostic Workup

1. The major purpose of the diagnostic workup is to exclude organic disease. To this end, the following procedures are recommended:
   a. CBC.
   b. Sedimentation rate.
   c. Urinalysis.
   d. Biochemical screening.
   e. Thyroid function tests (e.g., TSH; $T_4$; $T_3$ resin uptake or $T_3$ RIA, or both).
   f. Two-hour postprandial glucose or glucose tolerance test.
   g. Chest films.
   h. Electrocardiogram.
   i. HIV serology, if indicated.
   j. ANA.
2. If the initial workup is negative in a patient who is apparently well except for fatigue, usually organic disease can be excluded and no further workup is necessary. The patient should be kept under observation until systemic illness can reasonably be excluded. Patients with fatigue of physical origin sooner or later develop other symptoms or signs. Should these occur, further investigation is warranted.

# CHRONIC FATIGUE SYNDROME
### H. Harold Friedman

The chronic fatigue syndrome is a symptom-complex of unknown etiology that has received considerable attention recently. It is characterized by persistent or recurrent debilitating fatigue in association with other symptoms listed below under Diagnosis. It is found primarily in healthy, heterosexual teenagers and young adults, about three-quarters of whom are women. It has been attributed by some to a persistent mononucleosis infection due to the Epstein-Barr virus. However, this relationship has not been established. The diagnostic value of Epstein-Barr virus serologic tests in patients with the syndrome is doubtful. Treatment is unsatisfactory.

## Diagnosis

According to Holmes and coworkers (*Ann. Int. Med.* 108:387, 1988), to establish the diagnosis, a case of the chronic fatigue syndrome must fulfill major criteria 1 and 2 and the following minor criteria: 6 or more of the 11 symptom criteria and 2 or more of the 3 physical criteria; or 8 or more of the 11 symptom criteria.

### Major Criteria

1. A new onset of persistent or relapsing fatigue not previously present, sufficient to reduce daily activity by 50 percent or more, lasting at least 6 weeks.
2. Exclusion, by appropriate means, of other conditions that could produce similar symptoms, including malignancies, autoimmune diseases, infections, chronic

psychiatric illness, chronic inflammatory disease, neuromuscular disease, endocrine disease, drug dependency or abuse, side effects of medications or toxic substances, and chronic diseases.

## Minor Criteria

1. Mild fever (between 37.5°C and 38.6°C) or chills.
2. Sore throat.
3. Painful cervical or axillary lymph nodes.
4. Unexplained generalized muscle weakness.
5. Muscle discomfort or myalgia.
6. Prolonged (24 hours or more) generalized fatigue after previously tolerated exercise.
7. Generalized headaches unlike previous cephalalgia.
8. Migratory arthralgia without joint swelling or redness.
9. Neuropsychiatric complaints such as photophobia, scotomata, forgetfulness, irritability, confusion, inability to concentrate, difficulty in thinking, or depression.
10. Sleep disturbance (hypersomnia or insomnia).
11. Onset of the main symptom-complex in hours or a few days.

### Physical Criteria

These must be documented by a physician on at least two occasions, at least 1 month apart.
1. Low-grade fever (see Minor Criteria, 1).
2. Nonexudative pharyngitis.
3. Palpable or tender anterior or posterior cervical or axillary nodes (less than 2 cm in diameter).

   The differential diagnosis includes the conditions in Table 1-1. Convential laboratory tests listed in the Diagnostic Workup on page 7 are usually normal.

## FEVER OF UNKNOWN ORIGIN
### H. Harold Friedman

## Definition

Fever of unknown origin (FUO) is defined as continuous fever of at least 3 weeks' duration with daily temperature elevation above 101°F and remaining undiagnosed after 1 week of intensive study in the hospital (Petersdorf and Wallace), or as temperature greater than 100.5°F persisting for at least 3 weeks in patients in whom the history, physical examination, blood count, urinalysis, and chest films fail to indicate the diagnosis (Sheon and Van Ommen). Regardless of which of these criteria is employed, the diagnostic approach to FUO must be individualized for each patient. No hard-and-fast rules can be set, because each patient with cryptic fever presents a unique problem in diagnosis. The requirement of fever of 3 weeks' duration for the diagnosis of FUO is most important because it eliminates from consideration most viral and bacterial infections as well as other self-limited diseases associated with fever.

## Etiology

Most patients with FUO do not have rare diseases but usually suffer from common disorders that are difficult to diagnose because they present atypically. Most recently reported series of FUO reveal that infections comprise about 40 percent of cases; neoplasms (primary or metastatic), 30 percent; connective tissue diseases, 20 percent; and miscellaneous disorders, 10 percent. In approximately 10 percent of cases, the cause is unknown, but long-term follow-up studies in this group have shown that most patients had benign disorders that were simply undiagnosable at the time of the initial investigation. Table 1-2 lists most of the diagnostic entities encountered by Petersdorf and Wallace in several hundred patients with FUO.

## Diagnostic Clues

The type of fever curve, whether intermittent, remittent, or continuous, is of little or no help in the diagnosis of FUO.

### Infections

1. *Tuberculosis* is the most common infectious disease responsible for FUO. It may be disseminated without radiologic evidence of pulmonary involvement, and the tuberculin test may be negative. Funduscopic examination may provide the first suggestion of this disease if choroid tubercles are demonstrable. However, the diagnosis is usually made by smear and culture of gastric aspirates or by demonstrating tubercles in biopsies of the liver, lymph nodes, bone marrow, or pericardium. Sometimes only a therapeutic trial with antituberculotic drugs will establish the correct diagnosis.
2. *Infective endocarditis* may manifest itself initially as FUO, particularly if the patient has received antibiotics in the early stages of the disease. *Atrial myxoma* may mimic endocarditis because it can occur with fever, a heart murmur, and embolic phenomena. Angiocardiography and echocardiography help distinguish between the two.
3. *Urinary tract infections* rarely cause FUO unless associated with intrarenal or perinephric abscess or obstructive uropathy. Rare organisms causing FUO are diagnosed primarily by blood cultures.
4. *Liver abscess and subphrenic abscess* may initially appear as FUO without localized findings. Radioisotope scanning of the liver, CT scans, and ultrasonography are useful, safe procedures in diagnosing these entities. Arteriography may also be helpful in some situations.
5. *Miscellaneous causes of FUO,* in addition to bacterial infections, include some fungal pathogens, parasitic diseases, and such viral infections as infectious mononucleosis, anicteric hepatitis, and acquired immunodeficiency syndrome (AIDS).

### Neoplasms

Most patients with cancer have fever at some time during the course of their illness. The fever may be related to concomitant infection, localized obstruction by the tumor, surgery and postoperative complications, or the neoplasm itself. The diagnosis is most often established by biopsy of the bone marrow, liver, lymph nodes, or tumor masses. Neoplasms that are most frequently associated with fever are Hodgkin's disease, non-Hodgkin's lymphomas, leukemia and preleukemia, hepatoma, and hypernephroma. Carcinoma of the stomach, colon, pancreas, breast, and hepatic metastases are examples of other malignancies that may cause fever.

### Connective Tissue Diseases

It is not unusual for rheumatic fever, systemic lupus erythematosus (SLE), rheumatoid arthritis (particularly the juvenile variety), and polymyalgia rheumatica (temporal arteritis, giant cell arteritis) to present as FUO. On the other hand, scleroderma, dermatomyositis, and polyarteritis nodosa rarely appear in this manner. The clinical history, physical findings, and laboratory tests are more important than biopsy in establishing the diagnosis of connective tissue disease. One exception is temporal artery biopsy, which may establish the diagnosis of polymyalgia rheumatica.

## Miscellaneous Causes

1. Drugs are an important cause of FUO. A careful inquiry must be made in every case of FUO to determine whether the patient is taking any medications, because elimination of the offending agent may solve the problem and eliminate the need for extensive workup.
2. Multiple pulmonary emboli may cause FUO. Lung scans and pulmonary angiography will usually establish the diagnosis.
3. Regional enteritis, granulomatous disease of the colon, and ulcerative colitis may occur as FUO in the absence of abdominal complaints.
4. Patients who have altered immune responses due to disease (e.g., Hodgkin's disease, multiple myeloma) or chemotherapy not infrequently have fever due to infection with organisms unlikely to be found in immunologically competent individuals.

## Diagnostic Approach

1. Check the *history*.
    a. If other members of the family have been affected or are affected by a similar illness, exposure to a common etiologic agent may be involved or the disease may have a hereditary basis (e.g., familial Mediterranean fever).
    b. A past history of episodic illnesses over a period of years involving multiple organ systems suggests the possibility of connective tissue disease.
    c. The occupation of the patient may provide a clue to the cause of FUO. For example, a veterinarian, a butcher, or one engaged in animal husbandry may be suffering from a disease of animal origin.
    d. Inquiry about travel abroad is important because knowledge of the geographic locale where the patient has been may lead to a search for illnesses endemic to that area rather than those commonly found in the United States. For example, among United States military personnel in Vietnam, the causes of FUO have included such diseases as dengue, malaria, chikungunya, scrub typhus, and enteric diseases.
    e. A history of rodent bite during the 10 weeks before the onset of fever should suggest the possibility of rat-bite fever.
2. Rule out *habitual hyperthermia*. This usually occurs in young, psychoneurotic women, and is characterized by afternoon temperatures between 100° and 100.5°F, vague complaints, vasomotor instability, and a normal sedimentation rate. Removal of the patient from her stressful life situation or the administration of tranquilizers, or both, will result in the disappearance of the fever.
3. Rule out *factitious fever* (malingering). Clues to the diagnosis are a history of medical or paramedical training, complicated and inconsistent histories, absence of weight loss, the failure of the temperature curve to follow the normal diurnal cycle, excessively high temperatures (106° or 107°F, which is rare in adults), normal pulse and respiratory rates at the time of fever, and rapid defervescence unaccompanied by diaphoresis. If malingering is suspected, all temperatures should be taken by a nurse with a carefully checked thermometer, and the patient should be carefully observed throughout the procedure.
4. Perform careful and repeated complete *physical examinations*.
    a. Pay particular attention to the eyes, because ocular manifestations of sys-

**Table 1-2.** Common disease entities responsible for fever of unknown origin

I. Neoplastic diseases
  A. Tumors of reticuloendothelial system
    1. Leukemia
    2. Lymphoma, Hodgkin's disease
    3. Multiple myeloma (rare)
  B. Metastatic tumors
    1. From gastrointestinal tract
    2. From lung, kidney, bone
    3. Melanoma
  C. Solid localized tumors
    1. Kidney
    2. Liver
    3. Lung
    4. Pancreas
    5. Atrial myxoma
II. Infections
  A. Granulomatous infections
    1. Tuberculosis
    2. Coccidioidomycosis
    3. Histoplasmosis
    4. Actinomycosis
    5. Nocardiosis
  B. Pyogenic infections
    1. Right upper quadrant infections
      a. Cholangitis
      b. Cholecystitis (stone)
      c. Liver abscess
      d. Subphrenic abscess
      e. Subhepatic abscess
      f. Lesser sac abscess
    2. Abscesses secondary to bowel diseases
      a. Diverticulitis
      b. Appendicitis

II. Infections (continued)
  D. Other bacteremias
    1. Meningococcemia
    2. Gonococcemia
    3. Vibriosis
    4. Listeriosis
    5. Brucellosis
  E. Miscellaneous
    1. Malaria
    2. Infectious mononucleosis
    3. Cytomegalovirus disease
    4. Coxsackie B diseases
    5. Amebiasis
    6. Leptospirosis
    7. Trichinosis
    8. Q fever
    9. Acquired immunodeficiency syndrome (AIDS)
III. Connective tissue diseases
  A. Rheumatic fever
  B. Disseminated lupus erythematosus
  C. Rheumatoid arthritis
  D. Giant cell arteritis (temporal arteritis, polymyalgia rheumatica)
  E. Rare
    1. Scleroderma
    2. Dermatomyositis
    3. Polyarteritis nodosa
IV. Unclassified
  A. Drug fever
  B. Multiple pulmonary emboli
  C. Thyroiditis
  D. Sarcoidosis
  E. Hemolytic anemia
  F. Cryptic trauma

3. Pelvic inflammatory disease
4. Renal infections
   a. Pyelonephritis (rare)
   b. Perinephric abscess
   c. Intrarenal abscess
   d. Ureteral obstruction with infection
C. Subacute bacterial endocarditis

       G. Regional enteritis
       H. Granulomatous hepatitis
   V. Psychogenic fevers
       A. Habitual hyperthermia
       B. Factitious fever
   VI. Periodic fevers
       A. Familial Mediterranean fever
       B. Etiocholanolone fever
   VII. Undiagnosed fever of unknown origin

Source: Modified from R. G. Petersdorf and J. F. Wallace. Fever of Unknown Origin. In J. A. Barondess (ed.), *Diagnostic Approaches to Presenting Syndromes.* Baltimore: Williams & Wilkins, 1971. P. 305.

temic disease may provide the first clue to the diagnosis of obscure fever. An ophthalmologist may be of great help in interpreting ocular findings.

**b.** Examine carefully for lymphadenopathy, particularly in the area about the clavicles.

**c.** Hepatosplenomegaly occurs more frequently in neoplastic than in infectious diseases, and especially in the lymphomas.

**d.** Listen for bruits, which may provide evidence for malignant vascular tumors.

**e.** Check for sternal and bony tenderness, which may suggest myeloproliferative disease or metastatic tumor.

**f.** Check the navel, because intraabdominal neoplasms may metastasize early to the navel, where the presence is readily detected by palpation. Moreover, such metastases are easily biopsied under local anesthesia.

**g.** Examine the skin for nodules that also may represent the earliest manifestation of metastatic malignancy.

**h.** Rectal examination and proctosigmoidoscopy are indicated in all patients with FUO.

5. When there are symptoms or signs other than chills, fever, malaise, or weight loss (e.g., lethargy, disorientation, meningismus, rash, dyspnea, cough, cardiac murmurs, jaundice, visceromegaly, lymphadenopathy, dysuria or hematuria, arthritis or other joint manifestations, abdominal pain, nausea, vomiting, diarrhea), the initial investigation should be directed at those organ systems most likely to be the source of the FUO.

Depending on circumstances, perform most or all of the following laboratory tests. It may be necessary to do these tests serially. Surgical procedures, with the exception of easily performed biopsies, should be considered only after routine studies have failed to reveal the sources of FUO.

**a.** Routine laboratory tests.
   **(1)** CBC.
   **(2)** Sedimentation rate.
   **(3)** Urinalysis, and urine culture and sensitivity studies.
   **(4)** Stools for ova, parasites, occult blood, culture, and sensitivity studies.
   **(5)** Blood cultures: Take at least three sets of paired cultures from different sites. All specimens should be cultured aerobically and anaerobically and retained for several weeks.
   **(6)** Blood smears for malaria parasites if exposure to this disease within the previous year is possible.

**b.** Serologic tests.
   **(1)** Febrile agglutinins (rarely of help).
   **(2)** ASO and antistreptozyme titers to help in the diagnosis of rheumatic fever.
   **(3)** Rheumatoid factor.
   **(4)** ANA titer.
   **(5)** Mono test, heterophil agglutination, and Epstein-Barr antibody titer.
   **(6)** CEA.
   **(7)** Cytomegalovirus titer.
   **(8)** HIV antibody test.

**c.** Blood chemistries.
   **(1)** Biochemical screening and thyroid function tests.
   **(2)** Serum protein electrophoresis and immunoglobulins.

**d.** Miscellaneous tests.
   **(1)** Bone marrow core biopsy (not aspiration alone) and culture.
   **(2)** Gastric aspirate for acid-fast smear and culture.

**e.** Skin tests. Tuberculin, histoplasmin, coccidioidin, and possibly others, depending on circumstances.

**f.** Radiographic procedures.
   **(1)** Chest films.
   **(2)** IVP.
   **(3)** Barium enema and upper GI series, including small bowel study.

**(4)** Bone films to detect infection or neoplastic disease.

**(5)** Computerized tomography for suspected intraabdominal or retroperitoneal disease.

**g.** Ultrasonography, also for suspected intraabdominal and retroperitoneal lesions.

**h.** Radioisotope scanning procedures.

**(1)** Lung scan to detect pulmonary embolism.

**(2)** Liver scan to detect hepatic lesions.

**(3)** Bone scans to detect neoplastic disease.

**(4)** Gallium scan to detect occult infection.

**i.** Tissue examination.

**(1)** Biopsy of lymph nodes or readily accessible tumor masses.

**(2)** Needle biopsy of the liver, which often reveals the diagnosis if there is hepatic involvement.

**(3)** Biopsy of the skin and skeletal muscle in suspected connective tissue disease. (Usually this procedure is not very helpful.)

**(4)** Biopsy of the temporal artery in suspected polymyalgia rheumatica, which may establish the diagnosis.

**j.** Angiographic studies.

**(1)** Lymphangiography to detect lymphomas.

**(2)** Celiac aortography to detect hepatic, renal, and pancreatic tumors.

**(3)** Angiocardiography to detect atrial myxoma.

**(4)** Pulmonary angiography to detect pulmonary embolism.

**k.** Surgical procedures.

**(1)** Peritoneoscopy may be useful in detecting tuberculous peritonitis, peritoneal carcinomatosis, cholecystitis, and pelvic inflammatory disease.

**(2)** Exploratory laparotomy should not be done in FUO unless all noninvasive techniques have been exhausted and only if the clinical picture, roentgenographic studies, or laboratory findings point to the abdomen as the source of the fever.

**(3)** Bronchoscopy, bronchial brushing, culture, cytologic studies, and transbronchial biopsy should be done, and rarely, exploratory thoracotomy in the presence of unidentified pulmonary disease.

**l.** Therapeutic trials should be employed only as a last resort and only if they are reasonably specific. Shotgun mixtures of antibiotics, steroids, and other drugs are to be condemned because they usually solve nothing, confuse the clinical picture, and are not without hazard. Examples of more or less specific therapeutic trials include antituberculotic drugs for suspected tuberculosis; aspirin for rheumatic fever; heparin and anticoagulant therapy for pulmonary emboli; steroids for polymyalgia rheumatica, rheumatoid arthritis, or SLE; and penicillin and streptomycin for suspected bacterial endocarditis.

## UNEXPLAINED WEIGHT LOSS
### Harvey B. Karsh

Weight loss is often an early manifestation of many acute or chronic illnesses. It may occur in a broad spectrum of conditions, including endocrine or metabolic diseases, drug intoxication, neoplastic processes, and psychiatric disorders.

## History

Special attention should be focused on the following:

1. Documentation that weight loss has actually occurred.
2. An increased or decreased appetite.
3. The composition of the diet and the eating habits of the patient.

4. The presence of any gastrointestinal symptoms, regardless of how vague they might be.
5. A complete social and psychiatric history to elicit sources of anxiety, fear, and depression, or special situational problems.

## Weight Loss with Increased Appetite

Weight loss in spite of an increased appetite suggests the possibility of diabetes or hyperthyroidism.

## Conditions Associated with Accelerated Metabolism and Weight Loss

1. Neoplasms. Unexplained weight loss in middle-aged or elderly persons should suggest the possibility of occult malignancy. Neoplasms produce weight loss by increasing the metabolic processes of the host even in the absence of complicating anatomic, endocrine, or metabolic abnormalities.
2. Fever. Infections, neoplasms, cerebrovascular accidents, and metabolic disorders may be accompanied by fever. Because the basal metabolic rate increases by 7 percent with each degree of temperature rise, fever by itself can cause weight loss. Moreover, the anorexia, dehydration, and increased protein catabolism that commonly accompany any febrile illness may also contribute to the weight loss. Fever of unknown origin is discussed in the preceding section.
3. Congestive heart failure.
4. Chronic infections.
5. Excessive physical activity.
6. Periods of rapid growth.

## Conditions Primarily Associated with Anorexia or Decreased Food Intake

### Psychogenic Disorders

1. Anxiety and depression are among the most common causes of weight loss. The importance of psychological and emotional problems as causes of weight loss should not be underestimated. Depression, anxiety, hysteria, or serious psychosis may cause an unnoticed but nevertheless significant decrease in food intake. Correct diagnosis requires a thorough psychiatric and social history.
2. Anorexia nervosa.
   a. *Definition.* Anorexia nervosa is a psychogenic disorder characterized by loss of appetite and refusal to eat. It occurs predominantly in young women between 11 and 35 years of age.
   b. Signs and symptoms.
      (1) Weight loss occurs, varying from 10 to 50 percent of the premorbid weight.
      (2) Spontaneous or deliberate vomiting is a common occurrence.
      (3) Overactivity is usual and is out of proportion to the degree of cachexia.
      (4) Diarrhea may result from laxative abuse.
      (5) The patient may sleep poorly but awaken refreshed (unlike the depressed individual, who is always tired).
      (6) Acrocyanosis is often observed.
      (7) Pubic and axillary hair growth is normal.

**(8)** Bradycardia and hypotension occur commonly.
**(9)** Because of malnutrition, gonadal function is diminished. Decreased urinary estrogens, absence of cornified cells on vaginal smears, and low urinary gonadotropins are common findings. Urinary 17-ketosteroids may also be decreased. However, the plasma cortisol levels are normal, a finding that helps to differentiate anorexia nervosa from panhypopituitarism. Thyroid function is normal.

## Dietary Causes

With few exceptions, malnutrition is rare in the United States. However, the possibility of nutritional deficiencies should be considered in drug addicts, alcoholics, poor people, elderly people (particularly those living alone), and food faddists. Physicians, in the treatment of certain diseases by special diets, may sometimes inadvertently prescribe nutritionally deficient diets and thereby initiate or perpetuate weight loss.

## Affections of the Mouth and Pharynx

1. Mechanical. Ill-fitting dentures or a lack of dentures may so interfere with mastication that the quantity and quality of the food eaten is substandard.
2. Neurologic lesions. Neurologic disorders that affect the ability to chew or swallow food can result in an insufficient caloric intake and weight loss. Included in this group of diseases are such conditions as muscular dystrophy, strokes, amyotrophic lateral sclerosis, brainstem lesions, and syringomyelia.
3. Painful oral lesions.
   a. Nutritional diseases, including vitamin deficiencies.
   b. Painful lesions of the oropharynx due to connective tissue disease or other diseases.
   c. Candidiasis, which is often associated with the use of antibiotics.
   d. Gingivitis due to diphenylhydantoin or other drugs.
   e. Heavy-metal intoxication.

## Drug Effects

Drugs may cause weight loss as a by-product of their actions. Thus, digitalis and the amphetamines may cause anorexia. Drugs may induce anorexia, nausea, and vomiting by a direct effect on the gastrointestinal mucosa. Laxative abuse may result in malassimilation of necessary nutrients. Finally, some drugs may produce nutritional deficiencies, which in turn can cause anorexia, decreased food intake, and weight loss.

## Anorexia and Weight Loss as Symptoms

Anorexia and weight loss may be early or prominent symptoms in the following disorders:
1. Infectious diseases (e.g., tuberculosis).
2. Metabolic disorders.
   a. Hypopituitarism.
   b. Hyperthyroidism.
   c. Addison's disease.
3. Blood dyscrasias.
   a. Pernicious and other anemias.
   b. Lymphoma and leukemia.
4. Renal disease.
5. Liver disease.
   a. Acute hepatitis.
   b. Chronic hepatitis and cirrhosis.

6. Malabsorptive states (see Diarrhea, Chapter 5).
7. Malignancy.
   a. Carcinoma of the stomach.
   b. Carcinoma of the pancreas.
   c. Carcinoma of the colon.
   d. Other neoplasms.
8. AIDS

## Diagnostic Approach

1. It is manifestly impossible to investigate every possible cause of unexplained weight loss. Clues to the diagnostic approach should be sought in the history and physical examination.
2. When no obvious cause for weight loss can be discovered and when psychogenic disorders can be excluded, the initial workup should include, as a minimum, the following tests:
   a. CBC.
   b. Sedimentation rate.
   c. Urinalysis.
   d. Biochemical screening, serum electrolytes, and $T_4$ and $T_3$ resin uptake.
   e. Two-hour postprandial glucose or glucose tolerance test.
   f. Stools for occult blood, ova, and parasites.
   g. Chest films.
3. If the initial studies are unrevealing, further investigation is warranted in any patient who continues to lose weight without an adequate explanation. Consideration should be given to at least some of the following tests or procedures:
   a. Skin tests (e.g., tuberculin, histoplasmin).
   b. Serologic tests (syphilis, RA, LE, and ANA).
   c. Serum protein electrophoresis and immunoglobulins.
   d. X-ray studies (intravenous pyelography, complete GI series, bone survey).
   e. Tests to rule out endocrinopathies (e.g., Addison's disease, hypopituitarism).
   f. Tissue biopsy (bone marrow, liver, skin, and muscle).
   g. Radioisotope scanning procedures.
   h. Angiographic studies.
   i. Computerized tomography and ultrasonography when considered appropriate.
   j. HIV serology, if indicated.
4. In the elderly, unexplained weight loss is often multifactorial. Socioeconomic factors, such as loneliness and isolation, may lead to poor eating habits and malnutrition. Dementia, delirium, depression, drug reactions, and the presence of chronic diseases may be important etiologic factors.
5. Patients with unexplained weight loss should be kept under observation until systemic illness can be excluded. If the weight loss is due to physical causes, other symptoms and signs almost invariably develop over a period of time. As these occur, additional diagnostic studies should be undertaken.

## ANXIETY STATES
David H. Rubinstein

## Definition

*Anxiety* is a subjective feeling of apprehension, uneasiness, tension, or terror in response to danger. Anxiety should be distinguished from *fear,* which is an emotional reaction to a bona fide threatening situation. *Nervousness* and *worry* are terms commonly used by patients to describe anxiety.

*Phobic disorders* are characterized by the avoidance of certain situations that precipitate the symptoms of anxiety. There is a secondary constriction of normal life's activities that limit the individual's ability to function.

*Anxiety neurosis* is a chronic illness characterized by recurrent episodes of acute anxiety, often described as panic attacks.

*Generalized anxiety disorder* refers to persistent anxiety, worry, fears, ruminations, and anticipation of misfortune and has been continuous rather than intermittent.

## Etiology

Anxiety is probably the most common complaint encountered in practice. Similarly, anxiety neurosis is the most common neurotic syndrome seen clinically. Both anxiety and anxiety neurosis may accompany or be associated with almost any illness.

An anxiety state may be a component of other, sometimes more serious disorders, such as those listed below.

1. Psychiatric disorders (e.g., schizophrenia, depressive illness).
2. Disease of the central nervous system (e.g., postconcussion syndrome, vascular disease, degenerative disorders, seizures).
3. Endocrine and metabolic disorders (e.g., hyperthyroidism and hypothyroidism, hyperparathyroidism and hypoparathyroidism, hyperadrenocorticism, hypoglycemia, pheochromocytoma).
4. Drug effects (e.g., sympathomimetic agents, corticosteroids, alcohol).
5. Drug withdrawal syndromes (e.g., alcohol, barbiturates).
6. Miscellaneous conditions.
   a. Menopause
   b. Mitral valve prolapse (click-murmur syndrome).
   c. Porphyria.

## Clinical Features

### Anxiety

1. Subjective symptoms of apprehension, worry, difficulty in concentration, insomnia, irritability, "nervousness," and panicky feelings.
2. Somatic complaints such as giddiness, shakiness, restlessness, trembling, fatigability, cold clammy hands, dry-mouth, dizziness, lightheadedness, tingling in hands or feet, frequent urination, nausea, stomach upset, diarrhea, symptoms of the hyperventilation syndrome, palpitations, tightness in the chest, chest pain, and muscle aches.

### Phobic Disorders

1. Agoraphobia is the most common phobic disorder found in women. Agoraphobic individuals avoid being alone in public places, particularly supermarkets, public highways, tunnels, and bridges, or other situations where they must be confined or have to wait. They often fear that they will lose control or will die. As a result, they may become housebound.
2. Episodes of panic may accompany phobic disorders.

### Characteristics of Anxiety Disorders

1. Studies indicate that 10 to 20 percent of patients treated by general practitioners suffer primarily from symptoms related to functional anxiety. Anxiety disorders

affect women twice as frequently as men. The onset is usually during adolescence or early adult life. It seldom begins after the age of 35. Chronically anxious individuals in older age groups frequently experience an exacerbation of symptoms as they become physically incapacitated and helpless.

2. Anxiety has a persistent and fluctuating course. Ten to 12 percent of patients recover spontaneously. Fifteen percent deteriorate and experience substantial disability as a result of their symptoms, and the remainder are evenly divided between those who are symptomatic with mild disability, and those who are symptomatic without disability. Individuals who medicate themselves with alcohol or other substances clearly fare more poorly.

3. Unhappiness, depression, and demoralization are common in patients who experience anxiety. Anxiety is a debilitating symptom that causes one to feel that one is not in control of one's life and severely limits its forward progression.

4. Episodes of acute anxiety typically have an abrupt onset. There is a sense of foreboding, fear, and apprehension; a sensation of panic; and often a feeling of being seriously ill or that one's life is threatened. Some patients experience feelings of depersonalization. Symptoms such as labored breathing, smothering, palpitation, blurred vision, tremulousness, and weakness frequently accompany the apprehension and foreboding. The hyperventilation syndrome with tachypnea, breathlessness, circumoral paresthesias, numbness and tingling of the fingers and toes, and even carpopedal spasm is a common feature. Objective signs of distress such as tachycardia, sweating, tachypnea, tremor, hyperactive deep tendon reflexes, and dilated pupils may be seen. The frequency of attacks and their severity vary considerably from one patient to another. Episodes of anxiety usually terminate spontaneously.

5. Although most patients commonly have cardiorespiratory complaints, others suffer from the manifestations of a functional bowel syndrome. In fact, anxiety neurosis is the psychiatric disorder most commonly associated with this syndrome. However, functional enterocolonopathies may occur during the course of other psychiatric illnesses such as hysteria or depression.

6. Complications are seen far less frequently than in other psychiatric disorders. Judgment is not impaired. Suicide is a rare occurrence.

## Diagnostic Approach

1. The diagnosis of anxiety or anxiety neurosis can usually be established from the patient's history. The symptomatology is usually characteristic. Drug use and abuse should be excluded as possible causes of anxiety states. It is also important to be certain that anxiety is not a component of a more serious medical or psychiatric disorder and to be aware that it may coexist with such conditions.

2. A complete physical and neurologic examination is warranted to provide clues to the possible presence of central nervous system disease, endocrine disorders, cardiovascular disease, or other ailments.

3. The mental status should be evaluated in all patients with anxiety, to confirm the presence or absence of an underlying psychiatric disorder.

4. In addition to the physical, neurologic, and mental examinations, some diagnostic workup is probably indicated, if only to reassure patients that their symptomatology is not organic in origin. The procedures chosen depend on circumstances and, to some extent, on the symptomatology. Some or all of the following tests may be justified:
   a. CBC.
   b. Urinalysis.
   c. Biochemical screening.
   d. Thyroid function tests when thyroid dysfunction merits consideration.
   e. A 5-hour glucose tolerance test, if the symptoms are suggestive of hypoglycemia.

**f.** Urinary vanillylmandelic acid (VMA) determination to screen for pheochromocytoma in hypertensive patients with paroxysms of headaches, blurred vision, sweating, trembling, and pallor.

**g.** Chest films, an electrocardiogram, and possibly a treadmill study in suspected cardiac disease, especially when chest pain is a predominant symptom. Holter monitoring may be useful in determining whether or not palpitation is due to cardiac arrhythmia.

**h.** GI workup in patients with gastrointestinal somatization.

## DEPRESSION AND MANIA
David H. Rubinstein

### Definition

*Depression* is "exaggerated sadness coupled with pessimism." Pessimism is the essential feature that distinguishes depression from the ordinary "blues" or feelings of dejection that everyone experiences from time to time. Depression varies greatly in intensity, from mild dejection to profound despair, but characteristically involves a degree of sadness or pessimism, or both, that is out of keeping with life circumstances.

Grief, unlike depression, is a reaction to a real loss. The most significant loss that humans can sustain is the death of a spouse, close relative, or friend. Normal acute grief lasts 4 to 6 weeks and involves marked sadness, crying spells, preoccupation with the deceased (including feelings of anger and guilt), and a reduced interest in external affairs. The entire process usually occurs over a period of months. Delayed grief may occur months or years after the loss, sometimes on the anniversary of the death or loss.

Mania is characterized by an elevated, expansive, or irritable mood associated with hyperactivity, overinvolvement in activities, diminished need for sleep, pressured speech, and a flight of ideas. An exaggerated sense of well-being is usually present.

### Classification

There still does not exist an agreed-on method of classifying affective (mood) disorders. In the past, depressions were classified as endogenous or exogenous (reactive) depending on whether a precipitant could be identified. Another classification system distinguished neurotic depression, which was mild with no evidence of loss of reality testing, from psychotic depression, which was severe and included a depressed mood and signs and symptoms of depression, as well as loss of reality testing (e.g., hallucinations or delusions). However, the distinction between neurotic and psychotic depressive reactions was often difficult. In yet another dichotomy, agitated depression referred to disorders characterized by a great increase in movement, restlessness, and anxiety, whereas retarded depressions were characterized by a decrease in psychomotor activity, as well as a great deal of lethargy and hypersomnia. The following classification system has been found to be clinically useful:

**1.** A *major affective disorder* is a disorder of mood, found in individuals who have not had other psychiatric disorders, in which depression or mania is the predominant problem.

**a.** *Bipolar disorder—mixed type* has a tendency to recur, and there may be alterations in mood from depressive to manic or repeated episodes of mania. This is also referred to as the circular cyclothymic type of manic-depressive illness. The first manic episode of bipolar illness is likely to start before the age of 30. The first depressive episode may start at any age. Bipolar illness is more likely to occur in females and is likely to be familial. There is also a high incidence of alcoholism associated with bipolar illness. Those patients who are manic or have mania are classified as bipolar.

   **b.** *Bipolar disorder—manic type* and *bipolar disorder—depressed type* are disorders limited to a single or repeated episodes of mania or depression. Unipolar depressive illness may occur for the first time in the postpartum period. Depression that occurs for the first time in middle age or later is often referred to as involutional depression. Involutional melancholia refers to a specific entity that occurs in the elderly and is characterized by agitation, anxiety, delusional thinking of a dramatic nature (e.g., "I'm rotting"), obsessional concern with past misdeeds, and occasional delusions of a paranoid nature.

**2.** A *secondary affective disorder* is a disorder of mood that occurs in patients with a preexisting psychiatric illness other than depression or mania (e.g., the depression encountered in schizophrenia).

## Clinical Features of Depression

Depression is a clinical syndrome. The diagnosis should be suspected when patients exhibit the following:

**1.** A persistent mood of sadness, apathy, or irritability.

**2.** Feelings of unworthiness, hopelessness, guilt, suicidal thoughts, problems with memory, and concentration.

**3.** Physiologic or vegetative disturbances (e.g., anorexia, weight loss, sleep disturbances, fatigue, psychomotor retardation, emotional withdrawal and blunting).

   Depression may simulate, precede, accompany, or follow physical illness. Most depressed medical and surgical patients suffer from neurotic or reactive depressions. The incidence of depression is high in gastrointestinal disorders such as functional bowel syndrome, colitis, regional enteritis, hepatitis, cirrhosis, pancreatitis, and carcinoma of the pancreas. Depression is common in obesity, especially following weight reduction programs. Depression is particularly common in myocardial infarction and following cardiac surgery. Clinical depression may occur in any central nervous system disease, but most commonly in subdural hematoma, frontal lobe tumor, and chronic neuralgic illness such as multiple sclerosis or parkinsonism. It frequently accompanies Alzheimer's and Pick's disease. Depressive symptoms may simulate or coexist with metabolic or endocrine disorders. Diseases in this group include hypothyroidism, adrenal insufficiency, Cushing's syndrome, acromegaly, hyperparathyroidism, hyponatremia, hypocalcemia, and hypomagnesemia. Chronic drug abuse (e.g., barbiturates, opiates, bromides, tranquilizers) may produce depression. Prescribed drugs, such as reserpine, methyldopa, propranolol, L-dopa, steroids, and digitalis, also can cause depression. Systemic diseases associated with depression include connective tissue disease, lymphomas, rheumatoid arthritis, carcinoma of the lung, and disseminated carcinomatosis.

**4.** Cognitive changes, problems with memory and concentration, cognitive slowing.

### Subjective Symptoms

**1.** Apathy, lack of energy, tiredness.

**2.** Feeling sad or blue.

**3.** Crying spells.

**4.** Sleep disturbances, such as difficulty in falling asleep, early morning waking, and sometimes, hypersomnia.

**5.** Appetite disturbance (anorexia, hyperphagia).

**6.** Weight loss.

**7.** Constipation.

8. Diurnal variations in mood, typically worse in the morning with improvement as the day goes on.
9. Decreased sexual interest.
10. Loss of ability to enjoy things, loss of sense of humor.

### Objective Findings

1. Sadness, tearfulness, irritability.
2. Expressions of hopelessness, helplessness, guilt, and self-reproach.
3. Psychomotor retardation.
4. Inattention to personal hygiene, emotional withdrawal or blunting.
5. Difficulty in thinking and concentrating; problems with memory, including decreased retention or recall of past events; decreased attention span, ability to concentrate.
6. Auditory hallucinations sometimes present.
7. Delusions sometimes present, such as somatic or nihilistic delusions or delusions of sin and punishment, worthlessness, and poverty.
8. Suicidal intent or ideation; expressed wish to be dead or fear of dying, wish for things to be over or to escape from life.

## Clinical Features of Mania

### Subjective Symptoms

1. Marked optimism; inappropriate enthusiasm or altruism, or both.
2. Feelings of unmitigated power, energy, hypersexuality.
3. Feeling "entitled," or angry, and resentful toward those who try to set limits or oppose them.

### Objective Findings

1. Euphoria or expansive mood.
2. Excessive or inappropriate activity.
3. Pressured speech with rapid shifting of ideas.
4. Markedly social behavior often accompanied by inappropriate interactions with strangers, particularly in a person for whom this represents a significant change.
5. Poor judgment and impulsive behavior in business matters. Engaging in buying sprees.
6. Sexual promiscuity.
7. Delusions of grandeur or special powers; religious preoccupations.
8. Denial of the need for sleep.
9. Marked irritability, anger, and refusal to acknowledge that the behavior has changed or is abnormal.
   Mania may be associated with organic disease or drug-induced problems. Neurologic disease (e.g., multiple sclerosis) or endocrine disorders may mimic a manic episode. Amphetamines, methylphenidate, and scopolamine may also cause reactions that mimic mania.

## Diagnostic Approach

1. The history-taking and physical examination are directed at establishing the criteria for the diagnosis of depression and mania (i.e., disordered mood, cognitive changes, and physiologic disturbances, as outlined earlier in this section).
2. History. Inquiry should be made concerning the following:
   a. Past or present medical and psychiatric illness.

    **b.** Current medications, including over-the-counter and street drugs that may be responsible for a depressed or euphoric state.

    **c.** Alcoholism and drug abuse. Many patients resort to alcohol or drugs for relief from depression or mania. The risk of suicide is high among alcohol users.

    **d.** A family history of depression, nervous breakdown, highs, euphoria, and hyperactivity. The last three are associated with bipolar affective illness, which has been shown to have a genetic basis.

    **e.** A history of losses—death, divorce, separations from parents, children, siblings, lovers.

**3.** Physical examination is directed at a search for the stigmata of depression and mania and at detecting the presence or absence of organic disease. A careful neurologic examination and an evaluation of the mental status should be performed.

**4.** Workup. The major purposes of the diagnostic workup are to exclude organic illness as a cause of depression or mania and to determine the existence of organic disease that depression or mania may simulate, precede, accompany, or follow. The following guideline is suggested:

    **a.** CBC.

    **b.** Urinalysis.

    **c.** Biochemical screening.

    **d.** Serum electrolytes when indicated.

    **e.** Thyroid function tests when thyroid dysfunction is under consideration.

    **f.** Chest films.

    **g.** Electrocardiogram.

    **h.** GI workup when gastrointestinal symptoms need evaluation.

**5.** Depression should also be considered a diagnostic possibility under the following circumstances:

    **a.** Symptoms and signs that remain unexplained in spite of a complete workup.

    **b.** Symptoms and signs that do not respond to conventional treatment.

    **c.** Multitudinous complaints involving many organ systems for which no obvious cause is demonstrable.

    **d.** Unexplained chronic fatigue and lack of energy.

    **e.** Excessive weight loss or gain.

    **f.** Chronic alcoholism and drug abuse.

    **g.** Decline in sexual interest and performance.

**6.** A dexamethasone suppression test (DST) may help clarify the diagnosis of depression. One mg of dexamethasone is administered at 11:00 P.M. Samples of plasma are collected at 8:00 A.M., 4:00 P.M., and 11:00 P.M. More than 50 percent of patients with a major depressive episode "escape" from suppression. A plasma cortisol concentration of more than 5 μg in any sample is considered nonsuppression. A number of medications and illnesses may render the test invalid, including phenytoin, barbiturates, and meprobamate, all of which can enhance the metabolism of dexamethasone through hepatic enzyme induction. Patients with uncontrolled diabetes mellitus, febrile illness, and other acute illness may have increased pituitary adrenal activity reflected in nonsuppression. Psychotropic drugs, lithium, and neuroleptics do not interfere with the DST. Although there are false negatives with the DST, there are no false positives. The DST may clarify the diagnosis when the patient does not present with typical symptoms of depression.

**7.** In the evaluation of any depressed patient, it is important to determine to what extent the depression has impaired the patient's ability to cope with his or her environment. The degree to which interpersonal relationships are altered should also be assessed. The physician should inquire directly of any depressed patient about suicide and assess the risk. Many factors are associated with an increased risk of suicide: lethal plan, old age, male sex, isolation, and lack of personal resources. Psychiatric consultation and usually hospitalization are warranted in potentially suicidal individuals.

**8.** Once depression is diagnosed and classified, appropriate treatment should be initiated.

## ACQUIRED IMMUNODEFICIENCY SYNDROME (AIDS)

H. Harold Friedman

### Definition

The Centers for Disease Control (CDC) define the acquired immunodeficiency syndrome (AIDS) as an illness characterized by one or more opportunitistic diseases (diagnosed by reliable methods) that are at least moderately indicative of underlying cellular immunodeficiency, and absence of all known underlying causes of cellular immunodeficiency (other than infection with the virus presumed to cause AIDS) as well as the absence of all other causes of reduced resistance reported to be associated with at least one of those opportunistic diseases.

AIDS is caused by a specific retrovirus known as human immunodeficiency virus (HIV).

The syndrome primarily affects male homosexuals or bisexuals and intravenous drug abusers. It may affect some heterosexuals, blood product and transfusion recipients, and children born of AIDS-infected mothers.

Sexual contact, exposure to blood and blood products, particularly among intravenous drug addicts, and perinatal transmission are the major modes of HIV infection.

The disease is associated with significant morbidity and mortality. Its duration is variable.

### Laboratory Diagnosis*

The criteria for the diagnosis of AIDS are listed in Table 1-3.
1. Evidence for infection:
   When an individual has disease consistent with AIDS:
   a. A serum specimen from an individual 15 months of age or older, or from a child less than 15 months of age whose mother is not thought to have had HIV infection during the child's perinatal period, that is repeatedly reactive for HIV antibody by a screening test (e.g., enzyme-linked immunosorbent assay ([ELISA]), as long as subsequent HIV-antibody tests (e.g., Western blot, immunofluorescence assay), if done, are positive; or
   b. A serum specimen from a child less than 15 months of age, whose mother is thought to have had HIV infection during the child's perinatal period, that is repeatedly reactive for HIV antibody by a screening test (e.g., ELISA), plus increased serum immunoglobulin levels and at least one of the following abnormal immunologic test results: reduced absolute lymphocyte count, depressed CD4 (T-helper) lymphocyte count, or decreased CD4/CD8 (helper/suppressor) ratio, as long as subsequent antibody tests (e.g., Western blot, immunofluorescence assay), if done, are positive; or
   c. A positive test for HIV serum antigen; or
   d. A positive HIV culture confirmed by both reverse transcriptase detection and a specific HIV-antigen test or in situ hybridization using a nucleic acid probe; or
   e. A positive result on any other highly specific test for HIV (e.g., nucleic acid probe of peripheral blood lymphocytes).
2. Evidence against infection:
   A nonreactive screening test for serum antibody to HIV (e.g., ELISA) without a

*Source: SSA Pub. No. 68-0424500, September 1987.

**Table 1-3.** Criteria for the diagnosis of AIDS

1. Indicator diseases diagnosed definitively in the absence of other causes of immunodeficiency and laboratory tests for HIV
   Candidiasis of the esophagus, trachea, bronchi, or lungs
   *Cryptococcus,* extrapulmonary
   Cryptosporidiosis with diarrhea >1 mo
   Cytomegalovirus disease exclusive of liver, spleen, or lymph nodes in patients >1 mo of age.
   Herpes simplex virus infection causing a mucocutaneous ulcer >1 mo or bronchitis, pneumonitis, or esophagitis in patients >1 mo of age
   Kaposi's sarcoma in patients <60 yr of age
   Lymphoma of the brain (primary) in patients <60 yr of age
   Lymphoid interstitial pneumonia or pulmonary lymphoid hyperplasia, or both, in patients <13 yr of age
   *Mycobacterium avium* complex or *M. kansasii* disease, disseminated
   *Pneumocystis carinii* pneumonia
   Progressive multifocal leukoencephalopathy
   Toxoplasmosis of the brain in patients >1 mo of age
2. Indicator diseases diagnosed definitively regardless of other causes of immunodeficiency and laboratory evidence of HIV present
   All indicator diseases listed in Section 1
   Bacterial infections, recurrent or multiple, in patients <13 yr of age that are caused by *Haemophilus, Streptococcus,* or other pyogenic bacteria
   Coccidioidomycosis, disseminated
   HIV encephalopathy
   Histoplasmosis, disseminated
   Isosporiasis with diarrhea >1 mo
   Kaposi's sarcoma at any age
   Primary lymphoma of the brain at any age
   Non-Hodgkin's lymphoma of B cell or unknown immunologic phenotype, including small noncleaved lymphoma or immunoblastic sarcoma
   Mycobacterial disease exclusive of *M. tuberculosis,* disseminated
   *M. tuberculosis,* extrapulmonary
   *Salmonella* septicemia, recurrent
   HIV wasting syndrome
3. Indicator diseases diagnosed presumptively with laboratory evidence of HIV infection
   Candidiasis, esophageal
   Cytomegalovirus retinitis with loss of vision
   Kaposi's sarcoma
   Lymphoid interstitial pneumonia or pulmonary lymphoid hyperplasia, or both, in patients <13 yr of age
   Mycobacterial disease, disseminated
   *Pneumocystis carinii* pneumonia
   Toxoplasmosis, brain, in patients >1 mo of age
4. Indicator diseases diagnosed definitively in the absence of other causes of immunodeficiency and negative laboratory test results for HIV
   *Pneumocystis carinii* pneumonia
   Other indicator diseases listed in Section 1 and a T-helper/inducer (CD4) lymphocyte, count <400/mm$^3$

Source: Centers for Disease Control. Revision of the CDC surveillance case definition for acquired immunodeficiency syndrome. *M.M.W.R.* 36(Suppl.):1, 1987.

reactive or positive result on any other test for HIV infection (e.g., antibody, antigen, culture), if done.
3. Inconclusive evidence (neither for nor against infection):
   a. A repeatedly reactive screening test for serum antibody to HIV (e.g., ELISA) followed by a negative or inconclusive supplemental test (e.g., Western blot, immunofluorescence assay) without a positive HIV culture or serum antigen test, if done; or
   b. A serum specimen from a child less than 15 months of age, whose mother is thought to have had HIV infection during the child's perinatal period, that is repeatedly reactive for HIV antibody by a screening test, even if positive by a supplemental test, without additional evidence for immunodeficiency as described above (in 1.b) and without a positive HIV culture or serum antigen test, if done.

## Clinical Features of AIDS

The number of asymptomatic carriers of HIV exceeds the number of persons with AIDS or with late complications of the disease. Prospective studies, however, have shown that the rate of progression of the disease is high and increases with the duration of the infection.

A variety of clinical pictures and complications may be found in patients with AIDS. These are outlined below.
1. *Persistent generalized lymphadenopathy.* This condition occurs in approximately 50–70 percent of infected individuals. Other causes of generalized lymphadenopathy must be excluded by appropriate means.
2. *Hematologic manifestations.* Immune thrombocytopenia occurs in 5–15 percent of patients. It is characterized by low platelet counts (below 100,000/mm$^3$) and may be manifested by petechiae and bleeding episodes that are usually minor. Thrombotic thrombocytopenic purpura occurs infrequently. Anemia is a prominent feature of the disease and is usually normocytic normochromic.
3. *Acute retroviral syndrome.* The symptomatology is variable and tends to resemble a mononucleosis-like illness. The most prominent features are fever, malaise, sweats, myalgias, anorexia, nausea, diarrhea, lymphadenopathy, and pharyngitis. Some patients may have a truncal rash; others, neurologic abnormalities; still others, oral lesions. Hepatosplenomegaly is less common. Neurologic symptoms occur in a minority of patients.
4. *Constitutional symptomatology.* Although patients are often asymptomatic, a minority of patients complain of weakness, fatigue, low-grade fever, anxiety, or depression. In advanced disease, an *HIV wasting syndrome* may occur. This condition is characterized by severe weight loss, chronic diarrhea, or chronic weakness and fever in the absence of a concurrent illness other than the HIV infection. Such patients should be investigated thoroughly by clinical and laboratory means for the possible presence of opportunistic infections.
5. *Oral disease.* HIV infection has been associated with aphthous stomatitis and oropharyngeal and esophageal candidiasis. In the late stages of the disease, oral lesions are universally present and are often severe. *Hairy leukoplakia* is a late manifestation of the disease. Severe gingivitis and peridontitis have also been observed.
6. *Gastrointestinal disorders.*
   a. Esophagitis due to infections by *Candidia*, cytomegalovirus, and herpes simplex viruses occur commonly in disease of the upper GI tract. Odynophagia and dysphagia as well as retrosternal discomfort, nausea, and anorexia are often encountered. Esophageal ulcers are common.
   b. Cytomegalovirus gastritis, Kaposi's sarcoma, and lymphomas may be seen in the upper GI tract.
   c. Papillary stenosis and sclerosing cholangitis have been described in some patients.

**d.** Liver disease is a common accompaniment of HIV infection.
**e.** Enterocolitis due to bacteria, parasites, and viruses may cause symptoms such as bloating, nausea, diarrhea, and weight loss.

**7.** *Musculoskeletal complications.* Rheumatologic manifestations, including arthralgias, arthritis, the Reiter syndrome, a painful articular syndrome, and polymyositis are highly prevalent.

**8.** *Cutaneous lesions.* Dermatologic conditions that may occur are viral infections (e.g., herpes), dermatophytosis, Kaposi's sarcoma, herpes zoster, and molluscum contagiosum.

**9.** *Pulmonary disease.* Focal infiltrates, pleural effusions, mediastinal adenopathy, and interstitial infiltrates are common. Cavitary lung lesions may also be seen. Etiologic factors for these abnormalities include chiefly *Pneumocystis carinii,* but fungi, tuberculosis, Kaposi's sarcoma, *Cryptococcus neoformans,* lymphoma, and bacteria must also be considered.

**10.** *Neurologic manifestations.* A sensory peripheral neuropathy is a common finding. The Guillain-Barré syndrome, chronic inflammatory polyneuropathy, and multiple mononeuropathy may also occur. Other neurologic complications include aseptic meningitis, encephalopathy, and intracranial mass lesions. AIDS dementia is particularly devastating.

**11.** *Malignancies.* Kaposi's sarcoma is the most common neoplasm found in AIDS patients. Also seen are CNS and peripheral non-Hodgkin's lymphoma as well as Hodgkin's disease itself. Other neoplasms occur less frequently.

**12.** *Miscellaneous conditions.*
**a.** A variety of opportunistic infections are frequently complications of AIDS. The organisms involved include *C. neoformans,* cytomegalovirus, *Mycobacterium avium,* and especially *Pneumocystis carinii.* Toxoplasmosis, cryptosporidiosis, histoplasmosis, salmonellosis, and other infections are also seen.
**b.** Hyponatremia of multiple etiologies occurs in a majority of inpatients with AIDS.

## AIDS-Related Complex (ARC)

In addition to AIDS as described above, physicians have identified a group of individuals with signs and symptoms thought to be caused by the HIV virus. These individuals commonly have some of the following findings: recurrent fevers, lymphadenopathy, prolonged diarrhea, fatigue, weight loss, night sweats, and recurrent fungal, viral, or other infections (e.g., oral candidiasis). Laboratory findings may include a positive antibody test for the HIV, lymphopenia, T-cell reduction, T-cell ratio reversal, and skin anergy. The term "AIDS-related complex" (ARC) has been applied to this constellation of symptoms and signs.

## Clinical Significance of AIDS

The protean manifestations of AIDS merit consideration of the syndrome in the differential diagnosis of many of the entities discussed in the text. This is especially important because of the widespread prevalence of HIV infection.

## SLEEP DISORDERS
Paul M. Cox, Jr.
George E. Bokinsky

## Definition

Disorders of sleep can be divided into four types: (1) excessive daytime sleepiness, e.g., sleep apnea syndromes, narcolepsy; (2) inadequate sleep, e.g., insomnia; (3)

parasomnias, e.g., sleepwalking, teeth grinding; and (4) abnormal sleep/wake cycles, e.g., disordered sleep secondary to jet lag or shift work. Parasomnias usually do not present as the patient's complaint of sleep disorders; they are often diagnosed by the chief complaint and are not further considered here. Similarly, abnormal sleep/wake cycles usually are recognized by the individual and rarely are an etiologic problem presenting to the doctor. Occasionally they present as either insomnia or excessive sleepiness. This chapter, then, is artificially divided into sections of excessive sleepiness and inadequate sleep, but it should be recognized that other forms of disordered sleep must occasionally be considered.

## Excessive Sleepiness

### Etiology

Excessive daytime sleepiness may be caused by sleep apnea syndromes, narcolepsy, and frequently by insufficient nighttime sleep. The patient with sleep apnea may present not with complaint of excessive sleepiness but with complaints by the spouse of excessive snoring or interruptions of respiration, particularly if the patient has read in the lay press of sleep apnea syndrome.

### History

1. Patients with *sleep apnea syndrome* complain of excessive sleepiness. As with normal sleepiness, excessive daytime sleepiness is apparent in boring sedentary situations but may occur even during important tasks such as driving a car. Patients frequently do not recognize disordered sleep at night but their spouses may complain of excessively loud snoring or cessation of air flow, or both. These patients suffer effects of sleep deprivation and may complain of personality change, enuresis, myoclonus, or systemic hypertension. Patients frequently are middle-aged males with a history of weight gain. Alcohol intake frequently worsens the symptoms. Abnormalities of the upper airways, such as micrognathia and tonsil hypertrophy, may be gleaned on history.
2. *Narcolepsy* similarly presents as excessive sleepiness. Periods of daytime sleep are usually brief. These patients characteristically have cataplexy, which is a sudden onset of muscle weakness brought on by excitement or emotion, most commonly laughter. Some patients may undergo complete paralysis of the upper extremity muscles, but momentary attacks lasting less than a minute and causing the patient to drop something are more common. Most patients develop sleepiness several months before their first episode of cataplexy. Sleep paralysis, the inability to move during the onset of sleep, lasting up to ten minutes, is the third classic symptom. Hypnologic hallucinations, hallucinatory experiences at the time of onset of sleep or awakening, occur in 60 percent of patients and are considered the fourth element of the classic tetrad.

   Disturbances of memory and vision and changes in personality are also frequent complaints. Falling asleep during important activities such as driving or work is also common in this condition.
3. *Insufficient sleep.* The normal amount of sleep needed is variable, and many people chronically live on what is probably an inadequate amount of sleep. College students, house officers, individuals working at two jobs, young mothers whose children awaken frequently at night are often chronically sleep deprived. They may present complaining of excessive daytime sleepiness. Careful sleep history usually makes this diagnosis obvious.

## Physical Examination

1. *Obstructive sleep apnea syndrome.* Patients are usually considerably overweight. Hypertension is present in over half of these patients. (Conversely, obstructive

sleep apnea has been found in 20–50 percent of patients with essential hypertension). Structural abnormalities of the upper airway, e.g., micrognathia or tonsillar hypertrophy, are occasionally present. Subtle abnormalities of the uvula soft palate and posterior pharynx may be found. In patients with prolonged, severe obstructive sleep apnea, signs of cor pulmonale may be seen. These include distended neck veins, right ventricular lift and gallop, hepatomegaly, and peripheral edema.

2. Patients with narcolepsy and those suffering from insufficient sleep have a normal examination.

## Roentgenographic Findings

Patients with obstructive sleep apnea may demonstrate excessive soft tissue densities due to their obesity. Patients with cor pulmonale may show cardiomegaly. The chest roentgenogram is otherwise not helpful in diagnosis of sleep disorders.

## Laboratory Data

1. CBC. Erythrocytosis may be seen in patients with obstructive sleep apnea.
2. Arterial blood gases. Chronic hypoventilation, i.e., increased $PCO_2$ with low normal pH and metabolic alkalosis, may be seen in obstructive sleep apnea syndrome. Hypoxemia consistent with chronic hypoventilation or secondary to ventilation perfusion abnormalities associated with cor pulmonale may be present. More commonly, the arterial blood gases are normal.
3. Electrocardiogram. Patients with cor pulmonale show the characteristic findings of hypertrophy and right-axis deviation.
4. Urinalysis, biochemical screening, and ventilatory function tests are usually normal in patients with excessive sleepiness of any etiology.
5. Other procedures. Patients with suspected sleep apnea syndrome should undergo formal overnight testing in an accredited laboratory. EEG, ECG, oxygen saturation, respiratory effort, and air flow should be continuously monitored. The prevalence and length of apneas should be recorded as well as degree of hypoxemia and cardiac dysrhythmias. Duration and frequency of time in various stages of sleep should be recorded. Patients with suspected cataplexy should undergo the multiple sleep latency test. This test is performed during the day, and the patient is asked to try to sleep at two-hour intervals with measurement of onset of sleep latency and types of sleep.

The HLA types HLA-DR2 and HLA-DQwl are present in an overwhelming majority of patients with narcolepsy.

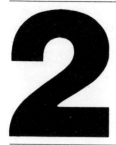

# Dermatologic Problems

## PRURITUS
### Kenneth H. Neldner

Itching sensations can be elicited only from a physical or chemical stimulation of cutaneous nerve receptors, located primarily in the region of the epidermal-dermal junction and around hair follicles. The stimuli may come from internal or external sources. It is currently believed that pain, temperature, and touch are all subserved by the same unmyelinated free nerve net as it terminates in the skin. Minimal stimulation of these fibers is believed to cause itching, whereas more intense stimulation of the same fibers induces pain.

Histamine and various endopeptidases (papain, trypsin, cathepsins, erythrocyte proteases, and lysosomal enzymes) are known chemical mediators of pruritus, but by unknown mechanisms. In its broadest sense, itching may be viewed as a uniform response to a wide variety of physical or chemical stimuli.

## Etiology

There are four general reasons for itching. These are discussed below in order of frequency.

### Itching Associated with a Visible Cutaneous Eruption

A complete discussion of itching skin rashes encompasses essentially the entire field of dermatology, because virtually any skin lesion may itch. This is beyond the purpose and scope of this text. Therefore, only the major categories and types of dermatoses that most commonly produce itching are summarized in Table 2-1.

### Itching Secondary to an Internal Disorder and Without a Visible Skin Rash

Itching without an associated skin rash is more difficult to evaluate. First it must be determined whether the patient has genuine pruritus or symptoms that are neurologic or psychosomatic in nature. A careful history and physical examination will usually establish the presence of any existing neurologic defect. Psychosomatic problems are more difficult to assess. The major categories of internal disorders associated with itching are summarized in Table 2-2.

The most common cause of itching in the patient without a rash is simple dryness of the skin, followed in order of frequency by obstructive biliary disease and lymphoma, particularly Hodgkin's disease and mycosis fungoides. Diagnostic workup should therefore concentrate initially on these areas and then proceed to less common possibilities, as the situation dictates.

1. Increasing *dryness* of the skin with age is common and may be considered a nor-

**Table 2-1.** The most common itching dermatologic disorders

A. Papulosquamous skin diseases
   1. Eczema (atopic, nummular, dysidrotic)
   2. Lichen planus
   3. Seborrheic dermatitis
   4. Psoriasis
   5. Pityriasis rosea
B. Vesicobullous diseases
   1. Dermatitis herpetiformis
   2. Erythema multiforme
C. Allergic reactions
   1. Contact dermatitis
   2. Systemic drug eruptions
   3. Urticaria
   4. Photoallergy
D. Infestations
   1. Bites (lice, fleas, scabies, bedbugs, mosquitoes, chiggers)
   2. Nematodes (creeping eruption, onchocerciasis)
E. Infection
   1. Bacterial (impetigo, folliculitis)
   2. Viral (exanthem, herpes simplex, varicella)
   3. Fungal (tinea capitis, tinea corporis, tinea pedis, *Candida*)
F. Environmental causes
   1. Wool, fiberglass, pollen, dust
   2. Miliaria (prickly heat)
   3. Sunburn
G. Miscellaneous conditions
   1. Purpura simplex
   2. Phototoxic reactions
   3. Urticaria pigmentosa
   4. Ichthyosis
   5. Juvenile rheumatoid arthritis
   6. Primary cutaneous amyloidosis
   7. Pruritus ani
   8. Pruritus vulvae

mal physiologic consequence of aging. It varies in severity from person to person. It is generally aggravated in the winter, especially in those geographic areas where prolonged heating decreases the humidity in the living and sleeping quarters. Dry skin pruritus is also called *senile pruritus, pruritus hiemalis,* or *asteatosis.*

2. Pruritus associated with *liver disease* nearly always implies the presence of an obstructive condition, because pruritus seldom occurs with jaundice secondary to hemolytic anemia and only rarely in infectious hepatitis. The constituent of bile responsible for itching has not been identified with certainty, but it generally has been accepted that elevated serum, skin, and skin surface bile acids were responsible for the pruritus of cholestasis (intrahepatic obstruction). However, recent studies have shown equally elevated serum and skin bile acid levels in patients with cholestasis who do not have pruritus. Liver function tests also correlate poorly with the presence of pruritus. The cause of pruritus in cholestasis therefore remains unknown. The clinical effectiveness of methyltestosterone, which relieves pruritus while often causing a rise in serum bile acids and worsening of cholestasis, tends to confirm the negative role of bile acids as causative agents for pruritus. Similarly, the effectiveness of cholestyramine or external biliary drainage in controlling pruritus indicates that some pruritogenic substance other

**Table 2-2.** The most common internal conditions associated with pruritus

A. Dry skin
B. Metabolic and endocrine causes
  1. Obstructive biliary disease
    a. Extrahepatic
      (1) Common duct stones
      (2) Common duct stricture
      (3) Carcinoma of bile duct or pancreas
    b. Intrahepatic
      (1) Biliary cirrhosis
      (2) Carcinoma of liver
      (3) Drug-induced cholestasis
      (4) Viral hepatitis
  2. Uremia
  3. Thyroid disease
  4. Hyperparathyroidism
  5. Diabetes mellitus
  6. Gout
C. Malignancy
  1. Lymphoma (Hodgkin's disease, mycosis fungoides, leukemia)
  2. Carcinoma
  3. Carcinoid
D. Parasitosis
  1. Hookworm
  2. Pinworm
E. Drug reactions
  1. Opium derivatives
  2. Histamine liberators
F. Miscellaneous causes
  1. Polycythemia vera
  2. Pregnancy

than bile acids is being removed. Intrahepatic obstruction may be induced by medications such as chlorpromazine, testosterone, and erythromycin estolate.

3. *Uremia* is a more common cause for itching in chronic renal diseases than in renal disorders producing acute nephropathy. The slow development of uremia generally correlates better with pruritus than do absolute levels of azotemia, although at least 75 percent of patients will have pruritus when BUN levels reach 100 mg/dl. The unrelenting itch of hemodialysis may at times become so severe as to be disabling. Topical capsaicin, a substance known to deplete substance P in peripheral sensory neurons, has been helpful in controlling the pruritus. This observation has raised the question about a role for substance P in other types of pruritus. Some hemodialysis patients develop prurigo nodularis papules, which they constantly excoriate to the point of bleeding. Treatment with the synthetic vitamin A derivative, etretinate, has helped these individuals, suggesting a currently unknown but possible role for vitamin A in the mediation of pruritic symptoms. Xerosis is also common among patients having hemodialysis, as is secondary hyperparathyroidism, adding to the list of problems that may induce pruritus in the uremic patient.

4. *Hypothyroidism* is commonly associated with generalized pruritus and is most likely related to the dry skin that characterizes this disease. *Hyperthyroidism* is seldom a cause for itching. When it does occur, it is believed to be related to the temperature changes of increased cutaneous circulation.

5. *Hyperparathyroidism* secondary to renal disease is the most common parathyroid disorder producing pruritus. Relief of itching with return of the elevated serum

calcium and phosphorus levels to normal following parathyroidectomy suggests that increased blood and tissue levels of calcium may be the pruritogenic stimuli, but the etiologic factors are not completely clear because not all hypercalcemic disorders are accompanied by pruritus.

6. *Diabetes mellitus* is a rare cause of itching, despite "common knowledge" to the contrary. The increased susceptibility of diabetics to cutaneous bacterial and yeast infections with secondary pruritus is a more common cause for itching than is the diabetes per se.

7. *Gout* rarely causes itching. When it does, the itching is presumed to be due to elevated blood and tissue levels of uric acid.

8. Of all the *malignancies* known to induce pruritus, Hodgkin's disease is the most common, and itching may be the first symptom in as many as 25 to 30 percent of the cases. Mycosis fungoides may also be preceded by itching in areas where characteristic skin lesions subsequently develop. Chronic leukemia is less commonly pruritic; itching is somewhat more common in lymphatic leukemia than in the granulocytic types. Carcinoma of any organ may produce itching, but this is most frequently associated with involvement of the stomach, pancreas, bowel, bronchi, esophagus, ovaries, and prostate gland. The carcinoid syndrome is characterized by flushing of the skin, but pruritus is rare.

9. Intestinal *parasitosis* with hookworm *(Ancylostoma duodenale* or *Necator americanus)* may produce generalized pruritus. The constitutional phase of the disease is preceded by evanescent skin lesions ("ground itch"), usually on the feet, at the sites where the *Ancylostoma* larvae penetrate the skin. Pinworm *(Enterobius vermicularis)* infestation is a common cause of pruritus ani, especially in children.

10. Subclinical *drug reactions* that do not result in urticaria or other rashes may be responsible for itching. These are particularly common in opium or heroin addicts and may occur in patients receiving morphine, codeine, or other histamine-liberating drugs, such as aspirin and polymyxin B.

11. Mild, generalized pruritus is a frequent complaint during *pregnancy* and, in some patients, is very severe and distressing. Approximately 65 percent of pregnant women have mild to moderate elevations in serum bilirubin level (0.75–3.0 mg/100 ml) during the last trimester, with a rapid return to normal after parturition. The degree of itching generally parallels the serum bilirubin level. If the pruritus does not disappear in the immediate postpartum period, underlying liver disease should be suspected.

12. *Polycythemia vera* is frequently associated with itching. Here, the itching is unique in that it is markedly aggravated after a hot bath. The combination of generalized pruritus and low serum ferritin (with normal hemoglobin values) should raise suspicions of occult carcinoma, particularly in males.

13. Prodromal itching of the anterior neck and upper trunk may at times (in about 40 percent of cases) precede an attack of childhood asthma. In some cases, recognition of this symptom allows institution of therapy that is able to abort the attack.

## Psychosomatic Pruritus

1. Neurotic excoriations (factitial dermatitis). The patient has multiple, dug out, superficial ulcerations of the skin and complains of severe, intractable pruritus. Most individuals freely admit to deep scratching and relate the intensity of the itching to nervous tension. Some are more evasive and deny that they had anything to do with the obviously self-induced lesions; situations of this type generally indicate a more severe underlying neurosis.

2. Psychotic states. The usual complaint is that "bugs" or parasites are crawling in the skin, producing intense pruritus. *Delusions of parasitosis* and *acarophobia* are the terms applied to this condition. Deep, self-inflicted excoriations and ulcerations are the rule. This is one of the most intractable and incurable forms of

pruritus. The patient readily reports that "bugs" are in his skin but adamantly refuses to accept any evidence or explanation to the contrary. Psychiatric treatment has been disappointing.

## Neurologic and Circulatory Disturbances

Any neurologic disease with manifestations of cutaneous paresthesias, hypoesthesia, or hyperesthesia may produce sensations in these areas that the patient interprets as pruritus. Neurologic examination in most instances quickly establishes the presence or absence of such a neurologic defect. Neurologic disease of this type is actually a rare cause of itching. Circulatory disturbances secondary to cardiovascular disease are also uncommon causes for itching. When itching is present, the lower extremities are most frequently involved, with the pruritus secondary to ischemic changes.

---

## Diagnostic Approach

---

1. Those patients with obvious skin lesions should be clinically and, if necessary, histologically evaluated in order to establish a diagnosis. A trained observer should be able to diagnose most dermatologic disorders with a high degree of accuracy. Patients with urticaria present special problems because of the diverse nature of the possible etiologic factors. Urticaria is therefore considered separately (see the next section).

2. Pruritus without an associated cutaneous reaction presents the most challenging diagnostic problem. The initial history and physical examination should include a specific evaluation for possible low-grade jaundice and generalized dryness of the skin.

3. The diagnostic workup then proceeds according to the results of the history and physical examination. In some instances, the clinical findings alone establish a diagnosis with certainty and no laboratory studies are necessary. At other times, extensive laboratory evaluation is required. The procedures that may be indicated are listed in Table 2-3. This list is neither complete enough to cover all possible exigencies nor is it to be considered routine workup for each and every case of pruritus of undetermined etiology. Each significant symptom or sign should be evaluated with an appropriate laboratory test, based on the clinical judgment of the examining physician.

4. Simple therapeutic measures may at times not only aid in diagnosis but also provide immediate relief for the patient. Hydration and lubrication of the skin by daily bathing for 15 to 20 minutes in a tub of tepid water, followed by the immediate application of any moisturizing lotion to the wet skin, will afford marked and lasting relief if the pruritus is related to simple xerosis. The addition of table salt to the water (1 cup per tub of warm water) is often beneficial. Relief obtained by such measures, in conjunction with a normal brief history and physical examination, often precludes further diagnostic workup.

## Role of Antihistamines

Even though histamine is the best known mediator of pruritus, therapy with conventional $H_1$-blocking antihistamines is generally disappointing. Combinations of $H_1$ and $H_2$ blockers have been recommended but in general offer little or no enhanced antipruritic effect. In general, the relief of pruritus achieved by any conventional $H_1$ blocker is in direct proportion to its degree of sedation, which in itself soon becomes an intolerable side effect of therapy. Newer, so-called nonsedating $H_1$ blocking antihistamines (terfenadine, astemizole, cetirizine) may offer some advantage by permitting much higher doses without the undesirable side effect of sedation.

**Table 2-3.** Procedures for evaluating pruritus of undetermined etiology

1. Hematologic studies
   a. Complete blood count
   b. Sedimentation rate
   c. Eosinophil count
2. Gastrointestinal workup
   a. Liver profile
   b. Cholecystography
   c. Serum amylase
   d. Stool for ova and parasites
   e. Liver biopsy
3. Endocrine evaluation
   a. Blood sugar and glucose tolerance tests
   b. Thyroid function studies
   c. Serum calcium and phosphorus
4. Genitourinary studies
   a. Urinalysis
   b. Blood urea nitrogen
   c. Serum creatinine
   d. Creatinine clearance
   e. Intravenous pyelogram
5. Evaluation for malignancy
   a. Lymph node biopsy
   b. Chest x-ray
   c. Bone marrow biopsy
   d. Upper GI examination
   e. Barium enema
   f. Proctosigmoidoscopy
   g. Mammograms
   h. Papanicolaou test
   i. Skull x-rays
   j. Pelvic x-rays
   k. Serum acid phosphatase
6. Miscellaneous studies
   a. Psychiatric evaluation
   b. Pregnancy test
   c. Blood and urine toxicology

# URTICARIA AND ANGIOEDEMA
Alan A. Wanderer

## Definition and General Information

Urticaria is characterized by transient erythematous, edematous pruritic wheals that affect the superficial layers of skin. The cutaneous wheals blanch on pressure, which is indicative of underlying edema. Angioedema is a condition with well-demarcated, nonpitting edema that involves deeper dermal tissues and mucosal membranes. The pruritus that accompanies urticaria is conspicuously absent in angioedema because of the paucity of sensory fibers in the deeper dermal tissues. Vasodilation, vasopermeability, and edema in urticaria and angioedema can develop from similar pathophysiologic mechanisms (e.g., IgE-mediated immune complexes, direct nonimmune mast cell degranulation, complement activation) that cause release or generation of biologically active mediators such as histamine, leukotrienes, prostaglandin $D_2$, and platelet activating factor.

Urticaria and angioedema are arbitrarily defined as acute if the symptoms last less than 6 weeks and as chronic if they persist longer than 6 weeks. Both symptoms may occur independently or in association with each other. Approximately 20 percent of the general population experience at least one episode of urticaria or angioedema, or both, during their lifetimes.

Most acute and chronic urticaria and angioedema are uncomplicated, but there are exceptions to this generalization. For example, urticaria or angioedema reactions secondary to hymenoptera stings, cold urticaria, and hereditary angioedema may be complicated by shock symptomatology. In addition, urticaria and angioedema are occasionally associated with systemic diseases such as infectious diseases, serum sickness, malignancies, collagen vascular disorders, and metabolic disorders.

## Etiology

A wide variety of causative factors have been implicated in the induction of urticaria and angioedema. The following list characterizes important diagnostic considerations.

1. Drugs. Since most medications have been associated with induction of urticaria or angioedema, it is essential that a careful drug history include prescription, nonprescription, and illicit drugs administered around the onset of the symptoms. Drugs taken as long as 1 month prior to the onset of symptoms may induce urticaria with serum sickness disorders (e.g., penicillin and other beta-lactam antibiotics). Examples of drugs most commonly associated with urticaria or angioedema include aspirin, antibiotics (e.g., penicillin and its congeners), and opiates.

2. Foods. Foods are frequently implicated as causes of acute and chronic urticaria or angioedema. Common offenders of acute urticaria or angioedema are fish, shellfish, nuts, and eggs. The causal relationship between foods and chronic urticaria or angioedema is more difficult to establish because of the vague temporal relationships between food ingestion and chronic symptomatology. Food additives such as metabisulfites, salicylates, and coloring dyes have also been implicated as causes of acute or chronic symptomatology.

3. Infection. There is ample evidence to suggest that viral infections can cause urticaria or angioedema. Urticaria can develop in the prodromal phase of hepatitis B virus infections as a result of immune complex deposition. Epstein-Barr and Coxsackie A and B viruses have also been associated with the onset of urticaria. Urticaria has been described with parasitic infestations such as giardiasis, amebiasis, and ascariasis. The association of chronic urticaria with *Candida albicans,* tinea, or occult bacterial infections (e.g., those involving the gall bladder, urinary tract, teeth, gums, and sinuses) remains poorly documented.

4. Inhalants. Inhalation of animal danders, pollens, foods, and chemicals can induce urticaria or angioedema. Occasionally, seasonal occurrences are observed in pollen-sensitive individuals who may also experience rhinitis or bronchospasm, or both.

5. Insect stings. The most common manifestation of hymenoptera stings is urticaria or angioedema, which may be localized or systemic. In general these reactions are mediated through IgE mechanisms. Urticaria or angioedema may also develop following stings or bites of spiders, fire ants, flies, and mosquitoes. Papular urticaria is frequently a manifestation of insect bites.

6. Contact urticaria. Substances that directly contact the skin can occasionally induce urtication. Typical urticaria-inducing contactants include animal dander or saliva, foods, drugs, and direct mediator-releasing substances from insects (e.g., moths, caterpillars) and sea nettles.

   **7.** Systemic disease. Urticaria and angioedema may be manifestations of the following systemic disorders:

     **a.** Connective tissue diseases (e.g., systemic lupus erythematosus, rheumatoid arthritis, dermatomyositis). This association is most likely complement-mediated.

     **b.** Neoplasms (e.g., lymphoma, leukemias, carcinomas). A rare association of acquired C1-esterase deficiency with lymphoma (Caldwell's syndrome) or carcinoma has been reported. Acquired cold urticaria may be associated with lymphoproliferative malignancies.

     **c.** Endocrine abnormalities (e.g., hyper- or hypothyroidism, with evidence of thyroid autoantibodies, hyperparathyroidism, diabetes mellitus, and menstrual cycle urticaria considered secondary to an autoimmune progesterone mechanism).

     **d.** Systemic mastocytosis or urticaria pigmentosa.

     **e.** Miscellaneous disorders.

       **(1)** Serum sickness (immune complex mediation) induced by heterologous serum, drugs, infectious illnesses.

       **(2)** Urticarial vasculitis (immune complex mediation) with and without hypocomplementemia.

   **8.** Psychogenic. The role of psychogenic factors as the sole cause of urticaria remains controversial. However, it is generally accepted that psychological problems can exacerbate chronic urticaria. There is currently no accepted personality profile that is characteristic of patients with urticaria.

   **9.** Genetic types. There are several rare types of urticaria or angioedema that are inherited by such autosomal dominant patterns as hereditary angioedema, vibratory angioedema, delayed cold urticaria, Muckle-Wells syndrome (urticaria, deafness, amyloidosis), familial localized delayed heat urticaria, and erythropoietic protoporphyria with solar urticaria. C3b-inactivator deficiency with urticaria is transmitted as an autosomal recessive disorder.

  **10.** Physical agents. This category includes urticaria or angioedema that is induced by physical agents such as thermal stimuli, pressure, vibration, and light energy. Approximately 15 percent of all urticaria and angioedema are induced by physical agents. The following is an outline of the various entities:

     **a.** Pressure.

       **(1)** Dermographism (immediate wheal and flare following pressure to skin).

         **(a)** Primary.

         **(b)** Secondary (secondary to drug reactions, insect stings, chronic mastocytosis).

       **(2)** Delayed dermographism (superficial wheal and flare evolves 4–6 hours after stroking skin).

       **(3)** Delayed pressure urticaria (deep painful swelling occurring 4–6 hours after pressure has been applied to a specific location). It is sometimes associated with constitutional symptoms such as fever, chills, and arthralgias. Most commonly occurs in young adult males.

       **(4)** Hereditary vibratory angioedema (autosomal dominant inherited disorder associated with development of angioedema following vibratory stimuli).

     **b.** Thermal stimuli.

       **(1)** Cold temperature.

         **(a)** Primary acquired cold urticaria (idiopathic onset of urticaria, angioedema, and occasionally shock immediately after exposure to cold temperature). Documented by positive immediate cold stimulation test (wheal develops immediately after application of 0°C stimulus to the skin). Some patients with a positive history of cold urticaria exhibit atypical responses to cold stimulation tests such as negative or delayed reactions. On occasion underlying diseases are associated with secondary acquired cold urticaria (e.g., cryoglobulinemia, infectious mononucleosis, syphilis, leukocytoclastic vasculitis, leukemia, and lymphomas).

**(b)** Familial types of cold urticaria (autosomal dominant inheritance).
   **(i)** Delayed cold urticaria.
   **(ii)** Familial cold urticaria. (This syndrome is misnamed, since the rash is nonurticarial and maculopapular in description. Fever, arthralgia, and leukocytosis also develop after cold exposure.)
**(2)** Heat.
   **(a)** Cholinergic urticaria (pruritic papular urticaria with heat, exercise, emotional stress).
   **(b)** Localized heat urticaria (immediate wheal develops after contact with warm temperature).
**c.** Solar urticaria. Urticaria develops immediately after exposure to sunlight. There are six types, each depending on the wavelengths of light that induce the urticaria. Erythropoietic protoporphyria (type VI) is a genetic abnormality of porphyrin metabolism. Differential diagnosis should exclude lupus erythematosus, photosensitizing agents, and polymorphic light eruption.
**11.** Miscellaneous factors.
   **a.** Aquagenic urticaria (urticaria develops after contact with water at body temperature).
   **b.** Episodic angioedema with eosinophilia and without cardiopulmonary involvement, differentiating it from hypereosinophilic syndrome.
   **c.** Exercise-induced anaphylaxis (pruritus, urticaria, angioedema, and collapse can develop during or immediately after exercise).
**12.** Idiopathic. Despite the best medical efforts, only 15 to 20 percent of all chronic urticaria or angioedema can be classified in one of the aforementioned categories.

## Diagnostic Approach

### History

**1.** Thorough history is essential and should include pertinent questions relevant to diet, drugs taken presently and during recent past (up to 1 month), environmental exposures, contactants, insect stings, activities such as exercise, relationship to physical agents, infectious illnesses, emotional stress, genetic patterns, and concomitant systemic illnesses. A complete review of systems should be included since a major objective of the evaluation is to exclude important underlying diseases.
**2.** The patient should maintain daily diary of skin lesions with particular emphasis on times of occurrence, foods and drugs ingested, and activities.

### Physical examination

**1.** Complete physical examination to include evaluation for systemic illnesses such as infectious illnesses (hepatitis, infectious mononucleosis), endocrinopathies (hyperthyroidism, hyperparathyroidism), vasculitis, serum sickness, neoplasms, and collagen vascular diseases.
**2.** Careful examination of skin lesions to definitively establish urticaria (wheals of typical urticaria persist less than 24 hours, as compared to urticarial vasculitis in which the wheals persist longer than 24 hours). It is important to delineate the type of urticaria. Relevant examples include cholinergic urticaria (papular urticaria); dermographic urticaria (linear wheals along paths of skin that have been scratched or rubbed); deep pressure urticaria (tender deep wheals over areas exposed to pressure such as the feet, buttocks, and hands); and urticarial vasculitis (wheals persist longer than 24 hours).

### Laboratory

**1.** Routine laboratory profile to include complete blood count, erythrocyte sedimentation rate, biochemical profile, and urinalysis.

2. Specific laboratory tests.
   a. Cold urticaria. Cold stimulation test (i.e., ice cube in plastic bag applied to forearm for 5 minutes) typically induces wheal formation. It is important to note that some patients may still have cold urticaria by history despite negative cold stimulation tests. Evaluation should include the following tests: cryoglobulins, syphilis serology, infectious mononucleosis panel, and antinuclear antibody (ANA).
   b. Other physical agents: dermographism, stroke skin with blunt object; solar urticaria, light testing with various wavelengths; cholinergic urticaria, methacholine skin test; heat urticaria, warm-water stimulation of forearm.
   c. Infectious illness evaluation. When pertinent, the following tests should be ordered: infectious mononucleosis panel, hepatitis B panel, stool for ova and parasites, miscellaneous (viral cultures, bacterial cultures of throat, blood, urine).
   d. Allergy evaluation. When appropriate, skin tests or radioallergosorbent tests (RAST) might be ordered for foods, inhalants, or insect venoms. In general, drug sensitivities cannot be accurately detected by these techniques, except for penicillin skin testing for major and minor antigenic determinants. There is no accurate RAST for drug sensitivities, including penicillin.
   e. Hereditary angioedema. Autosomal dominant pattern of angioedema (without urticaria), often triggered by trauma such as dental manipulation and occasionally associated with abdominal pain. Laboratory tests include complement level measurements (C2 levels are decreased during episodes of angioedema and C4 levels are always deficient) and decreased C1-esterase inhibitor (quantitative and functional assays).
   f. Immunologic evaluation for collagen vascular diseases, serum sickness, and urticarial vasculitis. When appropriate, the following tests might be ordered: ANA, native DNA binding, rheumatoid factor, immune complex assays (C1q binding, Raji cell), total complement levels, complement components for classic and alternative pathways, and skin biopsy to examine for evidence of leukocytoclastic vasculitis that is associated with urticarial vasculitis.
   g. Neoplasm evaluation is occasionally indicated. Specific examples include evaluation for (a) leukemia and lymphoma in cold urticaria with cryoglobulinemia and (b) Caldwell's syndrome (lymphoproliferative malignancies with angioedema). The latter is associated with decreased C1q levels and decreased C1-esterase inhibitor levels. C1q levels are normal in the hereditary forms of C1-esterase deficiency.

### Empiric procedures

1. Elimination diets or a simple three-day diet with rice and water to exclude ingestants as a cause of the urticaria. If no urticaria develops while the patient is on these diets, then suspect food should be individually added back into the diet. The patient should remain on a constant medication program in order to isolate the effect of diet.
2. Challenge procedures. The preferred technique is double-blinded challenges using dessicated foods in gelatin capsules. This procedure is not suggested for patients with IgE-mediated food sensitivities who might develop anaphylaxis.
3. Diagnostic trial with synthetic diets (Vivonex) for 1 week is also useful in eliminating ingestants as the cause of chronic urticaria or angioedema.

### Referral

Referral to an allergist or dermatologist may be appropriate.

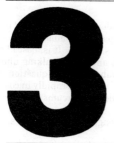

# Cardiovascular Problems

## CHEST PAIN
Phillip S. Wolf

Chest pain may have its origin in the heart; in the lungs or other organs of the chest; in the musculoskeletal structures of the thorax, neck, or shoulders; or in the upper abdominal viscera. The history, with particular attention to a detailed description of the pain and any associated symptoms, often provides most if not all of the essential information needed for a correct diagnosis. It is convenient for clinical purposes to classify chest pain into two categories: (1) recurrent, often paroxysmal, pain, which is mild or moderate in intensity, and (2) severe, prolonged pain, which is commonly associated with clinical evidence of acute, serious illness.

## Recurrent Chest Pain

Angina pectoris is the most important but not the most frequent cause of recurrent chest pain. Musculoskeletal disorders, as a group, are responsible for more cases of chest pain than any other disease entity. They account for most errors in the diagnosis of angina pectoris, although they may coexist with this condition. By meticulous attention to the history and examination of the chest wall, especially by palpation, it is often possible to resolve the diagnostic difficulties.

### Angina Pectoris

Atherosclerotic narrowing of one or more coronary arteries is the most common cause of angina pectoris. Other causes of angina include severe aortic stenosis, hypertrophic cardiomyopathy, pulmonary hypertension, and primary myocardial disease. However, on rare occasions typical angina may occur in the absence of apparent heart disease or demonstrable abnormality of the coronary arteries. Spasm of the coronary arteries currently is considered an established cause of angina both in patients with anatomically normal arteries and in those with underlying atherosclerosis. It is worth stressing that angina is uncommon in men below 35 years of age and in premenopausal women unless they have diabetes, hypertension, or hyperlipidemia.

CHARACTERISTICS OF ANGINAL PAIN

1. Anginal pain is "visceral" (poorly localized) and squeezing, oppressive, burning, or heavy in quality.
2. It is of brief duration, usually lasting from 2 to 10 minutes, only rarely longer or shorter.
3. It is usually moderate in intensity.
4. The pain is typically retrosternal, but it may occur in other locations. Even then, at least a portion of the pain is usually beneath the sternum. The pain may be

referred to the precordium, neck, lower jaws, shoulders, arms, back, and epigastrium. Radiation to the left shoulder and arm is especially common.

5. The pain is precipitated by effort or emotional stress, or both. It is most likely to occur after meals, on exposure to cold air or wind, and while walking uphill or climbing stairs. The pain often increases with recumbency. A key question to ask is, "Do you get discomfort behind your breastbone if you walk rapidly in cold air?"
6. Anginal pain can usually be excluded under the following circumstances:
   a. If it can be localized with one finger.
   b. If it consistently lasts less than 30 seconds or longer than 30 minutes.
   c. If the pain is sticking, jabbing, or throbbing.
   d. If it occurs exclusively at rest, with two exceptions: (1) angina preceding myocardial infarction and (2) a variant form of angina, described by Prinzmetal, that is characterized by pain at rest but not with exertion. Vasospasm of the coronary arteries is now considered the leading cause of this syndrome.
   e. If the intensity of the pain is consistently severe.

COEXISTENCE OF ANGINA WITH PAIN OF DIFFERENT ORIGIN

1. Anginal pain may coexist with chest pain due to musculoskeletal disease. When this occurs, a history of a second type of chest discomfort, different in character from anginal pain, may be elicited. The finding of tenderness on palpation of the chest wall confirms the musculoskeletal origin of this additional pain.
2. Preexisting disease of the neck, arms, shoulders, thorax, or upper abdomen may so condition the nervous system that if angina pectoris develops subsequently, ischemic pain may erroneously be perceived as arising from these structures. This explanation probably accounts for at least some cases of atypical angina.
3. Some patients with long-standing chronic coronary artery disease, especially after open-heart surgery, may develop chronic burning precordial pain that is associated with tenderness of the anterior thoracic wall. This condition, which has been termed *cardiac causalgia,* is of unknown etiology.
4. In a majority of patients, the diagnosis of angina can be established from the history alone. When doubt exists or diagnosis is difficult, the procedures listed below may be helpful.

DIAGNOSTIC APPROACH

1. Physical examination. Examination of the heart seldom provides the information needed for an unequivocal diagnosis of angina pectoris. However, the physical findings listed below provide supportive evidence for the diagnosis of angina, especially if they occur during an episode of pain.
   a. An audible or palpable fourth heart sound.
   b. A rise in blood pressure or pulse rate, or both.
   c. The appearance of the murmur of mitral regurgitation due to papillary muscle dysfunction.
   d. A palpable dyskinetic area or bulge at or around the cardiac apex.
   e. Paradoxical splitting of the second heart sound.
   f. Relief of pain by carotid sinus massage (the Levine test). The relief of pain appears to be related to slowing of the heart rate produced by carotid sinus pressure. In performing the test, to avoid influencing the patient's interpretation of the result, the physician should ask whether the maneuver has made the pain worse. A reply that the pain was not made worse but was relieved constitutes evidence in favor of the diagnosis of angina.
2. Use of nitroglycerin. Sublingual nitroglycerin relieves anginal pain in 3 minutes or less in a large majority of cases, provided the tablets are potent (capable of inducing headache and flushing or producing a burning sensation under the tongue). Failure of nitroglycerin tablets (especially if taken at 3- to 5-minute intervals) to relieve chest pain indicates either that the pain is not anginal or, if it is anginal, that it may represent unstable angina or myocardial infarction. On the other hand, a patient's statement that the pain diminishes 10 minutes or

more after taking nitroglycerin is evidence against, rather than for, the diagnosis of angina.

3. Electrocardiographic changes.
   a. No electrocardiographic changes are pathognomonic of angina pectoris. In fact, the resting ECG is frequently normal in patients with angina.
   b. During anginal attacks, S-T segment depression is the most commonly noted abnormality and is due to subendocardial injury and ischemia. However, this finding is nonspecific. If coronary artery spasm is present, S-T segment elevation (and, on occasion, increase in the R-wave amplitude) may be noted. S-T depression and T-wave changes have also been observed.
   c. Exercise testing increases the accuracy of the electrocardiographic diagnosis if the ECG is recorded both during and after exercise. The presence of at least 1 mm of flat or downsloping S-T segment depression that is 0.08 to 0.12 sec in duration is the major criterion for a positive result. Exercise testing may be performed by climbing stairs, walking a treadmill, or pumping a stationary bicycle.
   d. Exercise testing may be misleading in women under the age of 40 years. In this group, the incidence of coronary artery disease is remarkably low, but false-positive S-T segment depression is not uncommon.
   e. ECG changes of ischemia are probably much more common *without* anginal symptoms. "Silent ischemia" can be demonstrated by exercise or ambulatory ECG monitoring.
   f. The addition of radionuclide scanning with Thallium 201 has enhanced the accuracy of the exercise ECG. Scanning is especially useful when the exercise ECG is difficult to interpret (e.g., left bundle branch block, severe left ventricular hypertrophy, the Wolff-Parkinson-White syndrome) or when symptoms or ECG findings are not diagnostic with routine exercise testing.
4. Selective coronary angiography. Coronary angiography is currently the most accurate method for diagnosing coronary artery disease during life and for determining its severity. The procedure is not without hazard, but the risk is low in competent hands. As a general rule, the symptomatology of ischemic heart disease correlates exceedingly well with angiographic evidence of occlusive disease. Three exceptions are worthy of mention:
   a. In some individuals, angiography may disclose severe arterial obstruction in the absence of symptoms; thus, the presence of an obstructive lesion does not necessarily mean that it is causally related to chest pain.
   b. Spasm of proximal coronary arteries undoubtedly causes angina in some patients, but spasm is not always evident on angiography. Provocative maneuvers to induce spasm, including the intracoronary injection of ergonovine, have proven useful in some cases. In most cases, the absence of arterial narrowing on angiography helps to exclude angina as a cause of chest pain.
   c. In some patients, typical anginal symptoms occur with ECG and radionuclide evidence of ischemia but without atherosclerotic narrowing or demonstrable vasospasm. Termed "Syndrome X," the entity may represent inability of the coronary microcirculation to dilate with stress.

## Musculoskeletal Pain

1. The musculoskeletal structures of the neck, shoulder, and thorax are the most common sources of chest pain.
2. Anterior or posterior chest pain, or both, may result from involvement of the nerve roots of the cervical and upper thoracic spine by osteoarthritis, disk disease, or deformities. The radicular nature of and posterior component to the pain help to differentiate it from angina. The pain tends to occur at night. It may be precipitated by fatigue, incorrect posture, and movement of the involved segments but not movement of the body as a whole. It may also intensify with coughing or sneezing. The discomfort is usually dull and aching in character but is often

punctuated by brief sharp twinges of pain. The pain may last for hours at a time. Relief is often obtained through rest, analgesics, postural exercises, and local heat.

3. Costochondral and chondrosternal pain or swelling, or both (Tietze's syndrome), may simulate angina. The pain is usually well localized, but it may radiate across the chest and over to the arms. Tenderness to palpation over the involved articulations, especially with reproduction of the pain, is the clue to the diagnosis.

4. Rib pain in young people is usually the result of trauma. Fractures from trauma or hard coughing are easily recognized on examination, but other mechanical causes of rib pain may be subtle. For example, trauma may increase the mobility of the anterior ends of the lower ribs. The pain, which is described as sharp or burning, can be reproduced by local pressure. Rib tumors, when painful, are usually metastatic in origin.

5. Fleeting, jabbing, lancinating, or sticking pains are common in many normal individuals. They are easily differentiated from angina by their brevity and character and by the lack of any relationship to effort or emotional excitement. The cause of these pains is unknown.

6. The thoracic outlet syndromes (e.g., the scalenus anterior, costoclavicular, hyperabduction, cervical rib syndromes) may cause chest pain. Symptoms depend on whether neural or vascular structures are compressed at the thoracic outlet. Nerve compression is more frequent; pain and paresthesias are the leading symptoms. Demonstrable weakness is infrequent. Vascular compression is quite rare. Signs of venous obstruction of thrombosis may be present. Arm and head movements may reproduce the discomfort and pain. It is often difficult to evaluate the effects of various maneuvers because they may produce signs of neurovascular compression in some normal persons. Decreased ulnar nerve conduction is currently considered the most reliable objective method for demonstrating thoracic outlet compression. Angiography may be indicated in those patients with symptoms of vascular obstruction.

7. Disorders of the shoulder may produce pain that is referred to the chest. Although the pain may increase with effort, careful analysis usually reveals that aggravation of the discomfort is related specifically to shoulder movement and not to body motion. Local tenderness, pain on passive movements, and limitation of motion are commonly present.

8. Less common and usually obvious causes of pain in the chest are herpes zoster and superficial phlebitis of the thoracic wall or breast.

## Other Causes of Recurrent Chest Pain

1. The chest discomfort of angina may be mimicked by anxiety states. The discomfort may take various forms: (a) intermittent sharp, knifelike pains, (b) persistent precordial aching unrelated to effort, and (c) tight sensations in the chest. Typically, there is no constant relationship between the pain and exertion. The pain tends to appear some time after exertion or is associated with fatigue. The duration of the pain is variable. It may last for seconds, hours, or even days. Sighing respirations and symptoms due to hyperventilation are commonly associated. A statement that "the pain is coming from my heart" is almost a giveaway for the diagnosis of psychogenic pain.

2. Pain due to reflux esophagitis, with or without hiatal hernia, may closely simulate anginal pain. The discomfort is substernal and may radiate to the left arm or lower jaw. It may be precipitated by overeating, excessive alcohol intake, or consumption of highly seasoned foods. The pain is often nocturnal and most often triggered by recumbency. The patient may note a sour taste in his mouth. In severe cases, bending forward may cause the regurgitation of a mouthful of gastric contents. The pain may be relieved by assuming an upright position and by the ingestion of antacids. Reproduction of the pain with an acid infusion, demonstration of reflux by barium swallow, esophageal motility studies, and esophagoscopy with biopsy provide substantiating evidence for this diagnosis.

Diffuse esophageal spasm may occur in the absence of reflux. The pain, often described as a pressure or squeezing sensation, may be quite variable. It may be mild or severe, very brief or quite prolonged. Location is usually retrosternal, and radiation may occur into the jaws, neck, through to the back, or down the arms. Often the pain occurs with meals and may be associated with dysphagia for both liquid and solid foods. Relief in many cases is obtained with nitroglycerin. In several respects, then, the pain of diffuse esophageal spasm may mimic that of angina pectoris. Appropriate esophageal manometric and barium studies may be required for the diagnosis.

3. Pulmonary hypertensive pain may resemble angina in that it is precipitated by effort. The association of moderate or severe dyspnea and evidence of pulmonary hypertension are clues to the diagnosis. The response to nitroglycerin is not as clear-cut as it is in angina pectoris.

4. Patients with mitral valve prolapse often describe chest pain that is reasonably consistent for a given individual. Frequently the pain is left precordial, sharp, brief, and without a consistent relationship to effort. In other patients, the pain is located retrosternally, described as a sensation of heaviness or pressure, and related to effort. Whether there is any pathogenic relation of the pain to mitral prolapse is in dispute.

---

## Prolonged Chest Pain

---

Patients with severe, protracted chest pain may have serious underlying disease, such as myocardial infarction, dissecting hematoma (aneurysm) of the aorta, pulmonary embolism, and pericarditis. Therefore, immediate hospitalization of such patients for diagnosis and therapy is almost always indicated.

### Acute Myocardial Infarction

CHARACTERISTICS OF PAIN IN MYOCARDIAL INFARCTION

1. The pain in acute myocardial infarction is typically crushing, pressing, burning, aching, or viselike in quality. Although it may be mild or moderate in severity, it is more commonly quite severe.

2. If the patient has had angina previously, inquiry often discloses that the frequency and severity of the anginal pain were greater during the period preceding the acute attack.

3. The duration of the pain is variable. It may last from half an hour to several hours or longer.

4. The pain is typically retrosternal but may be in the precordium or other locations. Radiation of the pain to the anterior thorax, lower jaws, neck, shoulders, and arms is common. There is a tendency for it to be transmitted to the left shoulder and arm.

5. Symptoms of dyspnea, a cold sweat, and "indigestion" commonly accompany the pain.

6. In some instances, myocardial infarction is painless, but more often there are symptoms that the patient has overlooked or has attributed to "gas" or other nonspecific gastrointestinal complaints.

PHYSICAL FINDINGS

1. The patient may appear cold, diaphoretic, pale, cyanotic, and in obvious distress from the pain. Cardiogenic shock may be present in severe cases.

2. Physical signs of myocardial ischemia may be noted (see Angina Pectoris, p. 39).

3. Signs of congestive heart failure without peripheral edema may be noted on physical examination or in the chest roentgenogram.

4. An evanescent pericardial friction rub is not an uncommon finding.

5. Disorders of the heartbeat occur in almost all cases. Ventricular premature con-

tractions are the most common type of rhythm disturbance, but all types of arrhythmias, including conduction defects, may be seen.

DIAGNOSTIC APPROACH

1. The diagnosis of acute myocardial infarction is based primarily on objective evidence. Characteristic changes in the ECG and in serum enzyme activity, together with the clinical picture, establish the diagnosis.
2. The electrocardiographic diagnosis of myocardial infarction can be established with certainty in an appropriate clinical setting when abnormality of the initial 0.04 sec of the QRS complex (abnormal Q, QS, or R waves) is combined with characteristic S-T segment changes or typical T-wave abnormalities, or both. Unfortunately, ECG abnormalities that are usually considered diagnostic of myocardial infarction may sometimes occur in conditions such as left or right ventricular hypertrophy, cardiomyopathy, myocarditis, tumor of the heart, obstructive pulmonary emphysema, acute cor pulmonale, ventricular preexcitation, and left anterior fascicular block, and thus may lead to an erroneous diagnosis. It is also important to realize that the ECG may be normal or show only nonspecific abnormalities in myocardial infarction. Serial changes in the ECG may be significant, especially if the initial ECG is normal. It cannot be emphasized too strongly that a normal initial tracing does not necessarily rule out infarction.
3. Sometimes the diagnosis of infarction is obscured altogether as in left bundle branch block. Echocardiography is useful when the ECG is nondiagnostic. The finding on echocardiogram of a localized contraction defect of the left ventricle is diagnostic of infarction.
4. Elevated serum levels of enzymes released from necrotic cardiac muscle support the diagnosis of myocardial infarction. The serum creatine phosphokinase (CPK) test is most useful in this regard and has rendered other enzyme tests largely obsolete. The CPK level rises during the first 4 to 6 hours after myocardial infarction, reaches a peak in about 12 hours, and generally returns to normal levels in 36 to 48 hours. The degree of enzyme elevation roughly corresponds to the size of the infarct. Other conditions may elevate the level. These include muscle trauma, intramuscular injections, recent surgery, muscle disease, cerebral infarction, hypothyroidism, and cardioversion. Isoenzymes of CPK are useful in distinguishing between CPK of cardiac and noncardiac origin. The MB fraction is virtually specific for cardiac necrosis and may be detected in the serum within the first 6 hours after the onset of infarction.
5. Fever, leukocytosis, and an elevated sedimentation rate are nonspecific abnormalities commonly associated with myocardial infarction. However, a persistently normal sedimentation rate suggests that infarction has not occurred.
6. Acute pericarditis may occur as the presenting feature of acute myocardial infarction. There is a possibility of "silent" infarction causing pericarditis in middle-aged or elderly patients.
7. Patients with prolonged bouts of anginalike pain unaccompanied by signs of myocardial necrosis are considered to have unstable angina, which may herald the occurrence of myocardial infarction.
8. Patients with a myocardial infarction or angina pectoris frequently have a second, coexisting, cause of chest pain arising from the chest wall. Demonstration of marked chest wall tenderness usually suffices for the diagnosis.

## Dissecting Hematoma (Aneurysm) of the Aorta

Dissecting hematomas occur most frequently in hypertensive males between 40 and 70 years of age.

CHARACTERISTICS OF PAIN IN DISSECTING HEMATOMA

1. The pain, which is inordinately severe and often unbearable, is usually described by the patient as having a sharp, tearing, or ripping quality. Large, repeated doses of narcotics are often needed to relieve the pain.

2. The location of the pain correlates with the site of intimal rupture. When the tear is above the aortic valve, the pain is located in the anterior chest; when the rupture is distal to the left subclavian artery, the pain is referred to the back. The pain may radiate along the pathway of aortic dissection.

PHYSICAL FINDINGS

Usually the patient appears to be very sick but does not show signs of shock unless rupture through the aortic wall takes place. Dissection of the aorta may spread and occlude major arteries, resulting in characteristic findings:

1. Carotid or vertebral occlusion may lead to syncope, coma, hemiplegia, or blindness.
2. Interference with circulation to the arms or legs may cause vascular insufficiency of the involved limb, with loss of arterial pulsations.
3. Renal artery occlusion may cause acute hypertension and oliguria.
4. Mesenteric artery occlusion may produce infarction of the bowel, with abdominal pain and ileus.
5. Dissection at the base of the aortic root may extend into the aortic ring and cause acute aortic regurgitation.
6. Coronary artery occlusion, which occurs occasionally, may lead to myocardial infarction.
7. External rupture of the aorta into the pericardial sac usually results in cardiac tamponade and death. External rupture into other sites, such as mediastinum, peritoneum, or retroperitoneum, may occur, and also may terminate life.

DIAGNOSTIC APPROACH

1. The diagnosis of dissecting hematoma is often suggested by the clinical picture, provided it is considered in the differential diagnosis of severe chest pain.
2. The chest roentgenogram usually reveals widening of the aortic shadow in the mediastinum. Progressive widening of this structure in serial films is strongly suggestive of the diagnosis.
3. Aortography is the most precise method for diagnosing aortic dissection. Under ideal circumstances, the points of entry and exit of the dissection can be seen in the films. The location and extent of the dissection may help in deciding between surgical and pharmacologic management. The initial decision to perform aortography should be postponed until the diagnosis of myocardial infarction has been excluded. As a general rule, no harm is done to the patient with aortic dissection who is treated palliatively, but serious harm can come to the patient with myocardial infarction who undergoes aortography. It is inappropriate, however, to subject the patient to a variety of other diagnostic procedures such as cervical spine films, upper gastrointestinal or gallbladder roentgen studies since undue delay in making the diagnosis of dissection may result in fatality.
4. CT scanning with the use of intravenous contrast has emerged as safe and reliable in detecting dissection.
5. The ECG usually shows nonspecific abnormalities. Evidence of myocardial infarction indicates involvement of the coronary arteries by the disease process.

## Pulmonary Embolism

CHEST PAIN IN PULMONARY EMBOLISM

Chest pain is present in the majority of patients with pulmonary embolism. Most often, the pain is pleuritic in nature. Occasionally, severe retrosternal discomfort may occur, simulating the pain of acute myocardial infarction. Dyspnea accompanies the chest pain in most patients with pulmonary embolism. Less frequently associated symptoms are apprehension, cough, and hemoptysis. On examination, the respiratory rate exceeds 16 per minute in nearly all cases of embolism. Audible rales and an accentuated pulmonary closure sound are common. Sinus tachycardia is the usual rhythm.

DIAGNOSTIC APPROACH

1. The diagnosis of pulmonary embolism is usually suggested by the clinical setting in which it occurs. Embolism should be suspected whenever dyspnea and chest pain develop suddenly in patients who have been immobilized or bedridden for long periods of time because of surgery, trauma, hip fracture, congestive heart failure, or malignancy. The susceptibility to thromboembolic phenomena apparently also is increased in women taking oral contraceptives.
2. Chest roentgenograms are usually not helpful in the diagnosis. In a minority of cases, signs of pulmonary infarction (consolidation, pleural effusion, atelectasis) may occur. With extensive embolization, distention of the proximal pulmonary arteries or localized areas of decreased vascularity may be observed.
3. The electrocardiogram is of relatively little diagnostic value in most cases of pulmonary embolism. The most common findings are nonspecific T-wave changes (chiefly inversion) and nonspecific S-T segment abnormalities. Disturbances in rhythm are uncommon. The following patterns, if present, are strongly suggestive of acute cor pulmonale: an $S_1Q_3T_3$ pattern with T-wave inversion in the right precordial leads; an $S_1T_3$ pattern or T-wave inversion in lead III and the right precordial leads; or an $S_1Q_3T_3$ pattern with right bundle branch block. Unfortunately, signs of acute cor pulmonale are found in only about 25 percent of cases.
4. Arterial blood gases often reveal some degree of hypoxemia and are of supportive value in the diagnosis of embolism.
5. Lung scanning is the diagnostic method of choice and should be performed in any patient with suspected embolism. (Further details may be found in the section Acute Pulmonary Radiographic Abnormalities, Chapter 4.)
6. Pulmonary angiography is an accurate method for disclosing the presence of embolism, but because special techniques are required, angiography is less readily available than scanning. The procedure should be reserved for instances in which the information to be obtained is vital to proper diagnosis and treatment. Angiography may be indicated under the following circumstances: (a) when massive embolism is believed to be present and pulmonary embolectomy is contemplated. It is then essential to verify the diagnosis by angiography lest a seriously ill patient be subjected to unnecessary thoracotomy; (b) when a high suspicion of embolism exists and conventional studies fail to provide a diagnosis; (c) when the use of anticoagulants or other forms of therapy hinges on an accurate diagnosis.
7. Digital subtraction angiography (DSA) offers a new and safer alternative to selective pulmonary angiography when the diagnosis is in doubt.

## Acute Pericarditis

Nearly all patients with acute pericarditis have chest pain. Because only the lower portion of the external surface of the pericardium is pain-sensitive, much of the pain is presumably due to inflammation of the adjoining diaphragmatic pleura.

PAIN IN ACUTE PERICARDITIS

1. Three types of pain may occur in acute pericarditis:
    a. Pleuritic pain is the most common type.
    b. Steady, severe retrosternal pain of sudden onset, simulating that of myocardial infarction, may occur.
    c. The rarest type is pain at the cardiac apex felt synchronously with each heartbeat.
2. Characteristics of pericardial pain:
    a. The pain is commonly sharp. It is normally increased by breathing deeply, rotating the trunk, swallowing, or yawning—maneuvers that have no effect

on the pain of myocardial infarction. It is often worse in recumbency and is sometimes relieved by sitting up and leaning forward.

  **b.** The pain is most commonly located in the precordial region and may radiate to the neck or to the left shoulder and arm.

DIAGNOSIS OF ACUTE PERICARDITIS

**1.** The pericardial friction rub. On examination, the most important finding is the presence of a pericardial friction rub over the precordium. The rub is often very transient, but it may persist and may even last for weeks. Classically, it has a superficial quality and is grating or scratchy in character. It may have systolic, diastolic, and presystolic components. It is accentuated by deep breathing and may be heard only in certain body positions (e.g., with the patient sitting and leaning forward). Pericardial rubs are often quite changeable in character from minute to minute or hour to hour. When confined to either systole or diastole, a rub may be confused with a cardiac murmur. Repeated observation usually makes the distinction clear, because the friction rub either assumes a to-and-fro character or disappears.

**2.** Pericardial effusion. Acute pericarditis is often accompanied by pericardial effusion. The physical signs depend upon the amount of fluid and, in the case of tamponade, on the rapidity of its accumulation. Signs of pericardial effusion include an increased area of cardiac dullness and muffling of the heart sounds. Signs of tamponade include decreased systolic pressure with a narrow pulse pressure, tachycardia, pulsus paradoxus, and inspiratory elevation of the jugular venous pressure. Echocardiography has emerged as the simplest, safest, and most accurate method for the diagnosis of pericardial effusion.

**3.** Electrocardiographic changes. The electrocardiographic diagnosis of acute pericarditis is based primarily on the presence of sequential changes in the S-T segments and T waves in multiple leads. The QRS abnormalities of myocardial infarction are absent. Low-voltage and electrical alternans may occur when effusions are large. The cardiac rhythm is usually a sinus tachycardia, but atrial arrhythmias may occur. P-R segment deviations are seen occasionally.

**4.** Differential diagnosis of acute pericarditis and myocardial infarction. Because of the similarity in pain and, occasionally, in the ECG findings, it may be difficult to differentiate between acute pericarditis and myocardial infarction. The following points may be helpful:

  **a.** The presence of a pleuritic component to the pain favors pericarditis.

  **b.** The development of pathologic Q waves in the ECG occurs only with myocardial infarction.

  **c.** S-T segment abnormalities are more widespread in pericarditis than in infarction. When elevated, the S-T segment may be concave upward in pericarditis, whereas convex changes are more consistent with infarction. Reciprocal S-T changes are usually absent in the limb leads in pericarditis but are commonly present in infarction. In pericarditis, the T waves are usually not inverted until the S-T segment is isoelectric; in infarction, they begin to invert while the S-T segment is still elevated.

  **d.** Serum enzyme elevations are absent or minimal in acute pericarditis.

  **e.** A pericardial friction rub may occur in either condition but is far less likely in infarction. The rub is more persistent in pericarditis.

  **f.** Large pericardial effusions occur only in pericarditis.

## Other Causes of Prolonged Chest Pain

Pneumothorax, mediastinal emphysema, acute pancreatitis, acute cholecystitis, peptic disease, and perforated ulcer may sometimes cause severe chest pain. Usually, local symptoms, signs, radiographic studies, and laboratory findings provide the information needed for correct diagnosis.

## VENOUS PRESSURE
H. Harold Friedman

### Measurement

1. The peripheral venous pressure is measured most accurately by manometry. However, an adequate approximation of the venous pressure for clinical purpose can be obtained by inspection of the jugular pulsations.
2. Although internal or external jugular pulsations may be used to estimate venous pressure, the former are preferred for this purpose.
3. Right-sided pulsations are preferred for measurement because left-sided ones may be falsely elevated by kinking of the left innominate vein.
4. The reference level for bedside evaluation of venous pressure is the sternal angle.
5. The height of the jugular pulsations varies with the position of the chest. For this reason, the patient should be examined in a position that is optimal for revealing the venous pulsations.
6. The vertical distance between the top of the venous column and the sternal angle represents the venous pressure.
7. The upper limits for normal venous pressure at various degrees of body elevation are:
   a. Recumbent, 2 cm.
   b. 30 degrees, 3 cm.
   c. 45 degrees, 4.5 cm.
   d. Upright, at the level of the suprasternal notch.
   These values are less than those obtained by manometry because the true zero value is at the level of the right atrium.
8. When the findings on inspection are equivocal, the 1-minute abdominal compression test (hepatojugular reflux) may unmask latent elevation of the venous pressure.
   a. The abdominal compression test is considered to give a positive result if abdominal pressure for 1 minute causes a rise of at least 1 cm in the level of venous pulsations.
   b. A positive response is usually indicative of right-sided heart failure.
   c. Pure left-sided heart failure usually elicits a normal or, at most, an equivocal response.
   d. False-positive results may occur in severe emphysema, superior vena cava obstruction below the azygos vein, hypervolemia, restrictive cardiomyopathy, pulmonary embolism, and increased sympathetic stimulation.
9. The maximum normal antecubital venous pressure, as determined by manometry, is 12 cm when the zero level is located 5 cm below the sternal angle, and 1 cm when the zero level is 10 cm from the back.
10. The central venous pressure (CVP) can be determined by transvenous placement of a plastic catheter into the superior vena cava or right atrium. The CVP is primarily an indicator of right ventricular function. It reflects the approximate level of the pulmonary capillary or wedge pressure when right and left ventricular function are comparable, but not when the function of these chambers is different (e.g., left ventricular failure). The CVP may be elevated in congestive heart failure, circulatory overload, and when intrathoracic or intrapericardial pressure is increased. The CVP is low in hypovolemic states (e.g., shock). Serial determinations are useful in treating patients with hypovolemia and shock, and in monitoring fluid replacement therapy. The normal range for CVP is between 5 and 1 cm of water.

    Hemodynamic monitoring using the Swan-Ganz catheter permits measurement of the pulmonary capillary pressure (normal range, 5 to 12 mm Hg) and cardiac output (normal cardiac index, 2.7–4.3 liters/min/M$^2$). This procedure has largely replaced measurements of the CVP. This type of monitoring has found its greatest usefulness in the management of seriously ill patients with acute myo cardial infarction, cardiogenic shock, and severe left ventricular failure, in whom CVP measurements may be misleading.

## Abnormalities of Venous Pressure

1. Unilateral nonpulsatile distention of the neck veins usually is indicative of venous obstruction. Unilateral distention of the left jugular veins, however, may be caused by compression of the left innominate vein, a condition that is clinically unimportant.
2. Bilateral nonpulsatile neck vein distention associated with venous collaterals in the upper thorax is strongly suggestive of superior vena caval obstruction in the absence of heart disease, hepatic congestion, or venous engorgement in the lower half of the body.
3. Bilateral pulsatile neck vein distention associated with generalized elevation of venous pressure is commonly found in the following conditions:
   a. Right-sided congestive heart failure from any cause.
   b. Pericardial effusion with tamponade.
   c. Chronic obstructive pulmonary disease.
   d. Bronchial asthma.
   e. Pleural effusion.
   f. Hyperkinetic circulatory states.
   g. Tricuspid stenosis.
   h. Tricuspid regurgitation.
   i. Central circulatory congestion due to noncardiac causes.
4. Inspiratory distention of the neck veins (Kussmaul's sign), formerly considered to be pathognomonic of chronic constrictive pericarditis or cardiac tamponade, may also occur in severe right ventricular failure and the restrictive cardiomyopathies.
5. Expiratory increase in venous pressure may occur in some cases of bronchial asthma and chronic obstructive pulmonary disease.

## JUGULAR VENOUS PULSE
### H. Harold Friedman

## The Normal Jugular Venous Pulse

The normal visible jugular venous pulse (see Fig. 3-1) consists of three positive waves (A, C, and V) and two negative waves (X and Y). The A wave is normally the tallest wave, exceeding both C and V waves in amplitude. The X wave is usually deeper than the Y wave. The heart sounds are preferable to the carotid pulse for timing the venous pulsations at the bedside.

### The A Wave

The A wave is produced by right atrial contraction. It begins before $S_1$ and peaks just before or during this sound. If an $S_4$ is present, it coincides with the summit of the wave. It precedes the carotid pulse.

### The C Wave

The C wave is probably produced by right ventricular systole and the bulging of the tricuspid valve into the right atrium. Impact of the carotid pulse against the

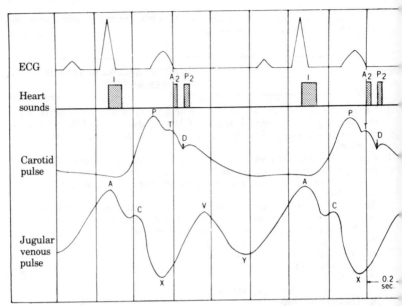

**Fig. 3-1.** Relationships between the electrocardiogram, heart sounds, arterial pulse, and jugular venous pulse. 1 = first heart sound; $A_2$ = aortic component of the second heart sound; $P_2$ = pulmonary component of the second sound; P = percussion wave; T = tidal wave; D = dicrotic notch; A, C, X, V, and Y = waves and troughs of the jugular venous pulse.

jugular vein may contribute to its genesis. It begins at the end of $S_1$ and peak shortly thereafter. It coincides with the upstroke of the carotid pulse.

### The X Descent ("Systolic Collapse" of the Venous Pulse)

The X descent is produced by right atrial relaxation and downward displaceme of the base of the heart. It begins with the downslope of the A wave and term nates in the X trough. Some authorities divide it into the X and X' descents, t C wave separating the two. The X trough occurs about 0.10 sec before $S_2$. The descent occurs during the peak of the carotid pulse.

### The V Wave

The V wave is produced by right atrial filling during right ventricular systo while the tricuspid valve is closed. It begins shortly before $P_2$ and peaks 0.06 0.08 sec after this sound. The peak of the V wave occurs after the dicrotic not of the carotid pulse.

### The Y Descent ("Diastolic Collapse" of the Venous Pulse)

The Y descent is produced by the rapid flow of blood into the right ventricle aft the opening of the tricuspid valve. It begins with the end of the V wave and en with the Y trough. The Y trough occurs about 0.20 sec after $P_2$. The Y desce comes long after the carotid pulse is felt.

## Abnormalities of the Jugular Venous Pulse

The types of abnormalities of the jugular venous pulsations and their causes are listed below.

### The A Wave

1. Large or giant A waves are caused by increased resistance at the tricuspid valve or increased resistance to right ventricular filling in the following conditions:
   a. Tricuspid stenosis or atresia.
   b. Ebstein's anomaly.
   c. Pulmonary stenosis.
   d. Pulmonary hypertension.
      (1) Primary.
      (2) Eisenmenger's syndrome (uncommon).
      (3) Mitral stenosis.
      (4) Acute and chronic cor pulmonale.
      (5) Tricuspid regurgitation (nonrheumatic cases secondary to pulmonary hypertension).
   e. Cardiomyopathy.
   f. Idiopathic hypertrophic subaortic stenosis.
   g. Aortic stenosis (some cases).
2. Decreased A waves are seen in the presence of a markedly dilated right atrium.
3. Absent A waves are seen in atrial fibrillation and atrial flutter (A waves replaced by flutter waves).
4. Cannon A waves are produced by fusion of giant A waves with C or V waves.
   a. Regular cannon waves.
      (1) Atrioventricular (AV) junctional rhythm.
      (2) First-degree AV block (some cases).
      (3) 2 : 1 AV block.
      (4) Atrial tachycardia (some cases).
   b. Irregular cannon waves.
      (1) Premature systoles.
         (a) Ventricular (frequently).
         (b) AV junctional (sometimes).
         (c) Atrial (rarely).
      (2) Complete AV dissociation.
         (a) Complete AV block.
         (b) AV junctional tachycardia (some cases).
         (c) Ventricular tachycardia (some cases).
      (3) Atrial flutter (difficult to detect).

### The X Descent

The X descent is decreased in atrial fibrillation. It is partially or completely obliterated by a regurgitant wave (called the CV, S, or V wave) in tricuspid regurgitation. It may be deeper than the Y descent in some cases of chronic constrictive pericarditis.

### The V Wave (Large V Wave)

1. Tricuspid regurgitation.
2. Right-sided heart failure.
3. Atrial septal defect (about 50 percent of cases).
4. Anomalous pulmonary venous drainage.

### The Y Descent

1. A slow, shallow Y descent is seen in tricuspid stenosis.
2. A rapid, steep Y descent is seen in constrictive pericarditis and in severe right sided heart failure.

## ARTERIAL PULSE
### H. Harold Friedman

### The Normal Arterial Pulse

Routine examination of the arteries should include palpation of the carotid, arm and leg pulses. The normal carotid pulse (see Fig. 3-1) consists of a brief upstroke a smooth dome-shaped summit, and a downstroke that is more gradual than the upstroke. The systolic percussion and tidal waves, as well as the dicrotic notch are not normally palpable, but they can be recorded. Most pulse wave abnormalities are detected best in the carotid arteries.

## Abnormalities of the Arterial Pulse

### Hypokinetic Pulse (Weak Pulse, Pulsus Parvus)

A small pulse signifies a narrowed pulse pressure. It is usually produced by low cardiac output in association with increased peripheral resistance. The causes are listed in Table 3-1.

### Hyperkinetic Pulse (Bounding Pulse)

A bounding pulse usually implies a widened pulse pressure. It is produced by varying combinations of increased stroke volume, increased cardiac output, and

**Table 3-1.** Causes of decreased pulse pressure*

Decreased cardiac output
    Congestive heart failure
    Shock
    Hypovolemia
    Acute myocardial infarction
    Cardiac tamponade
    Chronic constrictive pericarditis
    Cardiomyopathy and myocarditis
Peripheral vasoconstriction
    Shock
    Hypovolemia
Mechanical
    Valvular disease
        Aortic outflow obstruction
        Mitral stenosis or regurgitation, or both
    Aortic disease
        Coarctation of the aorta
        Aortic arch syndrome

*More than one mechanism may be operative.

**Table 3-2.** Causes of increased pulse pressure*

Decreased distensibility of the arterial system
    Atherosclerosis (most common)
    Hypertension
    Coarctation of the aorta
Increased stroke volume
    Normal
    Anxiety, exercise
    Complete heart block
    Aortic regurgitation
Increased cardiac output or decreased peripheral resistance, or both
    Fever
    Anemia
    Thyrotoxicosis
    Hyperkinetic heart syndrome
    Arteriovenous fistula
    Paget's disease
    Beriberi
    Cirrhosis of the liver

*More than one mechanism may be operative.

lowered peripheral resistance. The causes are listed in Table 3-2. A water-hammer pulse is an exaggerated type of bounding pulse. Corrigan's sign, as originally described, consists of visible abrupt distention and rapid collapse of the carotid pulse. It is therefore a sign detected by inspection, not by palpation. The sign is quite characteristic of aortic regurgitation.

### Pulsus Parvus et Tardus

This is a pulse of low amplitude that rises slowly to a late summit. It is usually found in valvular aortic stenosis. Although it may occur with less frequency in subvalvular aortic stenosis due to a fibrous ring or diaphragm, it is not found in idiopathic hypertrophic subaortic stenosis. The anacrotic pulse, a variant of pulsus parvus et tardus, in which a notch is palpable on the upstroke of the pulse wave, is indicative of severe aortic stenosis.

### Pulsus Bisferiens

Pulsus bisferiens is a twice-beating pulse in which both peaks occur during systole. The initial, or percussion, wave is brisk and forceful. The second, or tidal, wave is slower-rising and less prominent than the percussion wave. Pulsus bisferiens occurs most commonly in combined aortic stenosis and regurgitation, but it may occur in pure aortic regurgitation. Pulsus bisferiens is also characteristic of idiopathic hypertrophic subaortic stenosis.

### Dicrotic Pulse

A dicrotic pulse is a double-peaked pulse in which the initial wave occurs during systole and the final (dicrotic) wave occurs during diastole. It occurs in some fevers, notably typhoid fever, and occasionally in mild or moderate aortic regurgitation.

## Pulsus Alternans

Pulsus alternans is a condition in which the pulse waves during regular rhythm are alternately strong and weak. It may be detected by palpation but it is more accurately assessed by sphygmomanometry. To detect pulsus alternans, inflate the blood pressure cuff rapidly above the systolic pressure and then deflate it slowly until sounds are first audible. At this point, the beats are heard at one-half of the heart rate. When the cuff is deflated further, the rate doubles. There may be some variation in the intensity of the strong and weak beats. Pulsus alternans can be diagnosed only if the heart rate is regular. It is often accentuated when the patient is sitting or standing. Severe degrees may be palpable over the radial and other peripheral arteries.

Pulsus alternans is virtually diagnostic of left ventricular failure and is commonly associated with a ventricular ($S_3$) gallop rhythm. However, it may occasionally occur during or after paroxysmal tachycardia in an otherwise normal heart. Pulsus alternans must be differentiated from bigeminy produced by premature systoles. In pulsus alternans, the intervals between the strong and weak beats are equal. In extrasystolic bigeminy, weak ectopic beats occur prematurely and are followed by strong normal beats after pauses, resulting in ventricular cycles that are alternately short and long.

## Pulsus Paradoxus

Pulsus paradoxus is a condition in which the inspiratory decline in systolic pressure exceeds 10 mm Hg (maximum normal value during quiet respiration). To detect pulsus paradoxus, inflate the cuff rapidly above the systolic pressure and then slowly deflate it. The difference between the systolic pressures at which sounds are first heard only during expiration and later during both expiration and inspiration is a measure of the magnitude (in mm Hg) of the paradoxical pulse. Deep inspiration may cause a 10- to 15-mm fluctuation in the systolic pressure of a normal person but does not cause the radial pulse to disappear. Hence, disappearance of the radial pulse on deep inspiration suggests significant pulsus paradoxus.

Classic pulsus paradoxus occurs in cardiac tamponade and constrictive pericarditis, but it may also be found in chronic obstructive airway disease and occasionally in cardiomyopathy or shock. Pulsus paradoxus due to constrictive pericarditis or cardiac tamponade is sometimes associated with an inspiratory increase in venous pressure (Kussmaul's sign), whereas pulsus paradoxus due to pulmonary disease usually shows an expiratory increase in venous pressure.

---

## Pulse and Pressure Differences Between the Arms and Legs

---

Normally, with a standard cuff, the systolic blood pressure in the legs is about 20 to 40 mm Hg higher than that in the arms. With a large cuff (18 cm), the systolic blood pressure in the lower extremities is about the same as that in the upper extremities ($\pm$ 10 mm Hg). A large cuff is more accurate than a standard cuff for measuring the blood pressure in the legs. The femoral pulse should occur slightly earlier than the radial pulse and should be of equal or greater intensity. A diminished and delayed femoral pulse is a classic finding in coarctation of the aorta. Decreased femoral pulses may also occur because of occlusive disease in the terminal aorta or iliac arteries, aortic dissection, or aneurysm of the abdominal aorta. Decreased or absent popliteal and pedal pulsations with good preservation of the femoral pulses are indicative of occlusive peripheral arterial disease.

## Pulse and Pressure Differences Between the Arms

Normally there is a difference of less than 15 mm Hg of systolic blood pressure between the two arms. An aberrant radial artery is the most common cause of unequal radial pulses. Pulse and pressure differences between the arms may also be due to other causes:

1. Acquired disease.
   a. Subclavian steal syndrome.
   b. Aortic arch syndrome (pulseless disease, Takayasu's syndrome).
   c. Thoracic outlet syndrome.
   d. Arterial thrombosis and embolism.
   e. Aneurysm of the thoracic aorta.
   f. Dissection aneurysm.
   g. Incompressible brachial artery.
2. Congenital disease.
   a. Coarctation of the aorta.
   b. Supravalvular aortic stenosis. (In more than 50 percent of cases, the pressure difference between the arms exceeds 20 mm Hg, with the right arm pressure greater except in dextrocardia.)
   c. Patent ductus arteriosus.
   d. Anomalous subclavian artery.

# ARTERIAL HYPERTENSION
H. Harold Friedman

## Normal Blood Pressure

The maximum normal blood pressure is 140/90 mm Hg. In normal persons in the recumbent position, the popliteal blood pressure exceeds the brachial pressure by 20 to 40 mm Hg when determined by sphygmomanometry.

## Systolic Hypertension

### Definition

Elevation of the systolic pressure without concomitant elevation of the diastolic pressure constitutes systolic hypertension.

### Etiology

1. Decreased elasticity of the aorta due to aortic atherosclerosis (most common).
2. Increased cardiac output due to fever, anemia, thyrotoxicosis, hyperkinetic heart syndrome, arteriovenous fistula, Paget's disease, beriberi, or anxiety.
3. Increased stroke volume due to aortic insufficiency or complete heart block.
4. Coarctation of the aorta.

### Symptoms

Symptoms, if any, are produced by the underlying disease and are not attributable to the hypertension per se.

### Signs

Systolic hypertension is signified by a persistently elevated systolic pressure.

### Diagnostic Approach

1. Rule out coarctation of the aorta by checking the blood pressure and pulses in both the upper and lower extremities. If the blood pressure in the legs is 20 to 30 mm Hg less than that in the arms, or if the femoral pulse peak is delayed, or both, check further for evidence of aortic coarctation.
2. Rule out high-output states and conditions causing increased stroke volume.
3. If the foregoing conditions are excluded and the patient is middle-aged or elderly, aortic atherosclerosis is the most probable cause.

---

## Diastolic Hypertension

---

### Definition

Diastolic hypertension is defined as elevation of the diastolic pressure above normal values. It is almost always associated with concomitant elevation of the systolic pressure. The diagnosis of hypertension is not warranted unless blood pressure readings exceed normal values on at least three separate occasions after a 15- to 20-minute period of rest.

### Etiology

1. Primary, or essential, hypertension (90 percent of cases).
2. Secondary hypertension.
   a. Endocrine disorders.
      (1) Adrenal.
          (a) Aldosteronism (1 to 2 percent of cases).
          (b) Pheochromocytoma (0.1 percent of cases).
          (c) Cushing's syndrome.
      (2) Thyroid: hypothyroidism.
      (3) Pituitary.
          (a) Acromegaly.
          (b) Cushing's disease.
      (4) Parathyroid: hyperparathyroidism.
   b. Renal disease.
      (1) Renal artery lesions (7 percent of cases).
          (a) *Intrinsic:* atherosclerotic plaque (most common); fibromuscular hyperplasia; aneurysm, thrombosis, or embolism; arteriovenous fistula; arteritis.
          (b) *Extrinsic compression:* tumor involving renal pedicle, congenital fibrous band, retroperitoneal fibrosis.
      (2) Parenchymal (0.5 percent of cases).
          (a) *Unilateral:* congenital hypoplastic kidney; pyelonephritis (pyogenic, tuberculous); irradiation, trauma, renal neoplasm, unilateral renal vein thrombosis; obstructive nephropathy.
          (b) *Bilateral:* glomerulonephritis; pyelonephritis; polycystic disease; connective tissue disease; amyloidosis; gouty nephropathy; nephrocalcinosis; obstructive nephropathy.
          (c) Coarctation of the aorta.
          (d) Toxemia of pregnancy.
   c. Oral contraceptive agents.
   d. Miscellaneous causes: polycythemia, burns, lead poisoning, CNS lesions (increased intracranial pressure, brain tumors, bulbar poliomyelitis).

## Symptoms

1. The age and type of onset may provide clues to the etiology of hypertension.
   a. A gradual onset between the ages of 35 and 55 years is typical of essential hypertension.
   b. An acute onset in children or young adults suggests acute renal disease (e.g., acute glomerulonephritis).
   c. Moderate to severe hypertension in the young is usually indicative of chronic renal disease (e.g., chronic glomerulonephritis).
   d. A sudden onset in middle-aged or older persons suggests a renovascular cause.
   e. A rapid onset of severe, progressive hypertension, or sudden acceleration of preexisting hypertension, may herald the onset of a malignant phase in either primary or secondary hypertension.
2. Elevated diastolic blood pressure per se is asymptomatic except possibly for morning occipital headache.
3. Symptoms in patients with essential hypertension are nonspecific or are related to the cardiovascular, cerebral, or renal complications of the disease.
4. Some types of secondary hypertension, such as primary aldosteronism, Cushing's syndrome, or pheochromocytoma, may be associated with symptoms or signs that are strongly suggestive of its cause.
5. Muscular weakness in association with hypertension suggests coexistent hypokalemia.
6. Symptoms of muscle weakness (sometimes with paralysis) in association with polyuria, nocturia, polydipsia, tetany, and hypertension are strongly suggestive of primary aldosteronism.
7. Attacks of headache, blurring of vision, sweating, palpitation, nausea, trembling, and pallor with either paroxysmal or persistent hypertension are suggestive of pheochromocytoma.

## Signs

1. Delayed femoral pulses and blood pressures in the legs that are lower than those in the arms suggest coarctation of the aorta.
2. Decreased or absent femoral pulses may be indicative of occlusive disease in the abdominal aorta or iliac arteries or of coarctation of the aorta.
3. An abdominal bruit, audible anteriorly in the epigastrium or over the flank, is strongly suggestive of renal artery stenosis.
4. Bilaterally enlarged kidneys in patients with hypertension suggest polycystic disease.
5. An orthostatic drop in blood pressure suggests secondary rather than primary hypertension and is especially characteristic of pheochromocytoma.
6. The physical findings in some types of secondary hypertension (e.g., Cushing's syndrome) may be sufficiently characteristic to permit or at least suggest the correct diagnosis.
7. An assessment of the severity of the hypertension can be made from the degree of cardiac, cerebral, and renal involvement, and from the blood pressure readings:

   Mild: diastolic pressure 100 mm Hg or less.
   Moderate: diastolic pressure 100 to 120 mm Hg.
   Severe: diastolic pressure above 120 mm Hg.
   Malignant: diastolic pressure above 140 mm Hg.

8. The chronicity and severity of the hypertension may also be estimated by funduscopy. The normal arteriolar-venous (AV) diameter ratio is 3 : 4.

   Grade I (mild): AV ratio 1 : 2, no hemorrhages, exudates, or papilledema.
   Grade II (moderately severe): AV ratio 1 : 3, AV nicking, no hemorrhages, exudates, or papilledema.

Grade III (severe): AV ratio 1 : 4, hemorrhages or exudates, or both, but no papilledema.

Grade IV (malignant): AV ratio as above, marked arteriolar narrowing, hemorrhages, exudates, and papilledema.

## Initial Evaluation

The initial workup in patients with hypertension has a threefold purpose: (1) to
identify systemic complications of hypertension, (2) to establish an etiologic diagnosis, if possible, and (3) to screen for the fewer than 10 percent of hyperten-
sives with the potentially curable forms of the disease. Some workup is indicated
in every patient with hypertension. Under *ideal* conditions, every hypertensive
patient should have the comprehensive rather than the limited basic workup outlined in succeeding paragraphs. However, some selectivity is required because
neither funds, personnel, nor facilities are available for a complete evaluation of
every patient with hypertension. Furthermore, screening for the common causes
of curable hypertension can usually be done on clinical grounds with simple procedures.

LIMITED BASIC WORKUP

In patients with stable, mild, or moderate hypertension beginning after the age
of 35 years, many authorities believe that a satisfactory initial workup can be
limited to

1. Hematocrit.
2. Urinalysis.
3. Serum creatinine or BUN.
4. Serum potassium.
5. Electrocardiogram.
    Other tests that may be helpful include chest films, CBC, and a biochemical
    profile.

COMPREHENSIVE BASIC WORKUP

1. Urinalysis to screen for intrinsic renal disease. The urine usually shows no abnormalities in essential or renovascular hypertension and in primary aldosteronism unless the hypertension is severe, in which case there may be mild proteinuria or microscopic hematuria. On the other hand, it is rare to have primary renal
   disease without proteinuria and some abnormality of the urine sediment.
2. Urine culture and sensitivity studies to detect bacteriuria associated with pyelonephritis.
3. Biochemical screening, including
    a. Serum electrolytes (Na, K, Cl, and $CO_2$) to detect hypokalemia and alkalosis
       caused by primary aldosteronism, Cushing's syndrome, or other diseases.
    b. BUN and creatinine to screen for gross impairment of renal function.
    c. Serum uric acid to detect hyperuricemia, gout, or related gouty nephropathy.
    d. A 2-hour postprandial blood glucose or standard glucose tolerance test to de-
       tect diabetes mellitus or carbohydrate intolerance due to such other causes
       as pheochromocytoma, primary aldosteronism, or Cushing's syndrome.
4. Urinary vanillylmandelic acid (VMA) determination to screen for pheochromocytoma.
5. Urinary 17-hydroxycorticosteroid determination to screen for Cushing's syndrome.
6. An ECG for evidence of left ventricular and left atrial enlargement. Other abnormalities due to myocardial damage from associated coronary artery disease may
   also be discovered.
7. Chest films to estimate heart size, detect pulmonary complications, or diagnose
   aortic coarctation.
8. A rapid-sequence IVP to help identify unilateral disease of the renal parenchyma,

renovascular lesions, polycystic disease, or pyelonephritis. A normal result lends support to a diagnosis of essential hypertension.

9. Renal arteriography may be useful in evaluating renovascular hypertension and determining appropriate treatment.

## Subsequent Evaluation

NEGATIVE INITIAL WORKUP

Patients with mild to moderate hypertension that is familial and begins after the age of 35 years, with no abnormalities revealed by clinical history, examination, or initial limited or comprehensive workup, are assumed to have *essential hypertension* and should be treated accordingly. No further workup is necessary. When the initial workup suggests a potentially curable form of hypertension, additional studies are justified only if the results to be obtained will materially alter the treatment program. The evaluation must be tailored to each patient. Thus, a complete workup for pheochromocytoma is indicated if the clinical history and urinary VMA excretion suggest this diagnosis, because surgical removal of the tumor is necessary to effect a cure. On the other hand, a 65-year-old woman with a blood pressure of 160/100 mm Hg and no evidence of systemic complications does not need renal arteriography; even if renovascular disease were detected, surgical therapy probably would not be warranted.

ABNORMAL URINARY FINDINGS

1. If the urinalysis suggests *primary renal parenchymal disease* or if the BUN or serum creatinine is elevated, a creatinine clearance test should be performed to estimate the degree of renal function impairment and to provide a baseline for future studies. More comprehensive studies for the diagnosis of primary renal parenchymal disease are discussed in the section Proteinuria, Chapter 7.

2. The presence of abnormal urinary findings such as proteinuria, white cells, and white cell clumps or casts, together with bacteriuria, suggests the diagnosis of *chronic pyelonephritis,* although urinalysis may yield negative findings in this disease. Bacteriuria with over 100,000 colonies per milliliter of urine (from a clean-voided specimen) is considered significant. In chronic pyelonephritis, the IVP usually shows bilaterally shrunken kidneys with scarred and clubbed calyces.

---

# Hypokalemia
# and Hypertension

---

If the serum potassium level is low (3 mEq/liter or less) or borderline, further investigation for possible causes of hypokalemia and hypertension (listed below) is warranted. For practical purposes, if cases of essential hypertension treated with diuretics or other potassium-depleting drugs are excluded, the most common cause of hypokalemia in hypertensive patients is primary aldosteronism. Adrenocortical hyperplasia and other rare syndromes of adrenocortical dysfunction are uncommon causes of hypokalemia in patients with hypertension.

## Etiology

1. Essential hypertension with
   a. Vomiting and diarrhea.
   b. Diuretic therapy.
   c. Oral contraceptive or estrogen therapy.
   d. Steroid therapy.

**2.** Renal disease.
   **a.** Accelerated or malignant hypertension.
   **b.** Renovascular hypertension.
   **c.** Potassium-losing nephropathies (e.g., chronic pyelonephritis).
   **d.** Renin-secreting renal tumor.
   **e.** Liddle's syndrome.
**3.** Adrenocortical dysfunction.
   **a.** Primary aldosteronism.
      **(1)** Aldosterone-producing adenoma.
      **(2)** Cortical hyperplasia.
   **b.** Cushing's syndrome and the ectopic ACTH syndrome.
   **c.** Endogenous mineralocorticoid excess (some adrenocortical tumors).
   **d.** Exogenous administration of mineralocorticoids.
**4.** Pseudoaldosteronism (excessive licorice ingestion syndrome).

---

## Diagnostic Approach

---

The *first* step is to determine whether the potassium loss is the result of renal or extrarenal mechanisms. Extrarenal potassium depletion is easily recognized by the clinical picture and is correctable by replacement therapy with potassium salts. On the other hand, if there is renal potassium wasting, then diuretics, kidney disease (parenchymal or vascular), primary aldosteronism, or other rare forms of adrenocortical dysfunction may be responsible. Before proceeding with additional laboratory studies, it is well to recheck the history and physical examination for diagnostic clues.

**1.** History.
   **a.** Inquire specifically for possible causes of potassium depletion: Has the patient been taking diuretics, laxatives, steroids, estrogens, or oral contraceptive agents? Is there a history of vomiting or diarrhea? Has potassium intake been reduced?
   **b.** Be sure that the patient is not a licorice ingestor, because the glycyrrhizic acid in licorice may mimic the action of aldosterone by producing hypertension, alkalosis, and suppressed renin activity (but with low aldosterone secretion). Measurement of urinary aldosterone excretion will differentiate between primary aldosteronism and the syndrome of chronic licorice ingestion.
   **c.** Ask whether the patient has been on a low-sodium diet, because salt restriction may mask the hypokalemia of primary aldosteronism.
**2.** Physical examination.
   **a.** In primary aldosteronism, retinopathy is usually mild (Grade I or II) and edema is absent.
   **b.** A positive Trousseau's or Chvostek's sign in an untreated hypertensive patient is presumptive evidence of hyperaldosteronism.
   **c.** Lack of an abdominal bruit is an important sign favoring aldosteronism over renovascular hypertension.
   **d.** The Valsalva maneuver in primary aldosteronism does not elicit the characteristic hypertensive overshoot and bradycardia found in other types of hypertension.
**3.** Determining the mechanism of potassium loss.
   **a.** If the patient has been taking diuretics or other drugs that induce hypokalemia, these should be discontinued. Give 50 mEq of potassium (as the chloride) daily for 1 week. Stop the potassium chloride and recheck the serum potassium and sodium in 1 to 2 weeks. If the serum potassium is then normal, for practical purposes renal potassium wasting and the diagnosis of primary aldosteronism can be ruled out. On the other hand, if the serum potassium is borderline or low, proceed as in paragraph **b** below.
   **b.** If the serum potassium is borderline or low and there is no obvious cause for the hypokalemia, check for potassium wasting. Measure the 24-hour urinary

excretion of potassium while the patient is on a regular salt intake (as reflected in a urinary sodium level of approximately 100 mEq/24 hours). Urinary potassium excretion of less than 20 mEq/24 hours is strong evidence against renal potassium wasting and the diagnosis of primary aldosteronism, whereas a level of 60 mEq/24 hours or greater is strongly suggestive of renal potassium wasting.

  **c.** If the serum potassium is initially low and the studies outlined in paragraphs **a** and **b** above show negative findings, it can be assumed that the patient does not have renal potassium wasting or primary aldosteronism, and further investigation for this diagnosis is not warranted.

  **d.** If the preliminary results, as outlined in paragraphs **a** and **b** above, are suggestive of nondiuretic renal potassium wasting, the two most likely possibilities are primary aldosteronism and renovascular hypertension. At this point the determination of plasma renin activity and aldosterone excretion are the next steps indicated.

  **(1)** Plasma renin activity (PRA). The PRA test is done by comparing the plasma renin level under basal conditions with the level obtained after 4 hours of ambulation. The patient should be on a 20 mEq sodium diet for at least 4 days prior to the test. The normal response is a twofold or threefold rise in PRA after 4 hours of ambulation. Patients with primary aldosteronism show decreased plasma renin values, which typically fail to rise after activity. It must be remembered that about 25 percent of patients with essential hypertension have suppressed PRA, but aldosterone excretion is usually low or normal in these patients. PRA is decreased in patients with excessive production of deoxycorticosterone or corticosterone, and is normal or elevated in patients with secondary aldosteronism. The measurement of peripheral PRA 5 hours after the oral administration of 60 mg of furosemide is a somewhat simpler and more convenient screening procedure. However, the stimulation of renin activity is not as marked as that produced by a low-sodium diet.

  **(2)** Aldosterone excretion. Measure the quantity of aldosterone in a 24-hour urine sample after the patient has been on a sodium intake of at least 200 mEq per day. Increased aldosterone secretion after salt-loading is found in primary and secondary aldosteronism (it may also occur, rarely, in essential hypertension). When aldosterone excretion is increased, elevated PRA suggests renovascular hypertension, and low PRA suggests primary aldosteronism. Aldosterone secretion is reduced in the 17-alpha-hydroxylase and 11-beta-hydroxylase deficiency syndromes and in Liddle's syndrome.

  **(3)** Adrenal arteriography and venography. If the diagnosis of primary aldosteronism is established, adrenal arteriography or venography may be advisable in the preoperative evaluation of the patient for tumor localization. In some medical centers, tumor localization is attempted by catheterization of the adrenal veins bilaterally. Usually there is at least a twofold increase in the adrenal venous aldosterone levels on the side with the tumor.

## Summary of the Results of Various Tests for Hypertension with Hypokalemia

1. If aldosterone excretion is increased and PRA is suppressed, the diagnosis is primary aldosteronism due to an aldosterone-producing adenoma, nodular hyperplasia, or adrenocortical hyperplasia (glucocorticoid-remediable hypertension).
2. If aldosterone excretion is increased and PRA is normal or elevated, the diagnosis is secondary aldosteronism due to accelerated or malignant hypertension, renovascular hypertension, essential hypertension with diuretic therapy, or essential hypertension with oral contraceptive medications.

3. If aldosterone excretion is reduced and PRA is suppressed, mineralocorticoids other than aldosterone, such as deoxycorticosterone and corticosterone, may be responsible for the hypertension.

  a. The 17-alpha-hydroxylase deficiency syndrome is characterized by hypertension, hypokalemic alkalosis, hypogonadism, primary amenorrhea, little if any 17-hydroxycorticosteroids or aldosterone in the urine, and responsiveness to glucocorticosteroids.

  b. The 11-beta-hydroxylase deficiency syndrome is characterized by hypertension, hypokalemic alkalosis, sodium retention and edema, virilization in the female, precocious puberty in the male, reduced excretion of 17-hydroxycorticosteroids and aldosterone, and responsiveness to glucocorticosteroids.

## Abnormal Intravenous Pyelogram

The rapid-sequence IVP is a screening procedure for determining the role played by the kidney in hypertension.

1. If the kidneys are reduced in size and scarred and the calyces are clubbed, *chronic pyelonephritis* is probable.

2. If the kidneys are shrunken with normal calyces and pelves, *chronic glomerulonephritis* or *nephrosclerosis* is likely.

3. Grossly enlarged kidneys with spidery calyces are virtually pathognomonic of *polycystic disease.*

4. *Unilateral primary parenchymal disease,* not due to vascular impairment, is characterized by clubbed calyces and a thinned cortex on the affected side. In addition to the urographic findings, the evidence for unilateral parenchymal disease, rather than renovascular disease, as the cause of hypertension includes a history of urinary tract infections, decreased urine osmolality, and increased sodium concentration by split-function studies, normal renal vasculature by arteriography (except that the vasculature size will reflect the diminished function), and normal peripheral and renal plasma renin activity.

5. *Renovascular hypertension* is suggested by one or more of the following findings: (a) unilateral reduction in kidney size, exceeding 1.5 cm on the left or 1.0 cm on the right, (b) delayed appearance of the contrast medium on the affected side, (c) greater concentration of the radiopaque medium on the affected side when the contrast material finally does appear, and (d) notching of the pelvis or upper ureter on the affected side by collateral vessels. Even if renovascular hypertension is suggested by the urographic findings, it is unnecessary to do additional studies unless surgery is contemplated. Ancillary studies available for the diagnosis of renovascular hypertension in addition to the IVP are the radioactive renogram, determination of PRA, aortography, catheterization of the renal veins for PRA, and differential renal function tests.

  a. The radioactive renogram is a safe, easy test to perform. It is not a specific diagnostic study but provides a comparison of the blood flow to each kidney. Although positive renogram and IVP findings do not always coincide in the same patient, a combination of the two may identify renovascular disease in a larger number of cases than will either test alone.

  b. Digital subtraction angiography or aortography by the femoral route can be performed to visualize the renal arteries. The mere presence of anatomic renal arterial lesions does not establish their functional significance. Proof of their functional significance in the form of increased PRA should be obtained.

  c. PRA is usually increased in patients with renovascular hypertension both in the basal state and after 4 hours of ambulation.

  d. Some authorities believe that the best technique for confirming the diagnosis of curable renovascular hypertension is the determination of PRA in blood samples from the renal veins of both kidneys. A level of PRA on the involved side that is at least one and a half times greater than that on the uninvolved side is considered significant.

e. Split kidney function tests, employing bilateral ureteral catheterization, are usually performed prior to surgery, primarily to be certain that if nephrectomy is required, the remaining kidney will function adequately. The diagnosis of renal ischemia may also receive additional support. Split kidney function tests generally show impairment of renal function on the affected side unless there are segmental lesions that are too small to produce measurable renal function impairment. In the interpretation of the tests, a 50 percent or greater decrease in urine volume, a 15 percent or greater decrease in sodium concentration, a lowered glomerular filtration rate, and an increased creatinine concentration on the affected side are considered diagnostic of renal ischemia. Bilateral lesions may not be detected with this technique, and both false-positive and false-negative responses may occur.

## Increased Excretion of VMA

1. Urinary excretion of VMA that is twice the normal rate is virtually pathognomonic of *pheochromocytoma*. False-positive and false-negative results may be produced by interfering drugs.

2. Clinically, pheochromocytoma is characterized by one or more of the following features: paroxysmal or persistent hypertension; attacks of headache, blurred vision, sweating, palpitation, trembling, and pallor; hyperglycemia and glycosuria; orthostatic hypotension; a tendency to cholelithiasis; a familial incidence in some cases; and an association with such diseases as carcinoma of the thyroid gland, parathyroid adenoma, neurofibromatosis, and neuroectodermal diseases (e.g., Lindau-von Hippel disease and tuberous sclerosis). Ninety percent of pheochromocytomas occur in the adrenal gland, and of these about 10 percent are bilateral. Two percent of extramedullary tumors are multiple. Malignancy is present in fewer than 10 percent of cases.

3. If VMA excretion is increased, the diagnosis should be confirmed by assay of catecholamines or metanephrines, or both, in a 24-hour urine specimen.

4. If excretion of VMA, catecholamines, or metanephrines is normal in a case with a high index of clinical suspicion, urine should be collected for a short, carefully timed period during and immediately after an attack and examined for catecholamines.

5. Pharmacologic tests such as the phentolamine, histamine, tyramine, and glucagon tests are unnecessary and inadvisable because they are hazardous and less accurate than urine assays.

6. Extraabdominal location of the tumor can often be ruled out by physical examination of the neck and chest films. Computerized tomography of the abdomen is an excellent method for the localization of adrenal pheochromocytoma and may replace invasive procedures. However, invasive studies (arteriography and venography) together with the determination of catecholamine levels are indicated for the accurate localization of extraabdominal tumors.

7. All patients with suspected pheochromocytoma should be evaluated preoperatively by an expert.

## PRECORDIAL PULSATIONS AND MOVEMENTS
H. Harold Friedman

A great deal of useful clinical information is obtained by inspection and palpation of the precordium and chest wall. The apical impulse can be located and its characteristics defined. In addition, palpable sounds, murmurs, thrills and abnormal pulsations, and ventricular enlargement can be detected. For a complete examination, the patient should be examined while sitting, lying supine, and lying in the left lateral recumbent position. The heart sounds are the most useful reference points for timing cardiac pulsations.

## Apical Impulse

### Normal

1. The location of the apex beat is determined most accurately in the sitting position. The normal apical impulse lies in or about the fifth intercostal space inside the midclavicular line at a distance no greater than 10 cm from the left sternal border. The impulse is confined to a single area no greater than 2 or 3 cm in diameter.
2. The normal apex beat is a systolic outward movement of brief duration (from $S_1$ to before $S_2$) that has a light, tapping quality. A somewhat more forceful beat is not abnormal in tense or thin-chested individuals.
3. The outward thrust of the apex beat is accompanied by slight inward movement of the chest wall overlying the right ventricle.
4. The apical impulse may not be palpable in many normal individuals.

### Abnormal

1. Aside from its absence as a normal variant, the apical impulse may be impalpable because of disease (e.g., mitral stenosis, constrictive pericarditis). Thus, absence of the apex beat by itself has little diagnostic significance.
2. An apex beat that is not substantially displaced from its normal location but that is heaving, sustained (lasting from $S_1$ to $S_2$), forceful, and strong enough to lift the fingers against firm pressure, is indicative of left ventricular hypertrophy due to pressure loading (e.g., systemic hypertension, aortic stenosis). It is associated with increased systolic precordial retraction, producing the so-called *left ventricular rock*.
3. A sustained and abnormally bulging apical impulse, indistinguishable from the heave of left ventricular hypertrophy, may be encountered in myocardial infarction in the absence of hypertrophy.
4. An apex beat that is displaced laterally and downward is indicative of left ventricular dilatation, with or without hypertrophy.
   a. A sustained but weak apical impulse is indicative of dilatation.
   b. A hyperdynamic impulse, meaning one that is forceful, exaggerated, and abrupt (although prolonged beyond normal), is indicative of combined dilatation and hypertrophy due to volume overloading (e.g., aortic or mitral regurgitation, left-to-right shunt). A hyperdynamic impulse is also associated with a left ventricular rock.
5. Double apical impulses may be associated with an $S_3$ or $S_4$ gallop. In such cases, the ventricular impulse is systolic, and the additional impulse is diastolic.
6. Double apical thrusts, with both impulses occurring in systole, are strongly suggestive of idiopathic hypertrophic subaortic stenosis, but they may also occur in some cases of myocardial infarction, angina pectoris, left ventricular aneurysm, or the systolic click syndrome associated with prolapse of the mitral valve into the left atrium.
7. The presence of asynchronous cardiac impulses palpable at both the xiphoid and apex suggests combined ventricular hypertrophy.

## Left Parasternal Pulsations

1. A slight precordial lift may occur normally in children and young adults.
2. Bulging of the precordium in a child generally denotes long-standing right ventricular enlargement.

3. A localized, sustained, heaving lift in the lower left parasternal region is indicative of right ventricular hypertrophy due to pressure loading (e.g., pulmonary hypertension from any cause, pulmonary stenosis). The lift is associated with conspicuous systolic retraction of the chest further to the left, producing the so-called *right ventricular rock*.
4. A hyperdynamic impulse over a relatively large area parasternally is indicative of right ventricular enlargement due to volume loading (e.g., atrial septal defect). This impulse is also associated with a right ventricular rock.
5. A left parasternal lift may be palpable in the absence of right ventricular hypertrophy or pulmonary hypertension when the right ventricle is pushed anteriorly by a giant left atrium.
6. Marked right ventricular dilatation may displace the right ventricular beat leftward to the site of the normal cardiac impulse. In such cases, identification of the impulse as right rather than left ventricular in origin is supported by the presence of a right ventricular lift, an accentuated $P_2$, and the demonstration of a left ventricular impulse, or the thrill and murmur of mitral valvular disease, in the left axilla.

## Other Systolic Precordial Pulsations and Movements

1. A diffuse systolic depression of the precordium followed by a brisk diastolic rebound and a palpable or audible "knock" is characteristic of chronic constrictive pericarditis.
2. A diffuse systolic depression at the left side of the chest accompanied by an opposite pulsation at the right side is characteristic of tricuspid regurgitation.
3. Systolic depression of the midportion and right side of the chest may be found in marked aortic regurgitation.
4. Paradoxical sustained outward systolic movements, or bulges, are commonly palpable in patients with myocardial infarction or angina pectoris at some point medial to the apex beat. When present at the apex, however, they are indistinguishable from the apical thrust of a hypertrophied left ventricle. A bulge signifies the presence of ventricular asynergy or aneurysm.

## Pulsations in the Left Second and Third Intercostal Spaces

1. A faint, nonlifting, systolic pulsation may be normal in young people and patients with pes excavatum, and during tachycardia.
2. A systolic lifting pulsation in this area is indicative of pulmonary artery dilatation or increased pulmonary blood flow.

## Pulsations in the Second Right Intercostal Space

Pulsation in the second right intercostal space suggests dilatation of the aorta.

## Pulsations of the Sternoclavicular Joints and Sternum

1. Pulsation of the right sternoclavicular joint may indicate a right-sided aortic arch.

2. Pulsation of either sternoclavicular joint occurs in aortic dissection or aneurysm.
3. Systolic outward pulsation of the upper half of the sternum is generally due to aneurysm of the ascending aorta. Aneurysm of the transverse aorta is usually not associated with visible pulsations but may cause displacement of the trachea or a tracheal tug.

## Epigastric Pulsations

1. Epigastric pulsations may be helpful in the diagnosis of ventricular hypertrophy in patients with emphysema.
2. Pulsations in the epigastric region may originate in the aorta or result from an overactive or hypertrophied heart.
3. The pulsations of a hypertrophied right ventricle are palpable high in the epigastric area beneath the rib cage; those of a hypertrophied left ventricle are palpable under the left costal margin. To be indicative of hypertrophy rather than simple overactivity or displacement, such pulsations should have a significant downward thrust.

## Thoracic Arterial Pulsations

1. Visible arterial pulsations over the back of the chest occur frequently in coarctation of the aorta from an increased collateral circulation. They are seen best with the patient leaning forward and the back illuminated by a light from above shining obliquely downward.
2. Pulsations in the right lower neck beneath the sternomastoid muscle are usually due to kinking of the common carotid artery rather than to aneurysm.
3. Other abnormalities of the arterial pulse are described in the section Arterial Pulse, earlier in this chapter.

## Heart Sounds

The first sound and both components of the second sound, ejection sounds, the opening snap of mitral stenosis, pericardial friction rubs, and gallop sounds may all be palpable when present. They are identified by their characteristics and timing. Gallop sounds on occasion may be felt even when they are not heard. Left-sided gallops and the mitral opening snap may sometimes be felt more easily with the patient in the left lateral recumbent position.

## Thrills

Thrills are palpable vibrations associated with murmurs. The presence of a thrill indicates only that the accompanying murmur is loud. It has no other significance.

## HEART SOUNDS
### H. Harold Friedman

## Normal Heart Sounds

Usually only two heart sounds, called the first sound and the second sound, are audible in normal persons (see Fig. 3-1). The first sound ($S_1$) is ordinarily louder at the apex than at the base. The converse is true of the second sound ($S_2$). At the apex, $S_1$ is usually louder than $S_2$ but may be of the same or even lesser intensity than $S_2$. At the base, $S_2$ is louder than $S_1$. Decreased intensity of the heart sounds may be due to poor conduction of the sounds because of such conditions as a thick chest wall, emphysema, or pericardial effusion. Increased intensity of the heart sounds may occur normally in children or thin-chested individuals. In the discussion that follows, only cardiac factors influencing the intensity of the heart sounds are considered.

## The First Heart Sound ($S_1$)

1. The normal first heart sound is composed of audible mitral ($M_1$) and tricuspid ($T_1$) components.
2. *Increased intensity* of $S_1$ may be found in the following conditions:
   a. Sinus rhythm with a short P-R interval (0.08–0.12 sec).
   b. Hyperkinetic circulatory states.
   c. Mitral stenosis.
3. *Decreased intensity* of $S_1$ may occur when myocardial contractility is impaired or when hemodynamics are altered, as in shock, myocardial infarction, congestive failure, or terminal states. $S_1$ may be decreased in intensity in mitral or aortic regurgitation.
4. *Variation in the intensity* of $S_1$ is a common occurrence in arrhythmias such as atrial fibrillation, AV dissociation, ventricular tachycardia with AV dissociation, and complete AV block. The term *cannon sounds* refers to the very loud first sounds that occur intermittently in the last three conditions.
5. *Normal splitting* of $S_1$ is audible in 85 percent of normal subjects. $M_1$ and $T_1$ have about the same pitch and intensity and are heard with about equal loudness at both the apex and left sternal border.
6. *Wide splitting* of $S_1$ may result from mechanical delays in mitral or tricuspid valve closure (e.g., mitral stenosis, Ebstein's anomaly, atrial septal defect).
7. $S_1$ may be *masked* by a loud systolic murmur (e.g., mitral regurgitation).

## The Second Heart Sound ($S_2$)

The second heart sound ($S_2$) consists of aortic ($A_2$) and pulmonary ($P_2$) components. $A_2$ normally precedes $P_2$ and is the louder sound in adults. $P_2$ is usually audible in the pulmonary area; less commonly, it can be heard in the aortic area or left sternal border. It cannot normally be heard at the apex.

### Intensity

1. $P_2$ is usually louder than $A_2$ up to the age of about 20 or 30 years; in persons above this age, $A_2$ is louder than $P_2$.
2. *Increased intensity of $A_2$* occurs when the systemic arterial pressure is elevated, as in essential hypertension. It may also be accentuated in aortic dilatation or aneurysm and in some cases of aortic regurgitation. A tambourlike $A_2$ is characteristic of syphilitic aortitis.
3. *Decreased intensity of $A_2$* is commonly observed in hypotension, shock, and congestive failure. In valvular aortic stenosis, $A_2$ is usually diminished or absent.
4. *Increased intensity of $P_2$*, with $P_2$ louder than $A_2$, is found in pulmonary hypertension due to such conditions as mitral stenosis, left-sided heart failure, primary pulmonary hypertension, pulmonary emboli, and left-to-right shunts. In these conditions, $P_2$ is sometimes audible at the apex.
5. *Decreased intensity of $P_2$* or absence of $P_2$ is noted in pulmonary stenosis.
6. $A_2$ or $P_2$ may be masked by loud systolic murmurs (e.g., pulmonary stenosis and aortic stenosis, respectively).

## Splitting

NORMAL SPLITTING

1. Normal or physiologic splitting of $S_2$ into earlier $A_2$ and later $P_2$ components is heard best in the pulmonary area or along the left sternal border.
2. The maximum normal split between $A_2$ and $P_2$ is about 0.03 sec in expiration and 0.06 sec in inspiration.
3. In normal young adults, in the recumbent position, $S_2$ is either single or narrowly split during expiration, and is audibly and more widely split during inspiration. However, in the upright position, expiratory splitting of $S_2$ should not be audible.
4. In adults, audible expiratory splitting of $S_2$ in the upright position is, with rare exceptions, suggestive of organic heart disease.
5. $S_2$ is often single in both expiration and inspiration. This pattern is observed more frequently with advancing age and is quite common in normal adults above the age of 50 years.

NARROW PHYSIOLOGIC SPLITTING

Narrow physiologic splitting of $S_2$ due to early $P_2$, relative to $A_2$, is common in patients with severe pulmonary hypertension when right ventricular systole is not prolonged with respect to left ventricular systole.

WIDE SPLITTING

Splitting of $S_2$ that exceeds normal values may be caused by a delayed $P_2$, an early $A_2$, or a combination of the two.
1. The most common causes of wide splitting of $S_2$ with a *delayed* $P_2$ are as follows:
   a. Delayed activation of the right ventricle (e.g., complete right bundle branch block, left ventricular paced or ectopic beats).
   b. Prolonged right ventricular mechanical systole (e.g., valvular pulmonary stenosis with an intact interventricular septum, pulmonary hypertension, pulmonary embolism).
   c. Increased right ventricular stroke volume, as in left-to-right shunts (e.g., atrial septal defect, ventricular septal defect) and pulmonary insufficiency.
   d. Decreased impedance of the pulmonary vascular bed (increased hangout) as, for example, in normotensive atrial septal defect, idiopathic dilatation of the pulmonary artery, and mild pulmonary stenosis.
   e. Structural abnormalities such as pes excavatum and the straight back syndrome.
2. An *early* $A_2$ may result from decreased resistance to left ventricular ejection or decreased left ventricular stroke volume, as in ventricular septal defect or mitral regurgitation.

WIDE AND FIXED SPLITTING

1. The term *fixed splitting* (of $S_2$) refers to an already widely split $S_2$ that splits no further or splits by not more than 0.02 sec during inspiration in either the recumbent or sitting position.
2. Wide and fixed splitting of $S_2$ may be observed in atrial septal defects and some other left-to-right shunts, severe right-sided heart failure, acute massive pulmonary embolism, and cardiomyopathy.
3. The widely split $S_2$ of right bundle branch block is not fixed.

REVERSED OR PARADOXICAL SPLITTING

1. Reversed splitting of $S_2$ is rarely a normal finding. It results from delayed aortic closure so that $A_2$ follows rather than precedes $P_2$ during the entire respiratory cycle.
2. Usually the splitting narrows during inspiration and widens during expiration.

3. The most common causes of paradoxical splitting of $S_2$ are as follows:
   a. Delayed closure of the aortic valve.
      **(1)** Delayed electric activation of the left ventricle (e.g., complete left bundle branch block, right ventricular paced or ectopic beats).
      **(2)** Prolonged left ventricular mechanical systole (e.g., left ventricular outflow tract obstruction).
      **(3)** Decreased impedance of the systemic vascular bed (increased hangout) as in poststenotic dilatation of the aorta or patent ductus arteriosus.
   b. Early closure of the pulmonary valve. Early electric activation of the right ventricle as in the Wolff-Parkinson-White (WPW) syndrome, type B.

## Single Second Heart Sound

1. A single $S_2$ is a common normal variant in persons above the age of 50 years.
2. $S_2$ may be single because of changes in $P_2$:
   a. $P_2$ is faint or not detected (e.g., tetralogy of Fallot, tricuspid atresia, pulmonary atresia, pulmonary stenosis).
   b. $P_2$ is synchronous with $A_2$ (e.g., ventricular septal defect with Eisenmenger's syndrome, some cases of aortic stenosis, occasional instances of left bundle branch block, pulmonary hypertension).
   c. $P_2$ is masked by a systolic murmur (e.g., aortic stenosis).
3. $S_2$ may be single because of changes in $A_2$:
   a. $A_2$ is faint or not detected (e.g., aortic stenosis).
   b. $A_2$ is synchronous with $P_2$ (see paragraph **2b** above).
   c. $A_2$ is masked by a systolic murmur (e.g., pulmonary stenosis).
4. $S_2$ is single when there is only one semilunar valve (e.g., truncus arteriosus).

## Abnormal and Extra Sounds

The various abnormal and extra sounds that may be encountered are discussed below; their differential diagnoses are summarized in Tables 3-3 and 3-4.

### The Third Heart Sound (Ventricular Gallop, $S_3$)

NORMAL

1. The third sound ($S_3$) is commonly audible in normal children and young adults below the age of 30 years.
2. The normal $S_3$ is a soft, low-pitched sound that is usually localized to the apex. It is heard best with the bell of the stethoscope with the subject in the left lateral recumbent position. The sound is louder in expiration than inspiration.

ABNORMAL

1. $S_3$ is abnormal above the age of 30 years and probably at any age in the presence of heart disease.
2. $S_3$ occurs 0.12 to 0.18 sec after $A_2$ and coincides with the descending limb of the V wave of the jugular venous pulse.
3. $S_3$ may be accompanied by a palpable or visible apical shock or bulge.
4. A left-sided $S_3$ ($LS_3$) is caused by left ventricular disease or failure; a right-sided $S_3$ ($RS_3$), by right ventricular disease or failure. $LS_3$ is heard best at the apex; $RS_3$, along the left sternal border, the tricuspid area, and occasionally in the right supraclavicular fossa. $LS_3$ is louder in expiration; $RS_3$, in inspiration.
5. An $S_3$ sound may be the earliest sign of myocardial failure.
6. The intensity of $S_3$ is decreased by sitting or standing and increased by brief exercise.

**Table 3-3.** Differential diagnosis: $S_4$ preceding $M_1$ versus split $S_1$ ($M_1$ preceding $T_1$)

| Parameter | LS₄ preceding M₁ | RS₄ preceding M₁ | Split S₁ (M₁ and T₁) |
|---|---|---|---|
| Characteristics of sound | Faint, low-pitched sound (S₄) followed by higher-pitched sound (M₁) | Faint, low-pitched sound (S₄) followed by higher-pitched sound (M₁) | M₁ and T₁ about same intensity and pitch |
| Effect of pressure with stethoscope diaphragm | LS₄ more faint or inaudible | RS₄ more faint or inaudible | M₁ and T₁ may be more faint but sharper and clicky |
| Area of maximum audibility | Apex, especially in left lateral recumbent position, with bell chest piece; faint or absent away from apex | Lower left sternal border, with bell chest piece | Lower left sternal border and medial to apex but not lateral to it, with bell or diaphragm; equal intensity at apex and LSB |
| Interval between sounds | Usually 0.05 to 0.10 sec | Usually 0.05 to 0.10 sec | Usually about 0.03 sec |
| Precordial pulsations | Presystolic and systolic apical impulses | Right ventricular lift or heave | Single systolic apical impulse |
| Effect of respiration | LS₄ louder in expiration | RS₄ louder in inspiration | Splitting somewhat more evident in expiration |
| Effect of change in venous return | | | |
| Increase (e.g., leg raising) | LS₄ louder | RS₄ louder | Little or no effect |
| Decrease (e.g., sitting) | LS₄ more faint or inaudible | RS₄ more faint or inaudible | Little or no effect |

$LS_4$ = left-sided $S_4$, LSB = left sternal border, $M_1$ = first audible component of $S_1$, $RS_4$ = right-sided $S_4$, $S_1$ = first sound, $T_1$ = second audible component of $S_1$

7. An $LS_3$ is absent in pure or predominant mitral stenosis, but $RS_3$ may occur when there is pulmonary hypertension. If an $LS_3$ is heard in a patient with both mitral stenosis and regurgitation, it can be assumed that regurgitation is the predominant lesion.
8. $S_3$ must be differentiated from the second component of a split $S_2$, an opening snap, and an $S_4$ (see Table 3-4).
9. The pericardial knock, a diastolic filling sound occurring somewhat earlier than the usual $S_3$ (0.06–0.12 sec after $A_2$), is found in most cases of chronic constrictive pericarditis; it coincides with the end of the Y descent in the jugular venous pulse.
10. $S_3$ may coexist with $S_4$, producing a quadruple rhythm, whereas either sound alone, when combined with $S_1$ and $S_2$, produces a triple rhythm. When $S_3$ and $S_4$ coincide, the condition is called a summation sound, or gallop. Transient slowing of the heart rate by carotid massage may separate a suspected summation sound into its $S_3$ and $S_4$ components.

## The Opening Snap

1. The opening of the mitral or tricuspid valves is normally inaudible. Audible opening of an AV valve occurs when it is stenosed. The sound produced is called an opening snap (OS).
2. The OS of the mitral valve (OSMV) is virtually pathognomonic of mitral stenosis and indicates that the valve is pliable. The OS disappears when the valve becomes rigid, fixed, or calcified. It may also disappear in the presence of aortic insufficiency or when mitral regurgitation is the predominant lesion. Surprisingly, the OS persists after comissurotomy. It is audible both in sinus rhythms and in atrial fibrillation.
3. The OSMV is a high-pitched, snapping sound that occurs between 0.04 and 0.12 sec after $A_2$. The severity of mitral stenosis may be roughly estimated from the $A_2$-OS interval. As a rule of thumb, the stenosis is severe when the interval is short, and mild when it is long.
4. The OSMV is heard best at the lower left sternal border and at the apex, but it is also frequently audible at the base. The sound may be palpable as well as audible. Its timing coincides with the V wave of the jugular venous pulse. The intensity of the sound is not affected by respiration.
5. The mitral OS is associated almost always with a loud $S_1$ and frequently with a split $S_2$ and accentuated $P_2$.
6. An OS of the tricuspid valve (OSTV) may be heard in some patients with tricuspid stenosis. The auscultatory characteristics of this sound are similar to those of the mitral OS, but there are some differences. The OSTV is heard best over the lower end of the sternum or at the right lower sternal edge. The tricuspid $A_2$-OS interval is shorter than the mitral $A_2$-OS interval. The tricuspid OS is not appreciably affected by respiration. An OSTV is occasionally heard in atrial septal defects in the absence of tricuspid stenosis.
7. In severe MS, the $A_2$-OS interval may be so short that the OS cannot be clearly differentiated from the components of $S_2$. Under such circumstances, administration of phenylephrine may, by increasing the $A_2$-OS interval, separate the OS from $S_2$ enough to make it identifiable as a separate sound.

## The Fourth Sound (Atrial Sound or Gallop, $S_4$)

1. The fourth sound ($S_4$) occurs about 0.12 sec after the P wave, preceding $S_1$ by about 0.05 to 0.10 sec when the P-R interval is normal. $S_4$ sounds, also called atrial or presystolic gallops, are usually indicative of myocardial abnormality. Atrial sounds are not audible in atrial fibrillation.
2. $S_4$ is usually a soft, low-pitched sound; hence it is heard best with the stethoscope bell applied lightly to the chest wall. It may be inaudible with the diaphragm.
3. $S_4$ may be left-sided or right-sided in origin.

**Table 3-4.** Differential diagnosis of various heart sounds

| Parameter | Split $S_2$, $A_2$ preceding $P_2$ | Opening snap | $S_3$ | $S_4$ | Ejection sound |
|---|---|---|---|---|---|
| Characteristics of sound | $P_2$ soft unless accentuated | Relatively loud, high-pitched | Faint, low-pitched | Faint, low-pitched | Sharp, clicking |
| Interval between sounds | $A_2$-$P_2$, 0.03 to 0.05 sec during inspiration | $A_2$-OS, 0.04 to 0.12 sec | $A_2$-$S_3$, 0.12 to 0.18 sec; $S_3$-$S_1$, 0.18 sec | $S_4$-$M_1$, 0.05 to 0.10 sec; $S_2$-$S_4$, $> 0.20$ sec | $M_1$-ES, 0.04 to 0.09 sec; $M_1$-$T_1$, 0.03 sec |
| Area of maximum audibility | Localized to pulmonary area and LSB | Widespread; OSMV: 4LICS, apex, and LSB; OSTV: lower LSB; OSMV: loud, snapping $S_1$, at apex and $A_2$, $P_2$, and OS audible in pulmonary area | Localized: $LS_3$: apex in LLRP; RS3: LSB, tricuspid area, and supraclavicular fossa | Localized; $LS_4$: apex in LLRP, not transmitted; $RS_4$: lower LSB, sometimes lower RSB | Usually localized; PES: 2- and 3LICS; AES: apex, LSB, aortic area |
| Precordial pulsations | $P_2$ sometimes palpable if accentuated; other pulsations depend on underlying conditions | OS may be palpable; apical impulse often impalpable in pure mitral stenosis | $LS_3$ palpable or visible, or both; $RS_3$ may have right ventricular heave or lift | $LS_4$; presystolic and systolic apical impulses; $RS_4$: right ventricular heave or lift | ES not palpable; other pulsations depend on underlying conditions |

| | | | | | |
|---|---|---|---|---|---|
| Effect of respiration | Splitting increased unless fixed; P$_2$ louder on inspiration | OSMV louder on expiration; OSTV louder on inspiration | LS$_3$ decreased with inspiration; RS$_3$ increased with inspiration | LS$_4$ louder in expiration; RS$_4$ louder in inspiration | PES decreased and moves closer to S$_1$ with inspiration; AES not affected by respiration |
| Effect of change in venous return | | | | | |
| Increase (e.g., leg raising) | P$_2$ louder, split increased | Little or no effect | Louder | Louder | Little or no effect |
| Decrease (e.g., sitting) | A$_2$ louder, split decreased | Little or no effect | Fainter | Fainter | Little or no effect |

A$_2$ = aortic component of S$_2$, AES = aortic ES, ES = ejection sound, LICS = left intercostal space, LLRP = left lateral recumbent position, LS$_3$ = left-sided S$_3$, LS$_4$ = left-sided S$_4$, LSB = left sternal border, M$_1$ = mitral component of S$_1$, OS = opening snap, OSMV = OS mitral valve, OSTV = OS tricuspid valve, P$_2$ = pulmonary component of S$_2$, PES = pulmonary ES, RS$_3$ = right-sided S$_3$, RS$_4$ = right-sided S$_4$, RSB = right sternal border, S$_2$ = second heart sound, S$_3$ = third heart sound, S$_4$ = fourth heart sound, T$_1$ = tricuspid component of S$_1$

LEFT-SIDED S$_4$

1. Left-sided S$_4$ (LS$_4$) is usually heard best at the cardiac apex with the patient in the left lateral recumbent position.
2. It is usually associated with a presystolic apical impulse.
3. LS$_4$ may wax and wane with respiration, becoming louder during expiration or becoming audible only during this phase of respiration.
4. Maneuvers that increase venous return (e.g., leg raising, exercise) tend to increase the intensity of the sound; those that decrease venous return (e.g., sitting) have the opposite effect.
5. LS$_4$ has been reported to occur in some normal individuals over 50 years of age, but it is more commonly associated with one of the following conditions:
   a. Disorders characterized by decreased compliance of the left ventricle (e.g., systemic hypertension, aortic stenosis or insufficiency, cardiomyopathy).
   b. Acute myocardial infarction (LS$_4$ is heard in an overwhelming majority of cases).
   c. Attacks of angina pectoris.
   d. AV block, of varying degree.
   e. Hyperkinetic circulatory states (e.g., hyperthyroidism, anemia).
6. LS$_4$ is ordinarily not audible in mitral valve disease, but it may occur in acute mitral regurgitation due to ruptured chordae tendineae.

RIGHT-SIDED S$_4$

1. Right-sided S$_4$ (RS$_4$) is usually heard along the lower left sternal border and sometimes over the right internal jugular vein.
2. RS$_4$ is usually associated with a sustained left parasternal heave and a giant jugular A wave.
3. RS$_4$ may wax and wane during respiration, becoming loudest during inspiration.
4. Maneuvers that increase the venous return to the heart increase the intensity of S$_4$; those that decrease the venous return have the opposite effect.
5. RS$_4$ is heard in conditions in which there is either decreased compliance of the right ventricle or increased resistance to right ventricular filling:
   a. Pulmonary hypertension (e.g., atrial septal defect, ventricular septal defect, patent ductus arteriosus, pulmonary embolism, primary pulmonary hypertension).
   b. Pulmonary stenosis.
   c. Cardiomyopathy.

## Systolic Sounds

PULMONARY EJECTION SOUNDS

1. Pulmonary ejection sounds (PES) occur at the time blood is ejected from the right ventricle into the pulmonary artery. They follow M$_1$ by 0.04 to 0.09 sec (range 0.02–0.14 sec).
2. PES are heard best over the second or third left intercostal spaces. They are poorly heard or inaudible at the apex. They tend to decrease in intensity and move closer to S$_1$ during inspiration.
3. PES have a sharp clicking quality.
4. PES occur in most cases of pulmonary stenosis and in many cases of primary and secondary pulmonary hypertension.

AORTIC EJECTION SOUNDS

1. Aortic ejection sounds (AES) occur at the time of ejection of blood from the left ventricle into the aorta. Their timing is similar to that of PES.

2. AES, in contrast to PES, are usually heard best at the apex and have no respiratory variation. They may also be heard along the left sternal border and in the aortic area.

3. AES are present in almost all cases of congenital valvular aortic stenosis, but not in infundibular, supravalvular, or idiopathic hypertrophic subaortic stenosis. AES may be heard in some cases of rheumatic aortic stenosis and in occasional instances of aortic insufficiency, coarctation of the aorta, aneurysm of the ascending aorta, and the tetralogy of Fallot.

SYSTOLIC CLICKS

1. Clicks are systolic sounds. Although systolic clicks (SC) occur at any time during systole, they are more common in mid or late systole. They are usually single, but sometimes two or more sounds may be heard.

2. Systolic clicks are heard best in the midprecordium or at the apex, and may show respiratory or positional variation in intensity or even in timing from beat to beat.

3. Systolic clicks associated with mid or late apical systolic murmurs are indicative of mitral valve prolapse.

PERICARDIAL FRICTION RUB

1. The pericardial friction rub is a rough, scratchy sound, often quite changeable in character from day to day or even minute to minute, audible over the precordium in most cases of acute pericarditis but rarely in chronic constrictive pericarditis. The rub is usually louder on inspiration. The sound may have systolic, diastolic, and presystolic components. When two or three components are present, the diagnosis is made easily. When the rub is heard only during systole, it may be mistaken for a murmur or an extracardiac sound. With continued observation, the friction rub either assumes a to-and-fro character or disappears.

2. A pericardial friction rub should be differentiated from: (1) a *pleuropericardial friction rub,* which is usually louder at the apex, often associated with a left pleural friction rub, and markedly affected by respiration; and (2) the to-and-fro *crunching sound of mediastinal emphysema,* which is coarser in quality and often associated with crepitus of the soft tissues of the neck.

## HEART MURMURS
### H. Harold Friedman

Murmurs are related to several factors: (1) increased flow through normal or abnormal valves, (2) forward flow through narrowed or deformed valves, (3) backward or regurgitant flow through incompetent valves or septal defects, (4) more or less continuous flow through extracardiac and intracardiac shunts and narrowed or collateral vessels, and in vascular structures, and, less often, (5) vibration of loose structures within the heart. The following abbreviations are used in this section:

$A_2$ = aortic component of second heart sound
AES = aortic ejection sound(s) or click(s)
AR = aortic regurgitation
AS = aortic stenosis
ASD = atrial septal defect
CM = continuous murmur(s)
DM = diastolic murmur(s)
EM = ejection murmur(s)
ES = ejection sound(s) or click(s)
ICS = intercostal space
IE = infective endocarditis

|       |   |                                             |
|-------|---|---------------------------------------------|
| IHSS  | = | idiopathic hypertrophic subaortic stenosis  |
| IPS   | = | infundibular pulmonary stenosis             |
| JVP   | = | jugular venous pulse                        |
| LA    | = | left atrium                                 |
| LAE   | = | left atrial enlargement                     |
| LICS  | = | left intercostal space                      |
| LLRP  | = | left lateral recumbent position             |
| LLSB  | = | lower left sternal border                   |
| LRSB  | = | lower right sternal border                  |
| LSB   | = | left sternal border                         |
| LV    | = | left ventricle (ventricular)                |
| LVE   | = | left ventricular enlargement                |
| MR    | = | mitral regurgitation                        |
| MS    | = | mitral stenosis                             |
| OS    | = | opening snap                                |
| OSMV  | = | OS mitral valve                             |
| OSTV  | = | OS tricuspid valve                          |
| $P_2$ | = | pulmonary component of second heart sound   |
| PA    | = | pulmonary artery                            |
| PDA   | = | patent ductus arteriosus                    |
| PES   | = | pulmonary ejection sound(s) or click(s)     |
| PH    | = | pulmonary hypertension                      |
| PPH   | = | primary pulmonary hypertension              |
| PR    | = | pulmonary regurgitation                     |
| PS    | = | pulmonary stenosis                          |
| RA    | = | right atrium                                |
| RAE   | = | right atrial enlargement                    |
| RICS  | = | right intercostal space                     |
| RM    | = | regurgitant murmur(s)                       |
| RSB   | = | right sternal border                        |
| RV    | = | right ventricle (ventricular)               |
| RVE   | = | right ventricular enlargement               |
| $S_1$ | = | first heart sound                           |
| $S_2$ | = | second heart sound                          |
| $S_3$ | = | third heart sound                           |
| $S_4$ | = | fourth heart sound                          |
| SC    | = | systolic click(s)                           |
| SEM   | = | systolic ejection murmur(s)                 |
| SM    | = | systolic murmur(s)                          |
| SPH   | = | secondary pulmonary hypertension            |
| SRM   | = | systolic regurgitant murmur(s)              |
| T/F   | = | tetralogy of Fallot                         |
| TR    | = | tricuspid regurgitation                     |
| TS    | = | tricuspid stenosis                          |
| ULSB  | = | upper left sternal border                   |
| URSB  | = | upper right sternal border                  |
| VAS   | = | valvular aortic stenosis                    |
| VPS   | = | valvular pulmonary stenosis                 |
| VSD   | = | ventricular septal defect(s)                |

## Types of Murmurs

There are three basic types of murmurs: systolic, diastolic, and continuous. An SM begins with or after $S_1$ and ends before, at, or slightly beyond $S_2$. A DM begins with or after $S_2$ and ends before $S_1$. A CM begins in systole, continues through $S_2$ without interruption, and ends at some time in diastole.

## Systolic Murmurs

SYSTOLIC EJECTION MURMURS

1. *Mid systolic EM* are caused by normal or increased forward flow through either normal or abnormal right or left ventricular outflow tracts. They may be found in AS or PS, increased flow through a normal valve, ejection across a nonstenosed but deformed valve, dilatation of the aorta or PA, or combinations of these. The murmur of AS is the prototype of left-sided mid systolic EM, and the murmur of PS, of right-sided EM. Such murmurs begin after $S_1$ and end before $A_2$ if left-sided, and before $P_2$ if right-sided. The murmurs are of variable intensity, high- to medium-pitched, noisy, rough, or harsh in quality, and generally crescendo-decrescendo (diamond-shaped) in character.
2. *Early systolic EM* are primarily flow murmurs, beginning after $S_1$ and ending midway through systole. They tend to be decrescendo (kite-shaped) in character.

SYSTOLIC REGURGITANT MURMURS

SRM are due to flow from high- to low-pressure chambers or vessels. Thus they occur in MR, TR, VSD, and some aortopulmonary communications. RM may be classified according to their timing as pansystolic (holosystolic), early systolic, mid systolic, or late systolic. *Pansystolic RM* start with $S_1$ and end with or beyond $A_2$. They are typical of the aforementioned conditions. *Early systolic RM* start with $S_1$ but end in mid systole. They occur in some VSD, in tight MS with slight MR, and in TR from IE. *Mid systolic RM* begin after $S_1$ and end before or at $A_2$. They are usually found in MR due to papillary muscle dysfunction, although any type of SRM may occur in this condition. *Late systolic RM* start about mid systole, often with an SC, and end at or beyond $A_2$. They occur most often in nonrheumatic MR associated with prolapse of one or both mitral leaflets into the LA, but they may be found in rheumatic MR and in calcification of the mitral annulus.

## Diastolic Murmurs

DM may be classified as early diastolic, mid diastolic, or late diastolic (presystolic). *Early DM* are due to semilunar valve incompetence. *Mid and late DM* are due either to stenosis of the atrioventricular valves or to increased flow across these valves.

## Continuous Murmurs

CM begin after $S_1$, continue through $S_2$ without interruption, enveloping it, and end at some time in diastole before $S_1$. The murmur need not persist through all of diastole to be considered continuous. CM occur in extracardiac and intracardiac shunts but may be caused by flow through narrowed or collateral vessels or by increased flow in vascular structures.

---

## Description of Murmurs

---

Descriptions of murmurs should include their timing, intensity, pitch, quality, duration, location, and radiation. The most widely used system (Levine and Harvey) for grading the intensity of heart murmurs uses a six-point scale.

Grade 1: very faint.
Grade 2: faint.
Grade 3: moderately loud.
Grade 4: loud.
Grade 5: very loud.
Grade 6: loudest possible.

**Table 3-5.** The effects of physiologic and pharmacologic maneuvers on murmurs

| Murmur | Inspiration | Sudden standing | Sudden squatting | Vasodilators (amyl nitrite) | Vasopressors (phenyleph-rine or methoxamine) | Valsalva and post-Valsalva effect | Effect of miscellaneous maneuvers on murmur |
|---|---|---|---|---|---|---|---|
| Aortic stenosis | NSC | D | I | I | D or NSC | D, with delayed return of intensity of murmur | I after extrasystole or pause, and leg raising |
| Idiopathic hypertrophic subaortic stenosis | NSC | I | D | I | D | I | I after extrasystole or pause, sitting, standing; D after leg raising |
| Pulmonary stenosis | I | NSC | I | PS: I (most cases) Tetralogy of Fallot: D | PS: NSC Tetralogy of Fallot: I | D, with immediate return of intensity of murmur | |
| Aortic regurgitation | D | NSC compared with sitting | I | D Austin Flint murmur: D | I Austin Flint murmur: I | | I when sitting, when leaning forward, and in expiration |
| Mitral regurgitation Pansystolic | NSC or D | D or NSC | I | D | I | D, with later I | Beat after extrasystole or pause: NSC |

| | starts earlier; is longer | earlier; is longer | starts later; is shorter | starts earlier; is longer | | | Murmur starts later, is shorter |
|---|---|---|---|---|---|---|---|
| (click syndrome) | | | | | | | |
| Papillary muscle dysfunction | NSC | NSC | Variable | Variable | Variable | | D or NSC |
| Tricuspid regurgitation | I | D or NSC | I | I or NSC | NSC | | D, with later I |
| Ventricular septal defect without pulmonary hypertension | NSC | NSC | I | D | I | | NSC |
| Mitral stenosis | NSC or slight D; may reveal A₂-P₂-OS sequence | D | I | I | D; $A_2$-OS interval is widened | NSC | I after exercise and in left lateral recumbent position |
| Tricuspid stenosis | I | D | I | I | I | NSC | |
| Pulmonary regurgitation | I or NSC | | NSC | NSC | NSC | NSC | |

D = decreased intensity, I = increased intensity, NSC = no significant change in intensity

Source: Adapted from M. C. Dohan and M. G. Drisitiello, Physiologic and pharmacologic manipulations of heart sounds and murmurs. *Mod. Concepts Cardiovasc. Dis.* 39:121, 1970.

# Physiologic and Pharmacologic Maneuvers

Physiologic and pharmacologic maneuvers may have effects on the intensity of murmurs that may have some diagnostic significance. The maneuvers and their effects on various murmurs are summarized in Table 3-5. Use of these maneuvers is often helpful in the differential diagnosis of specific auscultatory problems (see Table 3-6).

Vasopressors increase peripheral resistance; vasodilators reduce it. Standing upright causes a decrease in venous return and a slight increase in heart rate and systemic arterial resistance. Squatting causes a transient increase in venous return and increased peripheral arterial resistance. Both of these effects increase the size of the left ventricle. The Valsalva maneuver obstructs venous return during the straining phase and diminishes the size of both the right and left ventricles.

# Diagnostic Approach to Murmurs

The diagnostic evaluation of any heart murmur involves first, a decision as to whether the murmur is innocent or organic, and second, if organic, a determination of the anatomic lesion and its cause. The workup of a patient with an organic murmur should include examination of the arterial and jugular venous pulses, inspection and palpation of the precordium and chest wall, and systematic auscultation of the heart, thorax, and related vascular structures. Also indicated in all cases are an ECG and chest films (preferably PA, lateral, and oblique views taken with a barium-filled esophagus). Cardiac fluoroscopy with image amplifi

**Table 3-6.** Maneuvers helpful in the differential diagnosis of similar murmurs

| Diagnostic problem | Useful maneuvers* |
| --- | --- |
| Mitral regurgitation versus tricuspid regurgitation | Respiration, amyl nitrite, vasopressor |
| Aortic stenosis versus idiopathic hypertrophic subaortic stenosis | Squatting, standing, Valsalva, amyl nitrite |
| Mitral regurgitation versus idiopathic hypertrophic subaortic stenosis | Squatting, standing, amyl nitrite, vasopressors |
| Aortic stenosis versus mitral regurgitation | Amyl nitrite, vasopressors, postextrasystolic beat |
| Aortic stenosis versus mid to late systolic murmur of mitral regurgitation | Standing, amyl nitrite |
| Mitral stenosis versus Austin Flint murmur | Amyl nitrite, vasopressors |
| Mitral stenosis versus tricuspid stenosis | Respiration, amyl nitrite, vasopressor |
| Pulmonary stenosis versus tetralogy of Fallot | Amyl nitrite |
| Pulmonary stenosis versus small ventricular septal defect | Amyl nitrite, vasopressors |

*The responses to these maneuvers are shown in Table 3-5.
Source: Adapted from M. C. Dohan and M. G. Drisitiello, Physiologic and pharmacologic manipulations of heart sounds and murmurs. *Mod. Concepts Cardiovas. Dis.* 39:121, 1970.

cation is invaluable in studying motion and dynamic changes as well as in the detection of valvular or other calcifications.

Based on the aforementioned procedures, it is possible to make the correct cardiac diagnosis in the vast majority of cases. When this is not possible or for other legitimate reasons (e.g., confirmation of a diagnosis, preoperative evaluation), apexcardiography, external recordings of the jugular and carotid pulses, phonocardiography, echocardiography, cardiac catheterization, and angiocardiography may be indispensable tools for diagnosis, differential diagnosis, or the study of cardiovascular hemodynamics. As a general rule, preference should be given to noninvasive techniques when the information yielded is comparable to that obtainable by catheter intervention. Because all of these supplementary techniques are highly technical and require special equipment, they usually are not performed by the nonspecialist in cardiology, and hence are not discussed here.

In the presentation that follows, primary consideration is given to the more frequent, uncomplicated murmurs encountered in adults, omitting discussion of many complex congenital or acquired lesions. The murmurs are described according to their timing and site of maximum intensity.

## Innocent Murmurs

Innocent murmurs are those not due to recognizable lesions of the heart. Although they may occur at any age, they are most common in children and adolescents. The characteristics of innocent murmurs in young people and their differential diagnosis are summarized in Tables 3-7 and 3-8. The aortic ejection murmur of middle and old age, although not innocent, is nevertheless benign. It is, so to speak, the innocent murmur of the elderly. It is discussed in paragraph **2d** below.

## Systolic Murmurs According to Site of Maximum Intensity

### Second Right Intercostal Space (Aortic Area): Mid Systolic Ejection Murmurs

1. Etiology.
    a. Left ventricular outflow obstruction.
        (1) Congenital aortic stenosis.
            (a) Valvular.
            (b) Subvalvular (discrete).
            (c) Supravalvular.
        (2) Acquired aortic stenosis.
            (a) Rheumatic.
            (b) Nonrheumatic.
        (3) Idiopathic hypertrophic subaortic stenosis.
    b. Aortic ejection murmur of middle and old age (probably due to aortic valve sclerosis).
    c. Transmitted murmur of mitral regurgitation.
    d. Aortic flow murmur in free aortic regurgitation.
    e. Supraclavicular arterial bruit.
    f. Coarctation of the aorta (some cases).
2. Diagnostic features.
    a. The murmur of AS is the prototype of left-sided SEM. When a crescendo-decrescendo, loud, noisy, harsh aortic EM, which is transmitted upward to the right and into the carotids, occurs in association with a thrill, a faint or absent $A_2$, and an anacrotic or small pulse with a delayed systolic peak, the diagnosis of AS is established. The presence of valvular calcification on fluoroscopy or x-ray is confirmatory.

**Table 3-7.** Innocent murmurs in young people and their differential diagnosis

| Innocent murmur | Maximum site and transmission | Features of innocent murmur | Organic murmur to be differentiated | Features of organic lesion |
|---|---|---|---|---|
| Pulmonary ejection murmur | 2LICS with radiation to LLSB and apex | Early to mid systolic, rough or blowing, low- to medium-pitched; increased in recumbency, held expiration, and after exercise; common in the straight back syndrome or pes excavatum; $S_2$ normally split; precordium quiet | Atrial septal defect | Murmur louder, longer, with wide fixed splitting of $S_2$; right ventricular impulse hyperdynamic |
| | | | Mild valvular pulmonary stenosis | Murmur louder, longer, harsher with thrill; $S_2$ widely split; sustained right ventricular lift |
| Vibratory murmur | Apicosternal region; may be widely transmitted | Early to mid systolic, medium-pitched, crescendo-descrescendo, vibratory, twangy, or groaning; louder with amyl nitrite; no significant change with vasopressors | Small ventricular septal defect | Murmur high-pitched, blowing, holosystolic, with thrill in 3LICS or 4LICS; when early systolic, often no thrill, but murmur is high-pitched, blowing; softer with amyl nitrite; louder with vasopressors |
| | | | Mitral regurgitation | Murmur holosystolic apical, transmitted to left axilla and scapula; softer with amyl nitrite; louder with vasopressors |

| | | | | |
|---|---|---|---|---|
| Supraclavicular arterial bruit | Maximum on the right side of neck, and louder above the clavicle than below it | Short, low-pitched early systolic; louder with slight compression of the subclavian artery; decreased or obliterated by marked compression of the subclavian artery or hyperextension of shoulders; sounds and precordium normal | Aortic stenosis | Murmur maximum in 2RICS or apex, often with thrill; $A_2$ decreased or absent; sustained left ventricular lift |
| Venous hum | Neck, especially on the right side with head turned away from side being examined | Continuous, low- to medium-pitched, peaking after $S_2$; decreases or disappears with recumbency; obliterated by compression of jugular veins; louder with amyl nitrite; softer or no change with vasopressors | Patent ductus arteriosus | Maximum over pulmonary area; not affected by position change or compression of jugular veins; peaks at $S_2$; softer with amyl nitrite; louder with vasopressors |
| Mammary souffle | RSB or LSB from 2ICS to 4ICS | Medium- to high-pitched, continuous, with systolic accentuation; occurs in late pregnancy and lactation, then disappears; obliterated by firm stethoscope pressure | Patent ductus arteriosus | See above |
| | | | Arteriovenous fistula of chest wall | Murmur louder, with thrill; usually not obliterated with stethoscope pressure; persists after pregnancy or lactation |

Source: Adapted from R. F. Castle, The innocent heart murmurs. *Rocky Mt. Med. J.* 69–45, 1972.

**Table 3-8.** Differential diagnosis of systolic ejection murmurs at left sternal border

**Part I**

| Parameter | Congenital pulmonary stenosis (uncomplicated) | Tetralogy of Fallot (uncomplicated) | Idiopathic dilatation of pulmonary artery | Atrial septal defect | Innocent murmurs |
|---|---|---|---|---|---|
| Clinical features | Murmur present from birth; growth and development normal; chubby, round facies typical | Cyanosis present at rest or after exercise; most common type of cyanotic congenital heart disease above the age of 4 years; dyspnea and squatting common | Asymptomatic in healthy young people | Asymptomatic; F>M; mostly young people | Normal in young people; also in straight back syndrome (SBS) and pes excavatum (PE) |
| Arterial pulse | Normal, or decreased if severe | Normal | Normal | Normal or small | Normal |
| Jugular venous pulse | Mild: normal A waves Moderate to severe: large A waves | Normal; large A waves occur if PS is severe and the VSD is small; large A and V waves in CHF | Normal | Usually normal; large A waves in PH or LV failure | Normal |
| Precordial pulsations | Valvular: sustained RV lift reaching to 3LICS; no impulse over 2LICS Infundibular: sustained RV lift, not reaching 3LICS | Slight RV lift below 3LICS | PA impulse palpable 2LICS; RV impulse not palpable | Hyperdynamic RV impulse: systolic pulsation of enlarged pulmonary trunk | Normal |

| | | | | | |
|---|---|---|---|---|---|
| Maximum thrill | Valvular: 2LICS or occasionally 3LICS Infundibular: 3LICS or more commonly 4LICS | Usually 3LICS | None | Usually absent, but may be felt over PA | None |
| Ejection sounds | Valvular: Mild: PES present or absent Moderate to severe: PES 2LICS, which decreases and moves toward $S_1$ with inspiration Severe: may be absent Infundibular: absent | PES rare because PS is usually infundibular; AES present in 2RICS only in severe PS or atresia | PES 2LICS | Absent unless PH is present | PES in SBS |
| Heart sounds | $S_1$: normal $S_2$: narrowly split in mild PS; widely split in more severe PS; widely split in infundibular PS $P_2$: valvular Mild: normal or increased Moderate to severe: decreased or absent Infundibular: usually absent $RS_4$: in moderate to severe PS | $S_1$: normal Mild: widely split $S_2$; $P_2$ decreased or absent Moderate: $P_2$ absent, $A_2$ loud Severe: $P_2$ absent, $A_2$ loud $RS_4$: absent | $S_1$: normal $S_2$: narrowly or widely split | $S_1$: normal, or loud and split with $T_1 > M_1$ $S_2$: wide, fixed splitting $P_2$: normal or increased and audible at apex $RS_4$: sometimes present $RS_3$: sometimes present | $S_1$: normal; may be loud in SBS or PE $S_2$: normally split; may be widely split with increased $P_2$ in SBS or PE $RS_4$: may be present in SBS or PE |

**Table 3-8** (continued)

**Part I**

| Parameter | Congenital pulmonary stenosis (uncomplicated) | Tetralogy of Fallot (uncomplicated) | Idiopathic dilatation of pulmonary artery | Atrial septal defect | Innocent murmurs |
|---|---|---|---|---|---|
| Systolic murmur | Harsh, long crescendo-decrescendo; Valvular Mild: ends before $A_2$ Moderate: ends with $A_2$ Severe: ends after $A_2$ Maximum: 2LICS or 3LICS, radiating upward and to the left Infundibular: maximum 3LICS or 4LICS Intensity increases with amyl nitrite; unchanged with vasopressors | Harsh, shorter than in VPS Mild: loud, late peak, ends at $A_2$ Moderate: loud, mid systolic peak, ends before $A_2$ Severe: short, early, faint If IPS, maximum in 3LICS or 4LICS If VPS (uncommon), PES with long systolic murmur Intensity decreases with amyl nitrite and increases with vasopressor | Shorter, maximum in 2LICS | Medium-pitched; short, or extends to $S_2$; usually maximum in 2LICS | EM: rough blowing; early to mid systolic, short, 2LICS Vibratory (Still's murmur): medium-pitched, groaning; in apicosternal region Cardiorespiratory: LSB or apex louder in inspiration; disappears with breath holding Murmurs widely transmitted |
| Other murmurs | Presystolic or PR murmurs occur, but are rare | Continuous murmur in pulmonary atresia | PR in some cases | Tricuspid diastolic flow murmur common in large shunts; murmur of PR in pulmonary hypertension | None |

|  |  |  |  | $P_3$ may be inverted in sinus venosus defect QRS: rSr′ in $V_1$ Secundum: RAD, CW loop in FP; Primum: LAD, CCW loop in FP | Normal |
| --- | --- | --- | --- | --- | --- |
|  |  |  | dominant R wave in $V_1$ |  |  |
| X-ray findings | Valvular: normal or decreased pulmonary blood flow; poststenotic dilatation of main PA and LPA Infundibular: PA not dilated | Dilated pulmonary trunk | Pulmonary vascularity normal or increased; *coeur en sabot* | Pulmonary plethora, small aorta; marked dilatation of main PA and RPA; dilatation of RA and RV | Normal |

**Part II**

| Parameter | Flow murmurs (high output states) | Primary pulmonary hypertension | Secondary pulmonary hypertension | Small ventricular septal defect (uncomplicated) | Coarctation of the aorta in adults (uncomplicated) | Idiopathic hypertrophic subaortic stenosis |
| --- | --- | --- | --- | --- | --- | --- |
| Clinical features | Hyperkinetic state; occurs at any age | Healthy, acyanotic young women; effort syncope, angina-like pain, dyspnea, fatigue common | Associated with left-to-right shunts (ASD, VSD, PDA) or mitral stenosis; cyanosis and clubbing common in congenital cases | Normal; usually recognized in childhood | Generally normal; M>F; arterial hypertension common | Mostly young adults, but occurs at any age |
| Arterial pulse | Bounding | Small; pulse pressure narrow | Normal | Normal | Small and delayed femoral pulse; blood pressure in arms greater than in legs; carotid pulses often prominent | Brisk and unsustained or bisferiens |

Table 3-8 (continued)

Part II

| Parameter | Flow murmurs (high output states) | Primary pulmonary hypertension | Secondary pulmonary hypertension | Small ventricular septal defect (uncomplicated) | Coarctation of the aorta in adults (uncomplicated) | Idiopathic hypertrophic subaortic stenosis |
|---|---|---|---|---|---|---|
| Jugular venous pulse | Normal | Large A waves | Large A waves | Normal | Normal | Normal or increased A waves |
| Precordial pulsations | Brisk LV impulse | Presystolic distention of RV RV lift 2 LICS: systolic impulse of dilated main PA, palpable $P_2$ and sometimes palpable PES | Depends on underlying lesion | Normal except for systolic thrill | Collaterals common around scapula LV impulse normal or sustained heave Pulsations of dilated ascending aorta often palpable in 2RICS or 3RICS | Sustained LV heave or double systolic apical impulse |
| Maximum thrill | None | None | Whether thrill is present depends on nature of primary lesion | Usually present at 3LICS or 4LICS near sternum; may be absent | Suprasternal common | LLSB or apex |
| Ejection sounds | None | PES in 2LICS and 3LICS, decreasing with inspiration | PES sometimes audible | Absent | AES commonly present and may be palpable; suggests bicuspid aortic valve | AES rare |

| | | | | | | |
|---|---|---|---|---|---|---|
| Heart sounds | S₁: normal<br>S₂: normally split as a rule | S₁: normal<br>S₂: normally split; may be widely split in RV failure<br>P₂: markedly accentuated<br>RS₄: may be present<br>RS₃: present in RV failure | S₁: normal<br>S₂: narrow, or widely split<br>P₂: markedly accentuated<br>OS and increased S₁ when MS is present<br>RS₄: common | S₁: normal<br>S₂: normally split as a rule | S₁: normal<br>S₂: single or normally split<br>A₂: accentuated<br>LS₃: common<br>LS₄: occasionally present | S₁: normal<br>S₂: usually single, but paradoxical splitting common<br>A₂: normal or decreased<br>LS₄: common |
| Systolic murmur | Short, early, maximum in 2LICS | Mid systolic EM in 2 LICS | Mid systolic EM in 2LICS | Soft, early, SEM; high-frequency; decrescendo or crescendo-decrescendo; ends in mid systole, maximum at 3LICS or 4LICS<br>Decreased by amyl nitrite and increased with vasopressors | Murmur most prominent at LSB and often transmitted to apex and along subclavian arteries; may be audible below clavicles on both sides<br>Murmur often louder posteriorly than anteriorly<br>Presence of AES and SEM in 2RICS and murmur of AR-bicuspid aortic valve | SEM maximum lower LSB or apex; may be pansystolic at apex<br>Murmur decreased or disappears with squatting or vasopressors; increased with Valsalva or amyl nitrite |

**Table 3-8** (continued)

**Part II**

| Parameter | Flow murmurs (high output states) | Primary pulmonary hypertension | Secondary pulmonary hypertension | Small ventricular septal defect (uncomplicated) | Coarctation of the aorta in adults (uncomplicated) | Idiopathic hypertrophic subaortic stenosis |
|---|---|---|---|---|---|---|
| Other murmurs | None | May have PR and TR | Diastolic flow murmurs (mitral or tricuspid) common PR and TR may occur In MS: mild diastolic, with presystolic crescendo accentuation | None | AR (see above) | None |
| Electrocardiogram | Normal | Normal axis or RAD; RAE; RVE | Biatrial and biventricular enlargement common in shunts | Normal | Normal or LVE | LVE; S-T-T changes; left or biatrial enlargement; abnormal Q waves |
| X-ray findings | Normal | Dilatation of main PA and its branches; RVE, RAE clear peripheral lung fields | Depends on primary disease, but pulmonary plethora, biatrial and biventricular enlargement common in shunts | Normal or slight LVE: little or no increase in pulmonary vasculature | Notching of ribs, especially in 3rd to 8th posterior ribs; retrosternal notching due to dilated internal mammaries | LVE; no poststenotic dilatation of aorta |

CCW = counterclockwise, CW = clockwise, FP = frontal plane, LAD = left axis deviation, RAD = right axis deviation

**b.** Isolated AS in persons under the age of 30 years is usually congenital, particularly if the valve is calcified. The valve is usually unicuspid. Above this age to about the age of 60 years, congenitally bicuspid valves predominate. Rheumatic aortic stenosis is almost always associated with mitral valvular disease and often with severe AR. Isolated rheumatic AS is rare. Calcific AS in the elderly is believed to be degenerative in origin. The murmur of AS must be differentiated from the benign nonobstructive aortic EM of middle and old age (see paragraph **2d** below).

**c.** The differential diagnosis of the various causes of AS is summarized in Table 3-9. It is especially important to differentiate between valvular AS and IHSS. Some important differences are as follows: The murmur of IHSS is medium-pitched and less rough than that of valvular obstruction. It is usually maximum at the LLSB or at the apex rather than in the 2RICS. The murmur, like that of AS, is ejection in type except at the apex, where it is likely to be holosystolic because of associated MR. Sudden squatting, the Valsalva maneuver, changes in position, amyl nitrite, and vasopressors may help differentiate between AS and IHSS when the auscultatory findings are similar. In IHSS, the thrill when present is maximum at the LLSB or at the apex, the ventricular impulse is sustained or double-peaked, the carotid pulse is brisk or bisferiens, $S_3$ and $S_4$ sounds are frequently audible, $S_2$ is single or paradoxically split, the murmur of AR is absent, and diagnostic abnormalities may be found in the ECG or echocardiogram, or on cardiac catheterization. IHSS must also be distinguished from MR due to other causes; for this purpose, compare the features of each in Tables 3-8 and 3-10.

**d.** The murmur of AS must also be differentiated from the benign nonobstructive aortic EM of middle and old age. The latter tends to be both less harsh and less intense than the murmur of AS. It shows little upward radiation but is commonly transmitted to the apex, where it may be louder than at the base. It retains the configuration of a mid systolic EM at all locations. The arterial pulse is normal unless the pulse pressure is increased by concomitant hypertension. The JVP, the apical impulse, and the heart sounds are normal. No extra sounds are audible. A thrill is rarely present. The diagnosis of this benign murmur is supported by the age of the patient, the presence of aortic dilatation or systemic hypertension, and the absence of murmurs of other valvular lesions. When the murmur is loudest at the apex, it may be mistaken for the murmur of MR, which differs in being higher-pitched, blowing, and pansystolic rather than mid systolic.

**e.** The differential diagnosis of the murmurs of AS and MR is discussed in Table 3-11.

**f.** In free AR, it may be difficult to determine whether a mid systolic aortic EM is due to flow or to coexisting AS. Favoring stenosis over flow are the absence of peripheral signs of AR, a normal diastolic blood pressure, and the harshness and late peaking of the murmur. Either murmur may be loud and may be associated with a thrill.

**g.** The differential diagnosis between aortic EM and innocent supraclavicular arterial bruits is given in Table 3-7.

**h.** The differential diagnosis of the murmurs of PS and AS is summarized in Table 3-12.

**i.** Coarctation of the aorta usually produces a basal SEM that may be heard in the 2RICS but that is more commonly heard better in the 2LICS or, rarely, at the apex. The murmur is heard as well or even better posteriorly in an area medial to the left scapula.

## Left Sternal Border: Mid Systolic Ejection Murmurs

1. Etiology.
   **a.** Right ventricular outflow obstruction.
      **(1)** Congenital pulmonary stenosis.

Table 3-9. The differential diagnosis of systolic ejection murmurs in the second right intercostal space

| Parameter | Congenital aortic stenosis | | | Acquired aortic stenosis | Idiopathic hypertrophic subaortic stenosis | Aortic valve sclerosis (nonobstructive) | Supraclavicular arterial bruit |
|---|---|---|---|---|---|---|---|
| | Valvular (75% of cases) | Subvalvular (discrete) | Supravalvular | | | | |
| Age | Youth | Youth | Youth | Adolescence to old age; rare below age 10 | Mostly young adults, but occurs at any age | Middle and old age | 10 to 20 years |
| Sex | | M : F = 4 or 5 : 1 | | M : F = 2 : 1 | Familial: M = F; Nonfamilial: M : F = 4 : 1 | M > F | M = F |
| Physical appearance | Normal | Normal | Typical facies | Normal | Normal | Normal | Normal |
| Arterial pulse | Small; slow rise to late systolic peak | Small; slow rise to late systolic peak | Right brachial and carotid greater than left; blood pressure in right arm greater than in left arm | Small; slow rise to late systolic peak | Brisk and unsustained, or bisferiens | Normal | Normal |
| Jugular venous A wave | Normal or increased | Normal or increased | Normal or increased | Normal or increased | Normal or increased | Normal | Normal |
| Apical impulse | Sustained heave | Sustained heave | Sustained heave | Sustained heave | Sustained heave or bifid impulse | Normal | Normal |
| Maximum thrill | 1st or 2nd RICS | 1st or 2nd RICS | Just beneath right clavicle and right neck | 1st or 2nd RICS | Lower left sternal border of apex | Uncommon; 1st or 2nd RICS | Supraclavicular |

| | | | | | | | |
|---|---|---|---|---|---|---|---|
| Aortic ejection sound | Common | Rare | Rare | Rare | Rare | Absent | Absent |
| Splitting of $S_2$ | Single or narrowly split; sometimes paradoxical | Single or narrowly split; sometimes paradoxical | Single or narrowly split; sometimes paradoxical | Single or narrowly split; sometimes paradoxical | Usually single, but paradoxical splitting common | Single or narrowly split | Normal |
| Intensity of $A_2$ | Normal or increased | Normal or increased | Normal or increased | Usually decreased or absent, sometimes normal | Normal or decreased | Normal | Normal |
| Audible or palpable $S_4$ | Uncommon in mild to moderate stenosis; common in severe | Uncommon in mild to moderate stenosis; common in severe | Uncommon in mild to moderate stenosis; common in severe | Uncommon in mild to moderate stenosis; common in severe and over age 40 | Common | Absent | Absent |
| Systolic murmur | Maximum 1st or 2nd RICS; harsh; ejection | Maximum 1st or 2nd RICS; harsh; ejection | Often maximum 1st RICS; harsh; ejection | Maximum 1st or 2nd RICS; harsh; ejection | Maximum lower left sternal border or apex, medium-pitched; ejection, but may be pansystolic at apex | Maximum 1st and 2nd RICS, but sometimes at apex; rough ejection; early peak, short duration | Maximum above rather than below clavicle; usually right-sided; rough ejection; early peak, short duration |

**Table 3-9** (continued)

| Parameter | Congenital aortic stenosis | | | Acquired aortic stenosis | Idiopathic hypertrophic subaortic stenosis | Aortic valve sclerosis (nonobstructive) | Supraclavicular arterial bruit |
|---|---|---|---|---|---|---|---|
| | Valvular (75% of cases) | Subvalvular (discrete) | Supravalvular | | | | |
| Murmur of aortic regurgitation | 10 to 20% of cases | 55 to 100% of cases | 25% of cases | Common | Absent | Absent | Absent |
| Effect of maneuvers on systolic murmur | | | | | | Maneuvers usually not performed | Maneuvers usually not performed |
| Sudden squatting | Increased | Increased | Increased | Increased | Decreased | | |
| Valsalva | Decreased | Decreased | Decreased | Decreased | Increased | | |
| Amyl nitrite | Increased | Increased | Increased | Increased | Increased | | |
| Vasopressors (phenylephrine or methoxamine) | Increased | Increased | Increased | Increased | Decreased or absent | | |
| Electrocardiogram | Left ventricular enlargement (LVE) with S-T changes | | | LVE, later with S-T-T changes; left atrial abnormality; may mimic anteroseptal myocardial infarction (MI) | LVE, S-T-T changes; left or biatrial abnormality; abnormal Q waves simulating MI common | Normal | Normal |

| X-ray findings | Concentric left ventricular hypertrophy (LVH); poststenotic dilatation of the aorta; valvular calcification common | Concentric LVH; poststenotic dilatation usually absent | Concentric LVH; poststenotic dilatation absent | Concentric LVH; poststenotic dilatation of aorta may be present; valvular calcification common, increasing with advancing age | LVH; poststenotic dilatation of aorta absent | Normal | Normal |

**Table 3-10.** Differential diagnosis of pansystolic regurgitant murmurs

| Parameter | Mitral regurgitation | Tricuspid regurgitation | Ventricular septal defect |
|---|---|---|---|
| Arterial pulse | Abrupt and collapsing | Reflects associated left-sided lesions | Brisk, bounding, or bisferiens |
| Jugular venous pulse | Normal | Large V waves with a rapid Y descent, often with systolic expansion of liver | Normal; large A waves in PH |
| Precordial pulsations | Hyperdynamic LV impulse; apical systolic thrill | Hyperdynamic RV impulse; diffuse systolic depression on left side of chest with opposite pulsation on right; systolic thrill LLSB | Hyperdynamic LV impulse; systolic thrill at 3LICS or 4LICS |
| Heart sounds | $S_1$: normal or decreased<br>$S_2$: wide expiratory splitting that is not fixed<br>$P_2$: often accentuated<br>$LS_3$: common<br>$LS_4$: rare<br>OS: rare | $S_1$: normal, increased, or decreased in tricuspid area<br>$S_2$: normal or wide splitting; paradoxical in early pulmonary closure<br>OS: rare<br>$RS_3$: common<br>$RS_4$: rare | $S_1$: normal<br>$S_2$: normal, or widely split with large shunts; with PH, $P_2$ increased and splitting normal or narrow<br>$LS_3$: often present<br>$LS_4$: absent |
| Systolic murmurs | Typical pansystolic, maximum at apex; high- to medium-pitched, blowing, and usually plateau-shaped. May be crescendo, decrescendo, or crescendo-decrescendo, radiation to left axilla and scapula<br>Mid or late nonpansystolic murmurs common in nonrheumatic types; may start with SC | Murmur is similar to that of MR but maximum at 4LICS or 5LICS; radiation to xiphoid, LRSB, and pulmonary area, but when RVE is marked, may be heard at apex | Harsh, plateau-shaped, maximum at 3LICS or 4LICS; with high VSD, may be maximum at 2LICS; the murmur may be early systolic rather than holosystolic when the VSD is small |

| | | | |
|---|---|---|---|
| Diastolic murmurs | Rumbling mid diastolic flow murmur may be heard at apex in pure, severe MR | Rumbling mid diastolic flow murmur may be heard at LLSB in pure, severe TR | A rumbling mid diastolic flow murmur may be heard at apex in large shunts. Murmur of AR indicates incompetence of medial aortic cusp |
| Effect of maneuvers on systolic murmur: | | | |
| Inspiration | Unchanged or decreases slightly | Increased | Unchanged |
| Amyl nitrite | Rheumatic: softer; Mid to late (click syndrome): softer, starts earlier, lasts longer; Papillary muscle dysfunction: variable effect | Increased | Small with PH: decreases; Large with hyperkinetic PH: louder; Large with pulmonary vascular disease: little change |
| Vasopressor (phenylephrine or methoxamine) | Rheumatic: louder; Mid to late (click syndrome): increased; Papillary muscle dysfunction: variable effect | NSC | Small: louder; Large: unchanged or paradoxical increase |
| Electrocardiogram | Atrial fibrillation common; LVE and LAE, and sometimes RVE | Atrial fibrillation usual; RVE and sometimes LVE | Small: normal; Large: LVE, RVE, LAE, RAE |
| X-ray findings | LVE and LAE | RVE, RAE, often with prominent great veins | Small: normal; Large: pulmonary plethora, large PA, LVE, RVE, LAE, RAE |

**Table 3-11.** Differential diagnosis of aortic stenosis and mitral regurgitation masquerading one for the other

| Parameter | Aortic stenosis | Mitral regurgitation |
|---|---|---|
| Arterial pulse | Small, delayed upstroke and peak | Brisk, collapsing |
| Precordial pulsations | Sustained LV heave; thrill over carotid arteries or 2RICS | Hyperdynamic LV impulse; apical thrill |
| Heart sounds | $S_1$: normal<br>$S_2$: usually decreased or absent; may be single, narrowly split, or paradoxically split<br>AES: may be present<br>$LS_3$: may be present in LV failure<br>$LS_4$: may be present | $S_1$: decreased or masked by murmur<br>$S_2$: normal or widely split<br>AES: absent<br>$LS_3$: commonly present without LV failure<br>$LS_4$: absent; present only in MR due to ruptured chordae |
| Systolic murmur | Ejection type regardless of location; transmitted to carotid arteries even with apical radiation<br>Murmur usually louder after long pauses (as in ventricular premature contractions or atrial fibrillation) | Holosystolic in pure rheumatic mitral regurgitation; usually transmitted to left axilla; radiates to base when posterior mitral leaflet is incompetent<br>Mid to late systolic murmur almost always maximal at apex<br>Murmur unchanged after long pauses |
| Phonocardiogram | Murmur ends before $A_2$ | Murmur ends at or after $A_2$ |
| Amyl nitrite | Murmur louder | Murmur softer |
| Phenylephrine | Murmur softer | Murmur louder |

**Table 3-12.** Differential diagnosis of murmurs of pulmonary and aortic stenosis

| Parameter | Pulmonary stenosis | Aortic stenosis |
|---|---|---|
| Effect of inspiration on murmur with patient standing | Louder | Fainter |
| Maximum site | Left sternal border | 2RICS or apex |
| Post-Valsalva effect | Immediate return of intensity of murmur | Delayed return of intensity of murmur |
| Effect of inspiration on ejection sound | Pulmonary ejection sound may decrease and move toward $S_1$ or disappear | Aortic ejection sound unchanged |
| $S_2$ | Usually widely split except in very mild stenosis, when splitting is narrow | Usually single or narrowly split; reversed splitting may be present in severe stenosis |
| $S_4$ | Right-sided $S_4$ often present | Left-sided $S_4$ often present |

      **(2)** Tetralogy of Fallot.
      **(3)** Acquired pulmonary stenosis.
         **(a)** Rheumatic fever.
         **(b)** Carcinoid syndrome.
  **b.** Idiopathic dilatation of the pulmonary artery.
  **c.** Atrial septal defect.
  **d.** Ventricular septal defect (some cases with small left-to-right shunts).
  **e.** Pulmonary hypertension.
    **(1)** Primary.
    **(2)** Secondary.
      **(a)** Left-to-right shunts.
      **(b)** Mitral stenosis.
  **f.** Coarctation of the aorta.
  **g.** Idiopathic hypertrophic subaortic stenosis.
  **h.** Pulmonary flow murmurs in hyperkinetic circulatory states (e.g., fever, anemia, thyrotoxicosis).
  **i.** Innocent murmurs.
    **(1)** Pulmonary ejection murmur.
    **(2)** Vibratory or Still's murmur.
    **(3)** Cardiorespiratory murmur.
**2.** Diagnostic features.
  **a.** As may be seen from paragraph **1** above, a large number of murmurs may have their sites of maximum intensity along the LSB. The murmur of VPS with an intact ventricular septum is the prototype of the SEM of pulmonary outflow obstruction, but similar murmurs may occur in other conditions. By attention to the various parameters listed in Table 3-5, including physiologic and pharmacologic maneuvers, it is often possible to distinguish between them. There will remain nevertheless a fair number of cases in which the diagnosis can be established only by cardiac catheterization.
  **b.** The differential diagnosis of innocent murmurs is considered in Tables 3-7 and 3-8.
  **c.** At times it may be difficult to distinguish between the murmurs of PS and AS. The differentiating features are listed in Table 3-12.

### Apex and Lower Left Sternal Border: Pansystolic Regurgitant Murmurs and Their Variants

**1.** Etiology.
  **a.** Mitral regurgitation.
    **(1)** Congenital: as an isolated lesion, part of an endocardial cushion defect, Marfan's syndrome, Ehlers-Danlos syndrome, IHSS, or anomalous left coronary artery arising from the pulmonary artery.
    **(2)** Acquired.
      **(a)** Rheumatic.
      **(b)** Nonrheumatic.
         **(i)** Papillary muscle dysfunction or rupture.
         **(ii)** Infective endocarditis.
         **(iii)** Ruptured chordae (rheumatic, infective endocarditis, trauma, unknown etiology).
         **(iv)** "Click" syndrome with prolapse of mitral leaflets into left atrium.
         **(v)** Calcification of the mitral annulus.
         **(vi)** Left ventricular dilatation (e.g., cardiomyopathy, aortic valve disease).
  **b.** Tricuspid regurgitation.
    **(1)** Rheumatic (organic or relative, or both).

      **(2)** Nonrheumatic.
         **(a)** Right ventricular dilatation (e.g., cardiomyopathy, severe left-sided heart failure).
         **(b)** Pulmonary hypertension.
         **(c)** Trauma.
         **(d)** Carcinoid syndrome.
    **c.** Ventricular septal defect.
      **(1)** Congenital.
      **(2)** Acquired (e.g., septal rupture in acute myocardial infarction).
**2.** Diagnostic features.
    **a.** The murmur of rheumatic MR is the prototype of the pansystolic RM. The murmur starts with $S_1$, which is typically decreased or masked by the murmur, and ends with or beyond $A_2$. It is high- to medium-pitched, blowing, and usually plateau-shaped, although it may be crescendo, decrescendo, or crescendo-decrescendo. $S_2$ is split narrowly when MR is mild, and widely when it is moderate or severe. An accentuated $P_2$ is common and a loud $S_3$ is often present. For practical purposes, a holosystolic murmur that is maximal at the apex, regardless of its characteristics, is virtually diagnostic of MR.
    **b.** The murmur of MR must be differentiated from the murmurs of TR and VSD (see Table 3-10). MR due to IHSS should be distinguished from MR due to other causes (compare Tables 3-8 and 3-10).
    **c.** The murmur of rheumatic TR should be distinguished from the usually co-existing murmur of MR. This may be difficult, but attention to the intensity of the murmur during inspiration and expiration usually provides the answer. The murmur of TR is louder in inspiration, whereas that of MR is unchanged or slightly diminished. Also, the former is louder at the LLSB, and the latter, at the apex.
    **d.** Sometimes the murmurs of AS and MR masquerade one for the other, as occurs when the former is louder at the apex or the latter is louder at the base. Table 3-11 should help in differential diagnosis between the two.
    **e.** Once the diagnosis of MR is established, its cause should be determined.
      **(1)** The congenital varieties, with the exception of IHSS, are usually found at an early age and are rarely problems in adult medicine.
      **(2)** Rheumatic valvulitis is by far the most common cause of MR, and a history of rheumatic fever or chorea can almost always be obtained.
      **(3)** MR due to IE is characterized by symptoms of systemic infection, embolic phenomena, and valvular vegetations.
      **(4)** MR caused by ruptured chordae tendineae is usually acute if the etiology is nonrheumatic, as in IE, trauma, or idiopathic cases. Rheumatic fever and IE account for about half the cases, but in about one-third the cause is unknown. In addition to the loud holosystolic murmur, distinctive features of ruptured chordae (in contrast to conventional rheumatic MR), include the sudden onset of dyspnea and pulmonary edema, sinus rhythm, minimal left atrial enlargement, mild cardiomegaly, and a fourth heart sound. Radiation of the murmur to the base and carotid arteries is produced by rupture of the posterior leaflet. When the anterior leaflet ruptures, the murmur radiates to the axilla, posterior thorax, and vertebral column.
      **(5)** MR due to rupture of a papillary muscle is most commonly caused by myocardial infarction. If the patient survives, congestive heart failure dominates the clinical picture. Survival depends not only on the severity of the MR but also on the state of the myocardium. Coronary and left ventricular angiography are indicated whenever MR is acute to assess the severity and possible causes of the lesion with a view to surgical intervention. The differential diagnosis between a ruptured papillary muscle and perforation of the interventricular septum in myocardial infarction is discussed in paragraph **(12)** below.

**(6)** MR due to papillary muscle dysfunction is common in coronary artery disease—both in angina pectoris and in myocardial infarction. The murmur is variable. It may be pansystolic or mid systolic (simulating an SEM), and it may change from time to time in the same patient. Atrial sounds are commonly audible. When the murmur is mid systolic, $S_1$ is often normal and SC may be heard.

**(7)** The mid systolic click-late systolic murmur syndrome is characterized by non-ejection SC, late SM, or both. The etiology is unknown in most cases, but the syndrome has been reported in patients with atrial septal defects, rheumatic heart disease, and papillary muscle dysfunction. Although the condition can occur at any age and in both sexes, the incidence is strikingly high (6 to 10 percent or more) in presumably healthy young women. The auscultatory findings are the result of prolapse of one or both mitral leaflets into the left atrium: the SC, to tensing of the redundant leaflets and elongated chordae tendineae; and the SM, to MR. The diagnosis can be confirmed by echocardiography, angiocardiography, or both. Complications are infrequent, but include ruptured chordae tendineae, infective endocarditis, ventricular arrhythmias, calcification of the valve, and sudden death (about 1.2 percent of cases). However, on an overall basis, the syndrome should be considered benign and is associated with a good prognosis.

**(8)** Nonrheumatic calcification of the mitral annulus is a not unusual cause of MR in elderly females. The hallmark of this condition is a J-, U-, or oval-shaped calcification at the site of the mitral annulus, demonstrated best by fluoroscopy under image amplification.

**(9)** MR or TR, or both, may occur in cardiomyopathy. In this condition, there are usually "unexplained" cardiomegaly and $S_3$ and $S_4$ gallops, accompanied by congestive failure. The RM of cardiomyopathy, whether mitral or tricuspid, tends to become fainter or vanish when failure ceases, whereas the murmurs of MR and TR due to other causes remain the same or become louder with restoration of compensation.

**(10)** MR may result from LV dilatation. The mechanism is not clear, but it may involve such factors as dilatation of the mitral annulus and papillary muscle dysfunction. The presence of a quiet precordium, marked lateral displacement of the cardiac apex, a nondynamic LV impulse, little left atrial enlargement, and a soft pansystolic murmur suggests LV dilatation rather than valvular disease as the cause of MR.

**(11)** TR is most often rheumatic and is more a functional than an anatomic lesion. Rheumatic TR is always associated with mitral and often with aortic valvular disease. Thus its cause is established by the company it keeps. In pulmonary hypertensive TR, there is usually good evidence of obliterative pulmonary vascular disease, persistent wide splitting of $S_2$ on expiration, and prominent A as well as V waves in the JVP (versus prominent V waves only in rheumatic TR). Traumatic TR is rare. TR is sometimes caused by the carcinoid syndrome (see p. 105).

**(12)** VSD is congenital but may sometimes result from rupture of the interventricular septum in myocardial infarction. A postinfarctional VSD must be distinguished from a papillary muscle rupture with a similar cause. With septal rupture, the murmur and thrill are usually maximum at the LLSB, with the clinical picture dominated by right-sided heart failure. In papillary muscle rupture, the murmur is usually not as intense and is loudest at the apex. A thrill is uncommon, and left-sided heart failure is the dominant clinical manifestation. Often the correct diagnosis can be made only by cardiac catheterization.

**(13)** Systolic whoops and honks are short, loud, somewhat inconstant, systolic murmurs, often preceded by systolic clicks, having auscultatory characteristics corresponding to the descriptive terms. Most whoops and honks are caused by MR.

## Diastolic Murmurs

### Early Diastolic Murmurs at the Base and Sternal Borders

1. Etiology.
   a. Aortic regurgitation.
      (1) Rheumatic fever.
      (2) Infective endocarditis.
      (3) Calcific aortic stenosis.
      (4) Senile aortic dilatation.
      (5) Disease of the aorta.
         (a) Dissecting aneurysm.
         (b) Arterial hypertension.
         (c) Marfan's syndrome.
         (d) Miscellaneous diseases.
      (6) Syphilis.
      (7) Congenital lesions.
         (a) Bicuspid aortic valve.
         (b) Coarctation of the aorta.
         (c) Ventricular septal defect.
         (d) Other congenital defects.
      (8) Postsurgical and posttraumatic.
      (9) Miscellaneous causes (e.g., ankylosing spondylitis, other rheumatoid variants).
   b. Pulmonary regurgitation.
      (1) Congenital.
         (a) Congenital pulmonary valve incompetence.
         (b) Absence of the pulmonary valve.
         (c) Idiopathic dilatation of the pulmonary artery.
      (2) Acquired.
         (a) Disease of the pulmonary valve.
            (i) Rheumatic.
            (ii) Postsurgical.
            (iii) Infective endocarditis.
         (b) Pulmonary hypertension.
            (i) Primary.
            (ii) Secondary: mitral stenosis (most common cause of PR), cor pulmonale, or Eisenmenger syndrome.
2. Diagnostic features.
   a. The murmur of AR is the prototype of the murmur of semilunar valve incompetence. The diagnosis is based on the presence of a high-pitched, blowing, but sometimes harsh or musical DM, beginning immediately after $A_2$ and lasting through most or all of diastole. The murmur is heard best at the 3LICS with the patient seated, leaning forward, and holding his breath in expiration. Transmission of the murmur is to the LSB, the apex, and sometimes to an area above the apex in the anterior axillary line. The murmur may also be audible in the 2RICS. Radiation of the murmur along the RSB rather than the LSB should suggest an uncommon cause of AR, such as disease of the proximal aorta or of the aortic valve, in association with dilatation and displacement of the aortic root. In the former category are such conditions as aneurysm, dissection, Marfan's syndrome, cystic medial necrosis of the aorta, and aneurysm of the sinus of Valsalva. The latter group comprises cases of aortic valve disease due to IE, trauma, VSD with AR, and syphilis. A musical murmur of AR is usually caused by eversion of an aortic cusp, most commonly of syphilitic or rheumatic origin. AR causes widening of the pulse pressure, except in mild cases, giving rise to peripheral signs such as a bounding or collapsing arterial pulse, pistol-shot sounds or double sounds (Traube's sign) over large superficial arteries, Duroziez's to-and-fro murmur, and capillary

pulsation; none of these findings is specific for AR. Pulsation in the 2RICS is usually due to dilatation of the aorta. Pulsation of the sternoclavicular joints suggests aortic aneurysm or dissection. The apical impulse is hyperdynamic, and in some severe cases may show a double outward movement in diastole. In marked AR, systolic depression of the midportion and right side of the chest may be seen. $S_1$ may be diminished or absent. $A_2$ is commonly accentuated but may be decreased when AS is present. An AES may be audible. Other murmurs that may occur in AR include an aortic SEM due to flow or concomitant AS (see p. 81), an apical holosystolic murmur due to anatomic or relative MR, and the rumbling Austin Flint mid diastolic murmur probably due to relative MS.

**b.** The murmur of PR, originally described by Graham Steell, must be distinguished from the murmur of AR, which has similar characteristics. Acquired PR is almost always due to dilatation of the pulmonary valve ring secondary to PH. In the presence of MS, the differentiation of AR from PR may be difficult or impossible. Aortic valvulography may be useful in establishing the diagnosis of AR but not in ruling PR in or out. Amyl nitrite may be of some help because it decreases the intensity of the murmur of AR but has no effect on the murmur of PR. In general, a basal DM should be attributed to AR if there are peripheral signs of AR, if AS is present, if the murmur is decreased with amyl nitrite, if LVE is noted, or if the aorta is large and pulsatile; and to PR if there is an accentuated $P_2$, if RVE but not LVE is present, if the murmur is unaffected by amyl nitrite, or if the lesion is secondary to PPH. PR may occur in the absence of PH following surgical treatment of VPS or IE, or from congenital incompetence of the pulmonary valve.

**c.** The Austin Flint murmur of AR must be distinguished from the murmur of MS, which is often associated with rheumatic AR. The patient with both AR and MS is more likely to be female, fibrillating, and having marked exertional dyspnea, hemoptysis, or both. Usually $S_1$ is accentuated, $P_2$ is loud, an OS is present unless the valve is calcified or inflexible, $S_3$ is absent, and the murmur is longer. An apical DM associated with calcification of the mitral valve should be attributed to MS whether an OS is present or not. In the absence of mitral valvular calcification or an OS, an apical DM should also be considered of stenotic origin if the SM of MR is audible. In contrast to the foregoing, the patient with the Austin Flint murmur is typically male, usually in sinus rhythm, with only moderate exertional dyspnea, and no history of hemoptysis. The murmur is early to mid diastolic and relatively short, $S_1$ is decreased, $P_2$ is commonly normal or only slightly accentuated, and $S_3$ is often present. No OS is audible. If a rheumatic origin can be excluded, an apical DM in AR should be considered an Austin Flint murmur. The Austin Flint murmur is decreased, and the murmur of MS increased, with amyl nitrite. In MS, the ECG is more likely to show RAD and RVE; in AR, LVE.

**d.** For practical purposes, AR is most commonly due to rheumatic fever, IE, calcific AS, or senile ectasia of the aorta, with rheumatic cases constituting about 75 percent of the total. Clues to the cause of AR may be found in the history, especially with respect to the time of discovery of the murmur. Murmurs beginning in childhood suggest a congenital origin; those discovered in the second or third decade are most often rheumatic; those found in the fourth or fifth decade or somewhat later are usually due to calcific disease of the aortic valve; and those discovered late in life are usually caused by aortic dilatation. A history of rheumatic fever is helpful when positive, but it is often absent in rheumatic cases. When mitral valvular disease coexists with AR, the cause is almost certainly rheumatic. A history of syphilis or of its treatment, a positive serology, calcification of the ascending aorta, and a tambour-like $A_2$ suggest a syphilitic origin. IE is diagnosed by the usual criteria for the disease. In the presence of familial disease, particularly if supported by appropriate clinical data, Marfan's syndrome, the mucopolysaccharidoses, and the Ehlers-Danlos syndrome should be considered as causes of AR. Ankylosing spondylitis and other rheumatoid variants sometimes cause AR. AR due to aortic dilatation is not associated with other valvular lesions, but systemic hypertension is a common accompaniment. It is probably the most common cause of AR in the elderly.

## Mid and Late Diastolic Murmurs at the Apex and Lower Left Sternal Border

1. Etiology.
   a. AV valve obstruction.
      (1) Mitral stenosis.
      (2) Tricuspid stenosis.
      (3) Atrial myxomas.
      (4) Left atrial ball-valve thrombus.
   b. Increased flow across the AV valves without obstruction (relative stenosis).
      (1) Mitral valve.
         (a) Active rheumatic valvulitis (Carey Coombs murmur).
         (b) Mitral regurgitation (some cases).
         (c) AR with the Austin Flint murmur.
         (d) Patent ductus arteriosus.
         (e) Ventricular septal defect.
      (2) Tricuspid valve.
         (a) Tricuspid regurgitation.
         (b) Atrial septal defect.
   c. Miscellaneous causes.
      (1) Hyperthyroidism.
      (2) Anemia.
      (3) Complete heart block.
      (4) Left ventricular dilatation secondary to hypertensive or arteriosclerotic heart disease, or both.
      (5) Atypical verrucous endocarditis.
      (6) Chronic or adhesive pericarditis.
      (7) Eisenmenger syndrome.
      (8) Primary pulmonary hypertension.
      (9) Coarctation of the aorta with aortic stenosis.
2. Diagnostic features.
   a. The murmur of MS is typically a low-pitched, rumbling, mid diastolic murmur with presystolic crescendo accentuation. The earliest murmur is usually a mid diastolic murmur, although sometimes it is only presystolic. In atrial fibrillation, the presystolic component disappears. $S_1$ is loud and sharp. $P_2$ is normal or accentuated, and an OS is present unless the valve is rigid, fibrosed, or calcified. $S_3$ and $S_4$ sounds are not present. The murmur is maximum at the apex and often confined to its vicinity. It is heard best with the bell chest piece at the site of the apical impulse with the patient lying in the left lateral recumbent position. When not clearly audible, it may become more discernible after exercise. The murmur is generally unaffected by respiration but may decrease slightly with inspiration. In pure MS, the apical impulse is often normal. An RV lift means PH or TR.
   b. When MS and MR are combined, SM and DM are usually audible, but $S_3$ and $S_4$ sounds and an OS are not heard. $S_1$ is usually decreased. If an $S_3$ sound is present, it can be assumed that MR is the predominant lesion. (See also paragraph **g** below).
   c. The differential diagnosis between the Austin Flint murmur and that of MS is discussed on page 105.
   d. The murmur of MS must be distinguished from that of left atrial myxoma, a condition in which, contrary to the situation in MS, the DM tends to vary with body position and an OS is not present. There is often a variable and at times

**Table 3-13.** Differential diagnosis of true and relative mitral stenosis

| Parameter | Mitral stenosis | Relative mitral stenosis |
|---|---|---|
| Right ventricular lift | Often present | Absent |
| Left ventricular lift | Absent | Present |
| Apical thrill | Sometimes present | Absent |
| Loud, sharp $S_1$ | Present | Absent |
| $P_2$ | Usually increased | Variable |
| OS | Present | Absent |
| $S_3$ | Absent | Present |
| Diastolic murmur | Rumbling; starts after opening snap; longer | Blowing; starts with $S_3$; shorter |

musical SM. Irregular clicks may be heard throughout systole and diastole. Fever and embolic phenomena are common. Left atrial myxoma can be diagnosed by echocardiography or angiocardiography.

  **e.** An atrial ball-valve thrombus may simulate MS but should be suspected if severe pulmonary congestion and embolic phenomena are associated with syncope, relief of symptoms in the upright position, murmurs changing with body position, tachycardia, and at times, episodes of coldness, cyanosis, and numbness of the hands and feet.

  **f.** The differential diagnosis of true MS and relative MS is summarized in Table 3-13. Also helpful in the diagnosis of relative rather than true MS is evidence of a primary condition capable of causing the relative stenosis (p. 103).

  **g.** The presence of a DM in patients with MR may raise the question of whether the DM is due to the MR itself or is the result of associated MS. Favoring pure MR as the cause of the DM is clinical evidence of severe regurgitation manifested by a large LV, a hyperdynamic apical impulse, wide splitting of $S_2$ on expiration, a soft $S_1$, and a DM that is loud and blowing and that starts with the $S_3$ sound. Favoring coexisting MS as the cause of the DM are the following: an earlier, longer, rumbling DM that begins after the OS, absence of $S_3$, normal splitting of $S_2$, a normal or increased $P_2$, calcification of the valve, and a normal-size or minimally enlarged heart.

  **h.** The murmur of TS is similar in its characteristics to that of MS. It differs in that it is maximal at the LLSB rather than at the apex and is louder on inspiration. The murmur of MS is unaffected or decreases slightly with inspiration.

  **i.** The carcinoid syndrome is commonly associated with stenotic or regurgitant lesions of the tricuspid and pulmonary valves. Systemic manifestations, such as cutaneous flushing and telangiectasia, intestinal hypermotility, bronchoconstriction, and hypotensive crises, in association with RV failure, are clues to the diagnosis. Confirmation may be obtained by finding increased urinary excretion of 5-hydroxyindoleacetic acid.

## Continuous Murmurs over the Thorax

**1.** Etiology and site of maximum intensity.
  **a.** Extracardiac shunts.
    **(1)** Patent ductus arteriosus (2LICS or immediately below left clavicle).

    **(2)** Pulmonary AV fistula: congenital or acquired (lower lobes or right middle lobe).

    **(3)** Systemic AV fistula (directly over the fistula).

    **(4)** Some cases of aortopulmonary septal defect (2LICS or 3LICS).

    **(5)** Postsurgical shunts in the tetralogy of Fallot (to the right or left of the upper sternum).

  **b.** Intracardiac shunts.

    **(1)** Sinus of Valsalva aneurysm with rupture into right atrium or ventricle (4LICS).

    **(2)** Coronary arteriovenous fistula with connection to the right atrium or ventricle (apicosternal region).

    **(3)** Small atrial septal defect with tight mitral stenosis: Lutembacher's syndrome (LLSB).

    **(4)** Total anomalous pulmonary venous drainage (ULSB).

  **c.** Arterial stenosis.

    **(1)** Coarctation of the aorta (posterior chest).

    **(2)** Pulmonary artery branch stenosis (SM or CM over site of stenosis).

    **(3)** Aortic arch syndrome (over affected vessel).

  **d.** Increased flow through normal or dilated vessels.

    **(1)** Jugular venous hum (neck, above the clavicle).

    **(2)** Mammary souffle (2LICS to 4LICS, or 2RICS to 4RICS).

    **(3)** Increased bronchial collateral circulation (posterior chest).

      **(a)** Truncus arteriosus.

      **(b)** Severe tetralogy of Fallot.

      **(c)** Other congenital malformations.

**2.** Diagnostic features.

  **a.** The murmur of PDA is the prototype of CM associated with extracardiac shunts. It starts with $S_1$, continues through $S_2$ without interruption, and fades steadily during diastole. Systolic accentuation of the murmur is quite characteristic. The murmur usually has a machinery-like quality. It is loudest in the 2LICS or immediately below the left clavicle. A thrill may be present. When PDA is associated with moderate to large left-to-right shunts, a DM due to flow may be heard at the apex. $S_1$ is usually normal. An $S_3$ sound is common. If PH develops, the diastolic component of the CM decreases or disappears, so that only an SM remains. $P_2$ becomes accentuated, a PES may be heard, and the murmurs of PR and TR may appear.

  **b.** When a patient has the clinical picture of a left-to-right shunt with PH and only an SM at the 2LICS or 3LICS, the diagnostic possibilities include PDA, VSD, ASD, and an aortopulmonary window.

  **c.** With CM, the location of the maximum site of the murmur may be of some diagnostic significance (see paragraph **1** above).

  **d.** Rupture of an aortic sinus with a right-sided communication is suggested by the sudden appearance of a CM in a young adult following trauma or exertion. The murmur is maximal at the LLSB.

  **e.** Coronary arteriovenous fistula with connection to the RA or RV is manifested by a superficial CM with diastolic accentuation, loudest in the apicosternal region, and is commonly associated with a thrill. The murmur is decreased by the Valsalva maneuver. In contrast, the CM of extracardiac shunts (e.g., PDA) shows systolic accentuation and is unaffected by the Valsalva maneuver.

  **f.** The to-and-fro murmurs of AS and AR, or of PS and PR, may be mistaken for CM. The chief differentiating point is that CM envelop $S_2$, but to-and-fro murmurs do not. By careful auscultation in to-and-fro murmurs, it will be found that the SEM ends before $S_2$ and the DM begins after $S_2$. There is thus a hiatus between the two murmurs, a condition that does not exist in CM.

  **g.** The characteristics and differential diagnosis of the jugular venous hum and the mammary souffle, both of which are innocent CM, may be found in Table 3-7.

## CARDIAC ENLARGEMENT AND THE CARDIOMYOPATHIES

Lane D. Craddock

### Cardiac Enlargement

Cardiac enlargement, with few exceptions, is a sign of organic heart disease. Its cause can usually be ascertained from the history, physical examination, and laboratory data (including the ECG, chest films, echocardiogram, radioisotope scanning, and angiocardiography). Assuming that artifactitious enlargement is excluded (e.g., cardiac displacement, transverse position of the heart, thoracic deformity, pericardial fat pads, cysts, faulty roentgenographic techniques) cardiomegaly, in actual clinical practice, is most often due to the conventional causes of heart disease—congenital malformations, coronary artery disease, hypertension, rheumatic fever, and pericardial disease. However, there remain a significant number of cases of cardiomegaly that are not due to the usual causes. Many of these appear to be the result of some type of cardiomyopathy. This section will consider briefly the more common causes of cardiac enlargement that are well known to the reader, but will consider in some detail the etiology, classification, clinical features, and differential diagnosis of the less well known cardiomyopathies.

In actual clinical practice, enlargement of the heart is usually detected by physical examination, electrocardiography (including vectorcardiography), radiographic techniques, or combinations of these methods, rather than by esoteric techniques. It is to be stressed that enlargement should rarely be missed by physical examination alone. Cardiac enlargement may be due to hypertrophy, dilatation, or a combination of the two. It may be generalized, or it may affect individual chambers in various combinations.

### Etiology

Generalized cardiac enlargement is most often due to congestive heart failure. Although initially, enlargement may take place in one or more of the heart chambers, eventual progression to involvement of all chambers is common. Thus, a patient with arterial hypertension may develop, successively, left ventricular enlargement and failure, enlargement of the left atrium, pulmonary vascular congestion, and finally, enlargement of the right ventricle and atrium. In other circumstances, a disease process may affect all chambers more or less simultaneously and thereby produce diffuse cardiomegaly (e.g., anemia, myocarditis, cardiomyopathy).

Individual chamber enlargement is usually a consequence of a single congenital or aquired lesion.

The major causes of cardiomegaly in the adult are listed below. It should be borne in mind that in some patients more than one etiologic factor may play a role.

1. Generalized cardiac enlargement.
   a. Congenital diseases.
   b. Acquired diseases.
      (1) Alcoholism.
      (2) Anemia.
      (3) Cardiomyopathy (see Table 3-14 for the various causes).
      (4) Coronary artery disease (late stage).
      (5) Hypertension (late stage).
      (6) Rheumatic fever (late stage or with multivalvular involvement).
      (7) Syphilis.

**Table 3-14.** Etiologic and clinical classification of the cardiomyopathies

Primary cardiomyopathy

Dilated (formerly referred to as congestive)
   Idiopathic
   Familial
   Peripartal

Hypertrophic (familial and nonfamilial)
   Obstructive
   Nonobstructive

Restrictive
   Endomyocardial fibrosis
   Endocardial fibroelastosis

Secondary cardiomyopathy*
   Connective tissue disease (e.g., systemic lupus erythematosus, scleroderma, dermatomyositis, rheumatoid arthritis)
   Neuromuscular disease (e.g., Friedreich's ataxia, myotonia atrophica, progressive muscular dystrophy)
   Vascular disease (e.g., ischemic cardiomyopathy)
   Metabolic disease (e.g., hyperthyroidism, hypothyroidism, hemochromatosis, glycogen storage disease, mucopolysaccharidoses, amyloidosis)
   Neoplastic disease (e.g., lymphomas, leukemia, metastatic carcinoma)
   Nutritional disease (e.g., beriberi, kwashiorkor)
   Myocarditis
      Viral
      Parasitic
      Protozoal
      Other
   Sarcoidosis
   Drugs, chemicals, and toxins (e.g., emetine, arsenic, carbon monoxide poisoning)
   Posttraumatic disorders

*Secondary cardiomyopathies usually give a clinical picture of congestive failure; less often, with symptoms resembling those of constrictive pericarditis. Ischemic heart disease may be seen clinically as a congestive or dilated cardiomyopathy, hence its inclusion in the classification.

       **(8)** Pericardial disease.
       **(9)** Neoplasm.
     **(10)** Endocrinopathies.
     **(11)** Incessant automatic supraventricular tachycardia in the young (rare).
  **2.** Left ventricular enlargement.
    **a.** Congenital or familial diseases.
       **(1)** Aortic stenosis.
       **(2)** Idiopathic hypertrophic subaortic stenosis.
       **(3)** Coarctation of the aorta.
       **(4)** Patent ductus arteriosus.
       **(5)** Tricuspid atresia.
    **b.** Acquired diseases.
       **(1)** Arterial hypertension.
       **(2)** Coronary artery disease.
       **(3)** Aortic stenosis, regurgitation, or both.
       **(4)** Mitral regurgitation.
  **3.** Left atrial enlargement.
    **a.** Congenital diseases.
       **(1)** Ventricular septal defect.
       **(2)** Patent ductus arteriosus.

       **(3)** Coarctation of the aorta.
       **(4)** Congenital mitral stenosis.
    **b.** Acquired diseases.
       **(1)** Left ventricular hypertrophy or dilatation.
       **(2)** Mitral stenosis, regurgitation, or both.
       **(3)** Infective endocarditis of mitral valve.
       **(4)** Left atrial myxoma.
       **(5)** Mitral valve prolapse (late stage or with rupture of the chordae tendineae).
**4.** Right ventricular enlargement.
    **a.** Congenital diseases.
       **(1)** Ventricular septal defects.
       **(2)** Atrial septal defects.
       **(3)** Transposition of the great vessels.
       **(4)** Tetralogy of Fallot.
       **(5)** Eisenmenger complex.
       **(6)** Anomalous pulmonary venous return.
    **b.** Acquired diseases.
       **(1)** Left ventricular hypertrophy or dilatation.
       **(2)** Mitral valve disease (especially stenosis).
       **(3)** Chronic obstructive pulmonary disease.
       **(4)** Primary pulmonary hypertension.
       **(5)** Tricuspid regurgitation.
       **(6)** Pulmonary vascular disease (especially pulmonary embolism).
       **(7)** Chronic alveolar hypoventilation (Pickwickian syndrome).
**5.** Right atrial enlargement.
    **a.** Congenital diseases.
       **(1)** Ebstein's anomaly.
       **(2)** Tricuspid regurgitation.
       **(3)** Atrial septal defect with large left-to-right shunt.
       **(4)** Valvular pulmonic stenosis.
       **(5)** Multiple pulmonary coarctation.
    **b.** Acquired diseases.
       **(1)** Right ventricular hypertrophy and dilatation (usually secondary to pulmonary hypertension).
       **(2)** Tricuspid stenosis, regurgitation, or both.
       **(3)** Right atrial tumors (most often myxoma).
       **(4)** Tricuspid valve prolapse (rare).

## Evaluation

**1.** It should be possible in the vast majority of cases, based on the history, physical examination, clinical picture, ECG, chest films, and appropriate ancillary techniques, such as echocardiography (including transesophageal), exercise stress when appropriate, cardiac catheterization, angiography, and radioisotope scanning, to determine both the mechanism (e.g., valvular stenosis, regurgitation) and the cause (e.g., rheumatic fever, arterial hypertension) of cardiac enlargement. A discussion of these procedures, their interpretation, and the criteria for the diagnosis of the various etiologic types of heart disease is beyond the scope of this text.
**2.** Should the cause of cardiac enlargement in any patient remain undetermined in spite of meticulous clinical and laboratory evaluation, careful consideration should be given to the diagnosis of a cardiomyopathy.
**3.** Primary consideration should also be given to the diagnosis of cardiomyopathy as the explanation of heart disease in patients with the diseases listed in Table 3-14.
**4.** The next section deals with various features and differential diagnosis of the cardiomyopathies.

## Cardiomyopathy

### Definition

The terms *cardiomyopathy, myocardosis,* and *myocardiopathy* refer to disease of the heart muscle. It is characterized anatomically by cardiomegaly due to hypertrophy or dilatation, or both, and functionally by a clinical picture consistent with congestive failure (congestive cardiomyopathy), cardiac hypertrophy with or without ventricular outflow obstruction (hypertrophic cardiomyopathy), or simulating constrictive pericarditis (restrictive or obliterative cardiomyopathy). All forms may involve systolic or diastolic dysfunction, or both.

### Etiology

Cardiomyopathy may be primary (idiopathic) or secondary. The primary cardiomyopathies are myocardial diseases of unknown cause, probably due to multiple causes and not related to any known systemic disorder. Immune mechanisms in dilated cardiomyopathy have received much attention recently, and studies strongly suggest a relationship, at least in some patients. Although a causative role has not been established, further work should clarify the issue. Secondary cardiomyopathies are those in which the myocardial involvement is secondary to a systemic illness even when the cause of this disease is not understood (e.g., amyloidosis). It should be noted that some authorities use the term *primary myocardial disease* to indicate any myocardial disorder, idiopathic or secondary, in which cardiac involvement is the major clinical manifestation. A combined etiologic and clinical classification of the cardiomyopathies is shown in Table 3-14. The author prefers this classification to that published by the WHO/ISFC in the August 1981 issue of *Circulation*.

### Clinical Features

DILATED CARDIOMYOPATHY

The clinical presentation is most commonly that of biventricular failure, although sometimes the picture of left or right ventricular failure predominates. Dyspnea orthopnea, paroxysmal nocturnal dyspnea, and dependent edema are thus common symptoms. Other presentations include syncope (due to arrhythmia or heart block), arrhythmia, embolic phenomena, and occasionally, angina. Sudden death is distressingly frequent. On physical examination, the usual signs of congestive failure may be noted. Cardiomegaly (predominantly left ventricular in most cases), reduced intensity of the heart sounds, regurgitant systolic murmurs, and gallop rhythm ($S_3$, $S_4$, or summation gallop) are characteristic. A decreased arterial pulse with a narrow pulse pressure is common. Cyanosis is rare.

HYPERTROPHIC CARDIOMYOPATHY

1. Obstructive (idiopathic hypertrophic subaortic stenosis).
   a. Patients in this group have left ventricular hypertrophy in association with muscular ventricular outflow obstruction. The disease is often familial and is common in young and middle-aged adults.
   b. Many cases are discovered before the onset of symptoms because of the detection, on routine examination, of left ventricular enlargement or a heart murmur, or both. Individuals with symptoms generally complain of exertional dyspnea, syncope, or angina.
   c. On physical examination it is observed that the apical impulse is typically forceful and often bifid, the arterial pulse is brisk and bisferiens, an $S_4$ is present, a systolic ejection murmur is audible at either the mid or lower left sternal border, and a mitral regurgitant murmur is often heard at the apex (see the preceding section, Heart Murmurs).

2. Nonobstructive.
   a. In addition to the aforementioned clinical patterns, there are patients with myocardial disease who present primarily with evidence of hypertrophy (usually concentric) of the left ventricle. A history of syncope, palpitation, angina, or dyspnea may be obtained. Most such cases are familial, although isolated nonfamilial cases do occur. There are no characteristic murmurs. An atrial gallop is commonly heard.
   b. Some of these patients eventually develop evidence of left ventricular outflow obstruction. It would thus appear that hypertrophic cardiomyopathy can exist with or without obstruction. Recent echocardiographic observations suggest that asymmetric septal hypertrophy is the pathognomonic anatomic abnormality and the common denominator of both the nonobstructive and obstructive forms.

RESTRICTIVE CARDIOMYOPATHY

1. A very small number of patients with myocardiopathy, notably those with diseases such as amyloidosis, leukemia, and polyarteritis nodosa, may have symptoms resembling those of constrictive pericarditis.
2. The major features are an elevated venous pressure, deep X and Y descents in the jugular venous pulse, severe right-sided heart failure, clear lung fields, and only moderate cardiomegaly.
3. Endomyocardial fibrosis and endocardial fibroelastosis are also primary cardiomyopathies. The former condition is seen almost exclusively in Africans; the latter, in children.

## Laboratory Studies

ELECTROCARDIOGRAM

1. The ECG is almost invariably abnormal in the cardiomyopathies.
2. Nonspecific S-T segment and T-wave abnormalities are common.
3. Almost any type of arrhythmia may occur, but ventricular premature systoles and atrial fibrillation are seen most frequently. Abnormalities of AV conduction are not uncommon.
4. P-wave abnormalities, especially left atrial and biatrial enlargement, are often present.
5. Left ventricular hypertrophy is quite common, but right ventricular hypertrophy is infrequent. All types of ventricular conduction defects, especially left bundle branch block and left anterior fascicular block, are often present. Ventricular preexcitation is a common accompaniment of familial forms of cardiomegaly.
6. Pseudoinfarction patterns occur frequently in idiopathic hypertrophic subaortic stenosis and amyloidosis.

CHEST FILMS

1. The chest x-rays usually reveal only cardiomegaly.
2. When congestive heart failure supervenes, evidence of pulmonary vascular congestion and pleural effusion may appear.

CARDIAC CATHETERIZATION

1. Cardiac catheterization is of greater value in ruling out valvular, congenital, and other types of heart disease than in establishing the diagnosis of a cardiomyopathy.
2. Hemodynamic studies may be helpful in differentiating between obstructive and nonobstructive forms of cardiomyopathy.
3. The finding of restricted filling (secondary to a noncompliant ventricle or a partially obliterated ventricular cavity, or both) supports the diagnosis of a restrictive cardiomyopathy, but it is also seen in constrictive pericarditis.

4. Coronary arteriography may be helpful in differentiating ischemic heart disease from other types of myocardial disease. A normal arteriogram excludes coronary artery disease as a cause of cardiomyopathy.

## Criteria for the Diagnosis of Cardiomyopathy

1. Cardiomegaly due to left ventricular or biventricular enlargement without evidence of valvular calcification.
2. An abnormal ECG.
3. The presence of an $S_3$ or $S_4$ gallop rhythm, or both.
4. Absence of sustained arterial hypertension and, almost always, absence of diastolic murmurs.
5. Exclusion of other causes of heart disease; rheumatic or other valvular disease, congenital heart disease, constrictive pericarditis, pericardial effusion, cor pulmonale, hypertensive heart disease, and coronary artery disease.

## Differential Diagnosis of Cardiomyopathy

CORONARY HEART DISEASE

Ischemia of the myocardium may produce a clinical picture indistinguishable from that found in other types of cardiomyopathy. An unequivocal, documented history of myocardial infarction or angina pectoris, or both, establishes the diagnosis of coronary artery disease. However, it should be recognized that typical or atypical angina may occur in cardiomyopathy. Ischemic cardiomyopathy is usually found in older patients. When it occurs in younger patients, the premature coronary heart disease is most often familial and is generally associated with abnormal serum lipid concentrations and abnormal lipoprotein electrophoretic patterns. Many such patients are diabetic or at least show abnormal findings on glucose tolerance tests. Physical findings are rarely helpful, although the presence of systolic precordial bulges due to ventricular asynergy or aneurysm is indicative of ischemic heart disease. The ECG may be helpful if diagnostic infarction patterns are present, but pseudoinfarction patterns are occasionally seen in cardiomyopathy. When it is not possible to distinguish between coronary heart disease and cardiomyopathy on clinical grounds, selective coronary arteriography, ventriculography, and hemodynamic studies may be of assistance.

CONGENITAL HEART DISEASE

Congenital heart disease is rarely a problem in differential diagnosis. Patient with hypertrophic cardiomyopathy and either left or right ventricular outflow obstruction may have murmurs mimicking aortic or pulmonary stenosis, respectively (see preceding section, Heart Murmurs, for further details). The correct diagnosis can be established by cardiac catheterization and angiographic studies. In rare instances, an Eisenmenger complex of long duration (e.g., with atrial septal defect) may show marked cardiomegaly without the identifying features of the congenital lesion and thus may be mistaken for a cardiomyopathy. However, cardiac catheterization will reveal the bidirectional shunting. Moreover, the associated arterial oxygen unsaturation will not be corrected by the administration of 100 percent oxygen. Sometimes the mitral regurgitant murmur of a cardiomyopathy may be mistaken for the murmur of a ventricular septal defect. Here again cardiac catheterization and angiocardiography will establish the correct diagnosis.

RHEUMATIC HEART DISEASE

The diagnosis of rheumatic heart disease is based on a history of rheumatic fever accompanied by a characteristic structural lesion of the heart (e.g., mitral stenosis) or on evidence of a characteristic structural lesion even in the absence of history of rheumatic fever. Rheumatic heart disease is often suspected as the cause of murmurs of mitral or tricuspid regurgitation in patients with congestive heart failure. When compensation is restored in such patients, murmurs due to cardiomyopathy tend to diminish or disappear, whereas rheumatic murmurs tend to become louder. The murmur of mitral stenosis is virtually diagnostic of rheumatic heart disease, although diastolic rumbles have been reported in a few patients with cardiomyopathy. Other diastolic murmurs (e.g., due to aortic insufficiency) virtually exclude cardiomyopathy. The presence of valvular calcification also eliminates cardiomyopathy. In doubtful cases, cardiac catheterization may be indicated.

HYPERTENSIVE HEART DISEASE

Occasionally confusion occurs between cardiomyopathy and hypertensive heart disease when the blood pressure is elevated. However, the arterial hypertension is much milder (diastolic pressure 90–110 mm Hg) in cardiomyopathy and is not sustained. It tends to disappear when congestive heart failure improves. In patients with systemic hypertension, it is usually possible to document a long history of elevated blood pressure with corroborative changes in the ocular fundi. In hypertensive heart disease, there is a rough correlation between the heart size and the severity and duration of the hypertension, whereas in cardiomyopathy the cardiomegaly is out of proportion to the mildness of the hypertension.

PERICARDIAL DISEASE

Patients with cardiomyopathy often have a clinical picture that may be confused with constrictive pericarditis or pericardial effusion. Some clinical features may be of assistance in the differential diagnosis. An apical impulse that is displaced downward and to the left favors myocardial rather than pericardial disease. The presence of the pansystolic murmurs of mitral or tricuspid regurgitation also supports the diagnosis of cardiomyopathy rather than pericarditis. Gallop rhythms are common in cardiomyopathy, although they must be differentiated from the early diastolic knock of pericarditis. In pericardial disease, there is a tendency to low voltage in the ECG; in cardiomyopathy, the findings are as described previously. Echocardiography, radioisotope scanning, cardiac catheterization, and angiocardiography may be of assistance in making the diagnosis. Sometimes the problem can be resolved only by exploratory thoracotomy. The differences in hemodynamics between restrictive cardiomyopathy and constrictive pericarditis are listed in Table 3-15.

PRIMARY PULMONARY HYPERTENSION

Primary pulmonary hypertension may be seen with cardiac enlargement and right-sided heart failure, simulating a cardiomyopathy. Clues to the diagnosis are an accentuated $P_2$, dilated pulmonary arteries and clear lung fields in the chest films, and electrocardiographic evidence of right ventricular enlargement.

HYPERKINETIC HEART SYNDROME

This is an uncommon entity. It is uncertain at present whether it should be regarded as a cardiomyopathy. The distinguishing features are a high cardiac output, an increased rate of ventricular ejection, slight cardiac enlargement, and a wide pulse pressure with brisk pulses.

## Differential Diagnosis of Primary and Secondary Cardiomyopathy

Because the clinical features of primary and secondary cardiomyopathy are similar, the differentiation is made only by excluding those systemic ailments known to produce myocardial disease. Some of the more important secondary cardiomyopathies and their distinguishing features are discussed below.

**Table 3-15.** Hemodynamics of myocardial and pericardial disease

| Parameter | Constrictive pericarditis | Cardiomyopathy |
|---|---|---|
| Left atrial pressure | Tends to equal RAP | 10 to 20 mm Hg > RAP |
| Right atrial pressure | Usually >15 mm Hg with prominent Y trough | Usually <15 mm Hg: normal if wedge pressure normal |
| Cardiac output | Tends to normal with normal AV difference | Usually low with increased AV difference |
| Right ventricular pressure | Consistent early diastolic dip | Early diastolic dip may disappear with therapy |
| Diastolic right ventricular pressure | Tends to equal or exceed ⅓ of systolic pressure | Usually does not equal ⅓ of systolic pressure |
| Pulmonary artery pressure | Systolic pressure usually <40 mm Hg | Systolic pressure often 45 to 65 mm Hg |
| Respiratory variation in pressures | Tends to be absent | Usually present |
| Diastolic pressure plateau | RAP = RVDP = PADP = PWP | PWP > RAP |

RAP = right atrial pressure, AV = arteriovenous, RVDP = right ventricular diastolic pressure, PADP = pulmonary arterial diastolic pressure, PWP = pulmonary wedge pressure
Source: N. O. Fowler, Pericardial Disease. In J. W. Hurst and R. B. Logue (eds.), *The Heart* (2nd ed.). New York: McGraw-Hill, 1970, P. 1267.

CONNECTIVE TISSUE DISEASES

The diagnostic features of these diseases are described in the sections Periphera▌ Joint Arthritis and Myalgia, Chapter 8.

NEUROMUSCULAR DISEASES

1. *Friedreich's ataxia* is characterized by ataxia, progressive skeletal deformities and speech disturbances, beginning in adolescence and terminating in congestiv▌ failure or infection within 20 years of its onset. Heart disease occurs in 30 to 5▌ percent of cases and may be the initial manifestation of the disease.
2. *Myotonia atrophica* is characterized by atrophy involving primarily the muscle▌ of the face, neck, forearms, and thighs, increased muscle tone, cataracts, prema▌ ture baldness, and gonadal atrophy. Although the neuromuscular defects are usu▌ ally apparent before evidence of heart disease appears, the latter may be see▌ first.
3. *Progressive muscular dystrophy* is characterized by weakness of the proxima▌ musculature of the extremities, a waddling gait, a "climbing up the legs" phenom▌ enon when arising from a sitting position, muscles that are hypertrophied or atr▌ phied, and skeletal deformities.

HYPERTHYROIDISM

Thyrotoxic heart disease is characterized by goiter, tachycardia, exophthalmo▌ warm moist skin, tremor, and arrhythmia, notably atrial fibrillation. The diag▌ nosis can be confirmed by thyroid function tests.

MYXEDEMA

Myxedema commonly causes pericardial effusion and is often associated with co▌ onary artery disease. Whether it can cause myocardial disease is disputed. Clin▌ ically, myxedema is suggested by cold intolerance; hoarseness; a low-pitche▌

voice; sluggishness, weakness, and fatigue; a dry, yellow, puffy skin; hair loss; a thick tongue; slow pulse; and decreased tendon reflexes. It is easily confirmed by determination of the serum $T_4$ level, the radioactive iodine uptake, or other thyroid function tests.

### ACROMEGALY

Acromegaly is associated with an increased incidence of clinical cardiovascular disease. Marked cardiac hypertrophy, particularly of the left ventricle, is a common finding. Hypertension and congestive heart failure are the major clinical manifestations. About one-third of patients have a diabetic glucose tolerance test. Typically, there is persistent elevation of plasma growth hormone levels that cannot be suppressed by an oral glucose load.

### HYPOPARATHYROIDISM

Clinical heart disease is uncommon in hypoparathyroidism. The major cardiac manifestations are electrocardiographic and result from the hypocalcemia. The changes noted include prolongation of the Q-T interval (due to lengthening of the S-T segment); sometimes with a prolonged P-R interval, nonspecific T-wave abnormalities; and changes in the QRS duration. Congestive heart failure may occur but responds to restoration of normal serum calcium levels. Sensitization of the myocardium by hypocalcemia to the effects of catecholamines may precipitate arrhythmias, angina, and even sudden death.

### PHEOCHROMOCYTOMA

Pheochromocytoma is quite rare. The usual clinical presentation consists of hypertension (sometimes paroxysmal), sweating, palpitation, headaches, pallor, and episodes of collapse. Cardiomyopathy with congestive failure may occur. The cardiomyopathy may be caused by focal cellular damage and fibrosis, possibly related to an imbalance between coronary blood flow and increased need. The diagnosis is based on finding excessive catecholamine production and demonstration of the tumor.

### HEMOCHROMATOSIS

This disease is characterized by a combination of liver disease, diabetes mellitus, hyperpigmentation of the skin, and heart disease.

### AMYLOIDOSIS

Amyloidosis is one of the less common causes of cardiomyopathy. It should be considered in any elderly patient with unexplained cardiac enlargement and congestive failure. Purpura, waxy skin deposits, peripheral neuropathy, macroglossia, and nephrosis are other features of the disease. The presence of a disease known to cause secondary amyloidosis (e.g., rheumatoid arthritis, ulcerative colitis, chronic suppuration, tuberculosis) should alert the physician to this type of cardiomyopathy. The diagnosis can often be established by gingival or rectal biopsy.

### NEOPLASMS

The presence of lymphoma, leukemia, or neoplasm should raise the question of secondary cardiomyopathy if the heart is enlarged or if it shows pericarditis. Arrhythmias are common.

### MYOCARDITIS AND PERICARDITIS

Myocarditis may occur in association with many viral, bacterial, rickettsial, and parasitic diseases. The clinical evidence of myocarditis generally appears as the initial manifestations of the systemic infection begin to subside. Fever is characteristic. Fatigue, dyspnea, palpitation, and precordial discomfort may occur. Cardiac enlargement, murmurs, tachycardia, arrhythmias, and conduction defects are commonly observed. Embolic phenomena may be evident. Cardiomyopathy with congestive failure may occasionally occur in the wake of the benign idiopathic pericarditis syndrome.

SARCOIDOSIS

Cardiomyopathy due to sarcoidosis should be considered in heart disease of obscure origin in young blacks. Tachycardia, cardiac enlargement, pericarditis, heart block, arrhythmias, and congestive heart failure may be noted. Cutaneous lesions, hilar and cervical adenopathy, and pulmonary infiltrates are common. Hyperglobulinemia and hypercalcemia may occur.

ALCOHOLIC CARDIOMYOPATHY

The consumption of large quantities of alcohol over a period of many years may cause myocardial disease in some individuals. The clinical spectrum is wide. Cardiac beriberi occasionally occurs in the alcoholic. It is manifested by moderate cardiomegaly, congestive failure, nutritional deficiencies, and responsiveness to thiamine. Beer-drinkers' cardiomyopathy, characterized by right-sided heart failure, massive cardiac dilatation, and other symptoms, is no longer seen since the addition of cobalt to beer was discontinued. The most common manifestations of alcoholic cardiomyopathy are cardiac dilatation and congestive failure, neither of which is responsive to thiamine. This type of cardiomyopathy may be observed in malnourished or obese, heavy drinkers.

DIABETIC CARDIOMYOPATHY

Diabetes mellitus is associated with a specific cardiomyopathy in the absence of large-vessel coronary artery disease. Noninvasive studies have shown alterations in systolic and diastolic function that may ultimately lead to congestive heart failure. These findings have been most prominent in diabetics with evidence of microvascular disease and hypertension. Pathologic studies have revealed myocardial hypertrophy and fibrosis with arteriolar and capillary basement membrane thickening in some patients. Autonomic neuropathy may play a role in the genesis of the left ventricular dysfunction.

## Diagnostic Approach to Cardiomyopathy

1. The diagnosis of cardiomyopathy should be considered in all cases of heart disease of obscure cause.
2. The diagnosis of cardiomyopathy is made by excluding other causes of heart disease and is based on the criteria listed earlier in this section (p. 112).
3. Once the diagnosis of cardiomyopathy is established, one must make every effort to distinguish between primary and secondary forms. In the examination of the patient, search carefully for systemic illness that may produce myocardial involvement. Each of the causes of secondary cardiomyopathy should be excluded. This can usually be accomplished through the history and physical examination supplemented by selected laboratory tests.
4. The following workup is suggested for cardiomyopathy:
   a. CBC.
   b. ESR.
   c. Urinalysis.
   d. Chest films.
   e. Electrocardiogram.
   f. Biochemical screening.
   g. Protein electrophoresis.
   h. Immunoglobulins.
   i. Serologic test for syphilis.
   j. ANA.
   k. Rheumatoid factor.

   **l.** Muscle enzymes (CPK, aldolase).
   **m.** $T_4$ or other thyroid function tests.
**5.** Other procedures sometimes needed to establish an etiologic diagnosis follow:
   **a.** Tissue biopsy (lymph nodes, bone marrow, skin, muscle, rectal mucosa, gingiva).
   **b.** Cardiac catheterization.
   **c.** Angiocardiography.
   **d.** Echocardiography (including stress echocardiography and transesophageal techniques).
   **e.** Radioisotope scans.
   **f.** Pulmonary function studies.
   **g.** Endomyocardial biopsy. Specimens of myocardium obtained by endomyocardial biopsy are utilized more commonly, both for establishing the diagnosis and determining the prognosis in cardiomyopathy. At present, the procedure is most useful in inflammatory disorders (e.g., myocarditis), infiltrative disease such as amyloidosis, and drug-induced toxicity. Studies in progress at present should, when completed, clarify its role.
   **h.** Magnetic resonance imaging. In the gated mode, it yields sharper delineation of the ventricular wall. Its use is increasing.

## PALPITATION AND DISORDERS OF THE HEARTBEAT
David Shander

### Definition

The term *palpitation* refers to any conscious sensation of cardiac activity. It is generally an unpleasant feeling. Palpitation is not necessarily an indication of the presence of heart disease or of any specific arrhythmia. It may occur even when the heartbeat is normal.

### Etiology

#### Normal

Palpitation may occur normally as a result of increased heart rate and vigor of myocardial contraction associated with physical activity or emotional stress. The cardiac rhythm is sinus tachycardia and needs no further discussion. Awareness of cardiac activity is common at night in many individuals who sleep on their sides. The heartbeat frequently is audible in the dependent ear and is probably the result of direct sound transmission to the ear. The sounds made by implanted synthetic prosthetic valves may cause annoyance when heard by the patient.

#### Neurocirculatory Asthenia (Cardiac Neurosis)

An awareness of the heartbeat occurs in some individuals in the absence of physical exertion or consciousness of any emotional stress. Such persons are usually neurotic and frequently have other psychosomatic complaints. The episodes of palpitation are commonly associated with shortness of breath, lightheadedness, and precordial pain. The respiratory difficulty is frequently described as an inability to "get enough air in" or a feeling of suffocation. There may be an overwhelming sense of terror, which tends to perpetuate the symptoms. In some instances, deliberate hyperventilation may reproduce all of the symptoms. It is well to remember that cardiac neurosis is often associated with real cardiovascular disease. Such patients are understandably anxious, and sometimes perceive minor symptoms out of proportion to their significance, precipitating an acute anxiety reaction associated with palpitation and breathlessness. Very loud murmurs of aortic stenosis, ventricular septal defect, and mitral regurgitation are sometimes heard by patients, especially when at rest.

### Palpitation Not Associated with Cardiac Arrhythmia

The conditions that may cause palpitation in the absence of arrhythmia are listed in Table 3-16.

### Palpitation Associated with Cardiac Arrhythmia

Cardiac arrhythmias, including premature contractions, paroxysmal and nonparoxysmal tachycardias, and marked bradycardias are the most common causes of palpitation. Some patients with artificial pacemakers have diaphragmatic or intercostal twitching produced by the pacemaker stimulus. This may be interpreted as palpitation. Other patients are aware of a change in cardiac activity when spontaneous beats are replaced by a pacemaker-induced rhythm.

### Premature Contractions

1. Many patients with premature contractions (Fig. 3-2) do not use the term *palpitation* to describe their complaint, but rather describe the premature systoles as flip-flop sensations in the chest, stoppage of the heart, or skipped beats.
2. Premature contractions may occur in the presence or absence of organic heart disease. They may be ventricular or supraventricular in origin. The clinical significance of such beats varies. Some are completely benign, whereas others may

**Table 3-16.** Causes of palpitation without arrhythmia

---

Noncardiac disorders
  Anxiety
  Anemia
  Fever
  Thyrotoxicosis
  Hypoglycemia
  Pheochromocytoma
  Aortic aneurysm
  Migraine
  Arteriovenous fistula
  Drugs (epinephrine, amphetamines, digitalis, nitrates, ganglionic blocking
    agents)
  Diaphragmatic flutter
Cardiac disorders
  Aortic regurgitation
  Aortic stenosis
  Patent ductus arteriosus
  Ventricular septal defect
  Atrial septal defect
  Marked cardiomegaly
  Acute left ventricular failure
  Hyperkinetic heart syndrome
  Tricuspid insufficiency
  Pericarditis
  Prosthetic valves
  Electronic pacemakers

---

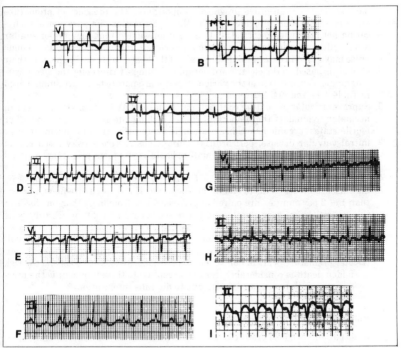

**Fig. 3-2.** Arrhythmias associated with palpitation. A. Atrial premature contraction (second beat) with aberrant ventricular conduction exhibiting the pattern of right bundle branch block. B. AV junctional premature contraction (second ventricular complex). The ectopic beat is similar in configuration to that of the conducted beats but is not preceded by a P wave. C. Ventricular premature contraction (second QRS complex). A sinus P wave deforms the T wave of the ectopic beat. D. Paroxysmal supraventricular tachycardia. Atrial activity cannot be identified. The QRS complexes are of normal duration. E. Paroxysmal atrial tachycardia with 2 : 1 AV block. F. Multifocal atrial tachycardia. Note the multiform P waves, the irregular P-P intervals, and the variable P-R durations. G. Atrial fibrillation with a moderate ventricular response. The P waves are replaced by small irregular oscillations, called f waves. The ventricular rhythm is irregular. H. Atrial flutter with alternating 2 : 1 and 4 : 1 AV conduction. The P waves are replaced by regular oscillations exhibiting a sawtooth pattern (F waves). I. Probable ventricular tachycardia. The QRS complexes are wide and bizarre. The T waves of the first, fourth, and seventh ventricular complexes are peaked due to superimposed independent atrial activity indicative of AV dissociation. An AV junctional tachycardia with aberrant ventricular conduction can produce the same appearance. The absence of fusion or capture beats or both does not rule out ventricular tachycardia.

have serious or even grave prognostic importance. The presence of premature beats in an ECG may provide a clue to the identification of a paroxymsal tachycardia not otherwise recorded. It is usually presumed that they are of similar origin. Although physical examination and close scrutiny of the jugular venous pulse may assist in determining the origin of the beats, the final diagnosis of their etiology is based on the electrocardiographic findings. Criteria for the electrocardiographic identification of the various types of premature beats are summarized in Table 3-17 and Fig. 3-2.

3. Supraventricular premature contractions (atrial and AV junctional) may occur in normal individuals. Other important causes include infectious disease and other febrile states, organic heart disease, particularly with atrial involvement (e.g., mitral valvular disease, pericarditis), chronic obstructive airway disease, and digitalis administration. Atrial premature beats are frequent precursors of atrial fibrillation, tachycardia, or flutter.

4. Ventricular premature beats are also frequently benign, but underlying myocardial disease or drug effects should be suspected if they occur frequently (more than 1 or 2 per minute), are paired or grouped, arise from more than one focus in the ventricles, are very closely coupled to the preceding beat, or are very wide (0.16 sec or more). Ventricular premature beats in myocardial infarction may be harbingers of ventricular fibrillation, especially if they encroach upon the vulnerable period (the region at or about the peak of the T wave). In general, ventricular premature beats in nonischemic conditions are less ominous and the risk of sudden death is considerably less. An exception to this statement is the presence of ventricular premature beats due to digitalis intoxication.

## Paroxysmal Tachycardias

Most patients who experience bouts of paroxysmal tachycardia complain of palpitation, yet some, surprisingly, are completely unaware of their existence. Paroxysmal tachyarrhythmias occur in normal individuals as well as in those with diseased hearts. Some are drug-induced; digitalis is the most notable offender in this group. Patients taking antiarrhythmic agents, especially of class I type, may be prone to arrhythmia exacerbation. These proarrhythmias may occur in as many as 30 percent of patients on such drugs.

Attacks of paroxysmal tachycardia may last from less than a minute to hours or days, and may be recurrent. As in the case of prematurities, paroxysmal tachycardias may be supraventricular or ventricular in origin. Prolonged episodes of paroxysmal tachycardia may give rise to faintness, lightheadedness, syncope, dyspnea, angina, or congestive heart failure. The clinical evaluation of paroxysmal tachycardia is summarized in Table 3-18. The electrocardiographic differential diagnosis is considered below.

## Bradycardias

Bradycardias may produce consciousness of the heartbeat when cardiac contraction is forceful as a result of increased stroke volume. Should the cardiac output decline, as a result of either very slow rates or weakened myocardial contractility, faintness or syncope may occur. The major causes of a slow pulse rate are sinus bradycardia, sinoatrial block, AV junctional rhythms, extrasystolic bigeminy, and AV block. Beta blockers, calcium channel blockers, digitalis, and amiodarone are cardiac drugs known to be associated with various types of bradycardia.

## Preexcitation Syndromes (Wolff-Parkinson-White; Lown-Ganong-Levine)

Paroxysmal supraventricular tachycardia occurs commonly with preexcitation. The ECG in the Wolff-Parkinson-White (WPW) syndrome demonstrates a short P-R interval due to prolongation of the QRS duration, the early portion of which is most prolonged and referred to as a delta wave. Secondary repolarization

**Table 3-17.** Electrocardiographic differential diagnosis of premature contractions

| Premature contractions | Initial deflection | P wave | P-R interval | QRS complex | Compensatory pause |
|---|---|---|---|---|---|
| Atrial (APC) | P wave | Premature; different from sinus P wave; usually upright but may be retrograde (inverted in leads II, III, and a VF, and upright in lead a VR) | Normal or prolonged | May be absent if APC is nonconducted; usually normal but may be wide and bizarre because of aberrant ventricular conduction or preexisting intraventricular block | Not fully compensatory unless sinoatrial (SA) node is suppressed by discharge of the APC |
| AV junctional (JPC) | P wave or QRS complex | Retrograde | 0.10 sec to negative; R-P interval variable; diagnostic if R-P interval $\leq$ 0.10 sec, even if QRS is abnormal | Usually normal but may be wide and bizarre because of aberrant ventricular conduction or preexisting intraventricular block | Not fully compensatory unless SA node is suppressed by discharge of the JPC or if sinus P is dissociated from a QRS that is not conducted back to the atria |
| Ventricular (VPC) | QRS complex | Sinus if dissociated from QRS; retrograde if ventricular impulse is conducted to atria | Absent if P and QRS are dissociated; if retrograde, R-P interval is >0.10 sec | Wide, bizarre | Fully compensatory unless retrograde conduction is present or beat is interpolated |

Note: It is not always possible by surface leads to distinguish absolutely between (1) VPCs and (2) JPCs with aberrant ventricular conduction.

**Table 3-18.** Clinical differential diagnosis of the tachycardias

| Tachycardias | Rate | | Regularity | Onset and termination |
|---|---|---|---|---|
| | Atrial | Ventricular | | |
| Sinus tachycardia | 100 to 150 but may be faster | 100 to 150 but may be faster | Regular | Gradual |
| Paroxysmal reentrant supraventricular tachycardia | 140 to 200 | 140 to 200 | Usually regular | Abrupt |
| Paroxysmal automatic atrial tachycardia | 100 to 180 | 100 to 180 | Usually regular | Usually abrupt |
| Paroxysmal atrial tachycardia with block | 120 to 250; usually 120 to 180 with 2 : 1 block | Variable | Regular or irregular | Gradual |
| Multifocal atrial tachycardia (chaotic atrial rhythm) | 100 to 180 | 100 to 180 | Irregular | Gradual |
| Atrial flutter | 220 to 350 | Variable; 2 : 1 block usually present if untreated | Regular or irregular | Abrupt |
| Atrial fibrillation | >350 | Variable | Irregular; if regular, indicative of advanced or complete AV block | Abrupt |
| Paroxysmal automatic AV-junctional tachycardia | 100 to 180; with AV dissociation, usually NSR | 100 to 180 | Regular | Usually abrupt |

| | Atrial mechanism | Ventricular rate | Regularity | Onset/termination |
|---|---|---|---|---|
| Nonparoxysmal AV-junctional tachycardia | Depends on atrial mechanism; AV dissociation often present | 65 to 130 | Regular | Gradual |
| Paroxysmal ventricular tachycardia | With AV dissociation, usually NSR; may have retrograde atrial activation | 140 to 200; may be slower with idioventricular or parasystolic ventricular tachycardia | Regular or slightly irregular | Abrupt |

| Response to carotid sinus massage | Physical signs | | Etiology |
|---|---|---|---|
| | Heart sounds | Jugular venous pulsations | |
| Gradual slowing, with return to previous rate | Normal | Normal | Physical or emotional stress; increased sympathetic tone; decreased vagal tone; drugs; hypoxemia; shock; hyperkinetic circulatory states; congestive heart failure; myocardial disease |
| No effect, or abrupt termination | S₁ usually constant in intensity | Normal or cannon A waves | Organic heart disease or normal subjects |
| No effect, or AV block may appear, P waves unaffected | S₁ constant in intensity | Normal | Most commonly associated with organic heart disease |
| May increase degree of AV block and slow ventricular rate; contraindicated in most situations | S₁ may vary in intensity | A waves at rapid, slightly irregular rate, exceed ventricular rate | Most often due to combination of digitalis excess and potassium depletion; may also occur in coronary heart disease, rheumatic heart disease, and pulmonary disease |

**Table 3-18** (continued)

| Etiology | Physical signs | | |
| --- | --- | --- | --- |
| | Jugular venous pulsations | Heart sounds | Response to carotid sinus massage |
| Acute and chronic pulmonary disease, especially with respiratory failure and hypoxia; organic heart disease may be associated | May not be visible | $S_1$ may vary in intensity | No effect, or gradual slowing |
| Almost always associated with organic heart disease; hypoxemia; shock; acute or chronic pulmonary disease | Flutter waves may be visible at multiples of ventricular rate | $S_1$ may vary in intensity if rhythm is irregular | May increase degree of AV block, slow ventricular rate, and reveal flutter waves |
| Almost always associated with organic heart disease (especially rheumatic or coronary heart disease); hyperthyroidism | Irregular pulsations | $S_1$ varies in intensity | Gradual slowing, with return to previous rate |
| Same as for paroxysmal atrial tachycardia | Regular or irregular cannon A waves may occur | $S_1$ constant; varies in intensity if AV dissociation is present | No effect, or abrupt termination |
| Digitalis toxicity; coronary heart disease, especially inferior infarction; rheumatic carditis; postcardiac surgery | Regular or irregular cannon A waves commonly present | $S_1$ constant; varies in intensity if AV dissociation is present | No effect, or gradual slowing, with return to previous rate; contraindicated in most situations |
| Coronary heart disease, especially myocardial infarction; congestive heart failure; drug toxicity (digitalis, quinidine, epinephrine) | Irregular cannon A waves when AV dissociation is present | $S_1$ varies in intensity; $S_2$ widely split | No effect |

changes are the rule. In the Lown-Ganong-Levine (LGL) syndrome a short P-R interval ($\leq$ 0.10 sec) is associated with a normal QRS duration and absence of delta waves. The recognition of preexcitation as a cause of supraventricular tachycardia is important because conventional forms of therapy may be ineffective.

## Sick Sinus Syndrome

A common cause of palpitation, dizziness, and syncope, at all ages (but most commonly in patients over 60) and in numerous clinical states, is the tachycardia-bradycardia syndrome commonly called the sick sinus syndrome (SSS). The term is somewhat of a misnomer because as many as half of these patients also have disease of other portions of the conduction system. A spectrum of arrhythmias is seen, including SA block, sinus arrest, sinus pauses, sinus bradycardia, supraventricular tachycardias, and AV conduction disturbances. Failure to elicit a tachycardia with 1 mg of atropine intravenously in a patient with sinus bradycardia suggests the possibility of the sick sinus syndrome.

# Diagnostic Approach

## History and Physical Examination

1. As a first step, disorders not associated with arrhythmia and neurocirculatory asthenia should be ruled out as causes of palpitation (see Table 3-16). This can usually be accomplished through the history, physical examination, and selected laboratory tests.
2. All patients in whom arrhythmia is suspected as the cause of palpitation should be evaluated for the presence or absence of heart disease. Chest films and an ECG should be included in such an evaluation.
3. In any patient complaining of palpitation, specific inquiry should be made as to whether the symptom is continuous when present or is related to isolated beats.
4. When rapid heart action is suggested by the history, additional features may help to distinguish between sinus and ectopic rhythms. A tachycardia with a rate above 140 per minute that starts and ends abruptly, and that can be terminated by vagal maneuvers performed by the patient (e.g., swallowing, coughing, breath-holding), suggests the diagnosis of paroxysmal rather than sinus tachycardia.
5. Cardiac arrhythmia is a not uncommon cause of syncope.
6. The use of coffee, tobacco, alcohol, and drugs should be quantified. It should be remembered that arrhythmias may be exacerbated in some instances by antiarrhythmic drugs.
7. Supraventricular arrhythmias, such as paroxysmal atrial tachycardia (PAT), are quite common in young women during pregnancy.
8. Associated symptoms or signs may provide clues to the presence of coexisting disease (e.g., hyperthyroidism, pheochromocytoma) that may be responsible for palpitation and dysrhythmia. Viral illnesses, especially influenza, may give rise to ventricular premature beats that may last for weeks or months after recovery.
9. During auscultation of premature beats, splitting of the heart sounds is wider with ventricular or aberrantly conducted beats than with premature beats in which the QRS complexes are of normal duration.
10. The jugular venous pulse may be of considerable help diagnostically (see Table 3-18).
11. The click-murmur syndrome of mitral valve prolapse is commonly associated with frequent premature contractions, both ventricular and supraventricular, and bouts of paroxysmal tachycardia. Palpitation is a common complaint. A careful physical examination and an echocardiogram may be helpful in diagnosis.
12. The hyperkinetic heart syndrome is an ill-defined condition consisting of a resting tachycardia associated with palpitation. It occurs in otherwise normal

healthy individuals and appears to be different from simple neurocirculatory asthenia.

## Electrocardiographic Findings

When a patient is seen during an arrhythmic episode, an ECG should be recorded at once. The diagnosis may then be obvious from the ECG. Not infrequently, however, particularly in paroxysmal tachycardias, the ECG may present diagnostic problems. Under such circumstances, attention to the points listed below may be helpful in unraveling the correct diagnosis. It is useful to divide paroxysmal tachycardias into those characterized by normal QRS duration and those in which the QRS duration is prolonged (0.12 sec or more).

1. Tachycardia with normal QRS duration.
    a. The supraventricular origin of a tachycardia is virtually established if the QRS complexes are of essentially normal configuration and duration. However, supraventricular tachycardia may be associated with abnormal QRS complexes. This variety is considered separately in paragraph 2 below.
    b. The identification of P waves or other atrial activity is crucial in diagnosing arrhythmias by ECG. Lead $V_1$ is often the most useful in this regard, but leads II, III, aVF, or $V_6$ may also be helpful. For this reason, a 12-lead ECG should be obtained whenever possible. Esophageal or intracardiac leads may be necessary in complex cases.
    c. A tachycardia is atrial in origin if it is initiated by a premature, ectopic P wave and followed by a QRS complex at a normal or slightly prolonged P-R interval.
    d. A tachycardia is AV junctional in origin if the P waves are inverted (retrograde) in leads II, III, and aVF, and upright in lead aVR; if the P-R interval is 0.10 sec or less; if retrograde P waves follow the QRS complexes; or if P waves are not detectable in the ECG.
    e. During a continuous tachycardia with unidentified or retrograde P waves, it is not possible to determine whether the tachycardia is atrial or AV junctional in origin. *Paroxysmal supraventricular* is then the appropriate term for this arrhythmia.
    f. Atrial flutter is recognized by the sawtooth appearance of the baseline (F waves) with an atrial rate usually greater than 250/min. Flutter waves may sometimes be separated by a flat baseline. F waves are usually best seen in leads II, III, and aVF, where they are usually inverted.
    g. Atrial fibrillation is characterized by absence of P waves, rapid irregular oscillations of the baseline (F waves), and an irregularity of the ventricular response (unless advanced or complete AV block or a nonparoxysmal AV junctional tachycardia is present). Fibrillatory waves may be fine or coarse in appearance, and when coarse may appear regular for brief periods, when they may be confused with flutter waves.
    h. Carotid sinus massage, vagal maneuvers, and cholinergic drugs are often helpful in the diagnosis. Vagal maneuvers other than carotid sinus pressure (e.g., eyeball pressure, induction of vomiting) are not recommended. Verapamil in a dose of 5 mg intravenously is the pharmacologic agent most commonly used at present to terminate supraventricular tachycardias. Recently, intravenous adenosine has been used successfully for the same purpose with less risk of hypotension. The use of a pressor agent (e.g., phenylephrine) to abruptly raise the systolic blood pressure is still a useful diagnostic, as well as a therapeutic intervention. Any of these interventions may slow or terminate or have no effect on supraventricular arrhythmias. Carotid sinus massage is the most widely used procedure. In sinus tachycardia, it generally produces a gradual slowing of the heartbeat, which usually reverts to its original rate after the pressure is released; sometimes sinus tachycardia is unaffected by this maneuver. Carotid sinus massage either terminates or has no effect on most paroxysmal atrial or AV-junctional tachycardias. In atrial flut-

ter, carotid sinus pressure increases the degree of AV block so that fewer flutter impulses are conducted to the ventricles. With a lesser number of ventricular complexes, the F waves are more clearly revealed, making this a very useful maneuver when the diagnosis of atrial flutter is uncertain. Carotid sinus massage should always be performed with caution, particularly in the elderly, and under electrocardiographic control. The procedure is contraindicated in cerebral vascular disease, heart block, and digitalis intoxication.

i. In patients with suspected sick sinus syndrome, the measurement of corrected sinus node recovery time (CSNRT) has been suggested. Atrial pacing is performed at 130 to 140 beats per min for 1 to 2 min. On cessation, the ensuing pause (before the first sinus beat) minus the prepacing P-P interval is suggestive of the sick sinus syndrome if it exceeds 525 msec. Unfortunately, false negative results are common.

2. Tachycardia with abnormal QRS duration ($\geq 0.12$ sec).

a. Tachycardia with abnormally wide QRS complexes may be supraventricular or ventricular in origin. All of the electrocardiographic manifestations of ventricular arrhythmia may be mimicked by supraventricular arrhythmia associated with QRS complexes that are abnormally wide as a result of aberrant ventricular conduction, bundle branch block, ventricular preexcitation, or hyperkalemia.

b. Tachycardias with abnormal QRS complexes are supraventricular in origin if they are initiated by premature, ectopic P waves, regardless of the configuration of the QRS complexes.

c. Tachycardias initiated by abnormal QRS complexes may be ventricular or AV junctional in origin. In the latter case, the QRS complexes may be bizarre because of the presence of the conditions listed in paragraph **a** above.

d. A tachycardia that occurs after a premature QRS complex and interrupts the T wave of the preceding beat (R on T phenomenon) is regarded as ventricular in origin.

e. The regularity of the tachycardia and its rate are of limited help in differential diagnosis.

f. The configuration of the QRS complexes may provide a clue, but it rarely permits absolute differentiation between aberrant ventricular conduction and ventricular ectopy. Favoring aberrant conduction are a triphasic RBBB pattern with an rsa′ pattern in $V_1$ and a qRS pattern in $V_6$. Favoring ectopy are monophasic or diphasic complexes, a qR or Rr′ pattern, a QS or rS pattern in $V_6$, a superior and rightward QRS axis in the frontal plane, an LBBB pattern with a wide R wave in $V_1$, or complexes that are positive in all of the precordial leads (preexcitation excluded) or negative in all of them. If the configuration of the QRS complexes during the tachycardia is the same as that during a known supraventricular rhythm, the tachycardia is considered supraventricular in origin.

g. In the presence of AV dissociation, an atrial arrhythmia can be excluded, and a ventricular rhythm is the most likely diagnosis, although a junctional mechanism with aberration or preexisting block is possible.

h. Retrograde conduction to the atrium may occur in AV junctional or ventricular tachycardias.

i. The most useful criterion for the diagnosis of ventricular tachycardia in the conventional ECG is the presence of early ventricular capture or fusion beats, or both. Absence of fusion or capture beats does not rule out ventricular tachycardia.

j. Because ventricular tachycardia is unaffected by carotid sinus massage, a response to this maneuver (such as termination of the tachycardia or slowing of the ventricular rate) is virtually diagnostic of supraventricular arrhythmia.

k. The most precise method available for differentiating between supraventricular and ventricular arrhythmias is the His bundle electrogram. With this recording, in supraventricular rhythms, an H deflection is seen to precede each QRS complex at a normal or prolonged H-V interval; and in ventricular rhythms, the QRS complexes are not preceded by H deflections. Esophageal or intracardiac leads may establish the diagnosis of supraventricular arrhythmia if a definite relationship between atrial and ventricular activity can be demonstrated.

l. Reversion of a tachycardia with wide QRS complexes to normal sinus rhythm with low voltage, direct current, cardioversion (10 watt-sec or less), or by a mechanical blow to the chest is suggestive of ventricular tachycardia. Similarly, reversion with lidocaine suggests a ventricular origin. Hence, these procedures may aid in diagnosis as well as therapy.

m. Wide QRS tachycardias may be monomorphic (all complexes of the same configuration) or polymorphic (changing complex configuration). Such tachycardias may be nonsustained or sustained (lasting more than 30 seconds). It is now recognized that sustained and polymorphic ventricular tachycardias are potentially more life-threatening than nonsustained and monomorphic forms. A unique polymorphic form exists, known as torsades de pointes, in which a rapidly occurring complex appears to rotate its vector about a point. Such rhythms are very malignant and are sometimes the result of the proarrhythmic effects of antiarrhythmic drugs or severe metabolic disturbances.

Recent studies have suggested that suppression of ventricular ectopy and asymptomatic nonsustained ventricular tachycardia, using antiarrhythmic agents, may not consistently reduce the risk of sudden death.

n. The diagnosis of arrhythmia may pose a real problem if the arrhythmia is not present at the time of examination. One solution, if the condition is not serious, is to ask the patient to return when the rhythm disturbance returns. However, if the episodes occur infrequently or are of brief duration even when frequent, it may not be possible to catch the patient during an arrhythmic episode. Under such circumstances, either the diagnosis must await a more propitious opportunity for examination, or the patient may be monitored.

## Electrocardiographic Monitoring

Patients with serious arrhythmia problems, particularly when associated with other cardiovascular symptoms and organic heart disease, should be monitored if the rhythm disturbance cannot be diagnosed in any other way. Monitoring can be performed either on an inpatient or an outpatient basis. In the hospital, radiotelemetry (if available) is the most suitable method for monitoring patients, because it permits them to be ambulatory. Direct connection to a nonportable unit is less desirable because the patient must be confined to bed. For outpatients, a portable apparatus is available that can tape-record continuously for 24 hours the patient's ECG while he goes about his normal activities. When the tape is later played back, the arrhythmias that occurred can be identified and reproduced on electrocardiographic paper to obtain permanent records. Exercise testing may elicit arrhythmias not present at rest or during normal activity and thereby provide a clue to the presence of symptomatic cardiovascular disease or indicate an increased risk of sudden death.

Small, portable, battery-operated devices are now available that allow the patient to record the heartbeat by placing the device on the chest. The electrocardiogram can then be transmitted by telephone to the patient's physician or to a central recording station. Many of the units have a memory capacity and can store fleeting arrhythmias for later transmission.

## Electrophysiologic Testing

In patients who have experienced life-threatening arrhythmias and episodes of sudden death with successful resuscitation, programmed electrical stimulation of the ventricles has been shown to be of value in subsequent management of the patient. The ability to induce sustained ventricular tachycardia, which is no longer inducible after administration of an antiarrhythmic agent, may be the best predictive test of antiarrhythmic effectiveness. Failing this, implantation of an automatic implantable cardioverter defibrillator (AICD) may be the only other fail-safe approach to sudden death from ventricular tachycardia or ventricular fibrillation.

## PERIPHERAL VASCULAR DISORDERS

Gilbert Hermann

## Introduction

The term *peripheral vascular disorder* applies to a variety of conditions that affect the arteries, veins, and lymphatics of the extremities. Disorders of the arterioles, capillaries, venules, and lymphatics, while they are occasionally clinically important, are not discussed because of their relative rarity.

The major problem for the clinician dealing with peripheral vascular disease is to distinguish between acute and chronic arterial occlusive disease on one hand and superficial and deep thrombophlebitis on the other. Fortunately, a careful history and physical examination coupled with appropriate diagnostic tests can almost always ensure a definitive clinical diagnosis.

## Arterial Disease

### Acute Arterial Occlusion

ETIOLOGY

1. Embolism. Intracardiac clots are the source of embolism in the vast majority of cases. Occasionally, smaller emboli can break off from clots or aggregated platelet fragments in the aorta or iliac arteries.
2. Thrombosis. Arterial thrombosis usually affects a major vessel previously compromised by atherosclerosis. Symptoms of chronic peripheral arterial insufficiency may precede the occurrence of acute arterial occlusion by many months.
3. Trauma. Acute occlusion may occur, either by direct disruption of the vessel secondary to the trauma or by elevation of an intimal flap and subsequent thrombosis secondary to trauma adjacent to the vessel.

SYMPTOMS

The symptoms of acute arterial occlusion occur fairly rapidly (1 to 2 hours), often in a previously asymptomatic extremity.

1. Pain. The pain may begin as numbness or tingling but progresses within a brief period of time to steady, severe pain.
2. Coldness.
3. Numbness.
4. Pallor.
5. Weakness.

PERTINENT PAST HISTORY

1. A history of myocardial infarction, particularly a recent one.
2. A history of rheumatic heart disease, with subsequent atrial fibrillation.
3. A history of trauma. It is important to note that a high-velocity missile passing near the vessel, even without disrupting the vessel, can by transmitted energy cause occlusion of the vessel secondary to intimal damage.

SIGNS

1. Temperature change. This can be best evaluated by gently feeling the affected extremity with the back of the hand rather than the fingers. This temperature change can best be determined by comparison with the opposite, uninvolved extremity. In general, sudden occlusion of a femoral artery results in a warm-to-cool temperature level at the knee or slightly below. Occlusion of the popliteal artery causes a temperature level in the distal leg at or above the ankle. As other branches begin to occlude, the temperature level ascends more proximally in the extremity.
2. Pulses. In general, the pulses are asymmetric with a palpable pulse in the unaffected extremity, while the same artery on the affected extremity has no pulsation. Occasionally, pulsations just proximal to a recent occlusion may be much more pronounced than those in a corresponding artery in the opposite unobstructed side. The posterior tibial artery is more consistent anatomically than the dorsalis pedis artery (98 versus 90 percent).
3. Color. The affected limb is usually paler than the unaffected extremity, particularly in the dependent position.
4. Sensation. The ability to feel pain or touch diminishes progressively as the duration of occlusion is prolonged.
5. Decreased muscle strength. This is often manifested by inability to move the digits of the affected extremity.
6. Cardiac arrhythmias. The presence of cardiac arrhythmia, particularly atrial fibrillation, favors embolic rather than thrombotic occlusion.

DIAGNOSTIC PROCEDURES

Although the diagnosis of sudden occlusion is usually made easily by history and physical examination, occasionally it is necessary to determine the extent of the occlusion and status of the proximal and distal arterial tree by other methods.
1. Duplex ultrasound is a valuable noninvasive technique for determining the point along the course of a major artery at which pulsatile flow either has ceased or is markedly diminished.
2. Arteriography. Although not necessary preoperatively in every patient with an acute occlusion, this procedure may provide important anatomic information.

## Chronic Arterial Occlusion

ETIOLOGY

1. Atherosclerosis. Primary, or associated with such generalized conditions as diabetes, hypertension, or hyperlipemia.
2. Arteritis (Buerger's disease). A disorder primarily affecting younger adults, characterized by involvement of the medium-sized arteries. Some believe the disease is actually a form of early atherosclerosis.
3. Vasospastic disorders.
   a. Raynaud's phenomenon. This condition is usually part of a symptom-complex associated with connective tissue or immune-related diseases. It presents only rarely as a primary disease.
   b. Drug-related disorders. Some drugs, such as the ergotamine preparation, can lead to severe vasospastic disorders.

SYMPTOMS

The symptoms listed below are usually related to large-vessel occlusion secondary to atherosclerosis, which is responsible for 90 to 95 percent of all chronic occlusive arterial disease.
1. Pain.
   a. Intermittent claudication. The character of the pain associated with peripheral vascular insufficiency is unique and should not be confused with leg or

buttock pain arising from skeletal or neurologic disease. Claudication is pain that typically begins after an increase in metabolic requirement (e.g., ambulation) and is relieved promptly with rest. It cannot be elicited by any other stimulus, such as palpation of the part or a change in its position.

  **b.** Rest pain occurs with far advanced vascular insufficiency and implies a pregangrenous state. Characteristically, the patient obtains some relief by dangling the affected extremity over the edge of the bed or by assuming a sitting position with both legs dependent.

2. Color. Red or violet color of the toes or foot on dependency implies moderate to severe arterial occlusive disease.
3. Temperature. This cannot be relied on as a definitive symptom, as many perfectly healthy patients complain of cold feet.
4. Ulceration. The ulcers may occur spontaneously or be secondary to minor trauma. The patients generally complain of pain in or around the ulceration.

PERTINENT PAST HISTORY

1. Diabetes mellitus.
2. Hypertension.
3. Family history of early complications of atherosclerosis.
4. Drug use, particularly of substances known to predispose to vasospastic problems.

SIGNS

1. Pulses. The presence or absence and quality of all peripheral pulses should be noted. This would include the carotid, brachial, radial, aortic, femoral, popliteal, dorsalis pedal, and posterior tibial pulses. Peripheral pulses may be normal in a patient with predominantly small-vessel disease, such as diabetes mellitus. Arteriosclerotic vessels generally feel hard and noncompressible.
2. Color. Dependent red or violet color is the most common color change noted.
3. Temperature. The temperature of the limb varies a great deal depending on the status of sympathetic activity. The ambient temperature obviously is a factor as well. A difference in temperature between the two limbs is significant.
4. Hair growth. Heavy hair growth on the distal extremities is evidence against the diagnosis of chronic arterial insufficiency. The absence of hair, however, may reflect a genetic characteristic and is not necessarily indicative of chronic ischemia.
5. Venous filling. The venous filling time can be estimated by having the patient assume the supine position and having the examiner elevate the patient's legs to 45 degrees for 1 to 2 minutes. The patient is then allowed to sit up with feet dangling over the edge of the examining table. There should be definite venous filling in 15 to 20 seconds. A venous filling time greater than one minute is definitely abnormal.
6. Ulceration. Ischemic ulcers generally occur on the lateral aspect of the lower leg, although they may occur in other sites. They are extremely tender to touch.
7. Abdominal bruits. When they occur over the abdomen, they are compatible with but not diagnostic of aortic or renal artery disease. Femoral or carotid bruits are abnormal and indicate arterial pathology.

DIAGNOSTIC PROCEDURES

1. Noninvasive evaluation.
    **a.** Pulse volume recorder (PVR).
    **b.** Duplex ultrasound.
2. Anatomic evaluation.
    **a.** Ultrasound. With modern technology, ultrasound can be useful for anatomic delineation of the aorta as well as some of the other large vessels.
    **b.** Arteriography. This is the most accurate method for determining the anatomic status of the peripheral arterial tree. Because this is an invasive procedure and carries some risk, it should be done only when reconstructive surgery is seriously considered as a treatment option.

## Venous Disease

### Superficial Phlebitis

SYMPTOMS

A rather rapid onset of pain over some portion of the course of the greater saphenous vein is typical, although superficial phlebitis can occur in any superficially varicosed vein. Occasionally, it can occur in the upper extremity following intravenous medication. No edema or systemic symptoms are observed.

SIGNS

A tender, red, swollen cord is palpable over the affected superficial vein. Occasionally the swelling takes the form of ovoid nodules. There is no edema, except along the course of the vessel. The arterial pulse is usually present and normal.

### Deep Phlebitis: Acute

ETIOLOGY

1. Trauma (e.g., following extensive pelvic surgery).
2. Stagnation of blood flow (e.g., elderly or debilitated patients, particularly in the setting of cardiac decompensation).
3. Changes in coagulability (e.g., malignancy).

SYMPTOMS

1. Sudden onset of thigh or lower leg edema, or both.
2. Pain that is aching in character, not related to exercise, and somewhat relieved by elevation of the affected extremity.
3. Bluish mottling of the skin, most marked in the dependent position.
4. Generalized malaise but no shaking chills.

SIGNS

1. Edema. The legs should be measured at the ankles, calves, and thighs bilaterally and the comparative findings recorded.
2. Tenderness, especially over the affected deep veins. Gentle palpation rather than forceful squeezing usually elicits this sign in a meaningful manner.
3. Dilated superficial veins.
4. Increased warmth of the affected extremity.
5. Mottling of the leg, particularly prominent in the dependent position.

DIFFERENTIAL DIAGNOSIS

1. Phlegmasia alba dolens with obliteration of the arterial pulses can be mistaken for acute arterial occlusion.
2. Rupture of the plantaris tendon or partial tear of the gastrocnemius muscle. Characteristically, the pain occurs suddenly while the patient is engaged in strenuous physical activity. Often, ecchymosis appears on the back of the calf following such a soft tissue injury.

DIAGNOSIS

1. Noninvasive methods.
   a. Duplex ultrasound.
   b. Plethysmographic techniques (e.g., impedance plethysmography, PVR).
2. Invasive diagnostic methods.
   a. Venography—most accurate.

## Deep Phlebitis: Chronic

SYMPTOMS

1. Swelling, most pronounced after prolonged upright position.
2. Enlarged superficial veins.
3. Ulceration of the lower leg.

SIGNS

1. Edema, usually confined to the lower leg.
2. Subcutaneous fibrosis: The skin is very thickened and brawny.
3. Stasis dermatitis.
4. Ulceration, usually on the lower third of the medial aspect of the leg; not as painful as ischemic ulcers.

DIAGNOSIS

1. A past history consistent with acute iliofemoral thrombosis, which is often postpartum or postsurgical.
2. Physical examination.
3. Venography.
4. Duplex ultrasound.

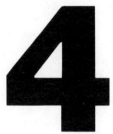

# Respiratory Problems

## DYSPNEA
Marvin I. Schwarz
Paul M. Cox, Jr.

### Definition

Dyspnea is the subjective complaint of shortness of breath. Other forms of breathlessness, such as sighing respirations and the subjective sensation of inability to take deep breaths, are thus not included in this discussion.

Other terms frequently confused with dyspnea but having distinctly different meanings include hyperventilation, which is excessive breathing with or without the sensation of dyspnea; tachypnea, which is rapid breathing; and hyperpnea, which is rapid and abnormally deep respirations.

Orthopnea refers to dyspnea in recumbency that is at least partially relieved by assuming an upright position. Paroxysmal nocturnal dyspnea (PND) is the term applied to attacks of severe breathlessness that generally occur at night and usually awaken the patient from sleep. Relief from or termination of the attack is frequently obtained when the patient sits up.

## Acute Dyspnea

### Etiology

1. The more common pulmonary diseases that are accompanied by acute dyspnea include pneumonia, pulmonary embolus, spontaneous pneumothorax, asthma, foreign body aspiration, noncardiac pulmonary edema (including noxious gas inhalation, high-altitude pulmonary edema, and neurogenic pulmonary edema), and the adult respiratory distress syndrome (fat embolization, shock lung).
2. The major nonpulmonary cause of acute dyspnea is cardiogenic pulmonary edema. Orthopnea and PND are commonly associated with cardiogenic pulmonary edema.
3. Acute hyperventilation syndrome is a relatively frequent neuropsychiatric cause of dyspnea.

### History

1. Pneumonia. Patients with pneumonia from any cause (viral, bacterial, or mycoplasmal) may have cough, sputum, pleuritic chest pain, fever, and chills after a prodrome of upper respiratory tract symptoms.
2. Acute pulmonary embolism. Patients with pulmonary embolism may have a characteristic clinical setting, such as prolonged immobilization, recent surgery, congestive heart failure, or recent trauma (particularly to the lower extremities). A predisposition to thromboembolism occurs in patients with a previous history

of thrombophlebitis, women taking oral contraceptives, individuals with sickle cell anemia or polycythemic states and individuals with congenital reduction in normally present anticoagulant proteins (antithrombin III, protein C, or protein S).

3. Spontaneous pneumothorax. Spontaneous pneumothorax is more likely to occur in young, tall, thin, individuals. The patient usually gives a history of sudden onset of chest pain and dyspnea brought on by strenuous exertion, coughing, or air travel. Predisposing factors include emphysema, recent chest trauma, and interstitial lung disease, particularly eosinophilic granuloma.

4. Acute bronchial asthma. Acute asthma may begin at any age but is more frequent in patients with a past or family history of atopic disease. The asthma may be seasonal and may be associated with specific events or inciting agents.

5. Foreign body aspiration. In the patient who has aspirated a foreign body, the history is usually obvious. The patient may not recall the event, however, especially if under the influence of alcohol or unconscious at the time or, as is frequently the case, the patient is a child and unable to relate any history.

6. Noncardiogenic pulmonary edema.
    a. Adult respiratory distress syndrome. Patients with this condition have insidious onset of dyspnea 24 to 72 hours after a severe, usually nonpulmonary, illness (e.g., hemorrhagic or septic shock, acute pancreatitis, multiple trauma, near drowning, overwhelming pneumonia).
    b. Noxious gas inhalation. There is usually a history of accidental exposure to a poisonous gas (e.g., chlorine, phosgene, smoke).
    c. High-altitude pulmonary edema. This condition usually occurs in young adults engaging in vigorous activity at a high altitude prior to acclimatization.
    d. Neurogenic pulmonary edema. This type of edema may be seen in epileptic patients during the postictal period and in patients with increased intracranial pressure.

7. Cardiogenic pulmonary edema. The patient usually has the characteristic symptoms of congestive heart failure—dyspnea, orthopnea, PND, nocturia, ankle edema—which may precede the acute dyspnea by days or weeks. Acute dyspnea may accompany the characteristic chest pain of acute myocardial infarction or be its sole manifestation. A previous history of heart disease should be sought. Occasionally, previously undetected mitral stenosis may be discovered after an initial episode of pulmonary edema.

8. Hyperventilation. This usually occurs in young people without other symptoms of cardiopulmonary disease, often in the presence of a recent emotional upset. Circumoral and carpopedal dysesthesias (tingling sensations) and carpopedal spasm may occur.

## Physical Findings

Tachycardia, tachypnea, cyanosis, and fever may be noted in patients with acute dyspnea.

1. Pneumonia. In the bacterial pneumonias, there are signs of consolidation, including bronchial breath sounds, increased tactile and vocal fremitus, and egophony. There may be an associated decrease in breath sounds and fine rales heard over the involved area. If a pleural effusion accompanies the pneumonia, the physical findings may include a pleural friction rub, decreased to absent breath sounds, decreased fremitus, and flatness to percussion. In contrast, the viral and mycoplasmal pneumonias characteristically show a paucity of physical findings. Sometimes only rales are heard.

2. Acute pulmonary embolism. Pulmonary emboli show a variety of physical findings. The examination may reveal such signs as rales heard over the involved area, a pleural friction rub, and evidence of pleural effusion. Splinting of the involved side may be present and manifested in elevation of the diaphragm and a generalized decrease in breath sounds. Cardiac examination may reveal signs of

right ventricular failure, including a right-sided third heart sound, the murmur of pulmonary regurgitation, or increased intensity of the pulmonary component of the second heart sound. Frequently, however, there are only the nonspecific findings of tachypnea and tachycardia.

3. Pneumothorax. The physical findings of pneumothorax are decreased breath sounds, increased resonance, and decreased fremitus on the involved side. There may be a shift of the trachea and heart to the opposite side. Distention of the neck veins may be visible if the pneumothorax is under tension, and hypotension may occur. Hamman's sign (mediastinal crunch) may be heard in the presence of a left-sided pneumothorax.

4. Bronchial asthma. Patients with asthma have hyperresonance to percussion and wheezing during their attacks. Prolonged expiratory phase is common. If bronchospasm is severe, the chest may be silent to auscultation.

5. Foreign body aspiration. A patient who aspirates a foreign body may have localized wheezing and decreased breath sounds on the involved side. There may be air trapping during expiration (hyperresonance to percussion on the affected side following forced expiration).

6. Noncardiogenic pulmonary edema.
   a. Adult respiratory distress syndrome. Clinical evidence of shock may be present. Conjunctival and axillary petechiae are commonly seen in fat embolism, and CNS changes are also common. Rales may be heard but are less prominent than in other forms of pulmonary edema.
   b. Noxious gas inhalation. Such patients usually have conjunctivitis, pharyngitis, acute bronchitis, and wheezing. Later on, diffuse, bilateral moist rales appear as the clinical picture of pulmonary edema evolves.
   c. High-altitude pulmonary edema. Fine, moist bibasilar rales are commonly audible, although there is no evidence of heart failure.
   d. Neurogenic pulmonary edema. The findings are as in paragraph c above in association with evidence of neurologic injury. Acute systemic hypertension may develop.

7. Cardiogenic pulmonary edema. There may be evidence of previous hypertension or heart disease. Cardiomegaly is suggested by lateral and downward displacement of the apical impulse. A third heart sound or summation gallop and murmurs may be heard. Examination of the lungs may reveal fine moist rales, particularly at the bases. Wheezes may also be heard. Peripheral edema, hepatomegaly, and distended neck veins suggest coexisting right-sided failure.

8. Hyperventilation. Fever and cyanosis are never present, and evidence of anxiety frequently exceeds the objective evidence for cardiopulmonary disease. Physical findings are normal except for tachypnea and occasionally tachycardia.

## Roentgenographic Findings

1. Pneumonia.
   a. Lobar consolidation with air bronchograms is usually present in bacterial pneumonia. Pleural effusion, which may be infrapulmonary or interlobar, is sometimes seen.
   b. Viral and mycoplasmal pneumonias may be lobar in distribution but are more likely to be diffuse and nonlobar in character. Pleural effusions occur less frequently than in bacterial pneumonias. Uncommonly, hilar adenopathy may occur.

2. Acute pulmonary embolism. The chest roentgenogram may be normal or may show evidence of splinting (a raised diaphragm and basilar atelectasis). Pleural effusion or pulmonary infiltrates may be seen after infarction of the lung. A lobar consolidation similar to bacterial pneumonia may be present. Vascular changes occur frequently in acute pulmonary embolism but are difficult to interpret. Vascular cutoffs and decreased blood flow may be demonstrated, particularly if previous x-ray films are available for comparison. With large central pulmonary emboli, a sausage-shaped dilation of the involved pulmonary artery may be seen.

Most patients with pulmonary embolism have normal chest x-rays or nonspecific findings.

3. Spontaneous pneumothorax. Findings on the chest roentgenograms are virtually diagnostic of pneumothorax if the films are examined carefully. Occasionally, a small pneumothorax is not seen unless inspiratory and expiratory films are evaluated. It is necessary to determine whether or not the pneumothorax is under tension. The classic findings of a tension pneumothorax are depression of the diaphragm on the affected side and shift of the mediastinum to the opposite side.

4. Bronchial asthma. In asthma, there may be radiologic signs of hyperinflation, such as flat diaphragm and increase in the retrosternal and retrocardiac air spaces. When an infectious process precipitates an asthmatic attack, evidence of pneumonia may be seen on the chest roentgenogram.

5. Foreign body aspiration. Rarely, the foreign body is radiopaque and can be visualized. The chest roentgenogram usually shows nothing abnormal. There may be evidence of unilateral air trapping, which is demonstrated best by fluoroscopy and expiratory films. Consolidation collapse of the lung distal to the foreign body may occur after a period of time.

6. Noncardiogenic pulmonary edema. Early in the course of noxious gas inhalation, neurogenic and high-altitude pulmonary edema, and the adult respiratory distress syndrome, the chest x-ray may be normal. Eventually, the films show evidence of pulmonary edema without cardiomegaly.

7. Cardiogenic pulmonary edema. The chest roentgenogram shows cardiomegaly except in mitral stenosis and some cases of acute myocardial infarction. Specific chamber enlargement is seen in valvular and congenital heart disease. An alveolar infiltrate showing a butterfly pattern is typical of this form of pulmonary edema. Distended veins to the upper lobes, Kerley's lines, and a peripheral or hilar haze, or both, may also be seen.

8. Hyperventilation. The chest film is normal.

### Laboratory Data

1. CBC. The hematocrit and hemoglobin values are normal in all of these conditions unless altered by coexisting disease. The white cell count is usually elevated, with a shift to the left, but it is rarely above 16,000 per cubic millimeter except in bacterial pneumonias. Asthma may be associated with a significant eosinophilia. Marked derangements in all formed blood elements may be seen in severely ill patients with acute adult respiratory distress syndrome (ARDS). Moderated thrombocytopenia is often seen in fat embolism, and severe thrombocytopenia is seen in the disseminated intravascular coagulation (DIC) that may accompany ARDS.

2. Urinalysis. Hematuria, proteinuria, formed elements, and casts may be seen in the pneumonias, congestive heart failure, and conditions associated with ARDS. All of these findings are nonspecific.

3. Serum electrolytes. A low serum sodium level may be seen in the infectious pneumonias. This may be associated with increased excretion of sodium in the urine.

4. Electrocardiogram. The classic pattern of acute myocardial infarction on the electrocardiogram may be diagnostic. Findings of right axis deviation, an $S_1Q_3T_3$ pattern, or right ventricular strain provide supportive evidence for the diagnosis of pulmonary embolism but do not distinguish this condition from other acute causes of dyspnea associated with increased pulmonary vascular resistance, such as severe airway resistance or hypoxemia. Atrial arrhythmias may be seen with any cause of respiratory failure.

5. Examination of the sputum.
   a. Gross examination. Pink frothy sputum is often seen in cardiogenic or noncardiogenic pulmonary edema. Blood streaking is usually not helpful. The presence of mucous plugs may suggest asthma. Grossly purulent sputum suggests a bacterial pneumonic process, whereas a mucoid sputum is seen more frequently in viral and mycoplasmal pneumonias.

    **b.** Gram stain. An adequate, freshly obtained sputum sample should be examined in patients with pneumonia. The gram stain should demonstrate large numbers of polymorphonuclear leukocytes. Only if a predominant or intracellular organism can be identified should it be tentatively considered the etiologic agent.

    **c.** Acid-fast stain. Acid-fast organisms should be sought carefully under oil immersion.

    **d.** Wright's stain. Eosinophilia may predominate in the sputum samples of asthmatic patients.

    **e.** Sputum cultures. Routine cultures for bacteria should be obtained. Facilities for culture of viruses, *Legionella,* and mycoplasmas are not usually available except in specialized laboratories.

**6.** Blood cultures. Blood cultures should be drawn from the febrile patient with acute dyspnea.

**7.** Arterial blood gases. Arterial blood gas results are of no value in differentiating among the various entities under consideration, but they are helpful in patient management because all of these conditions may include varying degrees of hypoxemia, hypercarbia, or both.

**8.** Serologic studies. Cold agglutinins may be elevated in mycoplasmal pneumonia. Rises in specific titers may be seen in viral pneumonias and pneumonia due to *Legionella pneumophila.*

### Further Studies

When the aforementioned studies are completed, the most likely diagnosis should be apparent and treatment instituted. If pulmonary embolism is a prime consideration, perfusion and inhalation lung scans should be performed. A pulmonary angiogram is needed if the lung scan is abnormal. Impedance plethysmography, Doppler examination, and venography of the lower extremities may be helpful in selected cases. If foreign body aspiration is suspected, early bronchoscopy is indicated. If asthma is the apparent diagnosis, treatment should be instituted and the workup completed when the patient's condition has stabilized. Severe hypoxemia or acute hypercarbia may require intubation and mechanical ventilation.

---

## Chronic Dyspnea

### Etiology

**1.** Pulmonary causes of chronic dyspnea.
    **a.** Chronic obstructive airway disease.
        **(1)** Emphysema.
        **(2)** Chronic bronchitis.
        **(3)** Chronic bronchial asthma.
    **Note:** Although there is usually considerable overlap among these three entities, the classic forms are described in the discussion that follows.
    **b.** Restrictive lung disease.
        **(1)** Interstitial lung diseases (the most common of which are sarcoidosis, rheumatoid lung, scleroderma lung, the pneumoconioses, histiocytosis X, lymphangitic carcinomatosis, and idiopathic fibrosing alveolitis).
        **(2)** Chest wall deformities (e.g., kyphoscoliosis and thoracoplasty).
        **(3)** Pleural fibrosis.
        **(4)** Alveolar-filling diseases (alveolar proteinosis, alveolar cell carcinoma, desquamative interstitial pneumonia, and alveolar microlithiasis).
        **(5)** Neuromuscular disease (e.g., myasthenia gravis, amyotropic lateral sclerosis).

**2.** Nonpulmonary causes of chronic dyspnea.
    **a.** Congestive heart failure and other low output states.

   **b.** Anemia.
   **c.** Hyperthyroidism.
   **d.** Upper airway disease.
   **e.** Obesity.
   **f.** Neurosis.

## History

1. Pulmonary causes.
   **a.** Chronic obstructive airway disease.
     **(1)** Patients with emphysema usually give a long history of steadily worsening dyspnea. There may be a family history of emphysema or other obstructive lung disease.
     **(2)** In chronic bronchitis, a productive cough is present for at least 3 months of every year for a consecutive 2-year period. Chronic bronchitis is usually associated with a long history of cigarette smoking, "smoker's cough," wheezing, and repeated pulmonary infections.
     **(3)** The history of patients with chronic asthma is similar to that of patients with acute asthma.
   **b.** Restrictive lung disease.
     **(1)** A complete discussion of all the causes of interstitial lung disease is beyond the scope of this text. In some conditions, diagnostic clues may be found in the history. In the connective tissue diseases, such as scleroderma, rheumatoid arthritis, and polymyositis, there may be a history or symptoms suggestive of the diagnosis. Sometimes, however, these diseases are first manifested by interstitial fibrosis, and the systemic manifestations develop later. Patients with eosinophilic granuloma may have a history of recurrent pneumothorax or diabetes insipidus, or both. Patients with sarcoidosis may have arthralgias and painful erythematous nodules on the shins. In the pneumoconioses, the occupational history is of prime importance. In lymphangitic carcinomatosis, symptoms caused by a primary carcinoma of the stomach, breast, prostate, lung, or other organ may be the presenting complaint.
     **(2)** In patients with thoracic deformities, the history is clear.
     **(3)** Patients with pleural fibrosis may give a history of previous tuberculosis, severe bacterial pneumonia, chest trauma, surgery for tuberculosis, or asbestos exposure.
     **(4)** Among the alveolar-filling diseases, alveolar proteinosis and alveolar cell carcinoma may have significant sputum production. In lipoid pneumonia, there may be a history of use of oily nose drops.
     **(5)** Neuromuscular diseases.
2. Nonpulmonary causes.
   **a.** Congestive heart failure. See Cardiogenic Pulmonary Edema under Acute Dyspnea.
   **b.** Anemia. Progressive dyspnea is a common symptom of anemia; it should be considered, particularly, if the patient complains of blood loss, pallor, and weakness.
   **c.** Hyperthyroidism. In thyrotoxic patients, dyspnea may be the predominant presenting symptom. Usually these patients have classic symptoms of thyrotoxicosis.
   **d.** Upper airway disease. Patients with upper airway disease may have a history of endotracheal tube intubation or tracheostomy. Occasionally bronchogenic carcinoma presents with tracheal obstruction. Such patients may complain of audible wheezing or upper airway rattling.
   **e.** Obesity. Corpulence is seldom the sole reason for a patient's complaint of dyspnea unless the obesity is severe or the weight gain rapid.
   **f.** Neurosis. See Hyperventilation under Acute Dyspnea. This is clearly a diagnosis of exclusion.

## Physical Examination

1. Chronic obstructive airway disease.
   a. Emphysema. Usually the emphysematous patient is thin and asthenic, the AP diameter of the chest is increased, and hypertrophy of the accessory muscles of respiration is visible. There is hyperresonance to percussion with depressed immobile diaphragm. Auscultation reveals decreased breath sounds and a prolongation of the expiratory phase of respiration. Faint expiratory wheezes may be heard.
   b. Chronic bronchitis. Chronic bronchitis is diagnosed by the history. The patient may have findings of airway obstruction. Patients with severe disease may be cyanotic or plethoric or have signs of cor pulmonale.
   c. Chronic bronchial asthma. Wheezing is one characteristic physical finding, and it may be associated with signs of hyperinflation of the lungs.
   d. Restrictive lung disease.
      (1) Interstitial lung disease. In interstitial fibrosis, clubbing is frequent. The chest examination may be normal except for dry inspiratory bibasilar rales. Signs of associated systemic diseases may be seen (e.g., arthritis, skin rash, lymphadenopathy, splenomegaly). Evidence of a primary carcinoma may be found in lymphangitic carcinomatosis.
      (2) Thoracic deformities. Kyphoscoliosis or a previous thoracoplasty is evident on inspection.
      (3) Pleural fibrosis. There may be diminished expansion of the chest wall. Dullness to percussion, decreased fremitus, and decreased breath sounds may be noted on the involved side.
      (4) Alveolar-filling diseases. There are no specific physical findings. Rales may be heard in occasional cases.
2. Nonpulmonary causes.
   a. Congestive heart failure. Elevated venous pressure, gallop rhythm, bibasilar rales, and dependent edema are the cardinal signs.
   b. Anemia. Aside from pallor, there are no specific signs of anemia, although there are specific signs associated with different causes of anemia.
   c. Hyperthyroidism. A goiter in association with tremor, moist skin, exophthalmos, hyperreflexia, and tachycardia is a classic sign of Graves' disease.
   d. Upper airway disease. Wheezing or stridor may be audible, and a tracheostomy scar may be present.
   e. Obesity. Excess adiposity is usually obvious on inspection.

## Roentgenographic Findings

1. Pulmonary causes.
   a. Chronic obstructive airway disease. Severe obstructive disease of any etiology is frequently accompanied by a normal chest x-ray.
      (1) The patient with emphysema may show bullous changes, evidence of hyperinflation of the lungs, and attenuation of the pulmonary vasculature on the chest roentgenogram.
      (2) Chronic bronchitis may be associated with roentgenographic evidence of cor pulmonale (right ventricular hypertrophy associated with pulmonary hypertension).
      (3) In chronic bronchial asthma, the chest roentgenogram may show signs of hyperinflation and sometimes diffuse fibrosis or chronic segmental fibrosis secondary to old infectious processes. Occasionally, evidence of mucoid impaction of the bronchi may be seen.
   b. Restrictive lung disease.
      (1) In the interstitial lung diseases, the chest roentgenogram demonstrates a linear, fibronodular, or fibroreticular infiltrate. Lytic lesions of the ribs or pneumothorax may be seen in histiocytosis X. Kerley's lines, pleural effusion, and mediastinal lymph node enlargement may be seen in lymphangitic carcinomatosis. A lung mass may also be demonstrable. In the

interstitial lung disease due to connective tissue disease, pleural effusion or scarring may be seen. In scleroderma, a mediastinal air-fluid level may be demonstrated when the esophagus is involved. Hypomotility and dilation of the esophagus due to scleroderma may be manifested by a mediastinal air-fluid level. In sarcoidosis, hilar lymphadenopathy may be present. Silicosis is usually a predominantly upper lobe disease, with multiple interstitial nodules that often coalesce. Cavitary disease due to superimposed myobacterial infection may be present. Asbestosis is a predominantly lower lobe disease—a linear interstitial pattern that may be associated with calcified plaques in the diaphragmatic pleura or lateral wall pleural thickening, or both.

   **(2)** In kyphoscoliosis, or after thoracoplasty, obvious skeletal deformity may be seen on the chest films.

   **(3)** In pleural fibrosis, the pleural line is thickened and may be calcified.

   **(4)** Alveolar-filling diseases demonstrate a characteristic acinar-filling pattern with air bronchograms, rosettes, and obliteration of the vascular markings. Early lipoid pneumonia and desquamative interstitial pneumonitis involve primarily the lower lobes.

**2.** Nonpulmonary causes.

   **a.** Congestive heart failure. The radiographic picture of congestive heart failure is described in the section on Acute Pulmonary Radiographic Abnormalities.

   **b.** Anemia. The chest roentgenogram is usually normal, although cardiomegaly may be present.

   **c.** Hyperthyroidism. The chest film is usually normal, although the heart may be enlarged.

   **d.** Upper airway disease. The chest roentgenogram may be normal, or there may be evidence of air trapping. The tracheal air shadow may be narrowed.

   **e.** Obesity causes no significant pulmonary parenchymal infiltration, although cardiomegaly may be present. Because of the adiposity, the lung parenchyma may appear diffusely infiltrated if the chest film is underpenetrated. Increased soft tissue is obvious.

## Laboratory Data

**1.** CBC. Erythrocytosis may be seen with any pulmonary cause of chronic dyspnea, if hypoxemia is present (erythrocytosis may also be seen in patients with sleep apnea or chronically high carboxyhemoglobulin, which may or may not be related to the cause of chronic dyspnea). Low hemoglobin and hematocrit values are the diagnostic features of anemia. Leukocytosis may be seen in patients with chronic airway disease who have superimposed infection; it may also be seen in chronic congestive heart failure. Lymphocytosis is common in thyrotoxicosis, anemia, and connective tissue diseases. Abnormalities of the white blood cells may be seen in certain types of anemia. Eosinophilia may occur in chronic asthma.

**2.** Urinalysis. Changes in urine sediment may be seen in the various connective tissue diseases, but these are nonspecific.

**3.** Blood chemistries. In severe chronic lung disease with alveolar hypoventilation, the serum bicarbonate level may be increased. Dilutional hyponatremia may be seen in congestive heart failure. The serum calcium value may be elevated in sarcoidosis. Serum creatinine and BUN may be elevated in renal failure due to connective tissue diseases.

**4.** Sputum examination. In chronic asthma, eosinophils are usually seen with Wright's stain. The periodic acid-Schiff stain is frequently positive in alveolar proteinosis. Sputum cytologic findings may be abnormal in alveolar cell carcinoma. In lipoid pneumonia, the Sudan III stain may be positive for fat-laden macrophages.

**5.** Electrocardiogram. In all forms of chronic pulmonary disease there may be evidence on electrocardiogram of right axis deviation, right ventricular enlargement and strain, atrial dysrhythmias, and right atrial enlargement. Evidence of left ventricular disease may be seen in chronic left-sided heart failure, and atrial and ventricular ectopy are common. Sinus tachycardia is frequently present in thy rotoxicosis and anemia.

6. Blood gases. In all pulmonary causes of chronic dyspnea, hypoxemia may b present. Hypoventilation ($PCO_2$ 45 mm Hg) is seen more commonly in chronic bronchitis and thoracic cage deformities. Hyperventilation (low $PCO_2$) may b seen in interstitial lung disease. Hypoxemia, with or without $CO_2$ retention, may be seen in congestive heart failure. Arterial blood gases are normal in anemia thyrotoxicosis, or upper airway disease, although $O_2$ content is low in anemia. I obesity there may be mild hypoxemia.

7. Serum protein electrophoresis. Electrophoresis occasionally shows a decrease o absence of alpha-1-globulin, particularly in younger patients with emphysema. I the alpha-1-globulin level is low, specific assays for alpha-1-antitrypsin defi ciency are indicated.

### Further Studies

From the foregoing data it should be possible to determine whether dyspnea is o pulmonary or nonpulmonary origin. Patients with pulmonary dyspnea shoul have pulmonary function studies performed. In chronic obstructive airway dis ease, the ventilatory functions show evidence of airway obstruction (e.g., dimin ished $FEV_1$ and MMEF), vital capacity may be normal or decreased, and there i usually an increase in the residual volume. In patients with a predominantl restrictive component (e.g., interstitial fibrosis, chest wall deformities, an pleural diseases), ventilatory function usually shows a reduction in vital capacit total lung capacity, and diffusing capacity, but good flow rates are maintained Lung biopsy may be indicated when the diagnosis of interstitial lung disease i not apparent from the clinical findings.

## WHEEZING
### Marvin I. Schwarz
### Paul M. Cox, Jr.

Wheezing is a common complaint in patients with pulmonary disease. It may b caused by any of the following:

1. Large airway obstruction.
   a. Laryngeal obstruction—tumor, vocal cord paralysis, inflammation, laryng spasm.
   b. Tracheal obstruction—stenosis, tumor.
   c. Foreign body aspiration.
2. Endobronchial tumors and granulomas.
3. Bronchial asthma.
4. Acute bronchitis.
5. Chronic airway obstruction.
6. Acute left ventricular failure (cardiac asthma).
7. Pulmonary embolism.
   Table 4-1 presents the differential diagnosis of wheezing.

## COUGH
### Marvin I. Schwarz
### Paul M. Cox, Jr.

### Acute Cough

All the causes of acute dyspnea, with the possible exception of pneumothora may also present with cough of acute onset or even with acute cough withou dyspnea. The most frequent cause of acute cough without dyspnea in a previously healthy patient is acute bronchitis. The diagnosis of acute bronchitis is based on evidence of a preceding upper respiratory infection, followed by cough productive of mucoid or purulent sputum. Myalgias, headaches, malaise, fever, and an influenzal syndrome may be associated. The physical examination usually reveals nothing abnormal except evidence of respiratory tract inflammation, including the presence of rhonchi on auscultation. The chest roentgenogram is normal. Laboratory abnormalities, if any, are nonspecific.

# Chronic Cough

## Etiology

Chronic cough is frequently found in the pulmonary conditions causing chronic dyspnea. However, patients with pure emphysema, thoracic wall deformities, and pleural fibrosis, as well as those with nonpulmonary causes of dyspnea, may not have associated cough. Additional causes of chronic cough are bronchogenic carcinoma, benign endobronchial tumors, and chronic granulomatous diseases, including tuberculosis, sarcoidosis, fungal diseases, and lung abscess. For discussion of bronchiectasis, an important cause of chronic cough, see the next section Hemoptysis.

## History

1. Bronchogenic carcinoma. Patients with bronchogenic carcinoma usually have a history of cigarette smoking of greater than 10 "pack-years." In addition to cough, they may have hemoptysis and weight loss. Exposure to asbestos or radioactive materials, such as in uranium mining, increases the risk of developing bronchogenic carcinoma, particularly in smokers.
2. Bronchial adenoma. Systemic symptoms are usually absent. Patients may complain of wheezing or give a history of recurrent pneumonia. Hemoptysis may be present.
3. Chronic granulomatous disease. Persistent cough may be the only symptom, but increased sputum production, hemoptysis, weight loss, fever, and night sweats are commonly associated. Patients with endobronchial sarcoidosis may have the same symptoms as those with fungal or tuberculous granulomatous disease. They may also have systemic symptoms such as arthralgias, arthritis, erythema nodosum, or skin rash. Erythema nodosum may also occur in histoplasmosis.
4. Lung abscess. Recent dental procedures, episodes of unconsciousness, and history of recent pneumonia due to staphylococci or gram-negative bacilli, in particular, are common antecedents. Halitosis, foul-smelling sputum, and fever are frequent complaints. There is often a history of excessive alcohol intake.

## Physical Examination

1. Bronchogenic carcinoma. In bronchogenic carcinoma, there may be evidence of recent weight loss. Lymphadenopathy may be present in the supraclavicular and infraclavicular areas. Bony metastases may be noted in the chest wall. Auscultation of the chest may reveal evidence of endobronchial obstruction manifested by localized wheezing, atelectasis, or pneumonia. Clubbing may be present. Evidence of metastatic disease may be noted in other organs, including the skin, liver, and brain.
2. Bronchial adenoma. In bronchial adenoma, abnormal physical findings are unusual. Occasionally, there is evidence of unilateral or localized wheezing. Evidence of atelectasis is sometimes found on physical examination.
3. Granulomatous diseases. These diseases may be present without abnormal physical findings. Because the distribution of such disease is usually apical and posterior, rales may be heard in these areas. When large cavities are present, char-

**Table 4-1.** Differential diagnosis of wheezing

| Disease | Clinical presentation | Laboratory findings | Chest roentgenogram | Associated clinical findings |
|---|---|---|---|---|
| Large airway obstruction: laryngeal stridor; tracheal stenosis; foreign body aspiration | Acute onset of dyspnea except in tracheal stenosis; previous history of intubation; atopic history in laryngeal stridor | | A narrowed air tracheogram and the demonstration of air-trapping on expiration films | Other allergic phenomena (e.g., urticaria). In laryngeal stridor wheezing heard over the major airways, obstruction to air flow greater on inspiration |
| Endobronchial tumors or granulomas | Gradual onset of dyspnea | Positive sputum cytologic findings or acid-fast smears; hypergammaglobulinemia and hypercalcemia with sarcoidosis | A hilar mass with or without lobar collapse; typical tuberculous infiltrates in the upper zone; bilateral hilar adenopathy with or without pulmonary infiltrates | History of tobacco consumption; weight loss, fever, cough; wheezing is localized |
| Asthma | Subacute or acute onset of dyspnea | Sputum and systemic eosinophilia: arterial blood gases demonstrate hypoxia and hyperventilation; $FEV_1$ reduced and responds to | May show hyperinflation or mucoid impaction | History of similar episodes and an atopic state |

| | | | | |
|---|---|---|---|---|
| | sputum. Other symptoms of URI | WBC with shift to the left | pneumonia develops | |
| Chronic obstructive pulmonary disease | Chronic cough, dyspnea, and sputum production | Purulent sputum with elevated WBC and shift to the left. Arterial blood gases may demonstrate hypoxemia and hypoventilation, or both; elevated hematocrit; $FEV_1$ diminished | May show evidence of emphysema and pulmonary hypertension | History of tobacco use; signs of cor pulmonale |
| Cardiac asthma | Acute onset of dyspnea, associated with paroxysmal nocturnal dyspnea and orthopnea | ECG may show evidence of acute myocardial infarction, ischemic changes, changes consistent with LVH, or P mitrale | Cardiac enlargement, diffuse alveolar filling; venous hypertension; Kerley's B lines; or left atrial enlargement | History of coronary, hypertensive, or rheumatic heart disease; physical exam may demonstrate a third heart sound gallop and systolic or diastolic murmurs |
| Pulmonary embolus | Acute onset of dyspnea, pleuritic chest pain, and cough | ECG may show evidence for acute right heart strain; arterial blood gases may demonstrate hypoxemia and hyperventilation; abnormal lung scan; positive angiogram | May be normal, or may demonstrate a pleural effusion, atelectatic lines, or an ill-defined pulmonary infiltrate | Evidence of lower extremity venous thrombosis |

URI = upper respiratory infection, LVH = left ventricular hypertrophy

acteristic cavernous breath sounds may be present. Sarcoidosis patients ma:
show evidence of arthritis, skin rash, erythema nodosum, or hepatosplenomegal
4. Lung abscess. Clubbing, halitosis, rales, and cavernous breath sounds may b
present.

### Roentgenographic Findings

1. Bronchogenic carcinoma. The chest roentgenograms of patients with broncho
genic carcinoma usually demonstrate a hilar mass or a single coin lesion. Me
diastinal lymphadenopathy may be present. If the tumor partially or totally oc
cludes a bronchus, evidence of volume loss in the form of elevation of th
diaphragm or a shift of the lung fissures and hilar structures may appear. An
other radiographic sign is pneumonia distal to the obstruction. Pleural effusio:
is often present and lytic lesions in the ribs occasionally may be seen. If there i
lymphangitic spread of the tumor, evidence of diffuse interstitial disease and Ker
ley's lines may be seen.
2. Bronchial adenoma. The most characteristic appearance of bronchial adenoma i:
that of a centrally placed, circumscribed mass with atelectasis distal to the lesion
A small number of cases may present as peripheral coin lesions.
3. Granulomatous diseases. Evidence of a primary complex (i.e., a calcified medias
tinal or hilar node on the same side as the calcified parenchymal lesion) may b
noted in tuberculosis. Posterior and apical infiltrative disease or cavity disease
or both, may be present. An apical pleural reaction and pleural effusion are com
monly seen. In the more chronic cases, there may be evidence of upper lobe vo
ume loss such as fibrotic streaking and retracted hilar structures. In sarcoidosi:
the roentgenographic findings are variable. Bilateral and symmetric mediastina
and hilar lymphadenopathy is the most common radiographic presentation. Thi
may be associated with alveolar or interstitial infiltrates, or both, early in th
course of the disease. Pleural disease or cavities are rarely seen. In the mor
chronic states of the disease, there is usually a diffuse interstitial infiltrate tha
may be linear or nodular, or a combination of the two. With further progressio
of the disease, bilateral upper lobe retraction with fibrotic streaking and cyst:
transformation may be seen.
4. Lung abscesses. These are seen radiographically as cavitary lesions, usually wit
air-fluid levels. An infiltrate may surround the cavity.

### Laboratory Data

1. CBC. Anemia may be seen in bronchogenic carcinoma, tuberculosis, fungus dis
eases, sarcoidosis, or lung abscess. The anemia may be hemolytic or, more fre
quently, have the characteristics of anemia of chronic disease. The white ce
count may be elevated in all of these disorders, particularly if there is an assoc
ated infectious process. Leukemoid reactions have been reported in tuberculosi:
2. Urinalysis. White blood cells with blood cell casts, proteinuria, and hematuri
may be seen singly or in any combination in patients with renal tuberculosis. I
the rare patients who have bronchogenic carcinoma associated with inappr
priate antidiuretic hormone (ADH) secretion, concentrated urine with high spe
cific gravity and increased osmolality may be found.
3. Electrolyte and serum enzyme abnormalities.
   a. Hyponatremia may occur in bronchogenic carcinoma with inappropriate AD
   secretion or, rarely, when adrenal insufficiency occurs as a result of adren:
   metastasis. Hyponatremia is also not uncommon in tuberculosis. Although
   may be secondary to inappropriate ADH secretion or adrenal insufficienc
   due to tuberculous involvement of the adrenal cortex, frequently no specif
   cause can be found. It usually disappears when treatment of the tuberculos
   is instituted.
   b. Hypercalcemia may be seen in bronchogenic carcinoma, sarcoidosis, and ce
   tain bronchial carcinoid tumors.

   **c.** In bronchogenic carcinoma, sarcoidosis, and tuberculosis, abnormalities of liver function may occur as a result of liver involvement.

**4.** Sputum examination. Sputum cytologic study may lead to diagnosis in carcinoma of the lung. Acid-fast stains are frequently positive in active tuberculosis, but they may be negative even when the culture is positive. Fungal organisms may be seen with special staining techniques. The sputum should be cultured for *Mycobacterium tuberculosis* and fungi. Gram stains may reveal the likely etiologic organism in lung abscess, but aerobic bacterial cultures should be obtained. Anaerobic cultures may be misleading because of contamination by anaerobes normally in oral secretions.

**5.** Electrocardiogram. Electrocardiographic evidence of pericarditis may be seen in tuberculosis, sarcoidosis, and bronchogenic carcinoma with pericardial involvement. In sarcoidosis, the electrocardiogram may rarely resemble that of myocardial infarction. Arrhythmias and atrioventricular conduction disturbances are seen occasionally.

**6.** Skin testing and serologic study. PPD-S (Tween stabilized, TU or intermediate strength): Greater than 10-mm induration at 48 to 72 hours is strong evidence of infection with tuberculosis. However, a positive result does not necessarily indicate active tuberculosis or prove that tuberculosis is the cause of the patient's symptoms. False-negative findings may be due to anergy, improper technique, and other factors that are poorly understood. A negative skin test finding does not rule out tuberculosis. First- and second-strength PPD are not useful in the diagnosis of tuberculosis and should not be employed.

**7.** Other diagnostic procedures.

   **a.** With fiberoptic bronchoscopes, bronchoscopy is a safe and relatively comfortable procedure. It should be performed whenever the aforementioned tests do not lead to diagnosis and to determine the extent and resectability of tumors. A biopsy should be done at the time. Bronchial brushings also may be obtained. Transtracheal and transcarinal needle aspiration may also be helpful to stage or diagnose tumors. Postbronchoscopy sputa for cytologic study, acid-fast and fungus stains, and cultures are probably not indicated routinely, although occasionally they may be positive even when bronchoscopy is negative. Bronchoscopy and "protected brush" sampling may be necessary in lung abscess to restore drainage and obtain cultures.

   **b.** Bronchography is no longer indicated in routine evaluation of the airways.

   **c.** Computerized tomography of the thorax is being found increasingly useful to detect or rule out mediastinal disease or to localize enlarged nodes to direct transtracheal needle aspiration or mediastinoscopy.

   **d.** Mediastinoscopy is useful for determining the resectability of bronchogenic carcinoma and for the diagnosis of sarcoidosis.

   **e.** In rare instances, the procedures listed above may not lead to a diagnosis. Diagnostic thoracotomy may then be necessary.

---

## HEMOPTYSIS
Marvin I. Schwarz
Paul M. Cox, Jr.

---

### Definition

Hemoptysis is the expectoration of blood or bloody sputum.

### Etiology

Some of the important causes of hemoptysis have been described in earlier sections. These include infectious pneumonias, pulmonary embolism, bronchogenic carcinoma, mitral stenosis, chronic obstructive pulmonary disease, and tuberculosis and other granulomatous diseases. Other causes of hemoptysis include bronchiectasis, pulmonary arteriovenous malformations, pulmonary sequestration idiopathic hemosiderosis, Goodpasture's syndrome, coagulation disorders, and in tracavitary fungus balls (aspergillosis). Bronchitis is the most common cause.

## History

1. Bronchiectasis. Characteristically there is a history of repeated episodes of pneu monia or bronchitis. Long-term production of foul-smelling sputum is a classic finding, but it is not always present. Sinusitis is common. There may be a history of pertussis, measles, or other causes of severe childhood pneumonia. Patient with cystic fibrosis may have a personal or family history of failure to thrive o meconium ileus. Patients with immune disorders may have had recurrent non pulmonary infections.
2. Pulmonary sequestration. The history may be similar to that of bronchiectasis In other instances, the patient may have been asymptomatic previously.
3. Idiopathic pulmonary hemosiderosis. This condition usually occurs in children and young adults. Cough and hemoptysis are the usual symptoms. Anemia is a common accompaniment and may cause the presenting symptoms.
4. Goodpasture's syndrome. The symptoms are similar to those in idiopathic pul monary hemosiderosis, although symptoms and signs of uremia also may be present. The symptoms of renal disease may antedate those of pulmonary dis ease, or vice versa.
5. Coagulation disorder. Patients with known coagulopathies or those undergoin anticoagulant therapy may have respiratory tract bleeding. Usually there is history of bleeding from other sites (e.g., the skin, gastrointestinal tract, th nares).
6. Intracavitary fungus balls. Aspergillomas are found only in patients with preex isting cavitary disease due to tuberculosis or other causes. They are more likel to be seen in older, debilitated patients.
7. Pulmonary arteriovenous malformations. A family history of pulmonary arterio venous malformations can be elicited in 60 percent of cases. Dyspnea is a commo complaint. In addition to hemoptysis, the patient may have experienced ep staxis, hematemesis, cerebral hemorrhage, melena, or unexplained anemia.

## Physical Examination

1. Halitosis and clubbing are frequent in bronchiectasis. Examination of the ches may reveal signs of chronic airway obstruction, but the most consistent finding are coarse, "sticky" bibasilar rales. In localized bronchiectasis, the findings ar confined to the area of involvement. Patients with Kartagener's syndrome hav a triad of bronchiectasis, sinusitis, and situs inversus. Patients with cystic fibro sis may have evidence of malnutrition.
2. In pulmonary sequestration, there may be localized rales over the site of seque tration.
3. In idiopathic pulmonary hemosiderosis, diffuse or localized rales may be hear Pallor secondary to anemia is common.
4. Patients with Goodpasture's syndrome demonstrate physical findings similar those of idiopathic pulmonary hemosiderosis; signs of uremia may be present.
5. Coagulation disorders frequently show evidence of bleeding from multiple site Ecchymoses or petechiae may be present. Examination of the chest may reve diffuse or localized rales.
6. An aspergilloma produces no characteristic physical findings, although finding of the preexisting condition (e.g., tuberculosis, lung abscess) may be present.
7. The physical findings associated with pulmonary arteriovenous malformatio include clubbing, cyanosis, and telangiectasis in the skin and mucous mem branes. On examination of the chest, continuous murmurs may be heard over th malformations.

## Roentgenographic Findings

1. In bronchiectasis, the chest roentgenogram may be normal, or evidence of basilar fibrosis, with or without cystic changes, may be noted. Localized changes are found in some cases. In more severe cases, the fibrotic and cystic changes may be diffuse. Cavity formation with air-fluid levels may be present. Situs inversus is evident in Kartagener's syndrome.
2. Pulmonary sequestration is shown radiographically as a circumscribed shadow, usually in the left lower lobe and continuous with the diaphragm. Air-fluid levels may be present if cavitation has occurred.
3. During the acute phase of idiopathic pulmonary hemosiderosis, evidence of diffuse or localized acinar-filling process may be seen. There may be resolution of these abnormalities or progression to an interstitial fibrotic pattern.
4. The roentgenographic findings in Goodpasture's syndrome are similar to those of idiopathic pulmonary hemosiderosis. The "butterfly" pattern of uremic pulmonary edema may be seen if the renal disease is severe.
5. The roentgenogram in hemoptysis due to coagulation disorders is similar to that of idiopathic pulmonary hemosiderosis and Goodpasture's syndrome.
6. An aspergilloma typically presents a round mass within a cavity. When the patient is placed in the lateral decubitus position, movement of the mass may be noted.
7. A pulmonary arteriovenous malformation appears radiographically as a sharply defined, round or oval, homogeneous mass 1 to 5 cm in diameter. It is usually in the lower lobes, and vascular structures may be continuous with the mass.

## Laboratory Data

1. CBC. This is usually normal in hemoptysis. Iron deficiency anemia may be seen in idiopathic pulmonary hemosiderosis and in Goodpasture's syndrome. Pulmonary arteriovenous malformations may have iron deficiency anemia secondary to recurrent bleeding, but more commonly, erythrocytosis secondary to chronic hypoxemia is seen. Massive hemoptysis rarely produces the picture of anemia due to acute blood loss, and other etiologies for the anemia should be considered.
2. Urinalysis. Urinalysis is helpful in the diagnosis of Goodpasture's syndrome and may demonstrate evidence of nephritis.
3. Blood chemistries. Laboratory findings of uremia may be present in Goodpasture's syndrome.
4. Examination of the sputum. Patients with Goodpasture's syndrome or idiopathic pulmonary hemosiderosis show hemosiderin-laden macrophages in their sputa.
5. Electrocardiogram. If pulmonary hypertension is present, there may be evidence of right axis deviation, right ventricular hypertrophy, and right atrial enlargement.
6. Other diagnostic procedures.
   a. Pulmonary function tests are of little value in differentiating between the various disorders. However, in bronchiectasis there may be evidence of obstruction to air flow. A patient with idiopathic pulmonary hemosiderosis or Goodpasture's syndrome may have a restrictive defect and reduction of the diffusing capacity.
   b. Bronchograms can be used to diagnose saccular bronchiectasis, but most authorities now consider computerized tomography equally sensitive and less invasive.
   c. Arteriography. In a patient with suspected pulmonary sequestration, aortography should be done.
   d. Biopsy. In patients with suspected Goodpasture's syndrome, a lung or renal biopsy should be performed, with immunofluorescent staining of the tissue. Patients with suspected idiopathic pulmonary hemosiderosis should have a lung biopsy.
   e. Serologic tests. Precipitating antibodies may be present in aspergillosis.

**f.** Coagulation screening should be performed when coagulopathies are suspected.

**g.** Miscellaneous studies. Sweat chlorides are elevated in cystic fibrosis. Increased fecal excretion of fat may be noted in cases of untreated cystic fibrosis and in some immune disorders. Serum globulin values are usually abnormal in immunologic diseases. Isolated deficiency of IgA may be associated with bronchiectasis or recurrent bronchitis.

**h.** Bronchoscopy should be performed when it is necessary to rule out intraluminal disease.

---

## CYANOSIS
Marvin I. Schwarz
Paul M. Cox, Jr.

### Definition

Cyanosis is a bluish color of the skin and mucous membranes, usually due to the presence of at least 5 g of reduced hemoglobin in the arterial blood. Although cyanosis frequently indicates arterial oxygen unsaturation, it reflects the degree of hypoxemia imperfectly. Not all cyanosis is related to the presence of increased amounts of reduced hemoglobin in the blood. Severe cyanosis, for example, may be due to the presence of abnormal pigments (methemoglobin or sulfhemoglobin) within the red blood cells.

### Etiology

Cyanosis may be classified as central or peripheral. Central cyanosis usually results from arterial hypoxemia caused by right-to-left cardiac shunt, pulmonary arteriovenous fistula, or acute or chronic pulmonary disease. It may occur in polycythemia vera in the absence of arterial oxygen unsaturation, because of the presence of an increased amount of reduced hemoglobin in the blood. In central cyanosis, both the skin and mucous membranes are blue. Polycythemia and digital clubbing are commonly present when cyanosis is severe and chronic. Peripheral cyanosis is caused by stagnant circulation through the peripheral vascular bed. Arterial oxygen saturation is normal unless cardiopulmonary disease is also present. The cyanosis primarily affects the exposed portions of the body, such as the hands, ears, nose, cheeks, and feet. Peripheral cyanosis may be caused by exposure to cold, nervous tension, reduced cardiac output, or vascular obstruction.

The most common cause of central cyanosis in the adult is pulmonary disease, especially chronic obstructive airway disease. Intracardiac right-to-left shunts are less common causes. Peripheral cyanosis is most commonly due to exposure to cold or emotional tension.

#### Central Cyanosis

1. Cyanotic congenital heart disease (e.g., tetralogy of Fallot, Eisenmenger's syndrome, trilogy of Fallot, tricuspid atresia, Ebstein's anomaly, transposition of the great vessels, pulmonary arteriovenous fistula).
2. Pulmonary disease.
   **a.** Acute (e.g., pneumonia, pulmonary embolism, atelectasis).
   **b.** Chronic.
      **(1)** Obstructive airway disease.
      **(2)** Restrictive lung diseases.

3. Hemoglobin abnormalities.
   a. Congenital.
   b. Acquired.

## Peripheral Cyanosis

1. Reduced cardiac output (e.g., congestive heart failure, cardiogenic shock, mitral stenosis).
2. Exposure to cold, including Raynaud's phenomenon.
3. Arterial obstruction.
4. Venous obstruction.

---

# History

## Central Cyanosis

1. Cyanotic congenital heart disease. There may be a history of cyanosis, dyspnea, heart murmur, syncope, squatting, congestive heart failure, or other cardiac symptoms dating from birth or childhood.
2. Pulmonary disease. The most common symptoms are dyspnea, cough, sputum production, wheezing, hemoptysis, and recurrent pulmonary infections.
3. Hemoglobin abnormalities.
   a. Congenital (deficiency of NADH diaphorase, hemoglobin M disease): A history of cyanosis from birth may be elicited in these types of methemoglobinemia.
   b. Acquired (methemoglobinemia, sulfhemoglobinemia): A history of exposure to chemicals or drugs may be obtained. The chief offenders are nitrates, nitrites, chlorates, quinones, certain aniline dyes, acetanilid, sulfonamides, and phenacetin.

## Peripheral Cyanosis

1. Decreased cardiac output. A history of mitral stenosis, myocardial infarction, or other heart disease usually can be elicited. In cases due to shock, evidence of hemorrhage, gram-negative sepsis, or other underlying disease may be obtained.
2. Exposure to cold (including Raynaud's phenomenon). A history of exposure to cold is usually obvious. In Raynaud's phenomenon, paroxysmal pain, pallor, and cyanosis, followed by redness, usually involving the fingers, occur upon exposure to cold or emotional stress.
3. Arterial obstruction. A history of antecedent intermittent claudication is often obtainable from patients with arterial occlusion. Diabetes predisposes individuals to arterial insufficiency. When arterial obstruction is embolic, the source is often a mural thrombus from mitral stenosis or myocardial infarction, or, in infective endocarditis, a bacterial vegetation.
4. Venous obstruction. There may be a long history of varicose veins, thrombophlebitis, edema, leg trauma, or immobilization.

---

# Physical Examination

## Central Cyanosis

There is bluish discoloration of the skin and mucous membranes.
1. Right-to-left shunt. Cardiac murmur(s) and evidence of right-sided cardiac enlargement are present.
2. Pulmonary disease. See Dyspnea, earlier in this chapter.
3. Clubbing is common in severe central cyanosis but is absent in cyanosis due to hemoglobin abnormalities.

### Peripheral Cyanosis

There is discoloration of only the distal extremities or nail beds.

1. Decreased cardiac output. Hypotension, tachycardia, cold moist extremities, decreased urinary output, and mental confusion are common. Signs of shock may be noted. Evidence of underlying heart disease may be present.
2. Raynaud's phenomenon. Evidence of underlying disease, such as scleroderma, systemic lupus erythematosus, and the cryoglobulinemias, may be noted unless the condition is idiopathic (Raynaud's disease).
3. Arterial obstruction. Signs of arterial occlusion are present (absent pulses, cool skin, skin mottling, and ulcers).
4. Venous obstruction. Signs of venous disease, such as varicose veins, edema, ulceration, and increased pigmentation of the skin, may be noted.

## Chest Roentgenographic Findings

Characteristic roentgenographic findings may be noted in certain types of heart disease and in pulmonary disease. Otherwise, chest films are of little or no diagnostic help in the evaluation of cyanosis.

## Laboratory Data

1. CBC. Erythrocytosis may be seen in right-to-left shunts and in the chronic pulmonary disease.
2. Urinalysis. This may be abnormal in Raynaud's phenomenon, which is associated with connective tissue disease and renal involvement. The abnormal findings include proteinuria, hematuria, and cylindruria.
3. Serum electrolytes and biochemical screening. The serum bicarbonate level may be elevated in a patient with chronic alveolar hypoventilation. The BUN may be elevated in circulatory collapse and decreased cardiac output and in patients with renal hypoperfusion. Acute hepatic injury may be reflected in abnormal liver function tests in patients with circulatory collapse. Liver function tests may also be abnormal in patients with cor pulmonale and chronic passive congestion of the liver. Serum levels of LDH, SGOT, and CPK may be elevated in patients with arterial and venous obstruction, because of skeletal muscle damage. In these patients, the serum bilirubin, serum proteins, and prothrombin time usually are normal.
4. Electrocardiogram. In patients with right-to-left shunt, the electrocardiogram may show findings related to the underlying disease. In patients with pulmonary disease, there may be evidence suggestive of chronic obstructive pulmonary disease with or without cor pulmonale. The electrocardiogram is usually normal in patients with Raynaud's phenomenon, but in those with connective tissue disease, evidence of pericardial or myocardial involvement may be noted. In patients with circulatory collapse, a pattern simulating myocardial infarction is sometimes seen.
5. Arterial blood gases. Hypoxemia is seen in all conditions causing central cyanosis except those with abnormal hemoglobins. Usually the arterial oxygen tension is normal in patients with peripheral cyanosis. Determination of $PO_2$ is thus useful in differentiating between central and peripheral causes of cyanosis. The arterial $PCO_2$ level is elevated in patients who are cyanotic from chronic or acute alveolar hypoventilation. Arterial saturation is low in patients with hypoxemia. Abnormal hemoglobins variably affect the apparent arterial saturation, depending on the method used.
6. Ventilatory function tests. Ventilatory function tests demonstrate a characteristic obstructive pattern in patients with chronic obstructive pulmonary disease. A

restricted pattern is observed in patients with interstitial fibrosing diseases of the lung. A restrictive or obstructive pattern, or both, may be seen in patients with left ventricular failure. DLCO is low in interstitial disease and emphysema and high in left ventricular failure.

7. Other procedures.
   a. Arterial blood gases drawn while the patient is breathing 100% oxygen often show large alveolar-arterial gradients (> 100 mm Hg) in patients with right-to-left shunts and pulmonary arteriovenous fistulas. Smaller alveolar-arterial gradients are seen in advanced obstructive or restrictive pulmonary disease. These are easily differentiated from shunts by the association of markedly abnormal ventilatory function test results.
   b. Cardiac catheterization and pulmonary angiography may be indicated for the diagnosis of congenital cyanotic heart disease and pulmonary arteriovenous fistulas.
   c. Mass spectroscopy of a hemoglobin sample is employed to confirm the diagnosis of methemoglobinemia or sulfhemoglobinemia. Determination of the $P_{50}$ by simultaneous measurement of $PO_2$ and $SO_2$ confirms the presence of abnormal hemoglobins.

## CONSOLIDATION COLLAPSE OF THE LUNG
Stanley B. Reich

### Definition

Occasionally, routine chest roentgenograms show consolidation collapse, or atelectasis, of the lung. This loss of volume of a segment, a lobe, or the whole lung is shown primarily by increased density of the area because of replacement of the air by fluid and displacement of the fissures because of the volume loss. Secondary changes include displacement of the hilum, elevation of the diaphragm, shift of the mediastinum, approximation of the ribs, and overinflation of the remainder of the lung, shown by alteration of vascular shadows. This condition is also called *atelectasis*, but *consolidation collapse* is a more precise and descriptive term.

### Etiology

1. The most serious cause is an endobronchial lesion, such as bronchogenic carcinoma, which causes absorption of air and collection of secretions. The symptoms and signs of infection or irritation may or may not be present.
2. Another cause is passive collapse secondary to adjacent disease, such as pleural effusion, pneumothorax, or thoracoplasty. These conditions usually can be identified easily on the roentgenogram.
3. Adhesive collapse occurs in conditions in which surfactant is diminished, as in the acute respiratory distress syndrome of infants or adults, or following cardiac bypass surgery. These entities usually can be recognized clinically, but radiographic studies are useful in following the progress of the disease.
4. Cicatrization as a result of prior infection and fibrosis may also cause this radiographic appearance. Patients may be asymptomatic at the time of examination but may recall the previous infection responsible for the condition.
5. Occasionally an acute or subacute inflammatory lesion or a pulmonary embolus may cause consolidation and loss of volume of a lung. Improvement and ultimate clearing of the involved lung may take from days to months.
6. Other causes include aspirated foreign bodies, intubation of the right mainstem bronchus, and atelectasis complicating surgery.

## Diagnostic Approach

1. As a first step, all prior films should be obtained if they are available. They may help in determining the time of onset of the disease process.
2. If the changes were present previously and are slowly progressive, a neoplasm must be excluded by bronchoscopy, bronchial brushing, cytologic study, and transbronchial biopsy.
3. If the lesion was present previously but has remained unchanged for a period of 6 months to 1 year, bronchoscopy, transbronchial biopsy with brushing for cytologic and bacteriologic study, and possibly CT scans are indicated to exclude an indolent neoplasm or a chronic inflammatory lesion with fibrotic changes.
4. If the lesion was present previously but has remained unchanged for a year or two, further observation with films taken at 2- to 3-month intervals is probably warranted if bronchoscopy is normal. During this time noninterventional investigation can be carried out (e.g., sputum, cytologic, and bacteriologic studies).
5. If the lesion was not present previously, it may be observed for a 2- to 3-week period while the usual clinical noninterventional investigation is pursued. If the lesion clears completely in that period, no further studies may be necessary except for follow-up films in approximately 3 months. If a residual infiltrate remains or if symptoms persist, it becomes necessary to do bronchoscopy, bronchial brushing, cytologic study, and transbronchial biopsy because neoplasms may show temporary improvement with clearing of an associated inflammatory reaction.
6. If pulmonary embolism is suspected, a lung perfusion/ventilation scan should be done to look for other areas of decreased vascular perfusion. If these are indeterminate, pulmonary angiography may be performed.

# ACUTE PULMONARY RADIOGRAPHIC ABNORMALITIES
William C. Earley

Acute pulmonary lesions often pose problems in differential diagnosis. Pneumonia, pulmonary edema, pulmonary infarction, atelectasis, and pulmonary embolism are the entities usually involved.

## Acute Parenchymal Infiltrates

Excluding neoplasm, parenchymal infiltrates are of three basic types: alveolar, interstitial, and mixed. This differentiation is frequently of considerable help in determining the cause of an infiltrate. On chest films, interstitial infiltrates are linear, linear-nodular, or nodular, with the nodules generally less than 5 mm in diameter. Alveolar infiltrates tend to be fluffy in appearance, with poorly defined borders; they commonly involve segments of lobes or entire lobes, and they frequently demonstrate air bronchograms.

Simply because infiltrates are seen on chest roentgenograms does not necessarily mean they are acute. For example, alveolar infiltrates, usually seen in acute processes, can also be seen in chronic processes such as alveolar cell neoplasm, sarcoidosis, and desquamative interstitial pneumonia. Similarly, interstitial infiltrates are often chronic and may be caused by disparate entities such as Hamman-Rich syndrome, connective tissue disease, granulomatous disease, eosinophilic granuloma, and fibrosis from chronic bronchitis and previous pneumonia. In all of the above instances, previous chest films for comparison and serial films for follow-up are of enormous help in arriving at an accurate diagnosis.

## Pneumonia

Although the radiographic patterns are quite variable and nonspecific, the following points may prove helpful in the diagnosis of pneumonia. Pneumonia due to aspiration may involve any or all segments of both lungs but is more generally seen in the most dependent portions of the lung. Thus, with the patient lying supine, the most dependent parts of the lung are the posterior segments of the upper lobes. Bacterial pneumonia is likely to present an alveolar pattern and involve segments of the lungs asymmetrically. Viral pneumonia tends to be interstitial in pattern and more symmetric and diffuse in distribution. It should be emphasized that these are generalities and that overlapping of patterns and exceptions may occur.

## Pulmonary Edema

Pulmonary edema is most commonly caused by left-sided heart failure, but it may also be the result of other conditions, such as iatrogenic fluid overloading, allergic reaction to medications (particularly blood transfusions), or the acute adult respiratory distress syndrome.

The lung changes in left-sided heart failure usually include the following: (1) pulmonary congestion, manifested by distended upper lobe veins; (2) interstitial edema, demonstrable primarily as narrow, linear strands perpendicular to the nearest pleural surface in the lower lobes; lamellar markings in the upper lobes; a hilar or peripheral haze or both; and at times, thickened interlobar fissures; and (3) alveolar edema, appearing typically as a fluffy infiltrate that tends to involve both lungs symmetrically but is nonetheless quite variable in appearance.

## Atelectasis

Atelectasis, or consolidation collapse of the lung, is discussed separately in the previous section. It is important to realize, however, that atelectasis is the most common postoperative respiratory complication. Plate, disk, or focal atelectasis is the variety most commonly encountered. The appearance of plate atelectasis is that of a rather thin, streaky density, usually located toward the lung bases. These densities are approximately perpendicular to the long axis of the body, but considerable variation is seen. Parenchymal scars from previous inflammatory disease or infarcts are the major differential possibilities. Large areas of atelectasis involving segments, lobes, or entire lungs are seen less frequently, but it is important to recognize them because they may represent serious disease. The major condition to be differentiated from lobar collapse, particularly in the lower lobes, is an encapsulated pleural effusion. The differentiation may be difficult or impossible, but two points may be helpful: (1) Signs of lobar collapse are usually not associated with encapsulated effusions, and (2) decubitus films may occasionally demonstrate fluid shifts with a change in body position.

## Pulmonary Embolism
## with Infarction

Pulmonary embolism that goes on to infarction may show an area of alveolar infiltrate near a pleural surface. Sometimes an infarct may be seen as a homogeneous density with its base adjacent to a pleural surface and its convexity directed toward the hilum. A resolving infarct may appear as a rather broad, streaky density, much like an area of plate atelectasis. The roentgenographic findings in infarction and infection may be identical, and the differentiation between the two entities cannot be made on the basis of chest films alone.

## Pulmonary Embolism
## Without Infarction

Pulmonary embolism without infarction frequently shows little or no abnormality in chest roentgenograms. Plain films may show pleural effusion, decreased vascularity of a lobe or a segment of a lobe, serial changes in the main pulmonary arteries due to alterations of blood flow, or a parenchymal infiltrate. None of these findings is specific for embolism.

A procedure that is sometimes useful in the diagnosis of pulmonary embolism is digital subtraction angiography. This procedure allows the visualization of peripheral arteries by the intravenous injection of contrast medium. For best results the patient must lie motionless during the injection of contrast medium and during filming. Heart motion during the procedure may cause problems, particularly on the left side.

Radionuclide lung scans have proved to be of great value in the diagnosis of pulmonary embolism. There are two types of scans: ventilation and perfusion. There are two varieties of ventilation scans. The most common ventilation scan is performed with xenon 133, a chemically inert gamma-emitting gas. Rapid-sequence images are made during inhalation, rebreathing, and washout of the gas. Normally, washout is complete in about 1 minute. These images show the areas of the lungs where there is no ventilation, delayed ventilation, and delayed washout. Areas of chronic obstructive pulmonary disease characteristically show mild delay in ventilation and a marked delay in washout. One problem exists with the xenon scan: the examination is routinely done in the posterior projection. If additional views done in different projections are desired for more accurate comparison with the perfusion scan, an additional dose of xenon is required.

The second variety of ventilation scan involves the use of very small particles of diethylene triamine penta acetic acid (DTPA) labeled with technetium 99m, a gamma-emitting isotope. The very small labeled particles of DTPA are given by inhalation. With this radiopharmaceutical, multiple views in different projections can be obtained, but the washout is not well evaluated. The ventilation scan usually precedes the perfusion scan.

The perfusion scan consists of an intravenous injection of myriads of small particles of albumin. The particles range in size from 10 to 100 microns and are labeled with technetium 99m, a gamma emitter. In effect, multiple, tiny radioactive-labeled emboli are being injected. The procedure is safe, and there are no contraindications. As with the ventilation scans, preexisting entities such as pneumonia, chronic bronchitis, emphysematous bullae, asthma, neoplasm, and heart failure can cause abnormalities in the perfusion scan.

When interpreting lung scans it is essential to have current chest films available for comparison. Areas in the lungs that ventilate normally but do not perfuse have a high probability of being caused by emboli.

## Lung Infiltrates in AIDS

The AIDS patient is more susceptible to the common bacterial pneumonias than individuals who are not immunologically compromised. The radiographic appearance of common infiltrates in the AIDS patient are often more severe and extensive than in the immunologically competent patient but are otherwise similar.

Listed below are some of the unusual infecting agents found in AIDS together with their most common radiographic appearances.

1. *Pneumocystis carinii* pneumonia (PCP). This infection is found in 80 to 85 percent of cases at some time during the course of the illness. Most commonly observed

**Table 4-2.** Perfusion and ventilation scans in the differential diagnosis of pulmonary lesions

| Disease | Perfusion scan | Ventilation scan |
|---|---|---|
| Embolism without infarction | No perfusion | Normal ventilation |
| Pneumonia | No perfusion | No ventilation |
| Embolism with infarction (infiltrate in lungs) | No perfusion | Decreased to no ventilation |
| Emphysematous bullae | No perfusion | Delayed ventilation; delayed washout |
| Chronic bronchitis | Decreased perfusion | Normal to delayed ventilation; delayed washout |

is a diffuse interstitial infiltrate, sometimes with an alveolar component, involving both lungs. The distribution tends to be symmetrical. Areas of hyperinflation and focal consolidation are not usually seen.

2. Histoplasmosis. The chest x-ray findings may resemble those seen in bacterial pneumonia, PCP, or tuberculosis.
3. Coccidioidomycosis. Nodular or interstitial infiltrates, or both, may be seen. Less common are cavitation and enlarged hilar nodes.
4. Cryptococcosis. The infiltrates may be diffuse or lobar with an alevolar or interstitial pattern. An occasional isolated nodule may occur.
5. Tuberculosis. Common findings are hilar and mediastinal lymphadenopathy and lower- and mid-lung infiltrates. Cavitation and apical infiltrates are rarely observed.

Table 4-2 lists the results of perfusion and ventilation scans in commonly occurring disease entities.

## THE SOLITARY PULMONARY NODULE

James H. Ellis, Jr.

### Definition

The solitary pulmonary nodule is usually defined in radiographic terms as a lesion that is single, round or ovoid, and less than 6 cm in diameter. It has distinct margins (i.e., it is surrounded by aerated lung parenchyma) and does not abut the chest wall, diaphragm, or mediastinum. It may or may not contain calcium. Although it is most often asymptomatic, cough, hemoptysis, or both may occur. Painful clubbing and endocrinopathy are extremely rare manifestations of solitary pulmonary nodules that subsequently prove to be bronchial carcinomas.

### Etiology

The most common causes of solitary pulmonary nodules are healed granulomas, primary pulmonary malignancies, pulmonary metastases, arteriovenous malformations, and pulmonary hamartomas.

The true incidence of such nodules is difficult to establish and varies greatly with such factors as the availability of routine or screening chest x-rays, the age of the population examined, and the incidence of endemic fungal infections (especially histoplasmosis and coccidioidomycosis). The same factors also influence the percentage of bronchial carcinomas in most reported series. For example, one mass x-ray screening program in 1949, involving 673,218 individuals in an area in which histoplasmosis was endemic, revealed only a 3 percent incidence of cancer in patients with solitary pulmonary nodules. (This was a period when the true frequency of bronchial carcinomas was lower than it is today.) On the other hand, the incidence of bronchial carcinoma was 63 percent in a series of highly selected "older" patients who had undergone thoracotomy for solitary nodules. In most series of patients with solitary nodules who have undergone thoracotomy, the reported incidence of bronchial carcinoma is about 36 percent.

## Diagnostic Approach

1. The primary problem confronting the physician when a solitary nodule is discovered is to determine whether nonsurgical measures or thoracotomy should be employed to establish the diagnosis. The decision, of course, depends on whether the lesion is benign or malignant. Benign nodules rarely require surgical removal. On the other hand, if the nodule is a bronchial carcinoma or adenoma it is potentially "curable" surgically, provided no metastases have occurred. Solitary pulmonary metastases from a primary extrapulmonary malignancy should seldom be removed and then only when the original tumor and other metastases have been controlled.

    Four factors generally determine the diagnostic approach: the age of the patient, the age and rate of growth of the lesion, the presence or absence of calcification within the nodule, and the patient's smoking history.

    a. Statistical studies indicate that below the age of 30, solitary nodules are infrequently malignant. Thereafter, the incidence of malignancy increases with advancing age.

    b. A second important consideration is the age and rapidity of growth of the lesion. If previous chest films can be obtained, the growth rate or stability of the patient's nodule often can be determined. An exhaustive search should be made for previous chest x-rays. Comparison of current and previous films may even obviate the need for invasive procedures and hospitalization. Earlier films are helpful because of the well-known and highly predictable growth rate of primary bronchial carcinomas. The "doubling time" of the nodule refers to the doubling in volume of the nodule. From the volume of a sphere ($V = 4\pi r^3$), it can be seen that a tumor doubles in volume when its diameter or radius increases by a factor of 1.26 (the cube root of 2). Thus, when a 10-mm nodule has increased in size to 12.6 cm (10 mm × 1.26), its volume has doubled. The mean doubling time of untreated primary bronchial carcinoma in a series of 41 patients was about 41.1 months for undifferentiated neoplasms, 4.2 months for squamous cell carcinomas, and 7.3 months for adenocarcinomas. The range of doubling times for primary bronchial carcinomas was 1 to 15 months. Single pulmonary nodules that double in size in less than 1 month are almost always either benign inflammatory lesions or, less often, solitary metastases of rapidly growing tumors such as chorionic carcinomas, testicular tumors, and osteogenic sarcomas.

    c. The presence of calcification within the lesion makes it extremely unlikely that the lesion is a primary bronchial cancer. Tomograms can often demonstrate calcium that is not seen on routine films. If there is uncertainty about the presence of calcification after tomography, the nodule should be managed as though it were noncalcified. A ring-shaped or target pattern of calcification is usually indicative of a histoplasmoma. A "popcorn" pattern is highly characteristic of a hamartoma. Both patterns are reliable signs of a benign lesion. Nodules with small "flecks" of calcium are most likely to be benign, but if the patient has other high risk factors, such as age over 35 years and a heavy smoking history, such nodules should be observed by repeated chest films at 1- to 3-month intervals.

**d.** Cigarette smoking is also an important consideration. The overwhelming majority of bronchial carcinomas occur in cigarette smokers. However, bronchial adenocarcinomas occasionally occur in nonsmokers, particularly in women. Alveolar cell carcinoma also does not bear a particularly specific relationship to smoking.

2. The workup of the patient can be performed on either an outpatient or inpatient basis. A complete history and physical examination plus routine laboratory tests, such as CBC, urinalysis, and biochemical screening, may suggest additional studies.

   A tuberculin stain test probably should be performed. Although a positive skin test confirms previous infection with the organism, it does not necessarily establish the cause of the nodule.

   Sputum specimens should be obtained for cytologic smears and cultures, for conventional pathogens as well as for acid-fast bacilli and fungi.

3. Bronchial carcinomas unfortunately metastasize early and extensively by hematogenous, lymphangitic, and direct extension. The latter mechanism is essentially ruled out by the definition of solitary nodule (i.e., surrounded by aerated lung parenchyma). Lymphatic extension outside of the thorax most frequently goes to supraclavicular and cervical lymph nodes. Occasionally, infraclavicular and axillary nodes are involved. Careful palpation of these areas is essential. Biopsy of any hard or enlarged nodes usually is indicated and, if positive, will abort the need for more invasive and risky tests. Hematogenous spread of bronchial carcinoma has a high incidence and a preference for organs with a rich blood supply, such as the brain, other areas of the lung, the liver, adrenals, bone, and even the skin (e.g., subcutaneous nodules). Except for pain from far advanced metastasis, bony involvement is often silent. Serum calcium, phosphorus, and alkaline phosphatase levels are not very sensitive screening procedures for bony involvement. Bone scans are much more sensitive indicators of bony metastasis and should be obtained before thoracotomy. Since bone scans sometimes give false positive results, an otherwise indicated thoracotomy should not be ruled out without careful consideration.

   Between 80 and 88 percent of patients with a solitary metastasis from an extrathoracic primary carcinoma give a history of previous diagnosis of the neoplasm. Most of the remainder have symptoms and signs or abnormal screening test results that suggest an extrapulmonary primary malignancy.

   If there is not evidence of extrathoracic cancer, then preoperative evaluation to determine if the patient can reasonably tolerate thoracotomy and lobectomy is indicated. This simply means careful attention to the cardiopulmonary history, particularly the patient's exercise tolerance. Current spirometry, arterial blood gas analysis, and an electrocardiogram are indicated. Ventilation/perfusion scanning, formal treadmill exercise, and cardiac catheterization are usually reserved for patients with unusual situations or borderline cardiopulmonary reserve.

4. Patients with a nodule of less than 1.5 cm in diameter seldom have mediastinal node involvement. Unless the hila are obviously enlarged on chest x-ray, mediastinoscopy does not seem necessary or indicated. On the other hand, the larger the nodule, the more likely it is that mediastinal node involvement will occur. Mediastinoscopy should be performed routinely, if possible, to avoid thoracotomy in patients who are beyond the stage of surgical cure. Most experts agree that contralateral, "high" ipsilateral, or subcarinal nodal involvement is a contraindication to thoracotomy. Positive nodes limited to "low" ipsilateral or intralobar positions, although certainly a poor prognostic sign, may not be an absolute contraindication to surgery, especially if combined with irradiation.

5. The most valuable diagnostic procedure is fiberoptic bronchoscopy performed under fluoroscopic control, provided the lesion is accessible to the bronchoscope. Bronchial brushing should be done, specimens collected for cytologic study and cultures, and a transbronchial biopsy obtained.

   Fiberoptic bronchoscopy with brush and transbronchial biopsy has a diagnostic accuracy of approximately 80 percent, with very acceptable morbidity and probably less than 0.1 percent mortality. Fluoroscopic-guided, percutaneous needle-aspiration biopsy approaches 80 percent accuracy for diagnosing malignant nodules, with a risk that is only slightly increased over that of bronchoscopic biopsy. The "borderline" patient and the conservative surgeon may be willing to accept the high risks of lobectomy even when cancer is present. Also, even when thoracotomy is not a consideration, a positive diagnosis helps in choosing therapy and increasing accuracy of prognosis.

6. If all studies including cultures are negative, radiologic studies should be performed 1 month later to determine the progress of the lesion. If after 1 month of study the cause of the nodule is undetermined, and the lesion has either remained unchanged in size or grown larger, surgical resection is indicated. If the lesion becomes smaller during the 1-month observation period, it is likely that the nodule represents an atypical inflammatory or embolic lesion rather than a neoplasm. Under these circumstances, a more conservative approach is probably warranted. It is then appropriate to continue chest films once a month for an additional 3-month period, and, when the lesion stabilizes, at intervals of 6 months or longer.

If investigation, including biopsy, proves the lesion to be benign, surgical removal is rarely necessary. However, if the etiology cannot be determined or malignancy is established, the lesion should be resected unless there are contraindications to its removal.

7. Major errors in the management of a solitary pulmonary nodule are failure to (a) follow a logical workup due to predetermined bias, (b) obtain old films, (c) provide a basic workup for metastatic disease, (d) observe the patient and nodule for 30 days when the lesion is new, (e) make any decision, and (f) recommend thoracotomy with conviction when indicated.

## MEDIASTINAL MASSES
John C. Riley

### The Mediastinum

The mediastinum is the extrapleural space within the thorax, lying between the lungs. It is bounded by the sternum anteriorly, the paravertebral regions posteriorly, the thoracic inlet superiorly, and the diaphragm inferiorly. The aerated lungs outline the structures within the mediastinum.

Division of the mediastinum into exact compartments is rather controversial, and newer definitions are proposed frequently. One of the most commonly used classifications divides the mediastinum into three compartments, as ascertained from the lateral chest radiograph. The anterior mediastinum is bounded by an imaginary line projected from the diaphragm and along the back of the heart and in front of the trachea to the neck. The posterior mediastinum is behind another imaginary vertical line that connects a point on each thoracic vertebra 1 cm behind its anterior margin. In between these two imaginary lines lies the middle mediastinum. Using this definition, the anterior mediastinum contains the thymus, ascending aorta, heart, and pericardium. The middle mediastinum contains the trachea, esophagus, hili and hilar lymph nodes, aortic arch, and numerous other lymph nodes and nerves. The posterior mediastinum contains a portion of the descending aorta and numerous nerves, including part of the sympathetic chain.

### Etiology

Each type of mediastinal tumor has a predilection for one of the three mediastinal compartments. Table 4-3 lists the common causes of mediastinal tumors and

**Table 4-3.** Sites of predilection of mediastinal masses in approximate decreasing order of occurrence

| Anterior mediastinum | Middle mediastinum | Posterior mediastinum |
| --- | --- | --- |
| Thymoma | Hiatal hernias | Neurogenic tumors |
| Teratoma | Lymph node disease (e.g., lymphoma, metastatic disease, sarcoidosis) | Aneurysm of descending aorta |
| Retrosternal thyroid | | Hernia (Bochdalek) |
| Lymphoma | Bronchogenic and tracheal tumors | Abscess |
| Aneurysm of ascending aorta | | Extramedullary hematopoiesis |
| Pericardial cyst and cardiac abnormalities | Bronchoenteric cysts | Anterior meningocele |
| Hematomas | Esophageal lesions other than hernias | |
| Parathyroid tumors | | |
| Hernias (Morgagni) | | |
| Mesenchymal tumors | | |

masses according to the region in the mediastinum in which they are most likely to be found. About 55 percent of mediastinal tumors occur in the anterior mediastinum, 30 percent in the middle mediastinum, and 15 percent in the posterior mediastinum. Approximately 50 percent of all mediastinal tumors are malignant.

The tumors most common in the anterior mediastinum include goiters, thymomas, teratomas, and lymphomas. The most common middle mediastinal tumors include diseases of the lymph nodes and bronchoenteric cysts. Although bronchogenic carcinomas may arise within the boundary of the mediastinum, they generally are regarded as parenchymal rather than mediastinal lung lesions. Neurogenic tumors are by far the most common posterior mediastinal tumors.

It is important to note that about 90 percent of middle mediastinal tumors are either primary or metastatic malignancies. Bilateral hilar lymph node enlargement is usually due to lymphoma but may occasionally be due to sarcoidosis. Unilateral lymphadenopathy is usually caused by a central or peripheral lesion of the lung, such as bronchogenic carcinoma or infection.

## Diagnostic Approach

1. The history and physical examination are usually of little value in the diagnosis of mediastinal tumors. The diagnosis is commonly established by routine chest roentgenograms. Symptoms such as cough, dyspnea, hemoptysis, and chest pain may be noted, but they are nonspecific. The occurrence of facial edema, hoarseness, nonpulsatile distention of the neck veins, or Horner's syndrome may suggest compression or displacement due to mediastinal structures. A history of anorexia, weakness, fever, and weight loss in association with generalized lymphadenopathy suggests lymphoma, Hodgkin's disease, or leukemia.
2. Routine PA and lateral chest films may be adequate for the detection and localization of mediastinal masses. Overpenetrated or high-KV films with Bucky technique are seldom used since computerized tomography (CT) is so widely available. Similarly, angled tomography of the hila is rarely used since CT has been so effective.
3. Barium swallow is occasionally useful if carcinoma of the esophagus is suspected. Chest fluoroscopy can occasionally be useful in evaluating for pulsatile lesions and a paralyzed hemidiaphragm.

**Table 4-4.** Differential diagnosis of pleural effusion

| Etiology | Characteristics of effusion | Clinical findings | Laboratory findings and diagnostic procedures |
|---|---|---|---|
| **Transudates: Protein less than 3 g/100 ml with normal serum protein concentration, LDH <200 IU, LDH ratio <0.6** | | | |
| Congestive heart failure | Usually right-sided but may be bilateral; may be localized to an interlobar fissure | Orthopnea, paroxysmal nocturnal dyspnea, tachycardia, cardiomegaly, gallop rhythm, murmurs, rales, peripheral edema | Chest films; electrocardiogram |
| Cirrhosis | Right-sided, occasionally left-sided or bilateral | Ascites, peripheral edema, physical signs of cirrhosis | Liver function tests; liver biopsy |
| Nephrotic syndrome | Bilateral or unilateral | Generalized edema; periorbital edema is characteristic; pallor | Cylindruria and proteinuria, hypoalbuminemia, hyperlipidemia |
| Meigs' syndrome | Usually right-sided, occasionally left-sided or bilateral; rarely, effusion is bloody; no malignant cells present | Benign or malignant ovarian tumor, rarely uterine fibroma; ascites always present | Removal of the tumor resolves the effusion and ascites |
| **Exudates: Protein greater than 3 g/100 ml with normal serum protein concentration, LDH >200 IU, LDH ratio ≧0.6** | | | |
| Bacterial or viral pneumonia (parapneumonic effusion) | Same side as infiltrate; polymorphonuclear leukocytes; no organisms seen; may be loculated | Pleuritic pain; friction rub may be present; may see recurrence of fever | Precedes clinical picture of pneumonia; usually resorbed within 2 weeks |
| Pulmonary infarction | May be serosanguinous; polymorphonuclear leukocytes | Pleuritic pain; friction rub, fever (<101°F); right ventricular heave; murmur of pulmonary insufficiency; increased $P_2$, right-sided $S_4$ or $S_3$ | Positive radioisotope scans; pulmonary angiography may also provide diagnosis |

| Disease | Pleural Fluid Findings | Clinical Features | Diagnosis |
|---|---|---|---|
| Tuberculosis | Lymphocytic pleural effusion; may be serosanguinous; acid-fast organisms rarely seen; increased cholesterol content if chronic | Usually pleuritic pain and fever in young adults; frequently asymptomatic | Positive skin test; pleural biopsy with histopathologic and bacteriologic studies |
| Rheumatoid arthritis | Polymorphonuclear leukocytes; glucose low; cholesterol may be elevated; LDH markedly elevated; complement low; low pH | More common in males; other systemic rheumatoid involvement (e.g., arthritis, subcutaneous nodules) | Positive serum rheumatoid factor; biopsy of subcutaneous nodule or synovium rarely indicated |
| Lupus erythematosus | Polymorphonuclear leukocytes; fluid glucose equals blood glucose; may be transudate if associated with heart failure or the nephrotic syndrome | Arthritis, skin rash, renal disease; superficial thrombophlebitis | Positive serologic results; urinary sediment abnormalities; renal or skin biopsy |
| Lymphoproliferative disorders | Polymorphonuclear leukocytes, lymphocytes, rarely eosinophils; occasionally transudate; rarely chylothorax | Night sweats, fever, pruritus; adenopathy; hepatosplenomegaly; chest roentgenogram may reveal hilar and mediastinal lymphadenopathy or parenchymal nodules or infiltrates | Lymph node, skin, pleural, liver, or bone marrow biopsy leads to diagnosis |
| Primary lymphedema | | Yellow fingernails, peripheral lymphedema; may follow upper respiratory illness | Normal cardiac, renal, and liver function |
| Myxedema | Frequently bilateral; may be transudate if associated with myocardial or pericardial disease | Clinical findings of myxedema; large heart on x-ray | Abnormal thyroid function test results |
| Subphrenic abscess | Polymorphonuclear leukocytes, occasionally a transudate ("sympathetic" effusion) | May follow ruptured viscus; amebic abscess; complication of abdominal surgery | Liver-lung radioisotope scan; CT scan or ultrasound |

**Table 4-4** (continued)

| Etiology | Characteristics of effusion | Clinical findings | Laboratory findings and diagnostic procedures |
|----------|------------------------------|-------------------|----------------------------------------------|
| **Exudates: Protein greater than 3 g/100 ml with normal serum protein concentration, LDH >200 IU, LDH ratio $\geqq$ 0.6** | | | |
| Peritoneal dialysis | No specific characteristics | Clinical picture is evident | Disappears following drainage of peritoneal cavity |
| Hydronephrosis | No specific characteristics | Picture of urinary obstruction | Disappears with relief of obstruction |
| Leakage through a subclavian vein catheter | Reflects characteristics of the intravenous fluid; may be transudate | | |
| Malignancy | Malignant cells; lymphocytes or polymorphonuclear leukocytes; major cause of hemorrhagic pleural effusions | History and physical findings of a primary or metastatic cancer; history of asbestos exposure in suspected mesothelioma | Pleural biopsy frequently positive |
| Pancreatitis | Polymorphonuclear leukocytes; high amylase; usually on left, but may be bilateral; occasionally it is transudate | Severe abdominal pain with radiation to back | Elevated serum and urine amylase |
| Pneumothorax | May contain inflammatory cells | Sudden onset of pain, dyspnea, cough; chest radiogram demonstrates an air-fluid level | |

| | | | |
|---|---|---|---|
| Chest trauma | May contain inflammatory cells; frequently hemorrhagic | | May be closed or open; chest x-ray may demonstrate fractured ribs or a pulmonary contusion |
| **Chylothorax** | | | |
| Chest trauma; lymphoma; postsurgical complication | Milky fluid; normal cholesterol; increased lipid content; positive Sudan III stain | Recent trauma or chest surgery; findings of lymphomatous disease | Lymph node biopsy indicated for palpable nodes |
| **Empyema** | | | |
| Bacterial, fungal, or tuberculous pneumonia; chest trauma; thoracic surgery; mediastinitis; lung abscess; ruptured subdiaphragmatic abscess | Polymorphonuclear leukocytes; may be lymphocytic in tuberculosis; organisms may be seen by Gram stain; may be loculated; low pH; grossly purulent | Fever, pleuritic chest pain, and findings associated with underlying etiology | Fluid culture positive (fungus, tuberculous, aerobic or anaerobic cultures); blood cultures occasionally positive |

LVH = left ventricular hypertrophy

4. Computerized tomography is used to evaluate any abnormal mediastinal lesion. The exact location (e.g., extrapleural, chest wall, mediastinum) may be established readily by this procedure, and critical information regarding the content of the lesions (fat, calcium, blood) may be obtained. CT is most often the definitive diagnostic tool for suspected mediastinal disease. Similarly, magnetic resonance imaging is especially useful in evaluating for vascular abnormalities such as aneurysms and dissecting hematomas. At this time, however, CT remains the primary and definitive method of evaluating the majority of mediastinal abnormalities.

5. Certain radiologic signs may provide clues to the causes of mediastinal tumors. These are discussed below.

   a. Content of the lesion. The presence of fat in the lesion suggests mediastinal teratoma, lipoma, fat pad, omental hernia, or hibernoma. Curvilinear calcifications suggest a cyst or aneurysm, but they may also be seen in thymomas or thyroid adenomas. An anterior calcified mass in a patient with myasthenia gravis is almost certainly a thymoma. A tooth is a sign of teratoma, and a phlebolith, of hemangioma. Gas in the mediastinum may occur in hiatal hernia, ruptured esophagus, or pneumomediastinum. Usually, these conditions can be easily differentiated from one another.

   b. Configuration of the mass. The configuration of mediastinal masses may have diagnostic significance. A huge esophagus, dilated from stricture, achalasia, or tumor, is likely to be long and broad and to contain an air-fluid level. Benign pericardial cysts, which are inseparable from the cardiac silhouette and occur most frequently in the anterior cardiophrenic angle, typically appear as sharply defined lesions of soft-tissue density. They may or may not transmit the cardiac pulsations. Thymic tumors in adults are irregular but smoothly outlined anterior mediastinal masses. Teratomas are usually well-defined structures containing hair, bone, or teeth. Substernal goiters merge with the soft tissues of the neck, move with swallowing, and tend to displace the trachea. Lymphomas may occur as frequently in the anterior as in the middle mediastinum and usually appear as dense, rounded masses. Bronchogenic cysts usually show as oval, sharply demarcated, soft-tissue densities that compress adjacent structures. Neural tumors in the posterior mediastinum may have a dumbbell or hourglass configuration.

   c. Change in size. The rapidity of growth of a mass is of limited diagnostic value because benign lesions may grow quickly and malignant ones slowly.

   d. Evidence of disease in other locations. It is almost certain that a mediastinal mass is metastatic in a young male with a testicular carcinoma. Enlarged mediastinal nodes are frequently found in lymphomas, leukemia, Hodgkin's disease, tuberculosis, and sarcoidosis. Paraspinal widening in a young child strongly suggests abdominal neuroblastoma.

6. In the presence of lymphadenopathy, skin tests for tuberculosis, histoplasmosis, coccidioidomycosis, and sarcoidosis may be indicated. Bone marrow examination and scalene or other lymph node biopsy may also be advisable.

7. Sputum cultures should be performed if tuberculosis or fungus disease is suspected.

8. If the diagnosis cannot be established on the basis of the foregoing studies, or if confirmation of a presumptive diagnosis is necessary, one or more of the following procedures may be indicated.

   a. Angiography is an accurate method of diagnosing vascular lesions of the mediastinum. MRI and CT, however, frequently give sufficient information so that angiography is not needed. Selective angiography (especially with digital subtraction techniques) is occasionally used in evaluating the postoperative neck and mediastinum for recurrent or persistent parathyroid adenomas.

   b. Echocardiography is the least expensive and least effective method of evaluating pericardial effusions and other cardiac and pericardiac abnormalities. Ultrasound is also occasionally useful in differentiating between cystic and solid masses.

**c.** Venography is useful when searching for anomalies or obstruction of the vena cava or azygous vein.

**d.** Radionuclide studies are valuable in the following cases:

**(1)** Radioactive iodine for thyroid goiters.

**(2)** Gallium scans for abscesses and neoplastic disorders.

**(3)** Monoclonal antibody techniques are being developed for diagnosis and treatment.

**e.** Bronchoscopy is of value in evaluating endobronchial lesions such as bronchogenic carcinomas. Bronchography is rarely used anymore.

**f.** Myelography is rarely useful in diagnosing posterior neural tumors and meningoceles. MRI, when available, is much better for these.

**g.** Computerized tomography remains by far the most effective tool in evaluating mediastinal lesions. The newer units can obtain high-resolution millimeter-thick slices, which are useful in evaluating the parenchyma of the lung. Dynamic CT with rapid IV contrast injection techniques and rapid slice acquisition is extremely useful in evaluating and differentiating vascular and nonvascular mediastinal lesions.

**h.** Magnetic resonance imaging is being used more commonly in patients with chest problems. The newer instruments using gradient techniques, cine–real time, and rapid three-dimensional acquired images are becoming the norm in many centers. MRI spectroscopy may soon provide insight into tissue specificity.

**9.** The final step in any approach to mediastinal tumors, unless the diagnosis has been established by other means, is a biopsy of the lesion by either thoracotomy or mediastinoscopy.

**10.** It is dangerous and inadvisable to "treat" a mediastinal tumor by observation. Every effort must be made to establish a diagnosis promptly to ensure proper treatment. If the lesion is malignant, it may be curable by surgery even though the resectability rate is low. An aggressive approach is also warranted in the diagnosis of benign lesions of the mediastinum because life-threatening complications may ensue if the lesion is not treated appropriately.

## DIFFERENTIAL DIAGNOSIS OF PLEURAL EFFUSION

Marvin I. Schwarz
Paul M. Cox, Jr.

The diagnostic features of pleural effusions are shown in Table 4-4. In the evaluation of a pleural effusion, it is important first to determine whether it is an exudate or transudate. If it is believed to be an exudate, additional diagnostic studies (e.g., cytologic study, culture, biopsy) must be undertaken. If the fluid is a transudate, attention should be directed to the underlying cause of the effusion (e.g., congestive heart failure, cirrhosis of the liver, nephrotic syndrome, hypoproteinemia). Exudates are characterized by one or more of the following features: a pleural fluid/serum protein ratio greater than 0.5, a pleural fluid lactic dehydrogenase (LDH) greater than 200 IU, and a pleural fluid/serum LDH ratio greater than 0.6. Transudates exhibit none of these abnormalities.

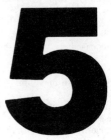

# Gastrointestinal Problems

## ABDOMINAL PAIN
### Sunder J. Mehta

Pain is the most common complaint of patients with gastrointestinal disorders. There is enormous individual variation in reaction to pain, and this important challenge to the physician can be met only by a thorough history and careful objective analysis.

## Types

Classically, abdominal pain is separated into three categories: visceral, parietal, and referred.

Visceral pain is felt at the site of primary stimulation. It is usually dull, aching, and poorly localized, and frequently difficult to describe. It may or may not be associated with referred pain. Parietal pain is a deep somatic pain that arises from irritation or inflammation of the parietal peritoneum or the root of the mesentery. It is more definite and easier to describe than visceral pain. Referred pain is pain felt at a site other than that stimulated, but in an area supplied by the same or adjacent neural segments.

The location of pain arising from specific organs is outlined in Table 5-1.

## Clinical Syndromes

The acuteness of abdominal pain determines the clinical approach to this important symptom and is therefore discussed under the separate headings of Acute Abdominal Pain and Chronic and Recurrent Abdominal Pain.

## Acute Abdominal Pain

Many diseases, some of which are nonsurgical, may cause acute abdominal pain (Table 5-2). The most common causes of acute abdominal pain are acute gastroenteritis, inflammatory disease (appendicitis, cholecystitis, diverticulitis, pancreatitis, salpingitis), renal and biliary colic, intestinal obstruction, and perforation of a viscus.

### Clinical Features

The salient findings of the more common conditions are outlined below. However, it must be borne in mind that many of these entities exhibit variant or atypical patterns.

**Table 5-1.** Location of pain from specific organs

| Organ | Location |
|---|---|
| Esophagus | Substernal; occasionally neck, jaw, arm, or back |
| Stomach | Epigastrium; occasionally left upper quadrant and back |
| Duodenal bulb | Epigastrium; occasionally right upper quadrant and back |
| Small intestine | Periumbilical; occasionally above the lesion |
| Colon | Below umbilicus, on the side of the lesion |
| Splenic flexure | Left upper quadrant |
| Rectosigmoid | Suprapubic region |
| Rectum | Posteriorly, over the sacrum |
| Pancreas | Epigastrium or back |
| Liver and gallbladder | Right upper quadrant, right shoulder, and posterior chest |

**Table 5-2.** Some important causes of abdominal pain

I. Pain originating in the abdomen
    A. Parietal peritoneal inflammation
        1. Bacterial contamination (e.g., perforated appendix, pelvic inflammatory disease)
        2. Chemical irritation (e.g., perforated ulcer, pancreatitis, mittelschmerz)
    B. Mechanical obstruction of hollow viscera
        1. Obstruction of the small or large intestine
        2. Obstruction of the biliary tree
        3. Obstruction of the ureter
    C. Vascular disturbances
        1. Embolism or thrombosis causing intestinal ischemia
        2. Nonocclusive intestinal ischemia
        3. Rupture of an abdominal aortic aneurysm
        4. Sickle cell anemia
    D. Abdominal wall disorders
        1. Distortion or traction of mesentery
        2. Trauma or infection of muscles
        3. Distention of visceral surfaces (e.g., hepatic or renal capsules)
II. Pain referred from extraabdominal sources
    A. Thorax (e.g., pneumonia, referred pain from coronary occlusion)
    B. Spine (e.g., radiculitis from arthritis)
    C. Genitalia (e.g., torsion of the testicle)
III. Metabolic causes
    A. Exogenous
        1. Black widow spider bite
        2. Lead and other poisoning
    B. Endogenous
        1. Uremia
        2. Diabetic ketoacidosis
        3. Porphyria
        4. Allergic factors (C′1-esterase deficiency)
IV. Neurogenic causes
    A. Organic
        1. Tabes dorsalis
        2. Herpes zoster
        3. Causalgia
    B. Functional

Source: Modified from W. Silen, Abdominal Pain. In G. W. Thorn, et al. (eds.), *Harrison's Principles of Internal Medicine* (8th ed.). New York: McGraw-Hill, 1976. P. 34.

1. Acute gastroenteritis.
   a. Anorexia, nausea, vomiting (common).
   b. Crampy, rather poorly localized abdominal pain and tenderness.
   c. Diarrhea (common).
   d. Fever and leukocytosis (common).
2. Acute appendicitis.
   a. Perforation is uncommon before 24 to 36 hours from the onset of symptoms. Initially, pain is diffuse epigastric or periumbilical, eventually shifting to the right lower quadrant (RLQ) of the abdomen.
   b. Nausea and acute loss of appetite are common; vomiting less so.
   c. Constipation or diarrhea is an inconsistent symptom.
   d. Tenderness, muscle spasm, and rebound tenderness in RLQ are frequently absent at the onset but become more evident after 24 hours.
   e. Fever is usually slight to moderate, especially during the first 12 hours.
   f. Moderate leukocytosis with neutrophilia is a late finding.
   g. With a retrocecal appendix, pain, vomiting, and RLQ muscular rigidity are less common.
   h. Plain x-ray of the abdomen may occasionally show a calcified appendolith. Ultrasound may be useful if perforation has occurred. Barium enema x-rays are not needed.
3. Acute cholecystitis.
   a. Previous history of fatty food intolerance, flatulence, postprandial fullness, and RUQ discomfort (common, but nonspecific).
   b. Steady, severe pain in RUQ or epigastrium.
   c. Tenderness, muscle guarding, and rebound tenderness (common). The gall-bladder may be palpable.
   d. Anorexia, nausea, and vomiting (common).
   e. Fever and leukocytosis (common).
   f. Radiopaque gallstones occasionally revealed by plain abdominal x-rays. Imaging of the gallbladder and biliary tree with either ultrasonography or iso-tope scanning with HIDA or PAPIDA is very helpful for a quick and accurate diagnosis. Oral cholecystography, although useful for the diagnosis of gall-stones, requires 12 to 36 hours to be completed. ERCP may be needed if acute cholangitis is suspected. Intravenous cholangiography is obsolete.
   g. Mild hyperbilirubinemia and bilirubinuria (common).
4. Acute diverticulitis.
   a. Lower abdominal pain, especially in the LLQ (common).
   b. Tenderness, muscle guarding, and rebound tenderness (common).
   c. Fever and leukocytosis (common).
   d. Constipation (common).
   e. Nausea, sometimes vomiting (common).
   f. Findings like those of acute appendicitis, but left-sided.
5. Acute pancreatitis.
   a. Common in alcoholics.
   b. Common in patients with cholelithiasis.
   c. May occur in hyperlipidemias.
   d. Abdominal pain variable, ranging from mild to severe, typically epigastric with radiation to the back. May be accompanied by prostration, sweating, and shock.
   e. Nausea and vomiting (common).
   f. Abdominal tenderness in epigastrium (common).
   g. Elevated serum or urinary amylase levels, or both (not pathognomonic). Elevated serum lipase (common).
   h. Hyperbilirubinemia and hypocalcemia may occur.
   i. Fever, leukocytosis (common).
6. Acute intestinal obstruction. The symptomatology depends on the site and completeness of the obstruction.
   a. Crampy abdominal pain (common).
   b. Vomiting (more common with obstruction of the proximal gut).

   c. Constipation; eventually complete inability to pass feces or flatus (common).

   d. Abdominal distention and tenderness (common).

   e. Hyperperistalsis and borborygmi are inconsistent symptoms.

   f. Radiographic evidence of bowel distended with gas proximal to the site of obstruction. Air-fluid levels common.

**7.** Perforated viscus.

   a. Most commonly produced by perforation of a peptic ulcer.

   b. Sudden onset of severe abdominal pain, aggravated by movement.

   c. Tenderness, abdominal rigidity, and rebound tenderness (common).

   d. Abdominal distention (uncommon initially).

   e. Obliteration of hepatic dullness (uncommon).

   f. Air demonstrable below the diaphragm in the roentgenogram (common).

   g. Hypotension and shock are common later on.

**8.** Mesenteric vascular infarction.

   a. Clinical setting often that of congestive heart failure, atrial fibrillation, or visceral hypoperfusion.

   b. Moderate to severe abdominal pain (common).

   c. Vomiting (inconstant).

   d. Bloody diarrhea (inconstant).

   e. Abdominal distention, tenderness, and rigidity in severe cases.

   f. Hypotension and shock in severe cases.

**9.** Acute salpingitis.

   a. Lower abdominal pain.

   b. Chills and fever.

   c. History of sexual exposure.

   d. Vaginal discharge.

   e. Adnexal mass(es).

   f. Demonstration of gonococcal infection or chlamydial infection.

## Diagnostic Approach

It is of the utmost importance to diagnose early. The most important question facing the clinician caring for a patient with severe acute abdominal pain is "Is prompt surgery needed?" Thorough history and physical examination are far more valuable than laboratory or radiologic tests. Surgical consultation should be promptly sought and analgesics withheld until the surgeon completes evaluation of the patient.

   All acute abdominal crises give rise to one or more of the following main symptoms and signs: pain, collapse, vomiting, or abdominal wall rigidity. Some main clinical presentations are as follows:

**1.** Abdominal pain by itself. Often this is the only symptom in the earliest stages of a number of serious conditions of simple intestinal colic, acute appendicitis, small-bowel obstruction, and acute pancreatitis.

**2.** Severe central abdominal pain with muscular rigidity (e.g., acute pancreatitis, ruptured aortic aneurysm, and mesenteric thrombosis).

**3.** Pain with vomiting and increased distention but no rigidity usually means intestinal obstruction.

**4.** Pain with constipation, increased distention, and perhaps vomiting may indicate large-bowel obstruction.

**5.** The presence of fever, tachycardia, perspiration, and hypotension suggests a serious disorder such as sepsis or a perforated viscus.

**6.** Severe abdominal pain with collapse and generalized rigidity of the abdominal wall usually means perforation of a viscus. Stomach and duodenum are more likely sites than colon.

**7.** Right hypochondrial pain and rigidity indicate acute cholecystitis or a perforated duodenal ulcer. Left hypochondrial pain and rigidity indicate acute pancreatitis, perforated gastric ulcer, or splenic rupture. Right lower quadrant pain, tenderness, and rigidity indicate acute appendicitis or tubo-ovarian disease or ileitis. Left iliac fossa pain, tenderness, and rigidity indicate diverticulitis. Hypogastric

pain and rigidity indicate perforated appendicitis, diverticulitis, or tubo-ovarian disease.
8. Pelvic, genital, and rectal examinations are mandatory. Pelvic inflammatory disease, a twisted ovarian cyst, or an ectopic pregnancy may be found. Torsion of the testicle may be uncovered in the male. Rectal examination may reveal an abscess or neoplasm.

HISTORY

1. In eliciting the history of pain, it is important to know its character, severity, localization, radiation, duration, frequency, times of occurrence, and the factors that alleviate or aggravate it.
2. Information about associated symptoms, both gastrointestinal (GI) and systemic, may be helpful in elucidating the cause of pain.
3. Careful inquiry should be made concerning the presence or absence of disorders that may cause referred abdominal pain (e.g., pneumonia, pericarditis, myocardial infarction, spinal arthritis).
4. Ask about symptoms that are associated with endogenous or exogenous metabolic causes of pain, as well as those of neurogenic origin (see Table 5-2).
5. Check the menstrual history. Midcycle follicular rupture is a frequent, harmless cause of abdominal pain. A history of a missed period followed by abdominal pain should suggest possible rupture of an ectopic pregnancy.
6. The family history may provide a clue to the cause of abdominal pain. Such familial disorders as hyperlipidemia, familial Mediterranean fever, thalassemia, sickle cell anemia, and acute intermittent porphyria are commonly associated with abdominal pain.
7. Anticoagulants may be responsible for intraabdominal or retroperitoneal hemorrhage and thereby produce abdominal pain.
8. A history of syphilis or gonorrhea may be helpful in elucidating the cause of abdominal pain.

ABDOMINAL EXAMINATION

1. Abdominal examination is of paramount importance.
   a. Inspect the abdomen for distention and visible peristalsis.
   b. Check for hernia at all potential sites.
   c. Abdominal auscultation, although valuable, is probably one of the least rewarding aspects of the physical examination, because perforation and strangulation of the gut can occur in the presence of normal peristalsis.
   d. Palpation of the abdomen must be thorough but gentle.
      (1) Check for masses, ascites, and splanchnomegaly.
      (2) Tenderness, rebound tenderness, and involuntary guarding are important signs of peritonitis.

PHYSICAL EXAMINATION

1. A complete physical examination is indicated.
2. The status of the cardiovascular and respiratory systems and the state of hydration of the patient should be evaluated.

LABORATORY STUDIES

Overreliance on lab tests often misleads the clinician. Useful tests include:
1. CBC.
2. Urinalysis.
3. Stool for occult blood.
4. SMA 12- or 22-type screens.
5. Serum and urinary amylase and lipase.
6. Chest upright and decubitus x-rays of the abdomen. Rarely, contrast studies of the GI tract may be indicated. Occasionally, abdominal ultrasound, abdominal CT scan, or HIDA scans are very useful in older patients.
7. Electrocardiogram.

**8.** Upper or lower endoscopy is rarely indicated.
**9.** Abdominal paracentesis may be useful.

Comments: As a general rule, the majority of severe abdominal pains that occur in previously healthy patients and last more than 6 hours are caused by diseases of surgical importance.

Laboratory examination, although important, rarely establishes the diagnosis. Leukocytosis should never be the sole deciding factor as to whether or not surgery is indicated. A peripheral white blood cell count greater than 20,000 per cubic millimeter may be seen with perforation, but also with pancreatitis. Conversely, the count may be normal with a perforated viscus. Routine urinalysis, serum electrolytes, and biochemical screening are of value in assessing the state of hydration and in ruling out renal disease, diabetes, or other complications. Serum amylase testing is overrated because disorders other than pancreatitis (e.g., perforated peptic ulcer, strangulated gut) may be associated with marked elevations.

Sometimes, a definite diagnosis cannot be made at the time of the initial examination. The possibility that a patient has an "acute abdomen" requires immediate consultation with a surgeon. If doubt exists, watchful waiting with repeated questioning and examination often indicates the proper course of action.

# Chronic and Recurrent Abdominal Pain

When pain has been present for weeks or months, the workup can be more deliberate and planned. The patient must be questioned carefully about the location, intensity, character, chronology, and setting of the pain; aggravating or alleviating factors; and associated signs and symptoms. Generally, it is the relationship in which pain occurs that is important. Each organ has its "usual" pain pattern—the location of pain being less useful information than its association with activity or the involved organ. Common pain patterns are described below.

**1.** Peptic ulcer disease. Epigastric pain, described as burning, gnawing, hunger, or aching, occurs 1 to 3 hours after a meal; about one-third of patients are awakened at night with pain. Most often it is quickly relieved with food or antacid, resulting in a pain-food-relief pattern. Some patients with gastric ulcer have increased pain after food, thus presenting a pain-food-pain-relief pattern. Pain is almost always episodic, lasting several days to weeks and is followed by a remission of months.
**2.** Biliary tract disease. Major symptoms include nausea, vomiting, and epigastric or RUQ abdominal pain that is steady (not colicky). Postprandial fullness, eructations, flatulence, and fatty food intolerance are nonspecific symptoms that are commonly associated with many other abdominal disorders.
**3.** Pancreatic disease. The pain is characteristically located in the epigastrium and tends to bore directly through to the back. Nausea and vomiting are commonly associated symptoms. The pain is constant, lasting for days, and is rarely colicky. Partial relief may be obtained by adopting the fetal position. A history of recent heavy alcohol ingestion or a past history of biliary tract disease is highly suggestive of pain of pancreatic origin.
**4.** Small intestinal disease. Characteristically located in the periumbilical region, the pain is crampy and may be associated with vomiting and changes in bowel habits. With proximal mechanical intestinal obstruction, vomiting occurs early in the clinical course; constipation and inability to pass flatus are more likely to occur with distal intestinal obstruction.
**5.** Irritable bowel syndrome. Abdominal pain is present at some time in most patients. It is generally located in the hypogastrium or LLQ. It rarely awakens the patient from sleep, unlike the pains previously discussed. The pain may be aggravated by food and is usually relieved by passage of flatus or a bowel movement. It may be associated with constipation or alternating diarrhea and constipation.

6. Colonic cancer. Abdominal pain is a common complaint with tumors proximal to the sigmoid. It occurs less frequently with rectal neoplasms and lesions of the distal portion of the sigmoid colon. It may be associated with a recent change in bowel habits. Bleeding per rectum is common. Mild anemia is common.
7. Miscellaneous causes.
   a. Chronic diverticulitis.
   b. Intermittent or chronic intestinal obstruction.
   c. Tuberculous peritonitis.
   d. Systemic diseases and intoxication (e.g., connective tissue diseases, lead poisoning, diabetes, porphyria, tabes dorsalis).
   e. Carcinoma of the pancreas.

### Diagnostic Approach

1. History.
2. Physical examination.
3. Characteristics of the pain.
4. Associated symptoms, especially weight loss and change in bowel habits.
5. Laboratory studies.
   a. CBC.
   b. Urinalysis.
   c. Stool examination for occult blood, ova, and parasites.
   d. Biochemical screening.
6. Gastrointestinal endoscopy (proctosigmoidoscopy, colonoscopy, upper GI endoscopy).
7. Roentgenographic studies.
   a. Plain films of the abdomen and chest films.
   b. Contrast studies of the gastrointestinal tract.
   c. Cholecystography.
   d. CT scan.
8. Abdominal ultrasonography.
9. Special studies for obscure pain.
   a. Urinary porphyrins.
   b. Hemoglobin electrophoresis.
   c. Abdominal angiography.
   Comments: Few disorders produce pain with distinctive pathognomic features. Clinical history usually only provides enough clues to supply some possibilities. Occasionally physical exam may provide the answer. Laboratory and radiologic studies are generally needed to confirm a tentative diagnosis.

## NAUSEA AND VOMITING
H. Harold Friedman

### Definition

Even though nausea and vomiting may occur independently, they are so closely related that they are considered together.

*Nausea* may be defined as the urge to vomit. *Vomiting* or *emesis* is the forceful expulsion of gastric contents. With few exceptions, nausea is a premonitory symptom of vomiting. *Retching* refers to the spasmodic respiratory activity that precedes emesis. Retching not followed by the expulsion of significant amounts of vomitus is often referred to as the "dry heaves." Vomiting should be distinguished from *regurgitation,* the term applied to the ejection of small quantities of gastric duodenal or esophageal contents not preceded by nausea and not accompanied by the abdominal muscular activity that characterizes the act of vomiting.

## Etiology

Nausea and vomiting are common manifestations of organic and functional disorders. The more common causes are listed in Table 5-3.

Nausea without vomiting may occur in uremia, x-ray therapy, alcoholism, liver disease, hypercalcemia, and pregnancy, and as a side effect of drug therapy (e.g., digitalis, opiates, antibiotics, oral contraceptives). Persistent nausea in otherwise healthy persons is frequently psychogenic in origin.

Vomiting may be due to any acute or chronic illness, or to a functional or nervous disorder. Vomiting may be the first sign of an acute abdominal emergency or of a serious systemic disease.

In everyday clinical practice, the most common causes of nausea and vomiting are acute gastroenteritis, febrile systemic illnesses, drug effects, and gastrointestinal disease.

## Clinical Features

1. Nausea and vomiting are rarely isolated phenomena. They are usually accompanied by other symptoms and signs.
2. Migraine headaches are commonly preceded or accompanied by nausea and vomiting.
3. The headache of intracerebral disease, notably that of increased intracranial pressure, is sometimes accompanied by vomiting that may be projectile in character.
4. Labyrinthine disease is typically manifested by vertigo, nausea, and vomiting.
5. Early morning vomiting before eating is seen in pregnancy, alcoholism, uremia, obstructive airway disease of heavy smokers, and sometimes, psychoneurosis.
6. Psychogenic vomiting is characterized by one or more of the following features:
   a. A lengthy history of vomiting.
   b. Maintenance of adequate nutrition despite the vomiting (except in anorexia nervosa).
   c. Vomiting during or shortly after meals.
   d. Surreptitious vomiting, often self-induced.
   e. Evidence of psychologic disturbances (e.g., anxiety, depression).
7. Delayed and recurrent vomiting 1 hour or more after meals, with large residues of gastric contents containing food particles, is usually indicative of gastric retention.
8. Esophageal obstruction is associated with regurgitation rather than vomiting.
9. The character of the vomitus may provide clues to an etiologic diagnosis.
   a. Odor. Vomitus with an acrid odor suggests the secretion of hydrochloric acid, easily confirmed by the laboratory. A fecal odor is characteristic of intestinal obstruction or gastrocolic fistula, but it is sometimes noted in paralytic ileus. A putrid odor is a sign of bacterial overgrowth of retained gastric contents or necrosis of a fungating gastric carcinoma.
   b. Contents. "Coffee ground" or bloody emesis is obviously of upper gastrointestinal origin. Bile usually appears in the vomitus when emesis is repeated. Its presence implies patency of the gastric outlet. Vomiting of bile is not uncommon following gastric surgery. The presence of food particles in vomited material is discussed in 7 above.
10. Persistent vomiting may have serious consequences (e.g., aspiration pneumonia, dehydration, electrolyte and acid-base disturbances, and hemorrhage due to tears at the esophagogastric junction).

**Table 5-3.** Causes of nausea and vomiting

A. Neurologic
1. Migraine
2. Labyrinthine disorders (Ménière's disease, motion sickness)
3. Cerebral lesions (especially if associated with increased intracranial pressure)
B. Psychogenic
1. Emotional and environmental stress
2. Surreptitious vomiting
3. Cyclic vomiting (infants and children)
C. Metabolic and endocrine
1. Renal failure
2. Metabolic acidosis
3. Drugs and chemicals
4. Electrolyte abnormalities (hyponatremia, hypercalcemia, hyperkalemia)
5. Hepatic failure
6. Hypothyroidism
7. Adrenal insufficiency
8. Pregnancy
9. Food allergy
10. Diabetes mellitus
D. Alimentary
1. Gastroduodenal
a. Peptic ulcer
b. Gastric outlet obstruction
c. Gastric atony
d. Postgastric surgery
2. Gastrointestinal
a. Gastroenteritis, including food poisoning
b. Appendicitis
c. Intestinal obstruction
d. Paralytic ileus
3. Hepatobiliary
a. Cholecystitis and cholelithiasis
b. Acute hepatitis
c. Cirrhosis of the liver
4. Pancreatic
a. Acute pancreatitis
b. Carcinoma of the pancreas
5. Peritoneal
a. Peritonitis
b. Carcinomatosis
E. Miscellaneous
1. Acute febrile illness
2. Myocardial infarction
3. Congestive heart failure
4. Chronic obstructive pulmonary disease
5. Reflex (e.g., renal, colic, salpingitis)

---

## Diagnostic Approach

---

1. The multiplicity of causes of nausea and vomiting makes it virtually impossible to follow a specific diagnostic approach.
2. Foremost in the evaluation of nausea and vomiting is the history. Special attention should be paid to the following:
   a. The temporal relationship between emesis and food intake; the character of the vomitus; and the onset, duration, and persistence of the nausea and vomiting.
   b. A past or present history of gastrointestinal disease or surgery.
   c. The presence or absence of specific gastrointestinal symptoms such as abdominal pain, hematemesis, melena, indigestion, heartburn, dysphagia, abdominal swelling, jaundice, diarrhea, and constipation.
   d. Inquiry concerning symptoms that would suggest a systemic illness or metabolic disorder capable of producing nausea and vomiting.
   e. Careful questioning about the use of medications that can cause nausea and vomiting.
   f. A history of weight loss.
   g. Background information about the patient's psychological and social history and of symptoms that may indicate a psychological disorder.
3. The physical examination may provide evidence of the organ system primarily involved.
   a. Fever may suggest infection but is nonspecific.
   b. Neurologic abnormalities, papilledema, and altered consciousness point to disease of the central nervous system.
   c. An alimentary origin is suggested by a history of abdominal pain and findings of tenderness, distention, splanchnomegaly, altered peristalsis, and abdominal masses on abdominal examination.
   d. Metabolic disorders may be suggested by the physical findings (e.g., in Addison's disease, thyrotoxicosis) usually required for the diagnosis of these conditions.
4. An isolated episode of emesis, or at most a few bouts of nausea and vomiting, associated with anorexia, malaise, aching, little or no fever, abdominal cramping, diarrhea, and negative physical findings, is virtually diagnostic of acute gastroenteritis. Little or no workup is necessary because the disease is usually self-limited. However, persistence of symptoms may mandate diagnostic studies. (See Acute Diarrhea, p. 185.)
5. The initial workup for all patients with *persistent or recurrent nausea and vomiting, or both,* should include:
   a. CBC.
   b. Urinalysis.
   c. Serum electrolytes.
   d. Biochemical screening.
   e. Serum and urinary amylase.
   f. Arterial blood gases (when an acid-base disturbance is suspected).
   g. Survey films of the abdomen.
   h. Chest films.
   i. Electrocardiogram.
6. If the gastrointestinal tract is believed to be at the root of the problem, as is most often the case with persistent and repetitive nausea and vomiting, additional tests are warranted. The procedures chosen should be based on the best clinical judgment of the physician. Such studies might include gastric aspirations, esophagogastroduodenoscopy, barium studies, cholecystography, and proctosigmoidoscopy. Stool examination for occult blood, ova, and parasites and stool cultures may be advisable. The presence of jaundice suggests a special approach. (See Jaundice, p. 203.)
7. The choice of other investigative procedures depends primarily on the clinical findings, but tests are sometimes performed for purposes of exclusion. Included

in this group are pregnancy tests in amenorrheic women, special studies to elu
cidate the cause of unexplained anemia, thyroid function tests in suspected thy
rotoxicosis, skull films, and other localizing procedures to rule out cerebral dis
ease.

## HEARTBURN (PYROSIS)
Barry W. Frank

### Definition

Heartburn, or pyrosis, is a painful or burning sensation located retrosternally o
in the subxiphoid region. The discomfort may radiate to the lateral anterior chest
jaws, and arms. Heartburn is frequently worse after meals and aggravated b
recumbency or bending forward. It is almost always relieved within 15 minute
by the ingestion of an antacid.

### Mechanism

Heartburn arises from alterations in the esophageal epithelium induced by th
reflux of acid and pepsin, or bile and pancreatic juice, or both. Motor abnormal
ties of the esophagus may contribute to its production. However, because pyrosi
may be experienced when esophageal motility is normal, it seems likely tha
chemical stimulation from esophageal reflux is the most important factor in it
pathogenesis.

### Gastroesophageal Reflux

The primary determinant of gastroesophageal reflux is the tone of the lowe
esophageal sphincter (LES). Although the LES cannot be identified anatomicall
its presence can be verified by physiologic means. Modern manometric method
have established that the LES possesses a resting tone that causes the intralu
minal esophageal pressure to exceed that of the stomach. Thus, in the norma
individual, an intact LES prevents the reflux of gastric contents into the esoph
agus, even when stomach pressures are high. Hiatal hernia has no significar
influence on LES pressure. The following are some of the complications of gastr
esophageal reflux:
1. Esophagitis (histologic alteration of the esophageal mucosa).
   a. With bleeding.
   b. With ulceration.
   c. With stricture.
2. Tracheal aspiration with chronic cough, pneumonitis, and fibrosis.

### Etiology

1. Gastroesophageal reflux due to an incompetent sphincter, with or without hiat
   hernia.
2. Medications.
3. Scleroderma, with involvement of the lower esophageal sphincter.
4. Barrett's syndrome (lower esophagus lined by columnar epithelium with ulcer
   tion at the transitional zone).
5. Tumor, by affecting sphincter function or altering motility.

## Diagnostic Approach

### Initial Evaluation

1. Upper GI series should be performed to detect intrinsic lesions of the esophagus and stomach. Unfortunately, reflux cannot be detected by this method in more than 25 to 35 percent of patients with heartburn.
2. Esophageal cineradiography with barium can be performed in order to follow the passage of swallowed barium through the esophagus. The patient should be examined in both the upright and the supine positions. Esophageal motility can be visualized, reflux observed, and small mucosal defects detected.
3. If the preceding studies show reflux without evidence of intrinsic esophageal disease, further tests are usually not necessary, and treatment may be instituted.
4. If the aforementioned studies are negative, the additional procedures listed below are indicated.
5. If x-ray studies show stricture, tumor, or an abnormal mucosal pattern, esophagoscopy and biopsy should be performed.
6. In the presence of persistent pyrosis unresponsive to treatment, further investigation is warranted.

### Subsequent Evaluation

1. Esophageal acid perfusion test (Bernstein test). The acid perfusion test determines whether the esophagus is sensitive to acid but does not necessarily prove that reflux is present. It is designed to reproduce the symptoms created by acid reflux. A nasogastric tube is passed into the midesophagus and positioned by fluoroscopy. With the patient seated upright, normal saline is administered via the nasogastric tube at a rate of 6 to 7.5 ml per minute. Then, without the patient's knowledge, 0.1 N HCl is substituted for the saline. This is perfused at the same rate until pain is produced or until 15 minutes have elapsed. The solutions are again interchanged without notifying the patient. The test is considered to give a positive result if heartburn is elicited by acid perfusion but not by saline. A high incidence of false-positive and false-negative results, ranging between 5 and 15 percent, makes it necessary to interpret the results with caution.
2. Esophagoscopy and biopsy. The newer, flexible endoscopes permit biopsy, suction, insufflation of air and fluid, and photography of the mucosa. The entire esophagus can be visualized. Endoscopy and biopsy make possible confirmation of tumors, strictures, or other lesions observed by x-ray. Esophagoscopy is also invaluable when radiologic studies are negative, because less evident lesions (e.g., esophagitis) may be detectable by this technique. It is ordinarily unnecessary to biopsy the esophagus in the presence of esophagitis. However, biopsy may be useful in revealing esophagitis when the mucosa is grossly normal in appearance.
3. Esophageal motility studies and measurement of the intraesophageal pH. Gastroesophageal reflux is demonstrated best by measurement of the intraluminal pH combined with simultaneous measurement of the intraesophageal pressure. To perform the test the patient swallows an assembly consisting of a pH electrode and three manometric catheters whose tips are placed 5 cm apart. The LES is located and its pressure characteristics noted. The motility of the esophagus is then recorded, and the reflux is measured by the pH electrode.
4. Continuous pH probe monitoring. Using an esophageal pH electrode, timed monitoring of esophageal pH from 1 hour to 24 hours can identify reflux in some patients not diagnosed by other means.
5. Esophageal scintigraphy. Using $^{99m}$Tc-sulfur colloid given orally, followed by feeding, reflux can be demonstrated as spikes of increased radioactivity above background counts.

# DYSPHAGIA
Barry W. Frank

## Definition

Dysphagia is nonpainful difficulty in swallowing. It is a subjective sensation experienced during the act of deglutition. There is usually a sticking sensation retrosternally as the bolus descends. In most instances, dysphagia is experienced at the same level as the lesion or above it, but not below it. *Odynophagia* is the term applied to painful swallowing. Dysphagia is a highly specific and significant symptom of organic disease. It should never be considered functional without an exhaustive evaluation. Dysphagia can be differentiated by a careful history from globus hystericus, which is a functional complaint. Globus hystericus is a sensation of a "lump in the throat." It is not necessarily associated with deglutition. The symptom is intermittent and is not associated with regurgitation. Foods and liquids can be swallowed without difficulty.

*Preesophageal dysphagia* is difficulty in emptying material from the oral pharynx into the esophagus. It occurs in disorders proximal to the esophagus, most often of neurologic or muscular origin. Esophageal dysphagia is usually the result of obstructive or motor abnormalities.

## Etiology

### Oropharyngeal Dysphagia

1. Loss of tongue function (myasthenia gravis, myotonia dystrophica).
2. Pharyngeal dysfunction (myasthenia gravis, vascular brainstem disease, dermatomyositis, hyperthyroidism).
3. Mechanical obstruction.
   a. Zenker's diverticulum.
   b. Tumor.
   c. Inflammatory stricture.

### Esophageal Dysphagia

1. Intraluminal obstruction.
   a. Esophageal webs.
   b. Lower esophageal ring (Schatzki's ring).
   c. Tumor.
   d. Lower esophageal sphincter spasm (hypertensive sphincter).
   e. Inflammatory stricture.
   f. Caustic stricture.
   g. Foreign body.
2. Extraluminal obstruction.
   a. Compression by tumors, enlarged lymph nodes, or substernal thyroid gland.
   b. Vascular abnormalities (aortic aneurysm, aberrant right subclavian artery, right-sided aortic arch).
3. Motility disorders.
   a. Achalasia.
   b. Scleroderma.
   c. Diabetic neuropathy.
   d. Diffuse esophageal spasm.
   e. Amyloidosis.
   f. Parasitic infection (Chagas' disease).
4. Miscellaneous causes.
   a. Infections (candidiasis).
   b. Crohn's disease.

## Symptoms

1. A detailed history may provide a significant clue to the etiology of dysphagia and hence aid in its evaluation.
2. Dysphagia of oropharyngeal disease is characterized by difficulty in moving a bolus of food from the mouth to the pharynx. There may be instant regurgitation of food through the nares, choking, and repetitive swallowing, particularly in neuromuscular disorders.
3. Esophageal dysphagia usually presents as a sticking sensation. It may be intermittent, as in the case of a lower esophageal ring, or progressive, as in the presence of a tumor. Regurgitation of undigested food may occur minutes to hours after a meal. Patients find that they must chew their foods thoroughly and that fluids may be required to "wash the food down." The time taken to eat frequently is prolonged.
4. The presence of weight loss suggests marked obstruction due to benign disease or a malignancy.
5. Respiratory symptoms, most often nocturnal, may occur from tracheal aspiration of esophageal contents. Esophageal disease should always be considered as a possible cause of recurrent unexplained pneumonia.
6. Heartburn suggests an inflammatory stricture or disease that involves the lower esophageal sphincter.
7. Raynaud's phenomenon suggests a connective tissue disease as the cause of dysphagia, which in turn is due to a motility disorder.
8. Halitosis and postprandial neck fullness should suggest the presence of a Zenker's diverticulum.

## Physical Examination

The physical examination is of little value in the diagnosis of dysphagia except in the presence of neuromuscular disorders, scleroderma, diabetes mellitus, cervical lymphadenopathy, or malnutrition.

## Diagnostic Approach

1. X-ray examination.
   a. A barium swallow is the most valuable procedure. It often reveals the cause and site of an obstruction, but a normal result should not deter further investigation, particularly by endoscopy.
   b. Cineradiography with barium, as described in the preceding section, Heartburn, is helpful in motility disorders.
   c. The addition of a marshmallow or a barium-soaked cotton ball is useful in an attempt to reproduce the dysphagia or define more precisely the location, type, and degree of obstruction.
2. Esophagoscopy and biopsy are essential in the diagnosis of esophagitis, strictures, rings, webs, and tumors.
3. When properly performed, exfoliative *cytologic studies* may be expected to yield the correct diagnosis in 95 percent of patients with esophageal carcinoma.
4. Esophageal motility study, as described in the preceding section, Heartburn, is essential to the diagnosis of motility disorders. It is the only technique that elucidates the status of the lower esophageal sphincter as well as the overall motility of the esophagus.
5. The esophageal acid perfusion test (Bernstein test) is of little value in the evaluation of dysphagia except when esophageal reflux is suspected.

## GASTROINTESTINAL BLEEDING
Andrew Mallory

### Definitions

*Hematemesis* is the vomiting of red blood or "coffee-ground" material. *Melena* is the passage of black, sticky stools. *Hematochezia* is the passage of fresh red blood per rectum. Upper gastrointestinal bleeding is defined as bleeding from a source proximal to the ligament of Treitz; lower gastrointestinal bleeding is from a source distal to this point.

### Etiology

Some causes of gastrointestinal bleeding are listed in Table 5-4.

### Clinical Features

Acute massive gastrointestinal hemorrhage results in the following hemodynamic changes: decreased cardiac output, rise in pulse rate, and drop in blood pressure. The latter is first detectable as an orthostatic change. A drop in systolic blood pressure of more than 10 mm Hg or an increase in heart rate of more than 20 beats per minute when sitting (with the legs "dangling") or standing usually indicates a loss of at least 1000 ml of blood. It should be remembered that the

**Table 5-4.** Causes of massive gastrointestinal bleeding in adults

| Area | Disease or disorder |
| --- | --- |
| Upper gastrointestinal tract | |
| Common | Ulcer (duodenal, gastric) |
| | Gastritis (stress, alcohol, drugs) |
| | Mallory-Weiss tear |
| Uncommon | Esophagitis |
| | Angiodysplastic or other vascular malformations (e.g., hereditary hemorrhagic telangiectasia) |
| | Gastric or esophageal carcinoma |
| | Duodenitis |
| | Hemobilia |
| | Aortoduodenal fistula |
| | Bleeding diathesis (including iatrogenic) |
| Lower gastrointestinal tract | |
| Common | Diverticular disease of the colon |
| | Angiodysplasia |
| | Inflammatory bowel disease |
| Uncommon | Colorectal carcinoma and polyps |
| | Ischemic bowel disease |
| | Meckel's diverticulum |
| | Postirradiation enteritis |
| | Hemorrhoids (common cause of minor bleeding; massive bleeding rare except in presence of portal hypertension) |

Source: Modified from L. B. Reller, et al. (eds.), *Clinical Internal Medicine.* Boston: Little, Brown, 1979. P. 197.

hematocrit may be normal and may grossly underestimate the amount of blood lost if volume readjustment to blood loss has not yet taken place. It may take as long as 24 hours for this phenomenon to occur.

Recovery of bright red blood from the stomach usually indicates a brisk rate of bleeding; recovery of dark blood indicates a slower rate of bleeding. However, fresh blood can be converted to dark-colored hematin in a highly acidic environment in a matter of seconds.

## Diagnostic Approach

### History

A carefully taken history usually helps to define both the site and cause of gastrointestinal bleeding.

1. Vomiting of blood or coffee-ground material localizes the source to the upper gastrointestinal tract.
2. A history of epistaxis or hemoptysis raises the possibility of sources other than the gastrointestinal tract causing bleeding in a patient with hematemesis.
3. Vomitus containing no gross blood or coffee-ground material in a patient with melena or rectal bleeding does not rule out an upper gastrointestinal source, because bleeding may have stopped before vomiting occurred or because bleeding into the duodenum may not have refluxed into the stomach. However, the presence of bile in the gastric aspirate indicates that reflux has occurred.
4. Melena usually means that the site of bleeding is proximal to the midtransverse colon.
5. Gross blood from the rectum usually means that the source of bleeding is located more distally in the large bowel. However, upper gastrointestinal sources may cause gross rectal bleeding if the hemorrhage is massive and bowel transit is rapid. Under these circumstances, the vital signs deteriorate rapidly.
6. Although there is a past history of ulcer disease in most patients with bleeding ulcers, bleeding may be the initial manifestation in up to 10 percent of cases of ulcer disease. Disappearance of ulcer pain often heralds the onset of bleeding.
7. A history of ingestion of particular drugs increases the likelihood of gastritis or ulcer disease. The evidence implicating salicylates is convincing. Other drugs, such as phenylbutazone, the nonsteroidal anti-inflammatory agents, and steroids, also may cause bleeding.
8. A history of cirrhosis of the liver increases the likelihood that esophageal varices are the source of the bleeding. However, in several studies approximately 50 percent of hemorrhages in cirrhotic patients were due to other lesions.
9. Stools may appear red in some persons after the ingestion of beets. Black stools may result from the ingestion of iron, bismuth-containing compounds (e.g., Pepto-Bismol), or charcoal.
10. A source of blood loss is often not found in the bleeding patient who is receiving anticoagulant therapy. A diagnostic workup is nevertheless indicated, especially in the patient who bleeds while his anticoagulation is in the "therapeutic range."

### Physical Examination

1. The initial examination may have to be limited in a patient with massive hemorrhage and deteriorating vital signs.
2. Particular attention should be directed to the following:
   a. Vital signs: for evidence of orthostatic pulse and blood pressure changes.
   b. Skin: for vascular spiders, palmar erythema, and jaundice in chronic liver disease; pigmented macules on the lips in the Peutz-Jeghers syndrome; telangiectasia on the face, palms, soles, or on the buccal or nasal mucosa in hereditary hemorrhagic telangiectasia; purpura or ecchymoses in bleeding diatheses; erythema nodosum in inflammatory bowel disease.
   c. ENT: for possible epistaxis.

   **d.** Abdomen: for hepatosplenomegaly, ascites, and caput medusae in cirrhosis; epigastric tenderness in ulcer disease or gastritis; the presence of a mass in Crohn's disease or malignancy.

   **e.** Rectal examination: to detect masses, hemorrhoids, or fissures; to confirm the presence of rectal bleeding or melena. It should be remembered that stools may remain tarry, and tests for occult blood may remain positive for several days after bleeding has stopped.

## Diagnostic Studies

**1.** Initial laboratory studies should include:

   **a.** CBC.

   **b.** Coagulation studies (prothrombin time, partial thromboplastin time, platelet count).

   **c.** Liver function tests.

   **d.** Electrolytes in selected cases, especially if vomiting or diarrhea has been present or if liver disease is likely.

   **e.** Serum creatinine, BUN, and blood glucose.

   **f.** Blood for typing and cross matching. At least 3 units of blood should be available at all times.

**2.** A large-bore (e.g., 24F) nasogastric tube should be inserted into the stomach even if only bright red rectal bleeding is present. The presence or absence of bile in the gastric aspirate should be noted. If no blood or coffee-ground material is recovered in 30 minutes, the tube can be removed. If blood is present, the tube should remain for purposes of lavage. Although lavage has not proved effective in lessening bleeding, it helps cleanse the upper gastrointestinal tract of blood and thus facilitates further diagnostic studies.

**3.** Additional procedures depend on the diagnostic facilities available to the physician.

   **a.** Panendoscopy is employed early in many patients with upper gastrointestinal tract bleeding. Its high accuracy, ease (at patient's bedside), safety, and therapeutic potential (injection, thermal) probably make it the procedure of choice. It is generally preferable to delay endoscopy until resuscitative measures restore vital signs and the stomach can be cleared of blood clots with a nasogastric tube. In many instances, the rate of bleeding slows during this period of time. Endoscopy can then be undertaken. However, if bleeding continues and especially if immediate surgery is contemplated, endoscopy may be performed.

      Panendoscopy is very safe in experienced hands. Relative or absolute contraindications are coma, an uncooperative patient, or the presence of severe cervical arthritis.

   **b.** Upper GI series is less sensitive than panendoscopy in diagnosing the source of upper gastrointestinal tract bleeding but may be better tolerated. It should not be done until the vital signs are stable. It is the procedure of choice when panendoscopy is unavailable or contraindicated.

   **c.** Arteriography is seldom necessary in the diagnostic evaluation of upper gastrointestinal bleeding. It is usually reserved for the patient with continuous brisk bleeding (at least 0.5–1.0 ml/min) after other diagnostic measures have failed. More commonly, however, patients with continued bleeding from the upper gastrointestinal tract and negative diagnostic studies are explored surgically after 5 to 6 units of blood have been transfused.

   **d.** Gastric or esophageal tamponade with a tube such as the Sengstaken-Blakemore may occasionally prove useful diagnostically as well as therapeutically in a patient with suspected varices.

   **e.** If bleeding appears to originate in the lower gastrointestinal tract (e.g., hematochezia with a negative nasogastric aspirate), proctosigmoidoscopy should be carried out promptly. If this procedure is unrevealing, a period of observation is usually recommended during which blood transfusions may be administered if indicated. If bleeding continues and the patient is hemodynamically stable, technetium 99m-labeled RBC scanning may prove useful in localizing the bleeding source. If positive, further identification and perhaps treatment can be offered by arteriography, or colonoscopy, or both. If negative, colonoscopy is usually indicated after adequate preparation.

  **f.** If bleeding is especially massive, prompt arteriography for localization and treatment (e.g., embolization, vasopressin infusion) should be done. Even if successful therapy cannot be carried out, localization of the bleeding source may greatly aid the surgeon should surgery become necessary. Colonoscopy carried out during massive lower gastrointestinal bleeding may on occasion prove useful, especially if the colon can be rapidly prepared by administration of an oral electrolyte solution beforehand.

---

# DIARRHEA
## Barry W. Frank

## Definition

Diarrhea may be defined as an increase in the fluidity, or frequency, or both, of the stool. The 24-hour stool weighs less than 300 g and contains about 150 ml of water. When daily stool weight exceeds 300 g (approximately 250 ml water) diarrhea is usually present. Whether acute or chronic, diarrhea results from or is associated with water and electrolyte malabsorption. There are four basic pathophysiologic mechanisms involved in the production of diarrhea. One or more of these factors may play a significant role in any given diarrheal state. They include the following: (1) abnormal intestinal motility, (2) increased vascular or mucosal permeability, resulting in fluid and electrolyte exsorption, (3) impaired intestinal absorption, and (4) intraluminal nonabsorbable osmotically active solutes. It is important to bear in mind that patients with inflammatory disease of the rectum may refer to the frequent passage of small quantities of blood and mucus as diarrhea.

## Acute Diarrhea

Acute diarrhea is usually of abrupt onset and short duration.

### Etiology

1. Infectious diarrhea.
    **a.** Bacterial: *Salmonella, Shigella, Campylobacter fetus, Vibrio cholerae,* enteropathogenic *Escherichia coli, Clostridium, Yersinia enterocolitica, Vibrio parahemolyticus.*
    **b.** Viral: enterovirus, hepatitis-associated virus, parvoviruslike agents, orbivirus, cytomegalovirus.
    **c.** Fungal: *Candida, Actinomyces, Histoplasma.*
    **d.** Protozoal: *Giardia lamblia, Entamoeba histolytica.*
    **e.** Helminthic: *Ascaris lumbricoides, Ancylostoma duodenale, Necator americanus, Trichuris trichiura, Strongyloides stercoralis.*
2. Toxic diarrhea.
    **a.** Bacterial toxins (food poisoning): staphylococcus, *Clostridium perfringens, E. coli, Clostridium botulinum, Bacillus cereus, Clostridium difficile, Pseudomonas.*
    **b.** Chemical poisons: arsenic, lead, mercury, mushrooms.
3. Dietary causes. Irritating foods, alcohol, drugs, food allergies, nonspecific food intolerance, nonabsorbable sugar substitutes (sorbitol, mannitol).

4. Miscellaneous causes. Appendicitis, diverticulitis, gastrointestinal hemorrhage, Schönlein-Henoch purpura, Stevens-Johnson syndrome, pseudomembranous enterocolitis, fecal impaction, ischemic colitis.

## Symptoms

The symptoms are usually abdominal cramps, urgency, tenesmus, nausea and vomiting, and watery stools with or without blood and mucus. Systemic symptoms, particularly fever and myalgias, may be present.

## Signs

The signs vary with the cause and severity of the disease, but diffuse abdominal tenderness and active bowel sounds are usually present. The temperature may be elevated. Involuntary guarding, localized tenderness, and rebound tenderness of the abdomen are rare.

## Diagnostic Approach

Acute diarrhea frequently is self-limiting. The etiology is generally established by the history and physical examination. However, immediate evaluation is necessary in the presence of severe abdominal pain, systemic symptoms, dehydration, bloody stools, or when symptoms persist beyond 24 hours. Under these circumstances, the following studies should be performed:

1. CBC.
2. Rectal swab for bacterial culture and sensitivity studies.
3. Immediate examination of a freshly passed stool for ova and parasites.
4. Serum electrolytes to aid in the diagnosis and management of dehydration.
5. Stool smears stained with Löffler's alkaline methylene blue for the presence of leukocytes. Fecal leukocytes are commonly present in bacterial infections and chronic inflammatory disease of the colon but are usually not seen in the stools of patients with diarrhea secondary to viruses, toxicogenic bacteria, and parasites.
6. Stool for *Clostridium difficile* titer when antibiotic-induced pseudomembranous colitis is suspected.
7. Sigmoidoscopic examination, which is helpful in the diagnosis of shigellosis, amebic colitis, and acute ulcerative colitis. It should be performed as a part of the immediate evaluation on any patient with bloody diarrhea.
8. A three-way abdominal x-ray examination should be obtained if there is bloating, severe abdominal pain, or obstructive-type bowel sounds upon auscultation, or if obstruction or perforation is suspected.

## Chronic Diarrhea

### Etiology

Table 5-5 lists the many causes of chronic diarrhea. Cases of diarrhea seen in office practice are caused most often by the following conditions: (1) functional disorders (irritable bowel syndrome, emotional diarrhea), (2) disease of the colon (diverticulitis, ulcerative colitis, Crohn's colitis, carcinoma), (3) disease of the small intestine (malabsorption syndromes, Crohn's disease), (4) diarrhea secondary to laxative abuse, and (5) gastrogenic diarrhea, including the postgastrectomy and postvagotomy syndromes. Other diseases are encountered less frequently. It is beyond the scope of this text to consider more than a few of these conditions.

**Table 5-5.** Causes of chronic diarrhea

A. Disease of the stomach
  1. Postgastrectomy (dumping syndromes)
  2. Postvagotomy
  3. Hypertrophic atrophic gastritis (Ménétrier's disease with hypoalbuminemia)
  4. Pernicious anemia with associated megalocytosis of the intestinal mucosal cells
  5. Zollinger-Ellison syndrome
B. Disease of the small intestine
  1. Inflammatory disease
    a. Crohn's disease
    b. Radiation enteritis
    c. Whipple's disease
    d. Collagen disease (polyarteritis, systemic lupus erythematosus, scleroderma)
    e. Amyloidosis
  2. Malabsorption diarrhea
    a. Gluten-sensitive enteropathy (nontropical sprue)
    b. Tropical sprue
    c. Disaccharidase deficiency
    d. Intestinal lymphoma
    e. Intestinal amyloidosis
    f. Intesetinal scleroderma
    g. Hypogammaglobulinemia
    h. Intestinal lymphangiectasia
    i. Pancreatic insufficiency
    j. Diarrhea of intestinal stasis (blind-loop syndrome, small bowel diverticula, postgastrectomy steatorrhea, intestinal pseudoobstruction)
    k. Small bowel resection with loss of absorptive surface
    l. Malabsorption associated with chronic skin disease (dermatitis herpetiformis, atopic dermatitis)
    m. Chronic giardiasis
C. Disease of the colon
  1. Ulcerative colitis
  2. Granulomatous colitis (Crohn's disease)
  3. Ulcerative proctitis
  4. Diverticulitis
  5. Colonic carcinoma
  6. Villous adenoma
D. Diarrhea in AIDS
  1. *Cryptosporidium* infections
  2. Amebiasis
  3. Giardiasis
  4. *Isospora belli* infections
  5. Herpes simplex infections
  6. Cytomegalovirus infections
  7. *Mycobacterium avium-intracellulare* infections
  8. *Salmonella typhimurium*
  9. *Cryptococcus* infections
  10. Candidiasis
  11. AIDS enteropathy
E. Miscellaneous causes
  1. Superior mesenteric artery insufficiency
  2. Addison's disease
  3. Diabetes mellitus associated with visceral neuropathy
  4. Endocrine tumors (carcinoid tumor, Zollinger-Ellison syndrome, nonbeta islet cell tumor of the pancreas with watery diarrhea, hypokalemia and hypochlorhydria, medullary thyroid carcinoma)
  5. Hyperthyroidism

**Table 5-5** (continued)

6. Drugs
   a. Antacids
   b. Antibiotics
   c. Hypotensive agents
   d. Cholinergic agents
   e. Cathartics
   f. Alcohol
   g. Quinidine
7. Functional bowel syndromes
8. Small bowel tumors
9. Eosinophilic gastroenteritis
10. Parathyroid disease
11. Biliary, gastric, or duodenal colic fistula
12. Infections
    a. Giardiasis
    b. Amebiasis
    c. Tuberculosis
13. Laxative abuse

FUNCTIONAL BOWEL DISORDERS

Patients with functional motility disorders ordinarily have a long history of intermittent or chronic diarrhea. Exacerbations usually are precipitated by emotional stress and anxiety. Diarrhea is most likely to occur in the morning or after meals. The stools may be large or small, semiformed or liquid, and mucus- or non-mucus-containing. Blood is not found in the stool unless produced by a complicating anorectal lesion. Systemic symptoms are absent, and nutrition is usually good. The diagnosis is made on the basis of history and by exclusion. The findings on physical examination, study of the feces, proctosigmoidoscopy, and barium enema are negative.

DISEASES OF THE COLON AND THE SMALL INTESTINE

1. Diverticulitis. Diverticula of the colon occur more frequently with advancing age; they are usually asymptomatic unless complicated by inflammation. The resulting diverticulitis may be manifested by acute attacks of left lower quadrant pain, tenderness, and fever. A palpable tender mass may be present. Constipation is usual, but diarrhea may occur with bloody stools. Symptoms may disappear after the acute episode subsides. In patients with low-grade inflammation, diarrhea is likely to occur intermittently, although it may be chronic. Crampy lower-abdomen pain is often a feature. The diagnosis is usually established by barium enema.
2. Ulcerative colitis. This is primarily a disease of youth, although it may occur at any age. Its course is characterized by remissions and exacerbations. During the acute phase, the diarrhea may be quite severe, with daily passage of as many as 30 or more bloody, mucus- and pus-containing stools. Fever, weight loss, abdominal griping, and tenesmus are common accompaniments. Complications include pericolitis, perforation of the bowel, malignant transformation, perianal disorders, arthritis, spondylitis, iritis, pericholangitis, and pyoderma gangrenosum. The diagnosis in over 90 percent of cases can be established by sigmoidoscopy and confirmed by rectal biopsy and barium studies. The sigmoidoscopic findings may be positive even when the contrast examination is negative.
3. Crohn's disease. This disorder occurs most frequently in adolescence and early adult life. Like ulcerative colitis, its course is marked by remissions and exacerbations. During acute attacks, there may be right lower quadrant pain, diarrhea, low-grade fever, and weight loss. The clinical picture of acute appendicitis is simulated in some patients. During periods of remission, constipation may be present

but with otherwise normal function. Fistula formation and intestinal obstruction are common sequelae. Nutritional deficiency and malabsorption are less frequent complications. The diagnosis is usually established by x-ray. Abnormality of the terminal ileum and skipped areas of involvement are typical. At times the clinical picture is indistinguishable from that of ulcerative colitis. Differentiating features that are helpful when present include sharp demarcation between diseased and healthy areas of bowel, absence of rectal and sigmoidal lesions in early cases, and evidence of involvement of all layers of the bowel wall.

4. Malabsorption. Diarrhea manifested by the passage of pale, bulky, greasy, frothy, foul-smelling stools, in association with evidence of nutritional deficiency and weight loss, suggests malabsorption. Fever, hypermetabolism, and significant loss of appetite do not occur. The diarrhea can usually be made to disappear in a 1- to 2-day period if oral feedings are withheld. The laboratory studies most useful in the diagnosis of malabsorption are listed below. Evidence of increased fecal excretion of fat is the most important factor in establishing the presence of steatorrhea. The differential diagnosis of various causes of malabsorption is beyond the scope of this discussion.

## Diagnostic Approach

HISTORY

The history may provide clues to the etiology of the diarrhea and the localization of the disease process.

1. Age. Diarrhea beginning in adolescence or early adult life suggests diseases such as ulcerative colitis, Crohn's disease, tuberculosis, and functional disorders. In middle age and in the elderly, carcinoma of the colon, diverticulitis, and pancreatic disease are among the more common causes.

2. Diarrhea patterns. Diarrhea alternating with constipation suggests carcinoma of the colon, diverticulitis, functional enterocolonopathies, excessive use of laxatives, and gastric disorders. Continuous diarrhea may be seen in ulcerative colitis, regional enteritis, intestinal fistulas, laxative abuse, and gastric disease. Intermittent diarrhea is a common feature of functional disorders, diverticulitis, allergies, and malabsorption.

   Relief of abdominal cramping by defecation suggests colonic disease; persistence after bowel movements suggests disease of the small intestine. Large-stool diarrhea suggests disease of the small bowel or proximal colon; small-stool diarrhea, involvement of the distal colon. Diarrhea with rectal tenesmus suggests inflammatory disease of the bowel combined with anorectal lesions. Diarrhea associated with abdominal distention should raise the possibility of partial obstruction.

3. Diurnal variations and relationship to meals. Diarrhea occurring primarily in the morning and after meals is found in gastric conditions, emotional disorders, Crohn's disease, and ulcerative colitis. Diarrhea that is not related to normal diurnal variations in colonic activity is often found in infectious disease. Nocturnal diarrhea is characteristic of diabetic neuropathy but is not specific for this diagnosis. When inflammatory disease of the bowel is severe, diarrhea may occur at night as well as during the day. Nocturnal diarrhea should always suggest an organic cause.

4. Weight loss. In the presence of undiminished appetite, weight loss suggests hyperthyroidism or malabsorption. Weight loss in association with fever and other systemic symptoms implies inflammatory disease of the bowel. Weight loss preceding the onset of diarrhea suggests carcinoma of the pancreas or other malignancy, tuberculosis, diabetes, hyperthyroidism, or malabsorption. Weight loss is uncommon in carcinoma of the colon until late in the course of the disease. Diarrhea without weight loss or other systemic manifestations is often functional in origin.

5. Characteristics of the stools. Watery stools with little fecal material occur commonly in psychophysiologic disturbances, severe inflammatory disease of the

bowel, and shortened intestines (after surgery). Semiformed, bulky, pale, foul-smelling, frothy, greasy stools bespeak malabsorption. Chronic bloody diarrhea with gripping abdominal pain and rectal tenesmus may result from amebic or bacillary dysentery, ulcerative colitis, Crohn's disease, and less often, other conditions. It should be remembered that in any diarrhea, bloody rectal discharge may occur from an associated proctitis or anusitis. Frequent, soft, nonfatty stools should suggest gastrogenic diarrhea. Stools that contain large amounts of mucus without pus or blood are a feature of functional bowel disorders. Semiformed or liquid stools with a greenish color because of excessive amounts of bile may result from excessive use of cathartics or from an infection. Voluminous, watery stools associated with hypokalemia suggest diarrhea produced by the abnormal production of gastrointestinal hormones (e.g., vasoactive intestinal polypeptide).

PHYSICAL EXAMINATION

There are few signs that have specific diagnostic value in chronic diarrhea. Evidence of weight loss, malnutrition, dehydration, and anemia point to disease of a serious nature. The physical examination may provide clues to specific diseases: reddish-purple flushing of the skin suggests metastatic carcinoid tumor; mucocutaneous pigmentation—Addison's disease or the Peutz-Jeghers syndrome; ecchymosis—malabsorption or Schönlein-Henoch's purpura; erythema nodosum or pyoderma gangrenosum—ulcerative colitis; Argyll Robertson pupils in the absence of syphilis—diabetic neuropathy; exophthalmos—Graves' disease; macroglossia—amyloidosis; lymphadenopathy—lymphoma; tuberculosis, metastatic carcinoma, or Whipple's disease; lymphedema—lymphangiectasia; peripheral arthritis or spondylitis—ulcerative colitis, regional enteritis, or Whipple's disease; uremic breath—renal failure; and clubbing—sprue or ulcerative colitis. In the abdominal and rectal examination, special attention should be paid to tenderness, masses, gaseous distention, bowel sounds, organomegaly, anal fistulae, and the presence of a rectal shelf or frozen pelvis. A palpable mass in the left lower quadrant should arouse suspicion of carcinoma or diverticulitis; on the right side of the abdomen, carcinoma and Crohn's disease. A palpable, stiff descending colon is common in ulcerative colitis and diverticulitis, but this may result from spasm.

PROCTOSIGMOIDOSCOPY

This procedure is indicated in all patients to detect rectal and colonic inflammatory disease, neoplasm, and parasitic disease.

RADIOLOGIC STUDIES

Roentgenographic examination is warranted in all patients. It should include plain abdominal films as well as a barium enema, upper GI series, and small bowel study. The routine abdominal films may reveal visceromegaly, partial obstruction, pancreatic calcification, and postoperative foreign bodies.

LABORATORY PROCEDURES

1. CBC to screen for anemia that may suggest blood loss, malabsorption, infection, or neoplasia. Eosinophilia suggests parasitic disease, allergic reaction, eosinophilic gastroenteritis, or neoplasia. Megaloblastic anemia suggests malabsorption of folic acid or vitamin $B_{12}$.
2. Stool, examined immediately for culture, ova and parasites, occult blood, and fecal leukocytes.
3. Serum electrolytes and BUN for electrolyte disturbances or uremia.
4. Serum protein electrophoresis to detect gastrointestinal protein loss, evidence of chronic inflammation, or hypogammaglobulinemia.
5. Serum carotene to screen for fat malabsorption. The results may be invalid if the patient has had either a limited or an excessive intake of vegetables.
6. Serum calcium, phosphorus, and alkaline phosphatase to detect parathyroid disease.

7. Thyroid function tests ($T_4$, $T_3$ resin uptake) to detect hyperthyroidism.
8. Fasting or 2-hour postprandial blood sugar tests to detect diabetes.
9. Serum folate and vitamin $B_{12}$ levels to detect deficiency that may be due to malabsorption.

SPECIALIZED TESTS IN THE EVALUATION OF CHRONIC DIARRHEA

The initial evaluation may well provide the proper diagnosis so that treatment can be instituted. Often, however, the initial evaluation only suggests the cause or the anatomic site of the lesion. More specialized procedures, such as those that follow, are then required.

1. Gastric analysis with pentagastrin stimulation. A nonbeta islet cell tumor of the pancreas should be suspected when diarrhea is associated with chronic peptic ulcer disease. In this entity, there is hypersecretion of hydrochloric acid resulting from the excessive production of gastrin. Gastric analysis should be performed before and after the subcutaneous injection of pentagastrin (6 μg/kg). The Zollinger-Ellison syndrome is usually associated with a baseline hydrochloric acid secretion above 15 mEq per hour and a ratio of basal to post-Histalog secretion of 60 percent or more. The diagnosis of nonbeta islet cell tumor is further supported by high serum gastrin levels.
2. Serum level of vitamin $B_{12}$ and a Schilling test. These may identify pernicious anemia associated with chronic diarrhea.
3. Seventy-two–hour fecal fat test. This test, although time-consuming, is invaluable in documenting a malabsorption problem as a cause of diarrhea. The patient must be on a diet containing a minimum of 80 g of fat per day. All feces excreted during a 72-hour period are collected and analyzed for lipid content. A normal individual should excrete no more than 5 to 7 g of fat every 24 hours. Increased fecal excretion of fat only indicates a significant abnormality in fat absorption; additional studies are necessary to establish its cause.
4. D-Xylose absorption. D-Xylose (25 g dissolved in 250 ml of water) is administered orally. The ability of the small intestine to absorb this carbohydrate is measured by determining the amount of xylose excreted in a 5-hour period. An abnormally low excretion of xylose (less than 5 g in 5 hours) suggests jejunal mucosal disease. The accuracy of the test is increased by measuring serum D-Xylose levels 2 hours after the oral dose is administered. The normal levels are less than 20 mg/dl.
5. Lactose tolerance test. This test is indicated when the history suggests that the diarrhea is related to milk intolerance. Following oral administration of lactose (100 g, or 1.75 g/kg of body weight for patients weighing less than 100 lb), patients with lactase deficiency show a rise in blood glucose to a peak of less than 30 mg/100 ml (expressed as glucose) associated with bloating, flatulence, cramps, and diarrhea. The most discriminatory finding using a noninvasive procedure is increased hydrogen excretion in the breath after a test dose of lactose.
6. Bentiromide test. This test is of value when pancreatic exocrine insufficiency is suspected. The principle underlying this noninvasive test is an adequate duodenal concentration of chymotrypsin to cleave para-aminobenzoic acid (PABA) from the synthetic peptide bentiromide. After a 500-mg oral dose of the peptide, PABA is released in the duodenum, absorbed, conjugated in the liver, and excreted in the urine. Normally there is less than 57 percent arylamine excretion in a 6-hour urine sample. Modifications of the test involving PABA levels have increased its accuracy.
7. Small bowel culture. A number of derangements of the gastrointestinal tract, such as multiple strictures, surgical blind loops, afferent loop partial obstruction, multiple jejunal diverticula, diabetic neuropathy, and scleroderma, may give rise to the intestinal stasis syndrome. The common feature is massive bacterial proliferation in the proximal small bowel. A sterile tube is passed into the stomach or the small intestine, and the aspirate is cultured on appropriate aerobic and anaerobic media. Cultures showing greater than 1 million colonies per milliliter of intestinal fluid should be regarded as abnormal.
8. Bile acid breath test. This procedure, not yet widely available, has been recom-

mended for the detection of intestinal malabsorption in the blind-loop syndrome with bacterial overgrowth and in ileal disease or resection. A test is considered positive if there is increased pulmonary excretion of $^{14}CO_2$ following the oral administration of glycine-1-$^{14}$C glycocholate.

9. Peroral small bowel biopsy. Many types of suction and hydraulic biopsy instruments are now available for procuring mucosal specimens to demonstrate histologic abnormalities peculiar to certain diseases. Extreme care must be taken to ensure proper orientation and processing of the biopsy material.

10. Dye-marker transit time. The time required for ingested food to be eliminated in the stool may at times be useful in correlating the symptoms with the laboratory evaluation. Ingestion of an intense dye (50 mg brilliant blue mixed with 350 mg methylcellulose) along with a regular meal provides a means of measuring the mouth-to-anus transit time.

11. Arteriography. Judicious use of celiac arteriography may be helpful in the diagnosis of arterial insufficiency, suspected tumors, or obscure submucosal abnormalities on routine barium studies.

12. Colonofiberoscopy. With the development of fiberoptic colonoscopes, endoscopic examination of the colon beyond the range of the rigid proctosigmoidoscope has become a reality. It may be decisive in establishing a correct diagnosis of colonic diarrhea in patients whose barium enema study is questionable and inconclusive.

13. To test for factitious laxative abuse, a stool specimen should be brought to a pH of 8.0. A maroon color indicates the presence of phenolphthalein, a common ingredient in laxative preparations. Urine tests are available to demonstrate the presence of aloes, senna alkaloids, and bisacodyl.

# CONSTIPATION
H. Harold Friedman

## Definition

Constipation may be defined as the passage of excessively dry, small (less than 50 g/day), or infrequent stools (less often than every other day). When a patient complains of constipation, it is well to ask what he means by the term, because the symptom may be imagined. For example, patients who equate good health with regularity of bowel movements often believe they are constipated even when stools are normal. Most patients, however, consider themselves constipated if they have hard stools, small stools, infrequent bowel movements, or stools that are difficult to expel.

## Etiology

The more common causes of constipation are listed in Table 5-6. Constipation results when filling or emptying of the rectum is impaired. Inadequate rectal filling may be a consequence of such diverse conditions as intestinal disease, systemic illness, functional bowel disorders, drug effects, and neurologic abnormalities. Emptying of the rectum depends on the integrity of the defecation reflex, which may be disturbed by anorectal disease, poor bowel habits, laxative abuse, neurologic illness, physical inactivity, old age, and other conditions.

## Clinical Features

### Chronic Constipation

1. Chronic habitual constipation with the passage of hard or infrequent stools is usually caused by improper eating habits, poor bowel habits, inadequate fluid

**Table 5-6.** Causes of constipation

A. Impaired rectal filling
   1. Dysfunction due to intrinsic gastrointestinal disease
      a. Narrowing of the lumen
         (1) Tumors (benign or malignant)
         (2) Inflammatory bowel disease
            (a) Crohn's disease
            (b) Ulcerative colitis
            (c) Chronic amebiasis
            (d) Diverticulitis
         (3) Irritable bowel syndrome
         (4) Congenital aganglionic megacolon (Hirschsprung's disease)
   2. Dysfunction secondary to systemic disorders
      a. Pregnancy
      b. Hypothyroidism
      c. Hyperparathyroidism and other hypercalcemic states
      d. Hypokalemia
      e. Diabetes mellitus
      f. Porphyria
      g. Lead poisoning
   3. Dysfunction secondary to drug effects
      a. Opiates
      b. Ganglionic blocking agents
      c. Anticholinergic drugs
      d. Nonabsorbable antacids
      e. Antidepressants
      f. Hematinics
      g. Diuretics
B. Impaired rectal emptying
   1. Segmental disturbances in the defecation reflex
      a. Anorectal disorders
         (1) Anal ulcer
         (2) Fissure-in-ano
         (3) Fistula-in-ano
         (4) Proctitis
         (5) Hemorrhoids
         (6) Increased anal sphincteric tone
      b. Neurologic disease
      c. Physical inactivity
      d. Weak abdominal musculature
      e. Old age
   2. Suprasegmental disturbances in the defecation reflex
      a. Poor toilet training
      b. Poor bowel and eating habits
      c. Laxative abuse
      d. Psychiatric disorders

---

intake, lack of exercise, medications, laxatives, or a combination of these factors. It may also occur in patients with irritable bowel syndromes, who often complain of alternating constipation and diarrhea, abdominal distress, and the passage of scybalous stools that may or may not contain mucus. Constipation is sometimes the manifestation of an anxiety neurosis or depression. In all of the foregoing conditions, the GI findings are negative. The diagnosis is made by exclusion.

  **2.** Chronic constipation may be due to rectal insensitivity, which in many cases appears to be the result of persistent suppression of the urge to defecate or laxative abuse. In such individuals, the desire for bowel movement often is lacking even when the rectum is filled with feces.

3. Chronic constipation may be associated with anorectal disease, such as fissures, ulcers, or hemorrhoids. The diagnosis is usually evident from the history, examination, and proctosigmoidoscopy.
4. Lifelong obstipation (severe refractory constipation) is sometimes due to megacolon.
5. Chronic constipation may also be due to a variety of gastrointestinal or systemic disorders, as outlined in Table 5-6.

### Acute Constipation

1. Constipation of fairly recent onset in a previously healthy individual, particularly if progressive, may be indicative of a serious disorder.
2. The most common cause of acute constipation, particularly in the elderly, is fecal impaction. The clinical setting is usually that of a feeble, weak, or debilitated individual, lying in bed and receiving frequent doses of sedatives or narcotics. It may also follow barium studies of the gastrointestinal tract. Soiling and involuntary passage of stools around the impaction may be interpreted erroneously as diarrhea. Rectal discomfort may be severe. The diagnosis is made by rectal examination.
3. Other causes of constipation of recent or acute onset are neoplasm of the rectum and large bowel, mesenteric vascular occlusion, painful anorectal lesions, drugs, intestinal obstruction, urinary tract disease, neurologic disorders, and systemic illness.

### Diagnostic Approach

1. Digital rectal examination is of major importance in the diagnosis of fecal impaction, anal and perianal disease, and lesions of the rectum. In a patient who is constipated at the time of examination, absence of stool in the rectum suggests a disorder of rectal filling rather than one of rectal emptying.
2. Habitual constipation of long duration does not require extensive workup if the patient is otherwise in good health. The diagnosis of its cause may be apparent from the history. The physical findings are negative, as are those of rectal and stool examinations. Proctosigmoidoscopy and barium enema should probably be done once to exclude organic disease.
3. When constipation is of recent origin, once fecal impaction has been excluded, a thorough investigation is warranted to rule out carcinoma of the rectum and colon. The digital rectal examination is an important procedure because about one-fourth of cancers are within reach of the examining finger. If rectal findings fail to explain the constipation, then stool examination for occult blood, proctosigmoidoscopy or colonoscopy, and plain abdominal films followed by barium enema, upper GI series, and small bowel study are indicated. If the GI workup is unrevealing, the systemic causes of constipation listed in Table 5-5 should be excluded by appropriate means.

### FUNCTIONAL BOWEL DISEASE
Sunder J. Mehta

Syndromes of functional bowel disease include nonulcer dyspepsia (NUD) and the irritable bowel syndrome (IBS). They are the commonest gastrointestinal disorders seen by primary care doctors and gastroenterologists. NUD is characterized by chronic or recurrent upper abdominal symptoms in the absence of peptic ulcer.

IBS comprises chronic abdominal pain or an abnormal bowel habit in the absence of structural or biochemical abnormality. About 20 percent of individuals have symptoms consistent with functional bowel disease, and about one-fourth of them seek medical care, generally before the age of 35 years.

## Etiology

The cause of the irritable bowel syndrome is unknown. The disorder is attributed to an abnormality of intestinal motility combined with a heightened pain response to bowel distention rather than to an increased volume of intraluminal gas. Paradoxically, decreased colonic motility is associated with diarrhea, and increased motility with constipation. The bowel musculature exhibits increased reactivity to parasympathomimetic drugs and cholecystokinin. Anxiety or depression is frequently associated with this disorder.

## Clinical Features

1. The syndrome is usually a chronic illness with frequent relapses, but the onset is abrupt in about one-fourth of the cases.
2. Symptoms generally recur throughout life. The diagnosis should be made with great caution in older patients who have not had symptoms at an earlier age.
3. The predominant clinical expression is irregularity of bowel function with or without abdominal pain. Most patients complain of frequent, small, loose stools rather than true diarrhea. Constipation is usually described as the passage of scybalous or pencil-like stools. There may be excessive mucus in the stools, but blood and pus are never present. A common pattern of defecation consists of the passage of a hard stool in the morning followed by several loose stools later in the day. Often, there is a feeling of incomplete evacuation following defecation.
4. Abdominal pain is present in the vast majority of patients. It is frequently ill-defined but is most often localized to the lower abdomen or left lower quadrant. Relief of pain may be obtained by the passage of flatus or feces.
5. Major triggering factors are stress and ingestion of food. Symptoms are related to the waking state.
6. Gaseousness, bloating, excessive flatulence, and dyspepsia occur commonly.
7. Vasomotor phenomena (faintness, flushing, sweating, palpitation) are noted frequently.
8. The occurrence of nocturnal pain or diarrhea, incontinence, fever, dehydration, and electrolyte disturbances suggests organic disease rather than an irritable bowel syndrome.
9. Physical examination is negative, but it may reveal tenderness over the colon.

## Diagnosis

The key to diagnosis is a good history. The diagnosis is generally one of exclusion, as there are no confirmatory tests.
1. Features that support the diagnosis of the IBS include the following:
   a. Onset below the age of 40 years, often in early adult life.
   b. Symptoms present for at least 3 months, most prominent during periods of emotional stress, and often associated with multiple complaints.
   c. Consistent pattern of symptoms, although they may vary in severity.
   d. Abdominal pain, typically increased after meals, and at least partially relieved by defecation.
   e. Discomfort typically felt during the day and at bedtime.
   f. Excessive mucus in the stools.

g. Negative physical findings except for tenderness, usually noted in the lower quadrants.

2. Features that militate against the diagnosis of the IBS include the following:
    a. Onset above the age of 50 years.
    b. Relatively short duration of symptoms.
    c. A steadily progressive downhill course, especially if associated with constitutional manifestations.
    d. Voluminous diarrhea (> 500 ml/day), weight loss, nocturnal symptomatology, rectal bleeding, and the presence of pus or fat in the stools.
3. As a group, patients are somewhat neurotic, anxious, or depressed.

## Diagnostic Approach

1. A careful history and physical examination, including pelvic and rectal examinations, should be performed to rule out organic disease. Careful inquiry should be made into the use of dairy- and sorbitol-containing products (sugar-free gum, pears, prunes, and apple juice).
2. Initial workup.
    a. CBC.
    b. Urinalysis.
    c. Stools for ova, parasites, and occult blood.
    d. Fecal smear for leukocytes. The presence of polymorphonuclear leukocytes indicates inflammatory bowel disease and practically excludes the diagnosis of functional bowel disorder.
    e. Proctosigmoidoscopy.
    f. Trial of milk-free diet as a crude screening procedure for lactose intolerance.
3. Subsequent workup. If symptoms persist and the initial workup is negative, additional studies are advisable to exclude malabsorptive states, inflammatory bowel disease, infections (e.g., amebiasis, giardiasis), and carcinoma of the colon.
    a. Barium enema, upper GI series, and small bowel study.
    b. Screening for malabsorption (see Chronic Diarrhea)—necessary.
    c. Colonoscopy—frequently needed in older patients.
    d. Lactose tolerance test or hydrogen breath test—rarely needed.
4. Other procedures. When the symptomatology is persistent or intractable and the workup is negative, additional investigation, such as abdominal CT scan, may be warranted. Having patients keep a 1-week diary of food intake, chronological occurrence, and symptoms can be useful.

## GASTROINTESTINAL GAS SYNDROMES
Sunder J. Mehta

1. Complaints of too much "gas" are a common clinical problem. The more common causes of indigestion, gaseousness, and flatulence are listed in Table 5-7. Surprisingly, patients with this complaint have normal volumes of bowel gas whose composition is no different from that of normal subjects.

    Clinically, three syndromes are seen: (1) excessive belching, (2) abdominal pain and bloating, and (3) excessive flatulence.
    a. Aerophagia, which is the excessive swallowing of air, is usually associated with abdominal fullness, gaseous eructations, and the presence of a large air bubble in the fundus of the stomach. Belching ordinarily relieves the discomfort. Pain is uncommon but when present may mimic coronary artery disease. Aerophagia is usually a habit, although it may be associated with organic disease. Many aerophagics are not aware that they are air-swallowers. Swallowed air that is not eructed passes down to the small bowel and colon. Should the air become trapped in the splenic flexure, left upper quadrant (LUQ) dis-

**Table 5-7.** Causes of indigestion, gaseousness, and flatulence

A. Functional or psychosomatic
B. Organic
  1. Disease of the esophagus
    a. Gastroesophageal reflux with or without hiatal hernia
    b. Achalasia
    c. Esophageal obstruction
  2. Disease of the stomach and duodenum
    a. Gastritis
    b. Gastric ulcer
    c. Duodenal ulcer
    d. Carcinoma of the stomach
  3. Disease of the biliary tract
    a. Cholecystitis
    b. Cholelithiasis
    c. Choledocholithiasis
  4. Disease of the pancreas
    a. Pancreatitis
    b. Carcinoma of the pancreas
  5. Disease of the intestines
    a. Malabsorptive states
    b. Intermittent intestinal obstruction
    c. Irritable bowel syndrome
    d. Abdominal angina
  6. Systemic illness
    a. Tuberculosis
    b. Heart disease
    c. Renal failure
    d. Chronic liver disease (e.g., cirrhosis)
    e. Diabetes mellitus

comfort, which radiates to the left side of the chest, left shoulder, and sometimes the left arm, may occur. This is the splenic flexure syndrome. Relief of the pain is characteristically obtained by defecation. The diagnosis is suggested by showing large amounts of air in the LUQ on plain abdominal x-rays.

  **b.** Abdominal pain and bloating. The primary problem is not too much gas but rather an irritable gut caused by some sort of mobility disorder that causes these patients to perceive pain when the gut is distended by gas.

  **c.** Flatulence is probably the result of a disturbance in bowel motility sometimes associated with an abnormal pain response to gaseous distention of the bowel. The possible routes by which gas may enter the gastrointestinal tract are air-swallowing, bacterial fermentation in the blowel, and diffusion from the blood. Food intolerance appears to play a role in the genesis of flatulence. Milk products may cause bloating, flatulence, and diarrhea in patients with lactase deficiency. Gluten-containing foods exacerbate the symptoms of nontropical sprue. Intolerance to fatty foods is a common occurrence in patients with biliary tract or pancreatic disease. Some food intolerances are undoubtedly allergic in origin, but in the majority of cases the mechanism is not understood. Flatulence is often a noteworthy, but never the sole, symptom of malabsorptive states or intestinal disease.

## Diagnostic Approach

This is similar to that discussed in the Functional Bowel Syndrome section. Identify the specific gas problem to see whether the patient is a belcher, a bloater, or a gas passer. Workup should be sufficient to convince the patient and physician that no organic gut lesion is overlooked.

# ABDOMINAL DISTENTION AND ASCITES
Barry W. Frank

## Abdominal Distention

### Definition

Abdominal distention may be defined as a sudden or gradual increase in the size of the abdomen. Distention may be persistent or intermittent.

### Symptoms

Abdominal distention may be entirely asymptomatic. More often, however, there is a sensation of fullness or pressure. Pain of varying severity may be noted. Other symptoms, such as vomiting, gaseous eructations, expulsion of flatus, post-prandial discomfort, constipation, localized pain, back pain, weight gain, shortness of breath, and edema, if present, may be clues to the etiology of the distention.

### Physical Examination

Detailed examination of the abdomen is essential and should begin with inspection. The presence and location of abdominal scars, the abdominal venous pattern, and the contour of the abdomen should be noted. Examination for flank fullness, shifting dullness, and a fluid wave should be made. Percussion aids in localizing abnormal areas of dullness, tympany, and resistance. Palpation defines enlarged organs, masses, areas of tenderness, and hernias. Auscultation reveals liver rubs, abnormal bowel sounds, and bruits. Pelvic and rectal examinations are essential to rule out pelvic disease.

### Etiology

LOCALIZED

1. Upper abdomen.
   a. Hepatomegaly.
   b. Splenomegaly.
   c. Renal enlargement by mass or cyst.
   d. Gastric distention secondary to mechanical or functional obstruction.
   e. Inflammatory mass.
   f. Abdominal wall hernia.
   g. Aortic aneurysm.
   h. Pancreatic cyst or tumor.
2. Lower abdomen.
   a. Uterine enlargement.
   b. Ovarian mass or cyst.
   c. Distention of the urinary bladder.
   d. Inflammatory mass arising from the sigmoid colon, cecum, or ileum.
   e. Abdominal wall hernia.

GENERALIZED

1. Ascites (discussed later in this section, p. 200).
2. Intestinal obstruction.
   a. Adynamic ileus.
   b. Mechanical obstruction.
   c. Idiopathic intestinal pseudoobstruction.
3. Large intraabdominal cyst.
4. Diffuse peritonitis from any cause.
5. Extreme constipation with fecal impaction.
6. Neurogenic obstruction (Hirschsprung's disease).
7. Large retroperitoneal mass.

## Diagnostic Approach

1. *Initial procedures.* In addition to the history and physical examination, a hemo-gram, urinalysis, liver function tests, and serum and urinary amylase determi-nations should be performed on every patient.
2. X-ray studies.
   a. Four-way abdominal films. Such films are indicated in virtually all cases, es-pecially if intestinal obstruction is suspected. With this procedure, evaluation of the size of the liver is inaccurate, but splenomegaly can be recognized. The kidneys are usually seen as well-defined shadows on each side of the spine at approximately the level of the third lumbar vertebra. The psoas shadows ex-tend obliquely and laterally toward the pelvis. Distortion of these shadows suggests retroperitoneal disease. A clearly defined line in the flank repre-sents the translucent area occupied by the properitoneal fat; this line is oblit-erated in the presence of abscess or infection. It is important to note the char-acter of the gas patterns in the intestinal tract. Fluid levels, abnormal calcium deposition, intraperitoneal air, and organ displacement are also im-portant. The nature and diagnostic implications of the many abnormalities that can occur are beyond the scope of this text, but proper interpretation is essential to accurate diagnosis.
   b. Barium studies of the gastrointestinal tract. When intestinal obstruction is suspected, regardless of its cause, barium x-ray studies should not be per-formed without consultation with the radiologist and not without detailed consideration of the clinical problem. Barium should not be used orally when perforation is suspected, when intestinal obstruction is complete, or when vomiting is persistent. Water-soluble contrast material, such as Gastrografin, should be used cautiously in patients susceptible to aspiration, to avoid pul-monary edema. In the hands of a skilled radiologist, barium enemas can be of great value in the diagnosis of colonic obstruction. If obstruction is not pre-sent, barium x-rays are indicated to look for intrinsic lesions or for displace-ment or alterations produced by extrinsic lesions. Unless the clinical history and physical examination strongly suggest the upper or lower gastrointestinal tract, a barium enema should be obtained first because it makes subsequent preparation for upper GI and small bowel series easier for the patient.
   c. Intravenous pyelogram. Retroperitoneal abnormalities often do not produce alterations of the barium x-rays. An intravenous pyelogram may be of value in defining renal pathology as well as disease in the retroperitoneum.
3. Liver scan. When distention occurs in the upper abdomen or when a right upper quadrant mass is present, a liver scan may be helpful in delineating the size and contour of the liver, or in revealing intrahepatic defects due to abscesses, cysts, or neoplasms.
4. Abdominal angiography. This diagnostic procedure may be of assistance in the diagnosis of suspected masses. Vascular abnormalities of significance include vascular occlusion, vessel displacement or straightening, and the presence of a vascular blush.

5. Ultrasonic scanning. This may be helpful in the diagnosis of intraabdominal and retroperitoneal cysts, pancreatic pseudocysts, pancreatic carcinoma, aortic aneurysms or other fluid-filled lesions, and solid tumors. The procedure is most effective for upper abdominal and pelvic pathology since intestinal gas significantly interferes with sound waves.
6. Computed tomography (CT). CT scans, if available, may be valuable in the detection and evaluation of intraabdominal and retroperitoneal masses and liver disease, and in the diagnosis of pancreatic disease, including carcinoma.
7. Laparoscopy. This relatively safe, simple procedure is being used more frequently as a method for internal inspection of the upper and lower abdomen. The technique involves three basic steps: induction of a pneumoperitoneum, insertion of the instrument, and inspection of the superficial structures of the abdominal cavity. Best seen are significant portions of the liver, the peritoneum, the anterior wall of the stomach, the uterus, and the ovaries. The ability to obtain biopsies is an added diagnostic dimension that may save the patient from the need for surgical laparotomy.
8. Paracentesis. See page 201.

---

## Ascites

---

### Definition

Ascites may be defined as an accumulation of fluid in the peritoneal cavity. The fluid is most often serous in nature.

### Symptoms and Physical Examination

See Abdominal Distention, page 198.

### Etiology

The most common causes of ascites are cirrhosis of the liver and congestive heart failure. Ascitic fluid may be a transudate or an exudate, or it may be chylous. The causes are listed below.

TRANSUDATIVE ASCITES

1. Prehepatic causes.
   a. Right-sided heart failure.
   b. Constrictive pericarditis.
   c. Venous occlusion.
      (1) Supradiaphragmatic occlusion of the inferior vena cava.
      (2) Budd-Chiari syndrome (hepatic vein occlusion due to thrombosis, tumor, or venous web).
      (3) Venooclusive disease secondary to hepatotoxins (e.g., seneciosis).
2. Hepatic causes.
   a. Cirrhosis of the liver.
      (1) Micronodular.
      (2) Macronodular.
      (3) Cardiac.
   b. Tumors of the liver (rarely).

EXUDATIVE ASCITES

1. Peritonitis.
   a. Ruptured viscus.
   b. Tuberculosis.
   c. Pancreatitis.

   **d.** Bile peritonitis.
   **e.** Pelvic inflammatory disease (rarely).
**2.** Tumors. Metastatic to the liver or peritoneum, or both.

CHYLOUS ASCITES

**1.** Trauma to the cisterna chyli in the abdomen.
**2.** Tuberculosis (occasionally).
**3.** Cirrhosis of the liver (occasionally).
**4.** Chronic inflammation, fibrosis, or hyperplasia of the major intestinal lymphatics.
**5.** Tumor involving the major intestinal lymphatics.

MISCELLANEOUS CAUSES

**1.** Meigs' syndrome (ovarian fibroma).
**2.** Myxedema.
**3.** Endometriosis.
**4.** Pseudomyxoma peritonei.
**5.** Anasarca with hypoalbuminemia.
**6.** Connective tissue diseases (rarely).

## Diagnostic Approach

**1.** Liver function tests. Because the most common cause of ascites is liver disease, the initial laboratory tests should include a serum bilirubin, alkaline phosphatase, SGOT, gamma glutamyl transpeptidase, prothrombin time, and protein electrophoresis. If acute or chronic hepatitis is suspected, the serum should be examined for the presence of antigens and antibodies as outlined in the section on Jaundice, page 203.
**2.** Diagnostic paracentesis. Diagnostic paracentesis is a valuable procedure with ascites because the character of the fluid is often helpful diagnostically. The procedure should be performed under sterile conditions. Ordinarily, 100 to 200 ml of fluid is adequate for the studies outlined below. It should always be performed if there is fever, abdominal pain, or both.
   **a.** Appearance of the fluid. Clear, straw-colored fluid is usually seen in liver disease or prehepatic obstruction. Bloody fluid suggests malignancy but may occur in nonmalignant liver disease. Turbid fluid implies infection or inflammation. Milky fluid is virtually pathognomonic of chylous ascites.
   **b.** Specific gravity. Ascitic fluid with a specific gravity greater than 1.017 is indicative of an exudative process.
   **c.** Protein content. Fluid with a protein content greater than 3.0 g/100 ml is found in exudates. When the protein content exceeds 4.0 g/100 ml, tuberculous ascites should be suspected.
   **d.** White cell count. White counts are often variable. However, when the count is greater than 900 per cubic millimeter, peritonitis is probable. A predominance of lymphocytes suggests tuberculosis.
   **e.** Amylase. Amylase levels above 500 units suggest pancreatitis or pancreatic ascites.
   **f.** Serum electrolytes. Electrolyte determinations are of little diagnostic value.
   **g.** Stains and cultures for bacteria. A Gram stain should be performed routinely to detect suspected or unsuspected infection of the peritoneum. Routine cultures for aerobic and anaerobic organisms, acid-fast bacilli, and fungi are advisable.
   **h.** Triglycerides. Although frank chylous ascites is detectable by the naked eye, a slightly turbid fluid may pose a diagnostic problem. The presence of chylous ascites is confirmed by finding elevated triglyceride levels in the fluid.
   **i.** Cytologic study. When intraabdominal malignancy is seen with "studding" of the peritoneum by tumor nodules and ascites, confirmation of the diagnosis can be obtained by histologic study of smears prepared from a centrifuged specimen of ascitic fluid.

3. Barium studies of the gastrointestinal tract. Contrast examinations are often necessary in the patient with ascites of unknown cause. In addition to disclosing intrinsic disease of the gastrointestinal tract and varices, displacement of the gut by extrinsic lesions may be revealed.
4. Liver scan. This test is most helpful in the diagnosis of space-occupying lesions of the liver and least helpful in determining liver size or liver function.
5. Abdominal CT scan or ultrasound studies. These may be helpful in the diagnosis of intraperitoneal masses, organ enlargement or displacement, and enlarged lymph nodes.
6. Needle biopsy of the liver. Percutaneous liver biopsy should be considered in most cases when liver abnormality is suspected as the cause of ascites. It is useful in establishing the histologic diagnosis in primary disease of the liver, in detecting malignancy, and in revealing hepatic manifestations of systemic disease (e.g., tuberculosis).
7. Selective angiography and retrograde venous catheterization. Selective arteriography of the hepatic and splenic arteries with delayed films to visualize the portal vein may be helpful in ascites of obscure cause. Retrograde venous catheterization may be useful in the diagnosis of cardiac and pericardial disease.
8. Peritoneoscopy. The introduction of pneumoperitoneum, insertion of a laparoscope, and inspection of the abdominal contents are useful for the direct visualization of the liver, gallbladder, pelvic organs, omentum, and peritoneal surfaces. Biopsies can be taken for histologic examination and culture. This procedure should be strongly considered when ascites is associated with a pelvic tumor, positive cytologic examination result, or suspected tuberculous peritonitis. With some exceptions, it should not be performed if the patient has undergone previous intraabdominal surgery.
9. Exploratory laparotomy. In the vast majority of cases, it is possible to discover the cause of ascites by means of the foregoing procedures. However, should the cause remain undetermined after adequate study, exploratory laparotomy may be necessary to establish a correct diagnosis.

## HEPATOMEGALY
### Andrew Mallory

## Definition

Hepatomegaly is defined as an enlarged liver. Defining only the location of the inferior edge of the liver on physical examination is inadequate in assessing liver size. Liver size can be best estimated on physical examination by gentle percussion in the midclavicular line during quiet breathing. The inferior margin may also be located by palpation. The normal range of size varies with height and sex. Hard percussion will result in smaller estimations. In one study, normal liver size was defined as $8 \pm 2$ cm for females and $10 \pm 2$ cm for males.

Liver scans and abdominal CT scans can also give useful indications of liver size. Plain films and barium studies are often misleading.

## Etiology

Common causes of hepatomegaly are listed in Table 5-8.

## Diagnostic Approach

### History

A history of heart failure, alcoholism, febrile illness, gallstones, foreign travel, diabetes, drug-taking, or symptoms suggesting malignancy is helpful. A family

**Table 5-8.** Causes of hepatomegaly

---

Venous congestion of the liver
    Congestive heart failure*
    Obstruction of vena cava or hepatic veins (e.g., tumor, thrombosis)
    Constrictive pericarditis

Obstruction of the common bile duct*
    Gallstones
    Tumors
    Pancreatitis

Infectious diseases
    Localized infections (e.g., amebic or pyogenic abscess)
    Diffuse infections (e.g., viral hepatitis,* tuberculosis, schistosomiasis)
    Hepatitis associated with systemic infections

Infiltrative diseases
    Fatty liver (e.g., alcohol,* diabetes)
    Amyloidosis
    Sarcoidosis
    Glycogen storage diseases

Neoplasms (e.g., primary, metastatic*)

Other
    Toxin- and drug-induced hepatitis (including alcohol*)
    Chronic persistent* or chronic active* hepatitis
    Cirrhosis (e.g., alcoholic,* postnecrotic, biliary)
    Wilson's disease
    Hemochromatosis

---

*Most common causes.
Source: L. B. Reller, et al. (eds.), *Clinical Internal Medicine.* Boston: Little, Brown, 1979. P. 211.

history of liver disease suggests Wilson's disease, hemochromatosis, or alpha-1-antitrypsin deficiency.

### Physical Examination

1. Inspection may reveal localized enlargement (e.g., abscess, tumor).
2. Auscultation may reveal a bruit (tumor), venous hum (portal hypertension with collateral flow), or friction rub (tumor).
3. Percussion (punch) may detect tenderness (hepatitis, biliary tract disease, congestion).
4. Palpation may reveal the firm liver edge of cirrhosis or the "rock hard" edge of malignancy. Nodularity suggests cirrhosis or tumor. Pulsations suggest tricuspid regurgitation. A palpable gallbladder suggests pancreatic carcinoma with bile duct obstruction.

### Laboratory Data

See Jaundice, next section.

---

## JAUNDICE
Andrew Mallory

---

## Definition

Jaundice is the yellow discoloration of the tissues caused by retention of bilirubin. When serum bilirubin exceeds 3 mg/100 ml, jaundice is usually present.

## Etiology

1. Increased quantity of bilirubin presented to the liver (e.g., hemolysis, transfusion of stored blood, hematoma with resorption).
2. Decreased hepatobiliary excretion of bilirubin.
   a. Defective uptake and transport of bilirubin by the liver cell (e.g., drug effects, Crigler-Najjar syndrome, possibly Gilbert's syndrome).
   b. Defective conjugation of bilirubin by the liver cell (e.g., Gilbert's syndrome, drug effects, breastfeeding jaundice).
   c. Defective excretion of bilirubin by the liver cell (e.g., drug effects, Dubin-Johnson syndrome, idiopathic cholestasis of pregnancy).
   d. Defective transport of bilirubin by the biliary system (e.g., common bile duct stone, pancreatic carcinoma, bile duct tumors).

   The examples given are conditions thought to arise exclusively from the mechanism stated. Many common causes of jaundice are due to combinations of these mechanisms. In clinical practice, the most common causes of jaundice are hemolysis, viral hepatitis, alcoholic liver disease, drugs, bile duct calculi, pancreatic carcinoma, and carcinoma metastatic to the liver.

## Clinical Features

### History

1. The insidious onset of anorexia, nausea, malaise, and fever in a young patient prior to the onset of jaundice suggests viral hepatitis.
2. Recurrent episodes of epigastric or right upper quadrant pain prior to the onset of jaundice in a middle-aged or elderly patient suggest biliary tract disease. These symptoms together with high fever and appropriate physical signs suggest cholangitis.
3. A long history of alcohol abuse is consistent with alcoholic liver disease.
4. Chronic weight loss and weakness preceding jaundice suggest malignancy. These symptoms when accompanied by depression, phlebitis, or epigastric pain point to pancreatic carcinoma.
5. The onset of jaundice in relation to the administration of certain drugs or anesthetic agents suggests drug-induced liver disease. The occupational history may suggest a toxin-induced liver disease.
6. A family history of jaundice raises the possibility of hemolytic disorders, Wilson's disease, Gilbert's syndrome, and alpha-1-antitrypsin deficiency.

### Physical Examination

Physical findings helpful in evaluating jaundice and the diseases suggested by these findings are listed below.

1. Spider nevi, gynecomastia, white nails, palmar erythema, and Dupuytren's contractures suggest cirrhosis.
2. Ascites, splenomegaly, dilated abdominal wall veins, and periumbilical venous hum suggest portal hypertension.
3. Kayser-Fleischer rings and neuropsychiatric changes suggest Wilson's disease.
4. Gray pigmentation suggests hemochromatosis.
5. Excoriations and xanthomas suggest primary biliary cirrhosis.
6. Severe left- or right-sided heart failure suggests passive congestion or hepatocellular ischemia.
7. Palpable nontender gallbladder suggests pancreatic carcinoma.

## Diagnostic Approach

**1.** Biochemical assessment.

    **a.** Serum aspartate aminotransferase (AST) and serum alanine aminotransferase (ALT) (formerly serum glutamic-oxaloacetic transaminase [SGOT] and serum glutamic-pyruvic transaminase [SGPT], respectively). AST is found in the following organs in order of decreasing concentration: heart, liver, skeletal muscle, kidney, and pancreas. ALT, although widely distributed in the body, is predominantly confined to the liver and is, therefore, more specific for liver disease. These two tests are sensitive indicators of hepatocellular necrosis. In general, levels greater than 10 times the upper limit of normal indicate acute hepatocellular injury as seen, for example, in viral hepatitis, drug- or toxin-induced hepatitis (other than alcohol), ischemic liver disease, or, transiently, cholangitis. Lesser elevations are nonspecific and may be seen with virtually any other form of liver injury, including cholestasis or infiltrative liver disease. Alcoholic liver disease is only rarely associated with AST elevations in excess of 10 times normal. AST/ALT ratio greater than two suggests alcoholic liver disease. In general, the degree of elevation of AST or ALT has little prognostic value.

    **b.** Serum alkaline phosphatase (SAP). This normally is derived from liver, bone, placenta, and intestine. The main clinical value of SAP is its sensitivity in detecting early intrahepatic or extrahepatic bile duct obstruction (often before jaundice develops) and in pointing to the presence of infiltrative diseases (tuberculosis, sarcoidosis) or space-occupying lesions (abscess, neoplasm). In addition, SAP helps differentiate hepatocellular from obstructive jaundice: high values (> 5 times normal) favor obstruction, and a normal SAP virtually excludes this diagnosis.

    SAP also rises in diseases of bone and in pregnancy. Greater specificity for liver disease can be provided by the serum gamma glutamyl transpeptidase, which is not elevated by bone disease or pregnancy. The serum 5-nucleotidase is also elevated in liver disease but not by bone disease, although it may increase in pregnancy. The heat-inactivation test is less helpful in assessing the source of SAP.

    **c.** Serum gamma glutamyl transpeptidase (SGGT). This enzyme is found in kidney, liver, and pancreas. Elevated values are most closely associated with SAP elevations. The main clinical value of this enzyme determination is its specificity for liver disease. In patients with elevated SAP due to bone disease or pregnancy, SGGT levels are usually normal.

    **d.** Serum bilirubin. An elevated serum bilirubin connotes either the presence of hepatobiliary disease, overproduction of bilirubin, or both. The direct-reacting (conjugated) bilirubin is specific for the presence of hepatobiliary disease and is a sensitive index of mild hepatic disease; elevations are found in more than 30 percent of patients with liver disease whose total serum bilirubin is normal. A mild increase in serum direct bilirubin results in urinary excretion of bilirubin: hence, a urine bilirubin determination may prove sensitive in detecting mild hepatic disease.

    The height of the serum bilirubin is of only limited diagnostic value in the individual patient. Elevations over 35 mg/100 ml generally indicate the presence of renal insufficiency in addition to hepatobiliary disease. Uncomplicated hemolysis seldom causes a total serum bilirubin of more than 5 mg/100 ml unless hepatobiliary disease is also present.

    **e.** Prothrombin time (PT). The PT reflects the activities of fibrinogen, prothrombin, and factors V, VII, and X. It is dependent on hepatic synthesis of these factors and intestinal absorption of vitamin K. Malabsorption of vitamin K occurs with impaired lipid absorption, as is commonly seen with bile salt deficiency secondary to prolonged cholestasis.

    The PT is helpful in assessing the extent of liver damage and in the prognosis. Little diagnostic significance should be given to a prolonged PT ($>$ 3 sec above control) unless it is measured at least 24 hours after parenteral injection of vitamin K. Hypoprothrombinemia related to bile salt deficiency will be corrected, whereas that secondary to hepatocellular disease will not.

  **f.** Serum proteins. The serum albumin concentration, like the PT, is a good indicator of hepatic functional reserve, but because of its half-life (20–26 days), changes are slow in reflecting liver damage. The alpha-1-globulins tend to be low in hepatocellular disease. An absent alpha-1-globulin suggests a homozygous alpha-1-antitrypsin deficiency. The gamma globulin concentration tends to increase with most forms of chronic liver disease. Marked increases (e.g., serum levels $>$ 3 g/100 ml) are suggestive of autoimmune chronic active hepatitis.

**2.** Serologic tests.

  **a.** Antimitochondrial antibody. Significant titers of antimitochondrial antibody are seen in over 85 percent of patients with primary biliary cirrhosis. Although not specific for this disease (e.g., elevated titers are occasionally seen with chronic active hepatitis), absence of the antibody is strong evidence against the diagnosis of primary biliary cirrhosis.

  **b.** Hepatitis antigens and antibodies.

    **(1)** Hepatitis A.

      **(a)** IgM hepatitis A antibody (IgMHAAb). This antibody is present in the serum at the onset of symptoms and usually disappears within 3 to 6 months.

      **(b)** IgG hepatitis A antibody (IgGHAAb). This antibody appears during convalescence and persists indefinitely.

    **(2)** Hepatitis B.

      **(a)** Hepatitis B surface antigen (HBsAg). This antigen is the first serologic marker to appear and usually disappears within 3 months.

      **(b)** Hepatitis B surface antibody (HBsAb). This antibody becomes detectable in the serum at a variable time after disappearance of the antigen and usually persists for life.

      **(c)** Hepatitis B core antibody (HBcAb). This antibody usually appears shortly after HBsAg and usually persists for life. It is present during the "window" between disappearance of HBsAg and appearance of HBsAb. IgM hepatitis B core antibody titers (IgMHB$_c$Ab) can also be determined. High serum titers usually are present early in the course of hepatitis B and disappear within 3 to 4 months.

      **(d)** Hepatitis Be antigen (HBeAg). This antigen appears within a few days of the appearance of HBsAg in most primary infections. It usually disappears just before the disappearance of the HBsAG in self-limited infections. Persistence of this antigen suggests chronic infection and is associated with a high degree of contagiousness. If this antigen does disappear from the serum, it is replaced by the hepatitis Be antibody.

    **(3)** Hepatitis C. Hepatitis C virus commonly causes both posttransfusion and community-acquired non-A, non-B hepatitis. The recently developed hepatitis C antibody assay has several limitations. It appears to be relatively insensitive and frequently requires 3 to 6 months to turn positive following an acute hepatitis C infection. It does appear to be more sensitive in detecting chronic hepatitis C virus infection.

    **(4)** Delta hepatitis. The delta agent is a defective virus that requires the presence of hepatitis B virus. Infection with this virus may occur simultaneously with hepatitis B or can present as a superinfection in an individual who is a chronic carrier of hepatitis B virus. Sensitive serologic assays for delta antibody are available.

**3.** Other tests.

  **a.** An upper GI series may reveal enlargement of the head of the pancreas.

  **b.** Ultrasound has become the procedure of choice for detecting gallstones within the gallbladder. Ultrasound and CT scanning are useful in detecting bile duct enlargement, pancreatic tumors, and space-occupying lesions in the liver.

**c.** A radionuclide biliary scan (e.g., HIDA scan) is especially useful in evaluating the patient with suspected acute cholecystitis. Visualization of the bile ducts but not the gallbladder on acute and delayed films suggests cystic duct obstruction.

**d.** Percutaneous transhepatic cholangiography and endoscopic retrograde cholangiopancreatography provide more detailed information regarding the cause of extrahepatic obstruction. With the latter technique, the pancreatic duct usually can be examined also. Choosing between these two procedures depends on such variables as blood coagulation studies, the general condition of the patient, the need to visualize the pancreatic duct, and local expertise.

**e.** Percutaneous liver biopsy is useful in diagnosing the cause of jaundice when the above tests have failed and in assessing the activity of disease (e.g., in chronic active hepatitis).

## General Comments

In most cases of jaundice, a detailed history and careful physical examination will establish the diagnosis. Biochemical tests usually serve to confirm the diagnosis. More sophisticated (and expensive) tests should be required only in the minority of cases, when the diagnosis remains in doubt.

# 6

# Hematologic Problems

## ANEMIA
Robert G. Chapman

### Definition

1. Anemia is a subnormal total red cell volume. The normal volume in males is 32 ± 3.5 ml/kg and in females, 25 ± 3.5 ml/kg. Persons living at elevations higher than 8000 to 9000 feet above sea level have an increased total red cell volume. Below this altitude, normal increases are of smaller magnitude and difficult to detect.
2. The total red cell volume can be measured with $^{51}$Cr- or $^{32}$P-labeled red cells or it can be calculated from the measured plasma volume and hematocrit reading. Simple tests measuring red cell concentration (hemoglobin and hematocrit values, red cell count) are usually used in place of the expensive and time-consuming total volume determinations. A normal plasma volume is assumed in evaluating the results.

### Normal Values

1. The normal hemoglobin concentration in males is not less than 14 g/100 ml; in females, it is not less than 12 g/100 ml. The normal hematocrit value in males is not less than 42 percent; in females, not less than 36 percent. The normal red cell count in males is not less than 4 million per cubic millimeter; in females, not less than 3.3 million per cubic millimeter. Of these, the red cell count is the least reliable. Automated determinations calculate the hematocrit value from the red cell count and the average individual red cell volume. Hematocrit readings done by this method are not as reliable as those measured directly by centrifugation. The ratio of hematocrit value to hemoglobin value is close to 3 : 1. Significant deviations from this ratio on automated counts should be questioned.
2. Dehydration, such as occurs in vomiting and diarrhea, may deplete the plasma volume and produce a rise in hemoglobin or hematocrit value without changing the total red cell volume. Pregnancy and congestive heart failure, on the other hand, have the opposite effect. When there is a rapid loss of blood, the hemoglobin and hematocrit values do not reflect the degree of blood loss until readjustment of the plasma volume has taken place. Therefore, under all of the foregoing circumstances, caution must be employed in using the hemoglobin and hematocrit values as indicators of the red cell volume.

### Causes of Anemia

#### Inadequate Erythropoiesis

1. Lack of essential nutrient (e.g., vitamin $B_{12}$, folic acid, iron).
2. Injury to the marrow (e.g., ionizing radiation).

**3.** Marrow inhibition (e.g., drug, immunologic agent).
**4.** Marrow replacement (e.g., neoplasm, fibrosis).
**5.** Hereditary defect.
**6.** Endocrine deficiency (e.g., hypothyroidism, hypopituitarism, renal failure).
**7.** Idiopathic ("refractory").

### Bleeding

**1.** Acute.
**2.** Chronic, with secondary iron deficiency.

### Hemolytic

**1.** Intracorpuscular defect.
  **a.** Abnormal hemoglobin (S, C, D, E, unstable).
  **b.** Defective globin synthesis (thalassemia).
  **c.** Defective heme synthesis (porphyria).
  **d.** Defective carbohydrate enzyme (G-6-PD, pyruvate kinase).
  **e.** Membrane defect (hereditary spherocytosis, elliptocytosis).
  **f.** Paroxysmal nocturnal hemoglobinuria.
**2.** Extracorpuscular defect.
  **a.** Secondary to:
    **(1)** Physical agent (e.g., water, thermal injury, microangiopathy).
    **(2)** Chemical agent (e.g., venom, drug).
    **(3)** Infection (e.g., malaria, septicemia).
    **(4)** Neoplasm (especially lymphoma).
    **(5)** Connective tissue disease (e.g., lupus).
    **(6)** Splenomegaly.
    **(7)** Isoimmunization (newborn, transfusion).
    **(8)** Paroxysmal cold hemoglobinuria.
  **b.** Primary, idiopathic (no underlying disease), usually autoimmune.

## Diagnostic Approach

**1.** In order to arrive quickly and efficiently at a correct diagnosis of the kind of anemia, a logical, stepwise procedure should be followed.
  **a.** Study the history and physical findings.
  **b.** Attempt to classify the anemia into hemolytic, blood loss, or bone marrow failure types, based on the pathophysiologic mechanism responsible for the red cell deficit.
  **c.** Perform more detailed tests and, at times, institute a therapeutic trial to determine the specific cause.
**2.** The initial laboratory evaluation reports hemoglobin, hematocrit, and red cell count and calculates the mean red cell volume (MCV), mean hemoglobin per red cell (MCH), and the mean concentration of hemoglobin in red cells (MCHC). These red cell indices have the following values normally: MCV 90 + 5 $\mu$M, MCH 30 + 2 pg, and MCHC 34 + 1 g per 100 ml of red cells. Values are the same for males and females. Listed below is a classification of anemias based on these indices.

| MCV | Etiology of anemia |
| --- | --- |
| Increased | Vitamin $B_{12}$ or folic acid deficiency due to pernicious anemia (lack of intrinsic factor), malabsorption, tapeworm, or drug (phenytoin [Dilantin], antifolate) |
| | Alcoholism and liver disease |
| | Refractory anemia |
| | Increased reticulocytes |

Normal     Acute blood loss
           Uremia
           Chronic disease
           Hemolysis, including hereditary spherocytosis
           Marrow failure (aplasia, x-ray or drug, invasion)
Decreased  Chronic disease
           Toxin (e.g., lead)
           Low MCHC (iron deficiency, thalassemia, sideroblastic,
             refractory)

3. Microscopic examination of the peripheral blood smear is an important supplement to the indices in evaluating red cell abnormalities. The smear should be examined in a systematic way for red cell size, shape, and color. The thin feathered edge is a good place to see polychromatophilic cells (reticulocytes) as well as platelet clumps and the larger white cells. Other features of red cell morphology are better evaluated in the body of the smear, just proximal to the feathered part, where cells are more evenly distributed but not overlapping. Red cell size varies mildly. Greater than normal variation (anisocytosis) is seen in some hemolytic anemias owing to the contrast between spherocytes and large reticulocytes. Size also varies due to fragmentation (schistocytes) seen in disseminated coagulation or abnormally functioning prosthetic heart valves.

   Red cell shape is normally round to slightly oblong. Abnormal variation in shape (poikilocytosis) is a prominent feature of thalassemia and, to a lesser degree, of severe iron deficiency. It is seen also in patients with extramedullary blood formation (myelogenous leukemia, myeloid metaplasia) or those without spleens. Red cells may lose their smooth surface to become burr- or spur-shaped echinocytes due to liver disease or, rarely, secondary to hereditary plasma lipid abnormalities (acanthocytes). They can be elliptical (hereditary elliptocytosis).

   Red cell color reflects the amount and distribution of hemoglobin within cells. Normally the central third of red cells is quite pale compared to the periphery, reflecting the cell's biconcave shape. The size of the pale center increases in both iron deficiency and thalassemia. This is also seen in a portion of the red cells in refractory anemias. An unusual hemoglobin distribution in liver disease (and hemoglobin C disease) gives the cells a targetlike appearance. This is due to the extra cell membrane surface area from uptake of extra unesterified cholesterol in liver disease. Other cell color abnormalities include distorted central pallor (stomatocytes), seen for both hereditary and alcoholic reasons, and basophilic cell inclusions. Fine blue stippling is seen in thalassemia (excess alpha chains), coarser stippling in toxic conditions (lead poisoning). Larger, round multiple Heinz bodies suggest drug damage in enzyme deficient cells, whereas single inclusions (Howell-Jolly bodies) are seen in the absence of a spleen. The presence of nucleated red cells suggests marrow stress or invasion by abnormal tissue and warrants bone marrow biopsy.

4. Anemia results from the inadequate formation of red cells, excessive blood loss, increased destruction of red cells, or a combination of these factors. Determination of the reticulocyte count and the serum bilirubin level, together with an assessment of the rate of development of the anemia, suggests the mechanism in most cases.

5. The reticulocyte count, better expressed as the number per cubic millimeter than as a percentage (normal is 30,000–80,000 per cubic millimeter), indicates the rate of red cell formation. As red cell formation increases, reticulocytes are released earlier from the marrow. Division of the reticulocyte number by a factor increasing from 1.0 to 2.5 as the severity of anemia increases has been suggested as a method to derive a red cell production index corrected for the distortion caused by this increasingly premature release. A high count, especially if there is no improvement in the anemia over a week or more, is good evidence for excessive red cell loss. A low count, especially in the face of anemia to which a normal marrow should respond, is very good evidence for bone marrow failure. It should be noted, however, that it takes 5 to 7 days after sudden hemorrhage or hemolysis

before reticulocytosis occurs. The marrow response to a hemolytic anemia may be blocked temporarily by an inflammatory process, resulting in a temporary depression of the reticulocyte count and a rapid worsening of the anemia.

6. The serum bilirubin (unconjugated) level, which normally does not exceed 0.8 mg/ 100 ml, is an indicator of red cell destruction. It is also affected by liver function. Increased red cell destruction (hemolysis) may raise the bilirubin level to 2 or perhaps 3 mg/100 ml but not higher unless liver function is also impaired. Mild hemolysis may not elevate the serum bilirubin at all. Hemoglobin loss from the body by hemorrhage or hemoglobinuria, of course, does not result in increased production of bile pigments. It should be remembered that anemia without increased hemolysis produces less than normal quantities of bilirubin. Hence, serum bilirubin levels in nonhemolytic anemias should be below 0.8 mg/100 ml.

7. Mild hemolytic disease with a normally functioning bone marrow may not cause anemia. This so-called compensated hemolysis may produce a reticulocytosis and possibly an elevated serum bilirubin level.

8. In the acutely ill patient who must be treated before a cause for anemia can be established, it is important to draw blood samples before therapy is begun. In all cases, the reticulocyte count and the serum bilirubin should be determined at the time of the initial hemogram. Blood samples should also be retained for the following tests: (a) serum iron and iron-binding capacity and serum ferritin, (b) serum haptoglobin, (c) serum folate and vitamin $B_{12}$ levels, (d) serum protein electrophoresis, and (e) hemoglobin electrophoresis. Because other red cell studies (e.g., fragility, autohemolysis, enzyme activity) require relatively fresh samples of blood, it is impractical to save blood for them. The first three tests listed are markedly affected by transfusion and by treatment with vitamin $B_{12}$ or folic acid. It is therefore essential to hold the pretreatment blood samples until it is decided whether these tests should be performed.

## Initial Evaluation

### History

Many facets of the history and physical examination are potentially helpful in the evaluation of anemia. Only the most important and useful ones are given here.

1. Any past anemia, the therapy employed, and the response to treatment should be reviewed in order to ascertain whether the present and the previous anemia are related. Chronic anemia or recurrent episodes of anemia over a period of years suggest a hereditary disease, whereas anemia of recent onset suggests an acquired disorder. Acceptance of any explanation for prior anemia must be predicated on objective evidence of an adequate response to specific measures. Anemia that is insidious in onset and gradual in development suggests bone marrow failure. Because of the relatively long life span of the red cell (4 months), failure of effective erythropoiesis takes some time to become apparent. Anemia that is rapid in its onset suggests either bleeding or hemolysis as a probable cause.

2. Inquiries should be made concerning diet, alcohol intake, medications used by the patient, and possible blood loss. An inadequate diet and excessive use of alcohol suggest possible folic acid deficiency. A review of the patient's medications is important because drugs may cause hemolysis, megaloblastic anemia, or bone marrow depression. Questions related to bleeding are especially important. Black stools, especially if they are foul-smelling and sticky, may indicate intestinal bleeding, unless the patient is taking iron. Previous subtotal gastrectomy, often for bleeding ulcer, is frequently associated with continued iron deficiency anemia due to either iron malabsorption or persistent bleeding. In women, menorrhagia may be responsible for excessive iron loss. This symptom is difficult to evaluate because many women do not know what "normal" bleeding is. As a rule of thumb, the use of one box (10) of napkins or tampons per period may be considered average; more than that probably represents excessive bleeding. Large menstrual

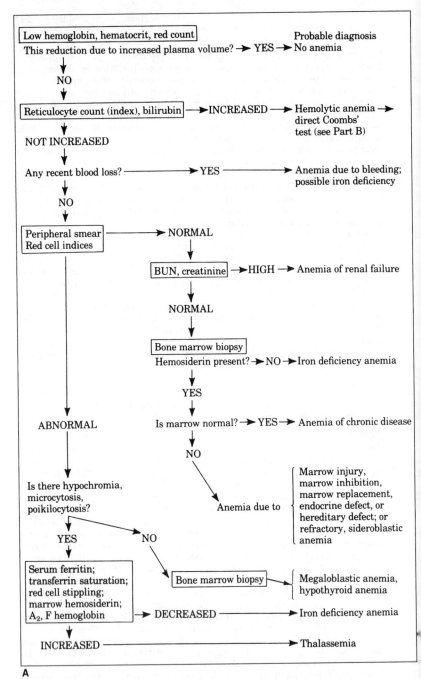

**Fig. 6-1.** A and B. Laboratory approach to the diagnosis of anemia.

blood losses may result in iron deficiency anemia. Measurements have shown that women who bleed heavily may lose about 1 pint of blood/period, representing a loss of about 200 mg of iron. Intensive exercise, especially distance running, is associated with mild anemia, possibly due to trauma or minor blood loss.

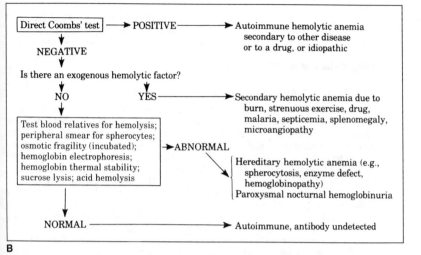

**B**

3. The family history is important in the hereditary anemias, especially in those with an autosomal dominant or sex-linked pattern. Inquiry should be made about anemia, jaundice, gallbladder disease, and splenectomy in blood relatives.

## Symptoms

1. Dyspnea, palpitation, and fatigue are common, although nonspecific, complaints.
2. Pallor may be noted by the patient or family, but frequently is missed by both.
3. Jaundice, similarly, may be present but overlooked.
4. Symptoms of postural hypotension are likely to occur when whole blood is lost rapidly.
5. Lifelong hemolysis may be asymptomatic except for the development of cholelithiasis at an early age and the occurrence of crises of abdominal pain or jaundice and weakness, or both.

## Physical Examination

The physical examination may be helpful in detecting anemia, bleeding, jaundice, or hemolysis, and perhaps its cause. Most often, however, the cause of the anemia is left unresolved by examination. Marked postural changes in pulse and blood pressure usually indicate rapid loss of whole blood. These signs may occur before changes in hemoglobin or hematocrit values become apparent. Estimation of the patient's state of hydration is necessary for the proper evaluation of these parameters. Pallor, of course, suggests anemia; when associated with jaundice, it may be indicative of hemolysis. Petechiae or purpura suggests the presence of a disorder that is also thrombocytopenic. Hemorrhages in the eyegrounds may occur in severe anemia from any cause. Glossitis is often seen in pernicious anemia or severe iron deficiency. Hemic murmurs are commonly heard in many severe anemias. Careful palpation for splenomegaly is important in all patients with anemia. Splenomegaly may be due to congestion (e.g., cirrhosis of the liver), hemolytic disorders, infections, connective tissue disease, or infiltrate or neoplastic disorders. The presence of lymphadenopathy suggests the possibility of infectious disease, connective tissue disorders, or infiltrative lesions. Assessment of proprioception, best determined by position sense in the toes, may provide a clue to spinal cord involvement in vitamin $B_{12}$ deficiency. Examination of the stool for occult blood is mandatory. A negative result, however, does not exclude the possibility of slight or intermittent bleeding. Iron therapy makes the stools black but does not invalidate the test for blood (Fig. 6-1A, B).

## Anemia Resulting from Bone Marrow Failure

### Diagnostic Approach

PERIPHERAL BLOOD COUNT AND SMEAR

1. Abnormality of peripheral blood cells other than red cells indicates a widespread marrow disorder. Vitamin $B_{12}$ deficiency and folic acid deficiency both produce thrombocytopenia and neutropenia. Hypersegmented neutrophils with more than five nuclear lobes occur commonly in both conditions. Pancytopenia may also occur in bone marrow injury or marrow replacement. The peripheral blood smear may also be helpful in differentiating between leukemia and neoplasm metastatic to the marrow. Although there are exceptions, the presence of immature white cells in the smear suggests leukemia, whereas a mature white cell population favors metastatic malignancy.
2. The red cell structure is not always abnormal in marrow failure anemia. Thus, in the anemia of renal disease, the red cells look normal, but there is a lack of polychromatophilic cells (reticulocytes on Wright's stain). Hypochromia (MCHC < 31 g/100 ml RBC) indicates hemoglobin deficiency, not iron deficiency. Its most common causes are iron deficiency and thalassemia. The presence of basophilic stippling in the large polychromatophilic red cells strongly favors the diagnosis of thalassemia over that of iron deficiency. The finding of similar blood smears in the patient's blood relatives, together with the demonstration of increased hemoglobin $A_2$ or F on hemoglobin electrophoresis, helps to establish the diagnosis of β-thalassemia. A mixed population of normal and hypochromic red cells is sometimes seen in untreated patients with poorly defined refractory anemias, some of which may terminate in acute granulocytic leukemia. Anisocytosis (abnormal variation in red cell size) is not a common feature of marrow failure anemia unless there is considerable poikilocytosis (abnormal variation in red cell shape). Marked poikilocytosis is a feature of thalassemia and, to a lesser degree, of iron deficiency. It may also be seen in severe vitamin $B_{12}$ or folic acid deficiency and in the hemoglobinuric hemolytic diseases (artificial heart valve–induced, paroxysmal nocturnal hemoglobinuria, hemolytic uremic syndrome), especially if iron deficiency becomes a secondary effect. Macrocytosis is good evidence for vitamin $B_{12}$ or folic acid deficiency.

BONE MARROW BIOPSY

Bone marrow biopsy is a most important procedure in the diagnosis of marrow failure anemia. Although marrow smears are useful in detecting the abnormal megaloblastic maturation of vitamin $B_{12}$ or folic acid deficiency, histologic sections of the marrow, obtained preferably by core biopsy rather than by aspiration, are of much greater value. Sectioned material is the only reliable method for evaluating general marrow cellularity and the distribution of cell types. Fibrosis and the serous fat atrophy of malnutrition or hypothyroidism can be detected only in sections. Packed tumor cells, which may not aspirate for smearing, are readily identified. Moreover, the reticulum cells, in which hemosiderin is stored, do not appear readily in aspirates. Thus, it is essential to have sectioned material, stained with Prussian blue, for the evaluation of iron stores. The bone marrow findings in various types of marrow failure anemia are as follows:

1. Generalized hypocellularity suggests a toxic injury to the marrow by drugs, chemicals, ionizing radiation, or possibly autoimmune mechanisms. It may also be seen in hypothyroidism or malnutrition.
2. Normal cellularity, except for a lack of erythroid tissue, suggests an immunologic cause, as may occur occasionally in thymoma; it may also be drug related.

3. Any cellularity with a lack of hemosiderin establishes the diagnosis of iron deficiency.
4. General hypercellularity of all marrow elements is seen in vitamin $B_{12}$ and folic acid deficiency. Patchy hypercellularity is also a finding in marrow fibrosis.
5. Hypercellularity with large numbers of abnormal cells is found in acute leukemia, lymphoma, multiple myeloma, and metastatic malignancy.
6. Hypercellularity due to increased erythroid tissue is observed in thalassemia and is often striking in the idiopathic refractory marrow failure anemias.

ROUTINE LABORATORY TESTS

1. Most important are renal function tests (BUN or serum creatinine). Marrow suppression, with its concomitant anemia, is a common occurrence in renal failure. Sometimes the anemia is severe before other symptoms and renal insufficiency are evident.
2. Mild anemia resulting from marrow suppression is also a frequent finding in chronic illness, such as rheumatoid arthritis or infectious disease. An increased sedimentation rate and varying degrees of diffuse hypergammaglobulinemia frequently are associated findings.

SPECIAL LABORATORY TESTS

1. Decreased blood levels of vitamin $B_{12}$ and folic acid may indicate which substance is lacking in a megaloblastic anemia. The normal values for vitamin $B_{12}$ and folate exceed 180 pg/ml and 6.5 ng/ml, respectively.
2. The serum iron and iron-binding capacity, from which the saturation of the iron-binding globulin is calculated, may help demonstrate inadequate iron stores. Saturation less than 16 percent is seen in iron deficiency anemia, especially when the hemoglobin is under 8 g/100 ml. Similar desaturation may also occur in a wide variety of inflammatory conditions (e.g., rheumatoid arthritis, infections). Serum ferritin determination (normal is 12–300 ng/ml) can be a more reliable indicator of iron stores in the presence of inflammation, but its level also rises in liver and other diseases. Bone marrow sections stained for hemosiderin are the most reliable indicators of iron stores. Lack of marrow iron in anemia is diagnostic of iron deficiency anemia.

X-RAY EXAMINATION

The demonstration of metastases suggests neoplastic marrow replacement as the cause of anemia. The finding of increased density of all bones is indicative of myelosclerosis, a condition in which fibrous tissue replaces the marrow. Chest films may show evidence of a thymoma, a tumor often associated with a lack of erythroid tissue in the marrow, resulting presumably from the effects of thymic humoral factors on red cell formation. The anemia is cured or relieved by removal of the tumor.

THERAPEUTIC TRIALS

Diagnosis by a well-designed therapeutic trial is appropriate in selected instances. In all trials, one agent at a time should be used. A rise in the hemoglobin and hematocrit values or an increase in the reticulocyte count is indicative of a positive response. When reticulocytosis is too slight to be detected, as may occur when the anemia is mild, one must rely on a rise in the hemoglobin and hematocrit values. Such changes are usually evident by the end of 2 weeks of treatment. A negative response does not necessarily preclude the possibility that the patient is deficient in the substance tested. For example, a patient with iron deficiency anemia may not respond to orally administered iron because of intestinal malabsorption or because a concomitant inflammatory process interferes with the marrow response to iron.

1. Therapeutic trials with vitamin $B_{12}$ or folic acid should employ very small doses (1 and 200 μg/day, respectively, administered parenterally) to avoid the cross-responsiveness of the marrow to these agents. However, when the patient is severely anemic, it is impractical to wait 1 or 2 weeks to observe the response to either folic acid or vitamin $B_{12}$. Therefore, large doses of both substances are often used simultaneously while waiting for the results of the serum folate and $B_{12}$ levels to be reported.

2. Some cases of refractory marrow failure anemia, with increased iron stores and significant numbers of ring sideroblasts in the marrow, may respond slowly to large doses of pyridoxine. Because no laboratory test is currently available to predict pyridoxine responsiveness, an empiric trial of this vitamin (daily oral dosage of 200 mg) is worthwhile in this type of anemia.

3. There are also other refractory anemias (presumably based on an immune mechanism, with a predominant incidence in older women) that respond to treatment with corticosteroids. A trial with steroid therapy is probably warranted in otherwise unresponsive refractory anemias.

SPECIFIC ETIOLOGY

Once a diagnosis of a specific deficiency anemia is made, the cause of the deficiency must be sought.

1. Folic acid deficiency may be the result of decreased intake, increased requirements, or interference with the metabolic activity of folic acid. It is usually the result of an insufficient intake of dietary sources (fresh green vegetables) because of poor diet, alcoholism, or intestinal malabsorption. Increased requirements of folic acid occur during pregnancy, and if intake is inadequate, a megaloblastic anemia may occur. Chronic hemolysis may also exhaust folic acid stores. Folic acid metabolism may be impaired by drugs such as diphenylhydantoin and methotrexate. In such cases, the megaloblastic anemia generally improves when the drug is stopped.

2. Dietary deficiency of vitamin $B_{12}$ occurs rarely. Although decreased intake may occur from intestinal disease or from competition for vitamin $B_{12}$ by intestinal organisms and parasites, it is usually caused by a lack of the gastric intrinsic factor that is essential for the absorption of the vitamin. This absorptive defect is demonstrable with the Schilling test. A small dose of cobalt 60–labeled vitamin $B_{12}$ is given orally; this is followed by the parenteral administration of a large amount of nonradioactive vitamin $B_{12}$. The urine is collected for 24 hours. Kidney function must be normal. If excretion of the labeled substance is normal, there is no indication for vitamin $B_{12}$ therapy. If excretion is low, the test should be repeated with the addition of intrinsic factor given orally. If the poor excretion in the first test is due to intrinsic factor deficiency, the result of the second test should be normal; if it is abnormal, other causes must be found for the malabsorption of the vitamin.

3. Iron deficiency in adults is rarely due to dietary deficiency alone. Intestinal malabsorption of iron is also an uncommon cause of iron deficiency, except in malabsorption syndromes or after gastrointestinal surgery. Bleeding is by far the most common cause of iron deficiency in adult men and postmenopausal women. In adult women, iron deficiency is most commonly due to unreplaced iron losses from menstruation or repeated pregnancies. When bleeding is occult, it is usually of gastrointestinal origin. Every effort must be made to demonstrate the source of the bleeding. Stools should be examined repeatedly for occult blood. Proctosigmoidoscopy and radiologic examination of the gastrointestinal tract are also indicated. Body iron stores can be estimated by assays for ferritin and serum iron. Prussian blue stains of bone marrow biopsies give the most reliable estimate of ferritin. If anemia is due to causes other than iron deficiency, ferritin is easy to find in the marrow. In iron deficiency, on the other hand, ferritin is absent. Serum

ferritin levels are less reliable measures of tissue iron stores but are still useful and much simpler to obtain. Levels at or below 12 ng/ml indicate iron deficiency, 13 to 20 ng/ml is borderline, and 20 to 300 ng/ml is normal. Serum iron itself can be measured, with normal levels being 50 to 150 μg/dl. The serum iron level as an indicator of iron stores is better evaluated by also determining the total serum iron binding capacity (TIBC) and expressing the result as the percentage of the TIBC that is saturated with iron. Levels below 16 percent saturation suggest deficient iron stores, but similarly low levels can be seen in inflammatory states, probably reflecting a block in the release of tissue iron into the plasma in such conditions. Elevation of TIBC above its normal 250 to 400 μg/dl supports a diagnosis of iron deficiency.

## Anemia Due to Bleeding

1. Bleeding may be rapid and massive or slow and hidden; it may be internal or external. Bleeding is most commonly external, arising from the gastrointestinal or genitourinary tract or from sites of trauma. When hemorrhage takes place internally into the body tissues, the red cell iron is usually recovered and used again in hemoglobin synthesis. The degradation of heme leads to increased bile pigment production and hyperbilirubinemia.
2. Routine blood counts may fail to indicate the degree of blood loss when hemorrhage occurs rapidly, because cells and plasma are lost together. Significant blood loss (over 500 ml) is suggested by symptoms and signs of postural hypotension or shock. Direct measurement of the total plasma or red cell volume provides the only accurate assessment of anemia in such cases.
3. Recovery from bleeding can occur when the bleeding is slow or controlled and tissue stores of iron are adequate. During recovery, a reticulocytosis is seen. The hemoglobin may rise as much as 1 g/100 ml per week.
4. Protracted bleeding results in exhaustion of the iron stores. Reticulocytosis then stops, and iron deficiency anemia develops. Hemosiderin is absent from marrow sections and serum transferrin iron saturation falls. Typical peripheral blood cell and serum iron changes may not be evident unless the anemia is severe (hemoglobin 8 g/100 ml).
5. Frequent testing of stools for occult blood is an excellent way to detect mild bleeding, but negative results do not rule out intermittent or a very slow rate of bleeding (< 4 ml of blood loss per day).
6. Aspirin ingestion is a frequent cause of low-grade bleeding. If continued long enough, iron deficiency anemia may result.
7. Menstrual blood loss is seldom rapid enough to cause either hypovolemia or acute anemia, but it may result in iron deficiency anemia, as mentioned previously.

## Anemia Resulting from Hemolysis

### Definition and Etiology

Human red blood cells have a normal life span of 120 days. A decrease in this life span for reasons other than bleeding is termed *hemolysis*. If the bone marrow is normal, it can compensate for a fourfold to sixfold decrease in the red cell life span and prevent anemia, producing what is called *compensated* hemolytic disease.

There are many causes of hemolysis. It is convenient to consider them in two categories: (1) intracorpuscular defects, nearly always hereditary, in which the red cell is abnormal from the time it is formed in the marrow, and (2) extracorpuscular defects, nearly always acquired after birth, in which the red cell is formed normally in the marrow but is injured by something in the circulation in which it lives.

The presence of an *intracorpuscular hemolytic disorder* is suggested by:

1. Evidence of a similar hemolytic disorder in a blood relative.
2. A history of lifelong anemia, recurring jaundice, or the development of gallstones before the age of 30 years.
3. A negative Coombs' test result.
4. Ancestry that is Jewish, Negro, Mediterranean, or Southeast Asian, because of the higher incidence of sickle hemoglobin, thalassemia, and glucose 6-phosphate dehydrogenase (G-6-PD) deficiency in specific populations.

Hereditary hemolytic disease may not be discovered until later in life, either because it is episodic (e.g., the drug-induced group with G-6-PD deficiency) or because it is well compensated until the vicissitudes of age compromise the marrow's ability to maintain compensation (e.g., hereditary spherocytosis).

*Extracorpuscular hemolytic disease* is frequently associated with an antierythrocytic antibody that is demonstrable by the direct Coombs' test. A positive Coombs' test result means only that the red cells are coated with gamma globulin; it does not necessarily imply that hemolysis is present.

A seldom used but very sensitive method for distinguishing intracorpuscular from extracorpuscular defects is the measurement of the survival of $^{51}$Cr-labeled compatible normal red cells in the patient. The life span of the donor cells is normal in patients with intracorpuscular defects but is shortened in those with extracorpuscular disorders.

## Hemolytic Anemia Due to Intracorpuscular Defects

LABORATORY TESTS

1. Peripheral blood smear.
2. Sickle cell preparation.
3. Hemoglobin electrophoresis for abnormal hemoglobin and for measurement of A and F hemoglobins.
4. Incubated sample for Heinz body formation or precipitation of unstable hemoglobin.
5. Screening for heat-unstable hemoglobin.
6. Tests for osmotic fragility (including incubation) and autohemolysis.
7. Enzyme screening for G-6-PD and pyruvate kinase (PK) deficiencies.
8. Urinary hemosiderin and sucrose lysis test; if positive, acid hemolysis test.

All of these tests should not be performed at once, because some, such as the acid hemolysis and osmotic fragility tests, are time-consuming and expensive. The peripheral smear should be examined carefully first, because it may provide excellent clues to the cause.

INTERPRETATION OF FINDINGS

1. Increased numbers of spherocytes with only mild to moderate anisocytosis, suggest hereditary spherocytosis. In most instances, blood smears of parents and siblings detect at least one other similar case.
2. Basophilic stippling, best detected at high magnification in the large polychromatophilic red cells, suggests abnormal RNA. This phenomenon is common in thalassemia and greatly helps to distinguish this disease from iron deficiency anemia, which produces an otherwise similar smear.
3. Sickling of the red cells may occasionally be seen in the smear, indicating the need for a sickle cell preparation and hemoglobin electrophoresis.
4. The presence of many target cells with little or no anemia, although not highly specific, suggests hemoglobin C abnormality, a condition in which mild hemolysis may occur.
5. Neutropenia occurs in the later stages of paroxysmal nocturnal hemoglobinuria (PNH). In addition, the continued loss of iron because of the hemoglobinuria may

lead to iron deficiency and to changes in the peripheral smear due to this type of anemia.

6. Howell-Jolly bodies in the red cells occur in the absence of splenic function, most often the result of previous splenectomy. However, they may also be seen late in the course of sickle cell disease when "autosplenectomy" has taken place because of repeated splenic infarctions.

7. Other red cell inclusions, some evident only with vital staining (methylene blue), may be seen in patients with abnormal unstable hemoglobins (e.g., Zürich, Köln).

8. If the peripheral smear suggests a specific disease, additional tests to support that diagnosis should be made:

   a. The autohemolysis test or incubated osmotic fragility test is indicated for the diagnosis of hereditary spherocytosis or enzyme deficiency. Increased hemolysis is almost always observed, but the addition of glucose before incubation does not always prevent it.

   b. Hemoglobin electrophoresis is performed for the measurement of $A_2$ and F hemoglobins in suspected thalassemia. Elevations of one or both of these hemoglobins may be seen in this disease. However, failure to find them increased does not exclude the possibility of thalassemia.

   c. Sickle cell preparation and hemoglobin electrophoresis are done for the diagnosis of sickle cell disease.

   d. Hemoglobin electrophoresis is required for the diagnosis of hemoglobin C disease.

   e. If PNH is suspected, the first tests should be a sucrose lysis test and an examination of the urine for hemoglobin and of its sediment for hemosiderin. Hemoglobinuria in PNH is intermittent, but, as in any condition with recurring hemoglobinuria, hemosiderin is present at all times in the shed cells of the urinary sediment. If the hemosiderin and sucrose lysis test results are positive, the diagnosis of PNH should be confirmed by a carefully performed Ham acid hemolysis test.

   f. The suspicion of an unstable hemoglobin may be confirmed by the examination of a heated (50°C) hemolysate for a precipitate or by incubating a methylene blue–stained red cell suspension to search for Heinz bodies or precipitate hemoglobin.

9. Red cell enzyme deficiencies do not produce any characteristic morphologic abnormalities in the peripheral smear. Those described so far are classified as hereditary nonspherocytic hemolytic anemia. An enzyme deficiency should be suspected if the problem appears to be intracorpuscular and no other causes of intracorpuscular hemolytic disorders are found. Although most frequently associated only with episodic hemolysis related to drug exposure or infection, some variants of red cell G-6-PD deficiency found in non-Mediterranean Caucasians may produce chronic hemolysis in the absence of exogenous factors. Because of its sex-linked inheritance, G-6-PD disease is expressed mainly in males. Screening tests for G-6-PD deficiency are available, but unfortunately they may be normal during the hemolytic episodes when many young red cells are present. Under such circumstances, the test should be repeated several months after recovery to confirm the diagnosis. Much rarer is the autosomally recessive red cell PK deficiency. Enzyme assays for red cell PK for the confirmation of this diagnosis are becoming more readily available.

10. The most common cause of intracorpuscular hemolytic anemia is hereditary spherocytosis (HS). Because of a membrane defect, the red cells in this disorder have a decreased surface area. The spherocytosis is the result of a decreased surface-to-volume ratio. The mean red cell diameter (not the volume) is decreased, and the mean corpuscular hemoglobin concentration is increased. Autohemolysis and osmotic fragility of the red cells, especially after incubation, are increased. No test is absolutely pathognomonic for the diagnosis of HS, but the demonstration of similar changes in a parent or sibling provides adequate proof in most cases. If splenectomy fails to eliminate evidence of hemolysis, the accuracy of a diagnosis of HS should be seriously questioned.

## Hemolytic Anemia Due to Extracorpuscular Defects

LABORATORY TESTS

1. Laboratory procedures that are useful in the evaluation of these disorders include the following:
   a. Peripheral blood smear.
   b. Plasma haptoglobin and perhaps, plasma hemoglobin.
   c. Urine hemosiderin.
   d. Fibrinogen and fibrin split products.
   e. RA factor and antinuclear antibody (ANA) test.
   f. More specific immunohematology tests in addition to Coombs' test.
   g. Donath-Landsteiner test and serologic test for syphilis.
   h. Various additional studies needed to detect underlying infections, neoplasms or other disorders.
2. The choice of tests for the evaluation of extracorpuscular disease depends to some extent on the clinical features. The history and physical examination are likely to be more helpful in evaluating these disorders than the hereditary diseases. A disease associated with acquired hemolysis may be evident before anemia becomes a problem. On the other hand, hemolysis may present a problem well in advance of other manifestations of the disease (e.g., SLE).
   a. The peripheral smear may be very helpful. Abnormalities of white cells and platelets may indicate the presence of another condition, such as leukemia or disseminated intravascular coagulation. The latter diagnosis is suggested by the occurrence of red cell fragmentation in the smear. Fragmentation is also seen in other conditions characterized by mechanical damage to the cell (e.g. abnormally functioning artificial aortic heart valves). Spherocytosis of the red cells suggests coating of the cells by antibody, but it may also result from thermal injury in burned patients. Spherocytosis, neutropenia, and varying degrees of thrombocytopenia may occur in systemic lupus erythematosus or in any condition in which the spleen is large enough to trap and destroy blood cells. In malaria, the parasites are seen within the affected red cells.
   b. When intravascular hemolysis is suspected because of red cell fragmentation in the peripheral blood or because of the occurrence of hemoglobinuria without hematuria, absence of haptoglobin and elevation of free hemoglobin levels in the plasma confirm the diagnosis. Plasma haptoglobin tends to be diminished in other hemolytic processes, but its complete absence in these conditions is rare. Significant intravascular hemolysis can often be detected by simple visual inspection of the patient's plasma for red hemoglobin or brown methemoglobin. As mentioned previously, the urine sediment contains hemosiderin in cases of recurrent hemoglobinuria. The loss of iron in the urine may be sufficient to cause the superimposition of iron deficiency on the original anemia. Intravascular hemolysis is accompanied by an elevation of the serum bilirubin, LDH, and SGOT levels. These findings may lead to confusion with liver disease. Mechanical injury to red cells in the feet of distance runners (march hemoglobinuria) can produce similar changes.
   c. When intravascular coagulation is suspected, fibrinogen levels and fibrin degradation products should be assayed. The finding of decreased fibrinogen levels and thrombocytopenia in association with red cell fragmentation is most suggestive of this disorder. An increase in fibrin split products helps to confirm the diagnosis. Other clotting factors also tend to be at low levels these may be measured for confirmation, if available. Prompt diagnosis and anticoagulant therapy are often needed to save the patient suffering from disseminated intravascular coagulation.
   d. Connective tissue diseases, particularly SLE and less frequently RA, are commonly associated with the presence of antibodies against the patient's own red cells and thus with a positive Coombs' test result. Because of this association, tests for ANA and rheumatoid factor should be performed on every patient with a Coombs'-positive hemolytic anemia. Negative test results do not

rule out the possibility of SLE, because the hemolytic disease may develop long before other manifestations of the disease appear.

   **e.** In addition to the Coombs' test, other immunologic studies can be done to characterize the protein coating of the damaged red cells.

      **(1)** The thermal characteristic of the antibody is important. The cold agglutinins found in infectious mononucleosis and mycoplasmal pneumonia may cause hemolysis. Although warm agglutinins are more common, they are less specific.

      **(2)** All Coombs'-positive hemolytic disorders may be classified into cold and warm agglutinin types. Unfortunately, this classification is often of little help in determining the cause of the autoantibody or in predicting the outcome of the illness.

      **(3)** An unusual but specific disease picture occurs in paroxysmal cold hemoglobinuria. This illness, which at times is associated with syphilis and diagnosed by the Donath-Landsteiner test, is characterized by episodes of brisk intravascular hemolysis and hemoglobinuria following exposure to cold.

   **f.** No attempt is made here to describe additional tests and procedures that might be helpful in establishing the cause of an acquired hemolytic anemia. Suffice it to say that a careful search for underlying disease is indicated in all such patients.

**3.** Coombs'-positive hemolytic anemias are regarded as primary or idiopathic if no evidence of an underlying disease can be found. The diagnosis of idiopathic acquired hemolytic disease is thus made by exclusion. However, such a diagnosis should remain tentative for at least a year or two because many such cases eventually turn up with a systemic disease such as SLE or a lymphoma.

## ERYTHROCYTOSIS (POLYCYTHEMIA)
John H. Saiki

### Definition

Erythrocytosis is defined as an elevation in hemoglobin and hematocrit values to levels greater than 18 g/100 ml and 54 percent, respectively.

### Etiology (Mechanisms)

**1.** Relative erythrocytosis. Red cell mass is normal and plasma volume is reduced (hemoconcentration), as occurs in dehydration and "stress" erythrocytosis (Gaisböck's syndrome).

**2.** Absolute erythrocytosis. Red cell mass is increased.

   **a.** Primary (autonomous proliferation). Polycythemia rubra vera.

   **b.** Secondary.

      **(1)** Increased erythropoietin production.

         **(a)** Associated with systemic hypoxia. Reduced $PaO_2$ (e.g., chronic lung disease, congestive heart failure, congenital heart disease with right-to-left shunts). Normal $PaO_2$ (e.g., impaired oxygen-carrying capacity of methemoglobinemia and hemoglobin M; impaired hemoglobin-oxygen dissociation with increased oxygen affinity, as in hemoglobin Chesapeake).

         **(b)** Associated with local renal hypoxia, as in renovascular disease.

         **(c)** Autonomous erythropoietin production (e.g., benign lesions—renal cysts, hydronephrosis, uterine fibroids; malignant lesions—hypernephroma, hepatoma, cerebellar hemangioblastoma).

      **(2)** Exogenous androgen administration.

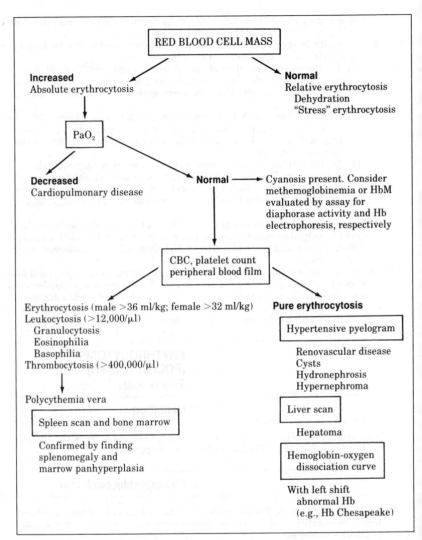

**Fig. 6-2.** Laboratory approach for evaluation of erythrocytosis.

---

## Diagnostic Approach

---

1. **History.** Careful inquiry regarding manifestations of chronic heart or lung disease, family history of high hemoglobin levels, chronic ingestion of androgens, and general well-being, appetite, weight loss, bleeding, and thrombotic problems.
2. **Physical examination.** Careful evaluation of cardiovascular and respiratory systems, hepatosplenomegaly, and evidence of cyanosis.
3. If no significant abnormalities are found via the history or physical examination, the following schematic laboratory approach is pursued (Fig. 6-2).
4. **Specific etiology.** Polycythemia vera, one of the myeloproliferative disorders, is

manifested as erythrocytosis, leukocytosis, thrombocytosis, panhyperplasia of the bone marrow, and extramedullary hematopoiesis with hepatosplenomegaly. Symptoms of fatigue, headache, pruritus, and occasionally, erythromelalgia are seen. Physical findings of plethora and hepatosplenomegaly are common. Complications of peptic ulcer disease, congestive heart failure from hyperviscosity, and thrombotic and bleeding problems are common and of major importance. The diagnostic criteria established by the National Polycythemia Vera Study Group are identified in the chart below:

### Diagnostic Criteria of Polycythemia Vera

**Category A**
1. Red-cell mass
   Male > 36 ml/kg
   Female > 32 ml/kg
2. Normal arterial
   $O_2$ saturation > 92%
3. Splenomegaly

**Category B**
1. Thrombocytosis
   Platelet count > 400,000/μl
2. Leukocytosis > 12,000/μl
   without fever or infection
3. LAP ↑ (> 100)
   without fever or infection
4. ↑ serum $B_{12}$ (> 900 pg/ml) or unsaturated
   $B_{12}$ binding capacity (> 2200 pg/ml)

The diagnosis of polycythemia vera is established with the following combinations:

1. $A_1 + A_2 + A_3$, or
2. $A_1 + A_2$ + any two from Category B.

## WHITE BLOOD CELL ABNORMALITIES
John H. Saiki

## Neutropenia

### Definition

Neutropenia (and its near synonym, granulocytopenia) is defined as an absolute neutrophil count of less than 1500 per cubic millimeter.

### Clinical Significance

1. Host resistance is related to the degree of neutropenia.
   a. More than 1500 neutrophils per cubic millimeter is associated with normal host resistance.
   b. 1000 to 1500 neutrophils per cubic millimeter is associated with mildly impaired host resistance.
   c. 500 to 1000 neutrophils per cubic millimeter is associated with moderately impaired host resistance.
   d. Less than 500 neutrophils per cubic millimeter is associated with markedly impaired host resistance.
2. The major consequence of neutropenia is vulnerability to infection. The usual clinical manifestations of infection are often absent because of the lack of granulocytes. Thus, pneumonia may be present without a significant infiltrate, meningitis may occur without pleocytosis, and pyelonephritis may be found without pyuria.
3. The three *most important* clinical problems seen with neutropenia are
   a. Aplastic anemia.
   b. Acute leukemia.

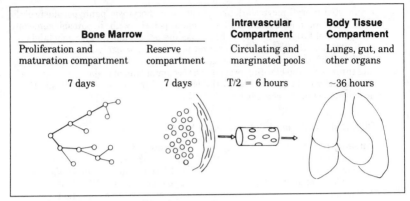

**Fig. 6-3.** Normal granulocyte kinetics.

    **c.** Drug-induced agranulocytosis.
       Each of these requires immediate therapeutic measures.
  **4.** Chronic neutropenias of varying severity (e.g., Felty's syndrome and chronic idiopathic neutropenia) are of minimal significance unless they are associated with recurrent infections.
  **5.** Neutropenia is commonly seen in association with anemia and thrombocytopenia; this is termed *pancytopenia*. The approach to pancytopenia is similar to the approach to neutropenia. All patients with aplastic anemia, and 25 percent of adults with acute leukemia, present with pancytopenia.

### Normal Granulocyte Kinetics

The highlights of granulocyte kinetics are illustrated in Figure 6-3. Granulocytes are produced and stored in the bone marrow, from which they are discharged into the vascular compartment. The cells are about equally divided between the circulating and marginated pools. Granulocytes eventually make their way into the body tissues but once there do not reenter the bloodstream.

### Mechanisms of Neutropenia

Neutropenia can result from either decreased production of neutrophils by the bone marrow or their accelerated removal from the blood by immune or consumptive mechanisms. Transfer of neutrophils from the circulating to the marginated pool may also result in low white cell counts.

### Etiology

  **1.** Proliferative defects (hypoproliferation).
    **a.** Marrow injury (e.g., radiation, drugs, paroxysmal nocturnal hemoglobinuria, hepatitis). Severe hypoproliferation of erythrocytes, granulocytes, and megakaryocytes is called *aplastic anemia*. This mechanism is of major importance.
    **b.** Marrow infiltration (e.g., acute and chronic leukemia, metastatic carcinoma, granulomatous infiltration). This mechanism is of major importance.
  **2.** Maturation defects (increased, but ineffective proliferation; defective cells are "screened out" and not delivered to peripheral blood): vitamin $B_{12}$ and folate de-

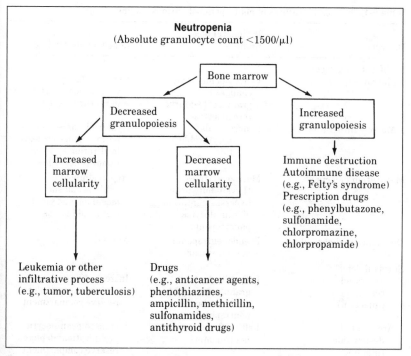

**Fig. 6-4.** Diagnostic approach to neutropenia.

ficiency. Neutropenia associated with this mechanism is seldom of clinical significance.
3. Distribution abnormality (increased margination): endotoxin. This mechanism is of little clinical significance.
4. Survival defects.
   a. Accelerated consumption (e.g., severe sepsis).
   b. Accelerated destruction (e.g., immune mechanisms, as seen with certain drugs and autoimmune diseases, and hypersplenism). This mechanism can be of major clinical significance when severe agranulocytosis occurs.

### Diagnostic Approach

1. See Figure 6-4.
2. Evaluation of the CBC, platelet count, and peripheral blood film is essential in all patients. A bone marrow aspiration is essential in all patients, except when the neutropenia is mild, stable, and clinically associated with a drug known to cause neutropenia (e.g., phenothiazines, antithyroid drugs, hydantoin analogues, and phenylbutazone). The peripheral blood film and bone marrow findings are illustrated in Table 6-1.
3. When aplastic anemia is identified, a history of exposure to drugs (chloramphenicol, phenylbutazone, hydantoin and analogues, sulfonamides, sulfonylureas, gold compounds, and quinacrine), insecticides (DDT, lindane, chlordane), and solvents (benzene) must be determined. Paroxysmal nocturnal hemoglobinuria and hepatitis are also associated with aplastic anemia and should be screened with a sugar water test and liver function tests, respectively.

**Table 6-1.** Diagnostic features of neutropenia of various origins

| Disorder | Peripheral blood findings | Bone marrow findings |
|---|---|---|
| **Proliferation defects** | | |
| Marrow injury | Pancytopenia; toxic changes in granulocytes; large reticulocytes | Hypocellularity; vacuolation of cytoplasm in precursor cells |
| Marrow infiltration | Pancytopenia; leukoerythroblastic reaction | Hypercellularity; reduced normal hematopoiesis; infiltration by fibrosis, tumor cells, or leukemia |
| Maturation defects | Macroovalocytes; Howell-Jolly bodies; hypersegmentation of granulocytes; pancytopenia | Hypercellularity; panhyperplasia; megaloblasts; giant metas and bands |
| Distribution abnormality | Pseudoneutropenia; normal smear | Normal |
| **Survival defects** | | |
| Accelerated consumption (infection) | Left shift; toxic granulation; Döhle's inclusion bodies; neutropenia | Increased granulocytic proliferation; depleted reserve compartment |
| Accelerated destruction (immune) | Left shift; neutropenia | Increased granulocytic proliferation; depleted reserve compartment |

## Leukocytosis

### Definition

Leukocytosis is defined as a white blood cell count in excess of 10,000 per cubic millimeter.

### Clinical Significance

Most frequently, leukocytosis is reactive to an inflammatory process. Most important is the differentiation between a reactive leukocytosis and leukemia.

### Diagnostic Approach

HISTORY

Patients with a reactive leukocytosis are symptomatic with fever and other manifestations of infection. Typically, the patient with chronic granulocytic or chronic lymphocytic leukemia is asymptomatic. Acute leukemia usually presents with weakness, fever with infection, and bleeding manifestations with epistaxis and bruising.

PHYSICAL EXAMINATION

Patients with chronic granulocytic or chronic lymphocytic leukemia usually appear perfectly well. Pallor, fever, and bleeding manifestations (petechiae and bruises) are characteristic of acute leukemia. Hepatosplenomegaly is commonly seen in both acute and chronic leukemia. Generalized lymphadenopathy is most characteristic of acute and chronic lymphocytic leukemia.

LABORATORY STUDIES

1. Evaluation of the peripheral blood film is the most critical procedure:

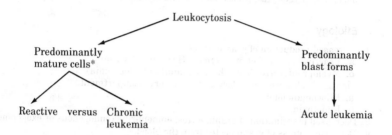

2. CBC and platelet count. The hemoglobin and hematocrit values are more likely to be normal or near normal in reactive leukocytosis and in the chronic leukemias. The platelet count is normal or elevated in reactive leukocytosis and chronic leukemia, but invariably it is markedly reduced in the acute leukemias. Mature leukocytes usually indicate a reactive process or chronic leukemia (see Neutrophilia). The presence of many blast forms is suggestive of acute leukemia.

3. Bone marrow aspiration. This contributes little to the diagnosis of a reactive leukocytosis or chronic leukemia and is seldom necessary for diagnostic purposes. However, it is often essential for the diagnosis of acute leukemia. The marrow in acute leukemia is hypercellular with greater than 30 percent blasts. Not uncommonly, leukemia is suspected, and the proportion of blast cells is only moderately increased. In this setting, close observation for a change in the percentage of blasts in both the peripheral blood and bone marrow allows the diagnosis of acute leukemia to be established.

4. Specific etiology. The chronic leukemias are discussed more appropriately under Neutrophilia and Lymphocytosis. Acute leukemia is further classified according to cell type. The specific cell types are identified by individual morphologic features (e.g., Auer rods in myeloblastic and monocytic leukemias) and by "the company they keep," which reflects maturation in any given cell line (e.g., the finding of promyelocytes in acute myeloblastic leukemia). Frequently, morphologic features are not conclusive and special stains are required (e.g., PAS positivity occurs in lymphoblastic leukemia). Serum and urinary lysozyme levels may be markedly elevated in acute monocytic leukemia. From a therapeutic standpoint it is important only to differentiate lymphoblastic leukemia from the nonlymphoblastic forms. Hyperuricemia is common in all acute leukemias. Disseminated intravascular coagulation may also occur in any of the acute leukemias, but especially in acute promyelocytic leukemia. Prothrombin time (PT), partial thromboplastin time (PTT), fibrinogen level, and fibrin/fibrinogen degradation products should always be determined.

## Neutrophilia

### Definition

Neutrophilia is defined as an absolute granulocyte count in excess of 7500 per cubic millimeter.

*See Neutrophilia, p. 227, and Lymphocytosis, p. 228.

### Clinical Significance

A neutrophilic leukocytosis is most frequently a nonspecific manifestation of inflammation. An absolute granulocytosis, when it is manifested as a leukemoid reaction, must be differentiated from chronic granulocytic leukemia. A granulocytic leukemoid reaction may be defined as an elevated granulocyte count associated with the appearance of immature granulocytic precursors in peripheral blood (i.e., myelocytes, promyelocytes, and myeloblasts).

### Etiology

1. Increased production of granulocytes.
    a. Reactive (e.g., infection, steroids, Hodgkin's disease).
    b. Myeloproliferative (e.g., chronic granulocytic leukemia).
2. Increased release of granulocytes from reserve compartment.
    a. Etiocholanolone.
    b. Endotoxin.
3. Decreased margination of granulocytes: epinephrine (endogenous or exogenous).
4. Decreased egress of granulocytes from the blood.
    a. Adrenal steroids.
    b. Prednisone.

### Diagnostic Approach

In the clinical setting, the practical problem is the differential diagnosis of reactive and malignant granulocytosis (see Table 6-2).

---

## Lymphocytosis

---

### Definition

Lymphocytosis is defined as an absolute lymphocyte count in excess of 4500 per cubic millimeter.

### Clinical Significance

Lymphocytosis is most common in childhood and is usually a nonspecific finding associated with viral infections. In the adult, lymphocytosis has greater specificity and therefore greater diagnostic value.

### Etiology

1. The etiologic mechanisms of lymphocytosis are not well known. Significantly, not all cases are a result of increased proliferation. In pertussis, the mechanism is thought to be related to a blockade of lymphocyte entry into lymph nodes.
2. Causes of nonactivated lymphocytosis (normal inactive small lymphocytes).
    a. Infectious lymphocytosis.
    b. Mumps.
    c. Varicella.
    d. Rubeola.
    e. Herpes simplex.
    f. Influenza.
    g. Tuberculosis.
    h. Pertussis.
    i. Other causes: the most important is chronic lymphocytic leukemia.
3. Causes of activated lymphocytosis (atypical or "turned-on" lymphocytes).
    a. Infectious mononucleosis.

**Table 6-2.** Differential diagnosis of chronic granulocytic leukemia
and leukemoid reaction

| Parameter | Chronic granulocytic leukemia | Leukemoid reaction |
|---|---|---|
| Clinical picture | Usually no symptoms, or symptoms related to splenomegaly | Often exhibit overt manifestations of underlying disease (e.g., carcinoma, infection) |
| Peripheral blood findings | Leukocytosis parallels spleen size; leukoerythroblastic picture with entire maturation "pyramid" of the granulocytic line; basophils increased; giant platelets | Leukocytosis unrelated to spleen size; myeloblasts rarely present; platelets normal in appearance; basophils not increased |
| Bone marrow findings | Hypercellular; megakaryocytes increased (early); myeloid: erythroid = 10 : 1; myelocyte dominates granulocytic series; basophils increased | Cellularity variable; megakaryocytes usually normal; myeloid: erythroid usually greater than normal: granulocytic "pyramid" intact; basophils not increased |
| Leukocyte alkaline phosphatase activity | Usually decreased or absent | Usually increased |
| Serum $B_{12}$ | Marked increase | Slight increase |
| Karyotype abnormality (Ph[1] anomaly) | Usually present | Absent |

    **b.** Infectious hepatitis.
    **c.** Toxoplasmosis.
    **d.** Cytomegalovirus (CMV).
    **e.** Posttransfusion syndrome.
    **f.** Drug-induced: para-aminosalicylic acid, diphenylhydantoin, mephenytoin.

### Approach

1. See Figure 6-5.
2. Lymphocytosis is not commonly seen as a clinical problem; it is usually a manifestation of an associated infection.
3. When it does exist as an isolated problem, evaluation of the peripheral blood film and determination of the CBC and platelet count are important.
    **a.** If the cells identified are blasts, then the diagnosis of acute lymphoblastic leukemia is made and confirmed by bone marrow aspiration.
    **b.** If the lymphocytes are small or medium-sized with many "activated" or "atypical" forms, then a monospot test, hepatitis B surface antigen (HB$_s$Ag), *Toxoplasma* immunofluorescence test, and CMV titer should be obtained in addi-

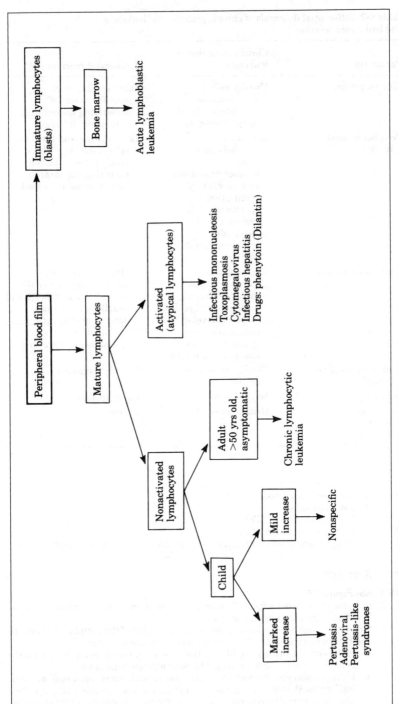

**Fig. 6-5.** Diagnostic approach to lymphocytosis.

tion to inquiry into clinical history (e.g., use of analeptic drugs, transfusion history, hepatitis, or recent history of an upper respiratory infection).
   **c.** If the lymphocytes are small and "mature" and the patient is an older, asymptomatic adult, the diagnosis of chronic lymphocytic leukemia is most likely. Evaluation for lymphadenopathy and splenomegaly, bone marrow aspiration for lymphocytic infiltration, and a serum protein electrophoresis for hypogammaglobulinemia will confirm the diagnosis.

## Basophilia

### Definition

Basophilia is defined as an absolute basophil count of more than 100 per cubic millimeter.

### Clinical Significance

Basophilia itself is seldom a clinical problem, but it may be a clue to diagnosis. Increases in the basophil count are particularly striking in the myeloproliferative disorders.

### Associated Conditions

1. Hypersensitivity states.
2. Myxedema.
3. Ulcerative colitis.
4. Myeloproliferative disorders.
   **a.** Polycythemia vera.
   **b.** Chronic granulocytic leukemia.
   **c.** Essential thrombocythemia.
   **d.** Myelofibrosis with myeloid metaplasia.

## Eosinophilia

### Definition

Eosinophilia is defined as an absolute eosinophil count of more than 500 per cubic millimeter.

### Clinical Significance

Counts between 500 and 1000 per cubic millimeter are nonspecific and should not be pursued as a clinical problem. Counts greater than 4000 per cubic millimeter have specificity.

### Associated Conditions

1. Allergic disorders (e.g., hay fever, bronchial asthma).
2. Parasitic infestation with tissue invasion (e.g., trichinosis).
3. Skin diseases (e.g., dermatitis herpetiformis).
4. Tumors (e.g., Hodgkin's disease).
5. Granulomatous disease (e.g., tuberculosis, coccidioidomycosis).
6. The hypereosinophilic syndromes.
   **a.** Eosinophilic leukemia.
   **b.** Fibroplastic endocarditis.
   **c.** Systemic vasculitis.

**d.** Löffler's syndrome.
**e.** Tropical eosinophilia.

## SPLENOMEGALY
### John H. Saiki

### Definition

Clinically, a palpable spleen represents an enlarged spleen. Enlargement must be confirmed by scan measurements.

### Clinical Significance

1. Splenomegaly most commonly is a secondary manifestation of an underlying disease, but may represent a primary lymphoma of the spleen.
2. Impaired gastric filling with early satiety may lead to weight loss. There may be increased susceptibility to rupture from trauma because of lack of protection by the rib cage.
3. Hypersplenism with cytopenia (single or multiple) occasionally is associated with increased susceptibility to infection and hemorrhage.

### Etiology

1. Congestion.
    **a.** Congestive heart failure.
    **b.** Portal hypertension.
2. Reactive hyperplasia.
    **a.** "Work hypertrophy" (e.g., hemolytic disease).
    **b.** Infections.
        **(1)** Bacterial (e.g., tuberculosis, infective endocarditis, brucellosis).
        **(2)** Viral (e.g., CMV, infectious mononucleosis).
        **(3)** Fungal.
        **(4)** Parasitic (e.g., malaria, toxoplasmosis).
    **c.** Connective tissue diseases (e.g., SLE, RA).
    **d.** Serum sickness.
3. Infiltrative diseases.
    **a.** Nonneoplastic.
        **(1)** Lipidosis (Gaucher's disease).
        **(2)** Sarcoidosis.
        **(3)** Amyloidosis.
    **b.** Neoplastic.
        **(1)** Lymphoproliferative disorders (acute and chronic lymphocytic leukemia and lymphoma).
        **(2)** Myeloproliferative disorders (polycythemia vera, chronic granulocytic leukemia, and myelofibrosis with myeloid metaplasia).
        **(3)** Metastatic tumor (extremely rare).

### Diagnostic Approach

1. See Figure 6-6.
2. History. Has the patient had a recent febrile illness to suggest an infectious cause? Does he have fever, sweating, itching, or weight loss, which represent the clinically important symptoms of lymphoma? Is there a history of congestive

heart failure or alcoholism to suggest passive congestion of the spleen? Is there a family history of anemia, splenomegaly, or splenectomy? Hereditary anemias (e.g., thalassemia minor) may be asymptomatic but associated with splenomegaly.

3. Physical examination. A very thorough examination for lymphadenopathy, hepatomegaly, and evidence of infection should be performed.

4. Confirmation of splenomegaly by spleen scan.

5. Initial screening studies.
   a. CBC, reticulocyte count, and platelet count.
   b. Serum bilirubin (total and direct), alkaline phosphatase, SGPT, SGOT, LDH, serum electrophoresis, acid phosphatase.
   c. ANA and RF.
   d. Serologic tests for fungi, complement-fixation test for toxoplasmosis, hepatitis test, monospot test, and heterophil antibody titer.
   e. X-rays: PA and lateral films of chest, flat plate of abdomen; barium swallow for evaluation of varices.
   f. Liver scan.
   g. Bone marrow aspiration and biopsy for culture, cytologic and histologic evaluation, staining for amyloid, fibrous tissue, bacteria (including acid-fast bacilli), and fungi.

6. If the patient has asymptomatic splenomegaly and the spleen is mildly to moderately enlarged (estimated < 400 g), continued observation at monthly intervals is a reasonable approach, particularly in the age group under 35 years. Primary lymphoma of the spleen is unlikely in this age group. If the spleen remains unchanged in size, the patient could be followed at progressively longer intervals. In the age group over 35 years without symptoms, close observation is imperative.

7. If the patient is symptomatic with fever, profuse sweating, anorexia, and weight loss, or if the patient remains asymptomatic, but documented enlargement of the spleen is noted, then further investigations are imperative. These include abdominal ultrasound, lymphangiography, and gallium scan. Even if results from these studies are negative, an exploratory laparotomy must be very seriously considered for diagnostic splenectomy, liver biopsy (core and wedge), and multiple lymph node biopsies.

## LYMPHADENOPATHY
John H. Saiki

### Definition

Lymphadenopathy is an abnormal increase in size or altered consistency of lymph nodes. It is a clinical manifestation of regional or systemic disease and serves as an excellent clue to the underlying cause.

### Etiology

1. Reactive.
   a. Infectious.
      (1) Bacterial (e.g., pyogenic, tuberculosis).
      (2) Viral (e.g., CMV, infectious mononucleosis).
      (3) Fungal (e.g., coccidioidomycosis).
      (4) Parasitic (e.g., toxoplasmosis).
   b. Noninfectious.
      (1) Sarcoidosis.
      (2) Connective tissue disease.
      (3) Dermatopathic.
      (4) Drug-induced (e.g., diphenylhydantoin).

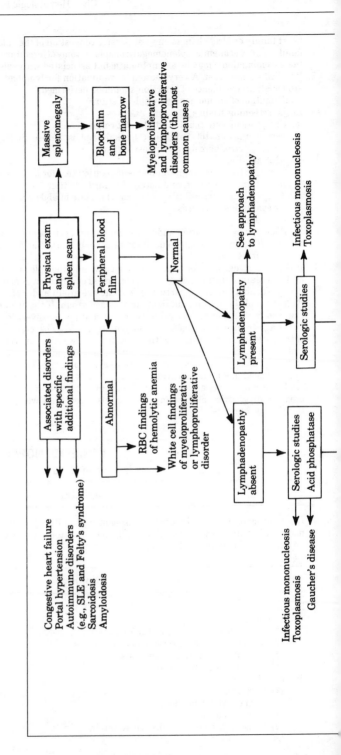

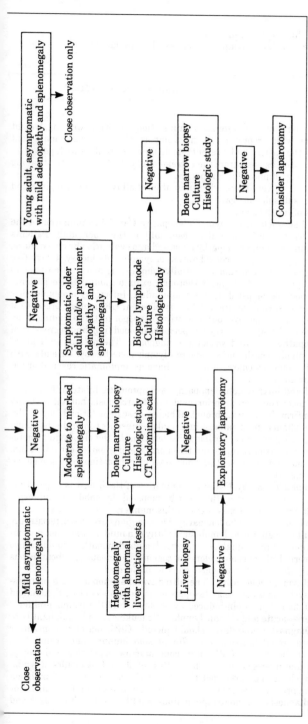

**Fig. 6-6.** Diagnostic approach to splenomegaly.

**2.** Infiltrative.
  **a.** Benign (e.g., histiocytosis, lipidosis).
  **b.** Malignant (e.g., primary lymphoma, metastatic carcinoma).

---

## Diagnostic Approach

---

**1.** See Figure 6-7.
**2.** History. Has the patient had systemic manifestations of fever, sweating, weight loss, and itching, which represent the most important symptoms of malignant lymphoma? Has the patient had a recent febrile illness or contact with pets (e.g., transmission of toxoplasmosis from the excrement of cats)? Is the patient taking analeptic drugs (e.g., diphenylhydantoin)?
**3.** Physical examination. Very thorough examination of all lymph node regions and evaluation for hepatosplenomegaly.
**4.** Specific regions of involvement.
  **a.** Cervical and supraclavicular lymphadenopathy. Careful examination of the head and neck region is imperative, especially in the older adult. Patients with unexplained lymphadenopathy must undergo evaluation by an ear, nose, and throat surgeon prior to consideration of lymph node biopsy. Thirty-five percent of head and neck tumors initially manifest as metastatic tumor to regional lymph nodes. Only after thorough examination of these patients should the node be biopsied. In the young adult, infectious mononucleosis must be given first consideration. A history of recent URI and the presence of splenomegaly are supportive, but a positive monospot test, the finding of activated "atypical" lymphocytes on the peripheral blood film, and regression of lymphadenopathy in 2 to 4 weeks are diagnostic. The patient with unexplained lymphadenopathy must undergo lymph node biopsy. Patients with malignant lymphomas characteristically have asymptomatic cervical or supraclavicular adenopathy.
  **b.** Mediastinal and hilar lymphadenopathy. Asymptomatic bilateral hilar adenopathy has been considered a priori evidence of sarcoidosis, but it is probably wisest to confirm this by transbronchial biopsy or scalene fat pad biopsy. Mediastinal lymphadenopathy almost invariably represents tumor. In the young adult, Hodgkin's disease is of prime consideration. In the older adult, metastatic carcinoma (usually lung) and thymoma are of greatest consideration. Full lung tomograms are essential, and biopsy by mediastinoscopy or mediastinotomy is imperative.
  **c.** Axillary lymphadenopathy. Careful examination of the breast is imperative. Unexplained axillary adenopathy must be biopsied. Lymphomas and, especially, occult breast cancer may occur in this manner.
  **d.** Inguinal and femoral lymphadenopathy. These regions are characteristically more difficult to evaluate, as lymphadenopathy of a mild degree is not uncommon in the normal individual. Asymmetric lymphadenopathy should arouse greater concern. If there is no evidence of regional cutaneous or subcutaneous inflammatory disease, then a biopsy must be performed.
  **e.** Generalized lymphadenopathy. Generalized lymphadenopathy is a manifestation of a systemic illness (e.g., toxoplasmosis, serum sickness, rheumatoid arthritis, diphenylhydantoin-induced hyperplasia, and the lymphoproliferative disorders—acute and chronic lymphocytic leukemia and malignant lymphomas). Diagnostic procedures should include CBC, platelet count, liver function tests, renal function tests, *Toxoplasma* immunofluorescence test, heterophil antibody titer, CMV titer, bone marrow aspiration and biopsy, chest x-ray, and liver-spleen scan. Regardless of above test results, a lymph node biopsy should be performed to rule out the presence of a lymphoma either as the primary disease or as an associated disease, and to confirm or aid in the diagnosis of a nonlymphomatous condition through cultures and

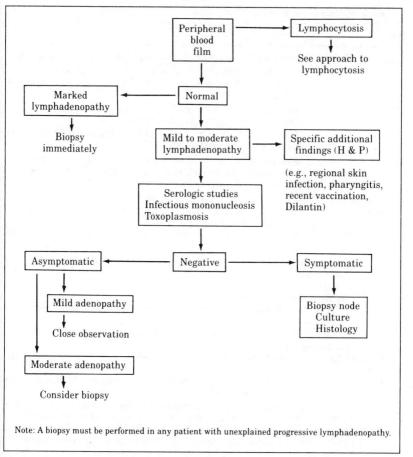

**Fig. 6-7.** Diagnostic approach to lymphadenopathy.

histologic evaluation. An exception to this approach would be the diagnosis of acute or chronic lymphocytic leukemia, established by the peripheral blood film or bone marrow.

5. **Specific etiology.** The malignant lymphomas: With a newly established diagnosis of lymphoma, the evaluation of extent of disease (to determine the clinical and pathologic stage [see Table 6-3] of the lymphoma) will determine the therapeutic approach. The following studies should be performed:

   **a.** History (especially symptoms of fever, sweating, and weight loss) and physical examination (especially lymph node areas, liver, and spleen).

   **b.** Hematologic studies: CBC and platelet count, reticulocyte count, Coombs' test, and bone marrow aspiration and biopsy (bilateral in the non-Hodgkin's lymphomas).

   **c.** Liver: Serum alkaline phosphatase and scan.

   **d.** Renal: Urinalysis, serum creatinine, and BUN.

   **e.** Lymph node regions.

      **(1)** External: Physical examination.

      **(2)** Mediastinal: Chest x-ray.

**Table 6-3.** Staging of the malignant lymphomas

| Stage | Criteria |
|---|---|
| I | Single lymph node region (I) or a single parenchymal lesion (I-E) |
| II | Two or more lymph node regions (II) or localized parenchymal disease with one or more node regions on the same side of the diaphragm (II-E) |
| III | Lymph node involvement above and below diaphragm (III) <br> Above plus splenic involvement (III-S) <br> Above plus localized parenchymal involvement (III-E) and when spleen is involved (III-SE) |
| IV | Disseminated foci of one or more parenchymal organs with or without lymph node disease. A single lesion in liver or bone marrow is defined as IV |
| Subclassification Symptoms | A—asymptomatic; B—symptomatic <br> Fever, sweating, and weight loss in excess of 10 percent of body weight within a 6-month period |

    **(3)** Retroperitoneal and mesenteric:
        **(a)** Hodgkin's disease: Lymphangiogram and CT scan of abdomen and pelvis.
        **(b)** Non-Hodgkin's disease: CT scan of abdomen and pelvis.
    **(4)** Spleen: Spleen scan, $^{99m}$Tc.
  **6.** Bone: Calcium, phosphorus, serum alkaline phosphatase, $^{99m}$Tc polyphosphate bone scan.
  **7.** Immunologic: Tests of humoral and cell-mediated immunity may be done but currently are not necessary for clinical staging.
  **8.** Exploratory laparotomy is carried out on most, but not all, patients with Hodgkin's disease. Only when findings might influence the therapeutic approach is this procedure done (i.e., patients with obvious clinical stage IV disease are not laparotomized). At laparotomy, multiple lymph nodes are biopsied (para-aortic, celiac axis, porta hepatis, splenic hilar, and any suspicious node identified by CT scan or lymphangiography). Both wedge and core biopsies of the liver are taken (core biopsies are most important), and splenectomy is performed (primarily for diagnostic purposes). Other benefits of splenectomy are that radiation therapy to the splenic area is no longer required and therefore radiation nephritis is averted, and hematologic tolerance to both radiotherapy and chemotherapy is improved. Silver clips should mark lymph node biopsy sites. The young woman should always have an oophoropexy. Exploratory laparotomy is rarely necessary for staging in the non-Hodgkin's lymphomas.

    Evaluation of the patient who has had a diagnosis of lymphoma in the past and received appropriate therapy should include periodic history taking, physical examination, and laboratory tests. The interval is proportionate to the duration of remission (i.e., the longer the remission, the longer the interval). After 2 years, 6-month intervals are appropriate and after 5 years, 12-month intervals are appropriate. Inquiry into feeling of well-being, appetite, weight loss, fever, sweating, itching, and recurrent lymphadenopathy is important. Physical examination should include weight, temperature, evaluation of all nodal areas, and examination of liver and spleen (if not surgically absent). Laboratory studies should include a CBC, serum alkaline phosphatase, chest x-ray, KUB of the abdomen for residual lymphangiogram dye, and other appropriate tests that previously demonstrated diseased areas of greatest involvement.

## BLEEDING AND CLOTTING DISORDERS

Jerome S. Nosanchuk

### Definition and Characteristics

Bleeding is defined as a breakdown in hemostasis. Hemostasis depends on vascular integrity, the number and quality of platelets, and plasma coagulation factors (procoagulants). Clotting requires the conversion of soluble plasma fibrinogen into an insoluble fibrin clot (Fig. 6-8). This conversion is mediated by a protease enzyme thrombin; the end product, fibrin, is rendered stable by factor XIII (fibrin stabilizing factor). Bleeding occurs when there is impairment of the hemostatic mechanism due to either defective synthesis or excessive utilization of clotting factors. Coagulation may also be impaired by circulating inhibitors of clotting factors or the proteolytic action of plasmin. The degree of bleeding is related to both the nature and the severity of the deficiency. A thorough history and physical examination are adequate to identify most bleeding disorders. The characteristics of bleeding in hemorrhagic disorders are given in Table 6-4.

Most operative and postoperative hemorrhage is due to inadequate surgical hemostasis. Patients with delayed bleeding or those whose bleeding is controlled initially but who subsequently bleed again are more likely to have intrinsic defects in coagulation factors than platelet abnormalities. This type of bleeding, especially if acquired, is more frequently due to multiple factors than to a single cause.

The final diagnosis of a coagulation disorder rests heavily on laboratory support (Fig. 6-8, Table 6-5). Functional deficiency or inhibition of a factor in the intrinsic pathway is generally detected by the activated partial thromboplastin time (APTT). Factors involved in the extrinsic system are usually detected by measuring the one-stage prothrombin time (PT). Both of these times are prolonged when fibrin formation is defective (e.g., low fibrinogen). Neither the PT nor the APTT detects abnormalities in factor XIII or platelets. It requires a significant reduction in any single factor to affect either the PT or the APTT. For example, pure factor VIII or IX deficiency must be reduced to a level that is 30 percent or less of normal before the APTT is prolonged. Paradoxically, severe deficiencies of factor II may not prolong the PT, because most reagent test systems are relatively insensitive to low factor II levels. However, a modest combination of multiple factor deficiencies usually prolongs the clotting times. Because clotting studies are very method-dependent, it is critical that samples be properly drawn using two-syringe or multiple vacutainer techniques and that the specimens be brought promptly to the laboratory for analysis. Consultation with the clinical hematology laboratory director or clinical pathologist is not only advisable but often mandatory for correct diagnosis and appropriate therapy.

### Evaluation of the Preoperative Patient

1. The most important initial step is to obtain an adequate history and physical examination. It is also important to ascertain whether the patient has experienced abnormal bleeding or bruising in the past. The site, extent, and duration of previous hemorrhagic phenomena, and the response to treatment, may be helpful. Specific questions should be asked concerning bleeding with minor injuries, lacerations, circumcision, tooth extraction, appendectomy, tonsillectomy, pregnancy, menses, and umbilical cord, as well as delayed bleeding and keloid formation. The patient should also be questioned concerning the use of drugs that may interfere with hemostasis (e.g., oral contraceptives, aspirin-containing med-

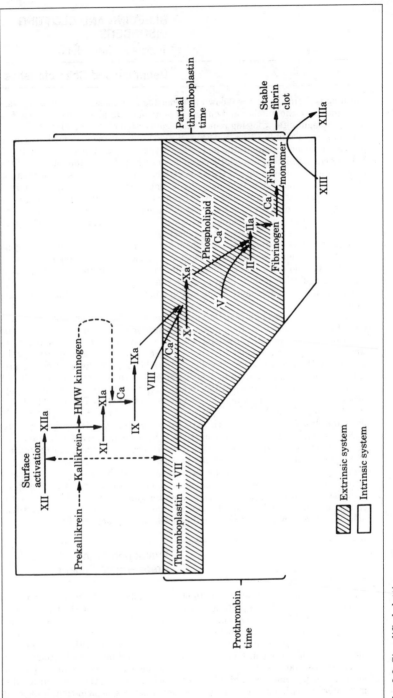

**Fig. 6-8.** Simplified clotting sequence.

**Table 6-4.** Characteristics of bleeding in hemorrhagic disorders

| Type of bleed | Definition | Location | Cause |
|---|---|---|---|
| Petechia | Smallest; punctate; about 1 mm in diameter | On extremities, usually absent over pressure point | Vascular or platelet abnormality |
| Purpura | 1 mm to 1 cm | Generally truncal, occasionally extremities | Vascular abnormality |
| Ecchymosis | Larger bleed with local extravasation | Soft tissues, joints | Factor deficiency or open blood vessel |
| Generalized | Diffuse or generalized ecchymosis | Large areas, mucous membranes, wounds | Disseminated intravascular clotting or primary fibrinolysis |

**Table 6-5.** Diagnosis of clotting deficiencies

| Deficient factor | Test | | | |
|---|---|---|---|---|
| | PT | APTT | Platelet count | Bleeding time |
| Fibrinogen (I) | A | A | N | N |
| Prothrombin (II) | A | A | N | N or A |
| Tissue thromboplastin (III) | | | | |
| Calcium (IV) | | | | |
| Labile factor (V) | A | A | N | N or A |
| (Not assigned) (VI) | | | | |
| Stable factor (VII) | A | N | N | N |
| Antihemophilic globulin (VIII) | N | A | N | N |
| Christmas factor (IX) | N | A | N | N |
| Stuart-Prower factor (X) | A | A | N | N or A |
| Plasma thromboplastin antecedent (XI) | N | A | N | N |
| Hageman factor (XII) | N | A | N | N |
| Fibrin stabilizing factor (XIII) | N | N | N | N |
| Prekallikrein (Fletcher factor) | N | A | N | N |
| HMW kininogen (Fitzgerald factor) | N | A | N | N |
| von Willebrand's (VIII$_{ag}$) | N | N or A | N | N or A |
| Thrombocytopenia | N | N | A | N or A |
| Functional platelet defect | N | N | N or A | A |
| Vascular defect | N | N | N | N or A |
| Antithrombin III | N | N | N | N |
| Protein C | N | N | N | N |
| Protein S | N | N | N | N |

N = normal, A = abnormal

icines, antibiotics, sodium warfarin [Coumadin], or heparin). A positive family history of bleeding suggests the presence of sex-linked or autosomal dominant disorders.

2. Knowledge of the patient's underlying disease may provide a clue to potential bleeding problems. A patient with significant hepatic disease, neoplasia, or uremia is at greater risk than a patient who is otherwise well.

3. The incidence of coagulation hazard is increased in some surgical operations. Cardiopulmonary bypass procedures and hypothermia may cause inactivation or destruction of clotting factors and platelets. Prostate surgery is associated with an increased frequency of fibrinolysis. The use of water rather than saline irrigation in bladder surgery can provoke hemolysis. Cardiovascular surgery, trauma, and other situations in which massive bleeding and replacement transfusion occur also have an increased potential for hemorrhage because of deficiencies in various clotting factors.

4. If, despite negative history and physical findings, a preoperative coagulation screen is still deemed necessary, the following studies are recommended. Negative findings with these tests virtually exclude the presence of a significant preexisting coagulopathy.
   a. APTT.
   b. PT.
   c. Fibrinogen.
   d. Platelet count.
   e. Bleeding time (preferably by a standardized template method).

5. Normal screening tests may occur in von Willebrand's disease, mild hereditary factor deficiencies, hereditary coagulation disorders (heterozygotic carriers), factor XIII deficiency, prekallikrein deficiency, some dysfibrinogenemias, some platelet function disorders, hemorrhagic telangiectasia, and vascular purpuras.

# Evaluation of a Bleeding Patient

The approach to the problem of a bleeding patient should be logical. A history and physical examination are mandatory. The following laboratory studies should detect the cause(s) and permit guidance in therapy for all but extremely rare coagulation defects.

1. PT and APTT. If abnormal, correction studies with pooled normal plasma, absorbed plasma, and serum reagent may be helpful.
2. Platelet count.
3. Fibrinogen level.
4. Bleeding time.
5. Fibrin split products.
6. Hemoglobin or hematocrit, or both.
7. Peripheral blood smear.
8. Clot for blood typing and antibody screen.
9. If excess heparin is suspected, either a protamine sulfate correction or a heparin resin absorption assay can establish the diagnosis.
10. Special studies, usually available only in larger laboratories, include specific factor assays, assays for inhibitors and antibodies, and platelet aggregation and antibody studies.

Most operative and postoperative bleeding is due to inadequate local control of a severed blood vessel. Once a patient begins to hemorrhage, it is mandatory to stop this bleeding because massive blood loss itself may deplete certain procoagulants. Only rarely are coagulation factor deficiencies responsible for this type of hemorrhage.

## Identifying the Cause
## of the Bleeding

Specific factor assays will be suggested by the laboratory consultant based on the preceding screening studies. Isolated deficiencies are usually hereditary, whereas those that are acquired frequently involve multiple factors.

### Hereditary Factor Deficiencies

1. Classic hemophilia (hemophilia A) or factor VIII deficiency, a sex-linked hereditary disorder, is the most common hereditary factor deficiency. It is detected by the presence of an abnormal APTT that is corrected by barium sulfate-adsorbed normal plasma and will not correct with known factor VIII–deficient plasma. It appears to be due to the production of normal amounts of nonfunctional factor VIII molecules because factor VIII antigen (VIII$_{ag}$) levels are normal. It should be noted that up to 40 percent of classic hemophiliacs have a negative family history for the disease.
2. Hemophilia B (Christmas disease), or factor IX deficiency, is less common. It also is a sex-linked, autosomally recessive inherited condition. The APTT is prolonged, but in contrast to hemophilia A, the abnormality is not corrected by barium sulfate-adsorbed plasma, although normal stored plasma or serum can correct the APTT.
3. The remaining numbered factor deficiencies are extremely rare.
4. Factor deficiencies must be confirmed by performing a specific factor assay using known factor deficient control material.
5. Although infrequent, acquired factor deficiencies can occur in a variety of diseases, including lymphomas, plasma cell dyscrasias, amyloidosis, and nephrotic syndrome.
6. Clotting factor inhibitors may be associated with some disease states, notably the connective tissue disorders. They also have occurred in ulcerative colitis, postpartum, and in association with some drug reactions. Occasionally, they occur in the absence of any identifiable disease. Special laboratory tests are necessary for their identification.

### Vascular Defects

Vascular disorders are poorly defined and not well understood. The etiology of vascular "fragility" is not always apparent. These patients have prolonged bleeding times. With the exception of vascular pseudohemophilia (von Willebrand's disease), the bleeding is rarely severe.

1. Classic von Willebrand's disease (VWD) exhibits autosomal dominant inheritance. It is characterized by a prolonged bleeding time, a decreased factor VIII level, decreased factor VIII antigen (in contrast to classic hemophilia in which VIII$_{ag}$ is normal), and failure of platelets to aggregate in the presence of the antibiotic ristocetin. Defective platelet adhesion is generally found. Numerous VWD variants have now been described. Type I VWD is important to identify since the drug DDAVP can be used to prevent bleeding in patients with this disease.
2. The factor VIII deficiency in von Willebrand's disease differs from that found in hemophilia A. Infusion of plasma concentrates causes a prolonged elevation of factor VIII levels in von Willebrand's disease but not in classic hemophilia, in which the factor VIII activity disappears rapidly. Similarly, the plasma from a classic hemophilia A patient corrects the von Willebrand patient's ristocetin aggregation defect.
3. Aspirin causes an exaggerated prolongation of the bleeding time in patients with von Willebrand's disease.

## Platelet Defects

Bleeding can occur because of too few or too many platelets. Platelets that are qualitatively defective may be unable to react normally in the clotting process even when present in adequate numbers. The normal platelet count is about 150,000 to 400,000 per cubic millimeter. One-third of the platelet mass is sequestered in the spleen. It takes 5 to 7 days for platelets to mature from megakaryocytes. The platelet survival time in the circulation is about 10 days. Transfused platelets survive 4 to 5 days in the absence of antiplatelet antibodies.

Platelets adhere to injured vascular endothelium by contact with subendothelial collagen. The adenosine diphosphate (ADP) released from the cytoplasmic granules of the platelets participates in the induction of aggregation and cohesion. Meanwhile, the phospholipids (platelet factor 3), and other cellular constituents that are discharged, activate Hageman factor (XII), which in turn activates the intrinsic clotting pathway. Thrombin and perhaps ADP cause consolidation of the platelet plug.

LABORATORY TESTS

1. If bleeding is thought to be due to a platelet abnormality, the following quantitative and qualitative platelet tests are indicated. The first three tests are available in most laboratories. The remainder may not be generally available.
   a. Direct examination of the stained smear.
   b. Platelet count.
   c. Bleeding time (template method preferred).
   d. Prothrombin consumption time with and without inosithin.
   e. Adhesion.
   f. Aggregation.
   g. Assay for platelet factor 3.
   h. Platelet sizing (volume).
   i. Clot retraction, while simple, is too nonspecific and takes too long. It is not recommended when a bleeding time can be obtained.
2. The probability of bleeding is related to the results of the quantitative and functional tests.
   a. Functionally normal platelets in numbers greater than 50,000 per cubic millimeter ordinarily prevent hemorrhage during surgical procedures.
   b. Major spontaneous hemorrhage is decidedly unusual with functionally normal platelet counts in excess of 20,000 per cubic millimeter.
   c. Spontaneous hemorrhage may occur with counts of 10,000 per cubic millimeter or less, but it is not unusual for patients with such levels and lower to go for long periods without serious complications, especially when the etiology of the thrombocytopenia is on an immune basis. The major threat at this low platelet level is intracranial hemorrhage, particularly in infants and young children. Patients with both anemia and thrombocytopenia are more likely to bleed than those with thrombocytopenia alone.
   d. In patients with depressed platelet counts, it may be important to have some idea of the functional integrity of the platelets. The best, most simple, readily available test of platelet function is the standardized (template) bleeding time. Studies of platelet adhesiveness and aggregation may sometimes be pertinent but are not widely available. These patients should be guarded from taking drugs that affect platelet function, particularly aspirin.

QUANTITATIVE PLATELET ABNORMALITIES

1. Definition. Thrombocytopenia is said to exist when the platelet count is below 100,000 per cubic millimeter. Thrombocytosis, usually a transient state, is present when the platelet count is greater than 400,000 per cubic millimeter. Thrombocythemia is a condition in which the platelet count exceeds 900,000 per cubic millimeter.

**2.** Etiology. The following is not an all-inclusive list.
  **a.** Thrombocytopenia.
    **(1)** Diminished or defective platelet production.
      **(a)** Congenital.
        **(i)** Wiskott-Aldrich syndrome.
        **(ii)** May-Hegglin syndrome.
        **(iii)** Chédiak-Higashi anomaly.
      **(b)** Acquired.
        **(i)** Aplastic anemia.
        **(ii)** Marrow infiltration.
        **(iii)** Radiation toxicity.
        **(iv)** Chemotherapy.
        **(v)** Direct toxicity to platelet production (e.g., thiazides, alcohol, estrogens).
        **(vi)** Cyclic thrombocytopenia (premenstrual).
      **(c)** Nutritional.
        **(i)** Vitamin $B_{12}$ deficiency.
        **(ii)** Folic acid deficiency.
        **(iii)** Iron deficiency.
      **(d)** Viral infections.
      **(e)** Paroxysmal nocturnal hemoglobinuria.
      **(f)** Splenic disorders.
        **(i)** Congestive.
        **(ii)** Neoplasms.
        **(iii)** Infiltrations.
        **(iv)** Infections.
      **(g)** Miscellaneous.
        **(i)** Heat stroke.
        **(ii)** Burns.
        **(iii)** Endocrine.
    **(2)** Increased platelet destruction.
      **(a)** Giant cavernous hemangioma (Kasabach-Merritt syndrome).
      **(b)** Infection (viral, bacterial, rickettsial, fungal, mycobacterial).
      **(c)** Disseminated intravascular coagulation.
      **(d)** Thrombotic thrombocytopenic purpura.
      **(e)** Hemolytic-uremic syndrome.
      **(f)** Drug-induced.
        **(i)** Immunologic (e.g., quinine, quinidine, heparin).
        **(ii)** Nonimmunologic.
      **(g)** Posttransfusion.
      **(h)** Idiopathic thrombocytopenic purpura.
      **(i)** Connective tissue disorders.
      **(j)** Extracorporeal circulation.
  **b.** Thrombocythemia.
    **(1)** Myeloproliferative disorders.
    **(2)** Chronic inflammatory states.
    **(3)** Acute inflammation.
    **(4)** Acute hemorrhage.
    **(5)** Iron deficiency.
    **(6)** Hemolytic anemias.
    **(7)** Malignant diseases.
    **(8)** Postoperative (especially splenectomy).
    **(9)** Drug-induced.
    **(10)** Postexercise.
  **c.** Thrombocytopenic purpura.
    **(1)** Acute idiopathic thrombocytopenic purpura (ITP) is usually a disease of childhood. Onset is usually preceded by infection (viral more frequently than bacterial). Spontaneous recovery within a 1- to 2-month period from onset is the general rule.

(2) Chronic idiopathic thrombocytopenic purpura is more often a disease of females between the ages of 20 and 50 years. Onset is usually insidious. The disease is characterized by the presence of a purpuric or petechial eruption. Splenomegaly is minimal if present at all. The platelet counts may range from 10,000 to 75,000 per cubic millimeter. Counts as low as 1000 per cubic millimeter may be seen. Bleeding is rare unless the platelet count falls below 20,000 per cubic millimeter. The number of megakaryocytes in the bone marrow is normal or increased, but the megakaryocytes are less granular and more basophilic than normal. These patients typically do not respond to platelet transfusions. Drug sensitivity, sepsis, TTP, disseminated intravascular coagulation, systemic lupus erythematosus, tuberculosis, sarcoidosis, and lymphoma must be excluded.

(3) Platelet sequestration (hypersplenism). Many conditions may cause splenomegaly with hypersplenism and thrombocytopenia.

(4) Other causes. Hemorrhage, multiple transfusions, and extracorporeal circulation may result in platelet losses and thrombocytopenia.

d. Thrombocythemia. Platelet counts above one million per cubic millimeter are likely to be dangerous. An exception to this is the thrombocythemia occurring after splenectomy for trauma or staging. Bleeding from the mucous membranes may occur, and thrombotic phenomena are common. The cause of the bleeding is presumed to be mechanical interference with the normal clotting mechanisms by the presence of excessive numbers of platelets and by the excessive release of platelet procoagulant factors.

QUALITATIVE PLATELET DISORDERS

1. Drug-induced. Drugs are the single most common cause of qualitative platelet defects, and aspirin is the single most common offender. Aspirin inhibits aggregation by irreversible acetylation of platelet cyclooxygenase (prostaglandins) One adult-dose aspirin may prolong the bleeding time for up to a week. Other drugs affecting platelet function include other anti-inflammatory drugs (except acetaminophen [Tylenol]), antibiotics, antidepressants, and many other miscellaneous agents.

2. Thrombasthenia (Glanzmann's disease). This is a rare disorder with autosomal recessive transmission characterized by a prolonged bleeding time and failure of the platelets to aggregate in the presence of ADP and thrombin. Bleeding occurs because platelets are unable to bind fibrinogen and hence to aggregate.

3. Thrombocytopathic purpura (platelet factor 3 deficiency). In this condition, the platelets lack clot-promoting activity because of defective phospholipid release The bleeding time is prolonged and aggregation of platelets by ADP and thrombin may be impaired.

4. Thrombocytopathy (Bernard-Soulier syndrome). This is a rare disorder characterized by a prolonged bleeding time, impaired aggregation by thrombin but not ADP, and normal phospholipid release. There are characteristically giant platelets with large, prominent, dense granules giving a pseudonucleated appearance

5. Paraproteinemia. Numerous manifestations of platelet dysfunction occur with myelomas and macroglobulinemias, which may be due in part to the protein covering the surface of the platelets.

6. Myeloproliferative disorders and leukemia. Multiple defects occur in these disorders.

7. Anemia, by itself, can cause a prolonged bleeding time in some patients. Correction of the anemia can correct the bleeding time.

## Acquired Disorders

VITAMIN K–DEPENDENT FACTORS

1. Factors II, VII, IX, and X are synthesized by the liver. All are dependent on vitamin K for their synthesis. Deficiencies in these factors are detected by measur

ing the prothrombin time. It should be noted that different methods of PT deter-mination exhibit different sensitivities to deficiencies in these factors.
2. Vitamin K is naturally synthesized by intestinal bacteria. It is absorbed only in the presence of bile salts because of its lipid solubility.
3. Depletion of vitamin K–dependent factors may occur in patients receiving anti-biotics (especially for "bowel preps"), in obstructive jaundice, malabsorption states (e.g., sprue), and hepatic parenchymal disease.
4. Parenteral vitamin K therapy can alleviate vitamin K deficiency unless hepatic cellular function is too severely compromised. In an emergency, more rapid rever-sal can be achieved with fresh frozen plasma.

LIVER DISEASE

1. Deficiencies may be noted in factors VII, IX, X, V, II, and I, in the order given. The degree of deficiency is related to the severity and duration of the hepatocel-lular disease.
2. Factor VIII paradoxically rises to extremely high levels.
3. Plasminogen and antithrombin III deficiencies may occur.
4. Fibrin split products are poorly cleared, thus predisposing to fibrinolysis.
5. Abnormal fibrinogens (dysfibrinogenemia) and antithrombin V may also be pro-duced.
6. Marrow platelet production may be depressed. Excessive sequestration of plate-lets may occur in the spleen, which may involve as much as 80 percent of the platelet mass in some hypersplenic states.

RENAL DISEASE

1. Uremic thrombocytopathy may occur when the BUN exceeds 100 mg/100 dl.
2. The thrombocytopathy is manifested by an adhesive abnormality that is correct-able by dialysis.
3. Urinary loss of procoagulants, especially factor IX, may occur.
4. In connective tissue disease with renal involvement, pathologic inhibitors of pro-coagulants may appear in the circulation.

MASSIVE TRANSFUSIONS

1. Bank blood is deficient in platelets and factor V. Factor VIII is also variably de-pleted. Clinical problems related to deficiencies in bank blood virtually never oc-cur unless at least 10 units of stored blood have been transfused.
2. Empiric replacement with fresh frozen plasma or platelets, or both, should not be instituted without first measuring PT, APTT, and platelet count. Where readily available, fibrinogen, FSP, plasminogen, and AT III should also be obtained. It is not uncommon for a previously healthy patient to receive 20 or more units of blood in less than 24 hours without requiring any component therapy.

REACTION TO HEPARIN THERAPY

1. Heparin is a naturally occurring substance; its greatest concentration is found in lung tissue. It interferes with clotting by a variety of actions: inhibition of factors V, IXa, and XIII; inhibition of the proteolytic activity of thrombin (antithrombin); increased inactivation of factor Xa; and, in large doses, inhibition of platelet ag-gregation.
2. Heparin prolongs the Lee-White whole blood clotting time, plasma or whole blood recalcification time, APTT, and even PT. The correlation of the heparin dosage with the results of these tests is imperfect.
3. No single test of heparin activity now available is clearly superior to any other. The optimum level of anticoagulation for heparin therapy varies with the indi-cation for use.

REACTION TO COUMARIN COMPOUNDS

1. Coumarin derivatives are drugs with similar mechanisms of action but with vari-able rates of absorption and duration of activity. Their principal action is inhibi-

tion of the hepatic synthesis of vitamin K–dependent factors (II, VII, IX, and X) either by interference with vitamin K transport in the liver or by direct competition with vitamin K. It is also possible that these compounds cause the liver to produce abnormal forms of factors II, VII, IX, and X, perhaps by interference with a late step in peptide chain formation.

2. Factor VII is depressed first by the action of these drugs. The PT is affected most by deficiency of this factor. Subsequently, factor IX (not measured by the PT) falls, followed by decline in factors II and X. The last two factors reach their lowest levels in about 5 to 10 days. Reversal of drug effects by intravenous vitamin K usually occurs in 6 to 12 hours, provided liver function is normal. However, factor II may remain depressed for some time after the PT and APTT become normal.

3. Coumarin drugs may prolong the APTT as well as the PT.

4. The PT is the test of choice for monitoring therapy with this group of drugs. The absolute PT compared to a control is more meaningful than "percent activity."

SURREPTITIOUS BLEEDING

Self-administered sodium warfarin (Coumadin), heparin, and aspirin have all been implicated in causing bleeding. Self-inflicted trauma has produced urinary tract, vaginal, rectal, upper gastrointestinal, and cutaneous bleeding. Patients with these manifestations usually have significant psychiatric disorders.

CIRCULATING ANTICOAGULANTS

Circulating anticoagulants are found most often in association with hemophilia A or systemic lupus erythematosus. In both instances the substances, which may be IgG autoantibodies, are active against factor VIII. Circulating anticoagulants that are active against other factors or that are found in other diseases have been described. Occasionally, circulating anticoagulants may occur in patients who are otherwise free of identifiable disease. Inhibitors can cause prolongation of either the PT or APTT. The lupus anticoagulant, which causes a prolonged PT or APTT generally does not cause clinical bleeding, but is associated with hypercoagulable states (see below).

## Defibrination Syndromes

CLASSIFICATION

1. Defibrination syndromes may be divided into three major categories: disseminated intravascular coagulation, primary fibrinolysis and therapeutic fibrinolysis.
   a. Disseminated intravascular coagulation (DIC) occurs when thromboplastin-like material enters the circulation in sufficient quantities to cause excessive deposition of fibrin in the microcirculation. The physiologic response to the fibrin deposition is extensive fibrinolysis, with the formation of soluble fibrin degradation products (fibrin split products). Some of the fibrin split products particularly fragments X and Y, are themselves potent anticoagulants.
   b. Primary fibrinolysis, in contrast, occurs in the presence of excessive plasmin which is a potent digester of fibrinogen. This disorder may also result in the production of fibrin split products.
   c. Therapeutic thrombolysis or thrombolytic therapy is a medically induced clot lysis using pharmacologic agents. It is used for coronary artery and selected peripheral vascular thromboses.

2. DIC is a relatively common hemorrhagic disorder. It constitutes more than 90 percent of the defibrination syndromes. It is often associated with a treatable predisposing disease such as bacteremia, abruptio placentae, retained dead fetus incomplete abortion, burns, and snakebite. Other less directly treatable cause include transfusion reactions, giant hemangiomas, surgical manipulations, and carcinoma.

**3.** Primary fibrinolysis is rare. It is associated most frequently with prostatic adenocarcinoma and cirrhosis of the liver.

DIAGNOSIS OF ACUTE DIC AND PRIMARY FIBRINOLYSIS

**1.** The clinical situation is generally urgent. Bleeding is extensive and characteristically occurs from multiple sites such as the mucous membranes, incisions and wounds, needle puncture sites, the gastrointestinal tract, and the genitourinary tract.

**2.** In both diseases the pathophysiologic process is essentially the conversion of plasma to serum in vivo. Thus, variable depressions of plasma fibrinogen level, platelet count, and procoagulants are seen. The PT and APTT are usually prolonged. The fibrin split products (FSP) that are produced can be measured directly or estimated from the thrombin time. Measurement of D-dimer may be helpful.

**3.** The tests listed below (shown with "typical" results) are recommended for the diagnosis of diffuse intravascular clotting. All but the last three tests are widely available and generally can be completed within one hour. Other tests are useful but less available.

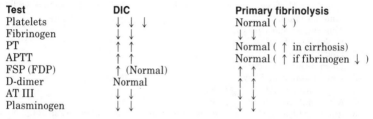

| **Test** | **DIC** | **Primary fibrinolysis** |
|---|---|---|
| Platelets | ↓ ↓ ↓ | Normal ( ↓ ) |
| Fibrinogen | ↓ ↓ | ↓ ↓ |
| PT | ↑ ↑ | Normal ( ↑ in cirrhosis) |
| APTT | ↑ ↑ | Normal ( ↑ if fibrinogen ↓ ) |
| FSP (FDP) | ↑ (Normal) | ↑ ↑ |
| D-dimer | Normal | ↑ ↑ |
| AT III | ↓ ↓ | ↓ ↓ |
| Plasminogen | ↓ ↓ | ↓ ↓ |

**4.** Comments.
   **a.** Fibrinogen is considerably elevated in women during the third trimester of pregnancy and in many males and females under stress. Thus, in such individuals a "normal" fibrinogen level may actually represent a depressed one when compared to fibrinogen concentrations in the prehemorrhagic state.
   **b.** Not all cases show all of the features of the respective disorders; for example, the PT or APTT may be relatively normal.
   **c.** The red blood cell structure in advanced DIC is often abnormal, with the formation of schistocytes and helmet cells. However, DIC may occur in the absence of these changes.

**5.** Additional studies.
   **a.** Measurement of D-dimer may be useful.
   **b.** In both DIC and primary fibrinolysis, factor V is depleted. Assay for this factor may not be readily available.
   **c.** Factor VIII is low in both of these entities. However, factor VIII, like fibrinogen, is a stress factor and may be elevated before or concomitant with the bleeding episode. Thus, a normal level may be misleading. Low levels may occur in liver disease.
   **d.** Cryofibrinogen may be detectable in DIC, but its determination is time-consuming. It is useful only retrospectively.
   **e.** Antithrombin III is depleted in DIC according to some, but not all, methods.
   **f.** Plasmin and plasminogen assays are decreased.
   **g.** Plasma paracoagulation tests (ethanol gelatin and protamine sulfate precipitation) for fibrin monomers—increased in DIC but not fibrinolysis—have proved unreliable.

THROMBOLYTIC THERAPY

**1.** Although PT, APTT, and TT are frequently ordered prior to administration of therapy, there are no guidelines to adjust therapy based on values obtained.

**2.** When postthrombolytic clotting parameters are measured, they are markedly prolonged. There are no established criteria, however, to adjust therapy based upon the results.

3. There may be some value to obtaining coagulation studies if concurrent heparinization is anticipated.

TRANSFUSION THERAPY

Although there is insufficient space here to adequately review this subject, the primary purpose of blood transfusion is for oxygen-carrying capacity. Most patients do not need transfusion for an acute bleed without a hemoglobin of less than 8 gm/dl unless they are in shock or have angina or known cardiac disease. Component therapy—platelets, fresh frozen plasma, factor concentrates, or albumin—should not be administered without good indication and documentation.

## Hypercoagulable State

Patients with a hypercoagulable state usually have a clinical history of one or more thrombotic episodes. Laboratory studies to support the clinical diagnosis of hypercoagulability or to identify patients at risk from this disorder are often unrevealing. However, one or more of the following abnormalities may be found in some patients.

1. Abnormally short APTT.
2. High platelet count.
3. Low AT III level.
4. Low protein C activity.
5. Low protein S activity.
6. Spontaneous platelet aggregation.
7. Abnormal thrombin generation time.
8. Abnormalities in thromboplastin generation and thromboelastography (occasionally).
9. Circulating platelet microaggregates.

PROTEIN C DEFICIENCY

1. Heterozygous manifests venous thromboemboli or warfarin-induced skin necrosis, or both.
2. Homozygous produces purpura fulminans neonatalis.
3. Acquired (liver disease, DIC, adult respiratory distress syndrome, postsurgical) causes venous thromboemboli.

PROTEIN S DEFICIENCY

1. Heterozygous is associated with venous and possibly arterial thromboemboli.
2. Homozygous is associated with venous thromboemboli.
3. Acquired (liver disease, pregnancy, DIC, nephrotic syndrome, SLE) causes venous thromboemboli.

ANTITHROMBIN III DEFICIENCY

1. Autosomal dominant inheritance with AT III levels of 25 to 50 percent of normal.
2. Frequently manifests thrombophlebitis and pulmonary emboli.
3. Pregnancy, oral contraceptives, surgery, trauma, and infection predispose to thrombosis.
4. Because of low AT III level, patients appear to be heparin resistant and require large amounts of heparin to prolong APTT.

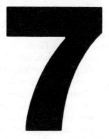

# Renal, Electrolyte, Blood-Gas, and Acid-Base Problems

## RENAL AND URINARY TRACT DISORDERS

S. Robert Contiguglia
Jeffrey L. Mishell
Melvyn H. Klein

In the approach to diseases of the kidney and urinary tract, it is important to differentiate between primary renal disease and renal disease that is secondary to a systemic disorder. A strong effort should also be made to determine the anatomic localization of the lesion (e.g., the glomerulus, tubules, interstitium, vascular system, lower urinary tract). Special attention should be paid to those diseases that are either preventable or treatable.

Kidney and urinary tract disease may be discovered in a number of ways.

1. In many cases, a renal abnormality is suspected because the patient's complaints are directly related to the urinary tract or urine formation. Examples of such symptoms are frequency, dysuria, burning on urination, urgency, colic, polyuria, nocturia, hematuria, oliguria, and anuria.

2. Disease of the urinary tract may also become evident because of the nonrenal manifestations of a systemic illness that involves the kidney secondarily. Examples of such conditions are as follows:
   a. Metabolic diseases (e.g., diabetes mellitus).
   b. Connective tissue diseases (e.g., systemic lupus erythematosus, polyarteritis nodosa, scleroderma).
   c. Infectious diseases (e.g., gram-negative sepsis, tuberculosis, malaria, infective endocarditis).
   d. Cardiovascular diseases (e.g., hypertension, congestive heart failure).
   e. Infiltrative diseases (e.g., multiple myeloma, lymphoma).

3. Occasionally patients have symptoms and signs of renal failure (e.g., uremia, anuria, hypertension, edema) without any prior knowledge of kidney disease.

4. Finally, some patients are discovered to have renal diseases because of the finding of laboratory abnormalities (e.g., proteinuria, microscopic hematuria, abnormal renal function tests, electrolyte and acid-base disturbances) during the course of a routine examination or an investigation for another purpose.

## Frequency, Urgency, and Dysuria

### General Considerations

1. This triad of symptoms is most often associated with infection of the urinary tract. However, care must be taken to evaluate each symptom, because any one may represent conditions other than urinary tract infection.

2. Psychoneurotic water drinkers and patients with polyuria from any cause may complain of frequent voiding with an increased urine flow. In contrast, bladder inflammation may cause frequency without an increase in urine flow.
3. Urgency is most often caused by bladder inflammation, although a full bladder caused by increased urine flow may also cause this symptom. The urgency of urinary tract infection is more compelling; moreover, it is paradoxical because only small amounts of urine are passed at each voiding. External compression of the bladder by masses, as in pregnancy, may also generate the feeling of urgency.
4. Dysuria is suggestive of urethral inflammation, which may be a manifestation of urinary tract or genital infection. Some patients may complain of burning during febrile states.

### History

1. A history of recurrent urinary tract infections suggests underlying anatomic or physiologic abnormality of the urinary tract.
2. Other causes of this triad of symptoms, particularly genital infections, should be excluded.
3. The presence of chills and fever suggests systemic involvement. These symptoms are usually seen with upper urinary tract involvement.
4. The back pain often associated with this triad of symptoms strongly suggests upper urinary tract involvement.

### Physical Examination

1. A complete physical examination is indicated.
2. The presence of costovertebral angle tenderness is compatible with renal inflammation. Suprapubic tenderness suggests cystitis. However, neither of these findings needs to be present to diagnose urinary tract infection.
3. Because abnormalities of the urethral meatus and along the course of the urethra may cause dysuria, specific attention should be given to these areas during examination.
4. An acutely inflamed prostate gland may cause urethral symptoms. Hence this gland should be examined carefully in all males with urinary symptoms.

### Laboratory Findings

1. Pyuria and bacteriuria are consistent with the diagnosis of urinary tract infection. Leukocyte casts are pathognomonic of renal parenchymal infection.
2. Urine culture and sensitivity tests should be done. Positive cultures recovered from catheterized or suprapubic puncture specimens are significant. Bacteriuria with over 100,000 colonies/ml of urine (from clean-voided specimens) is considered abnormal.
3. Urethral discharge, if present, should be examined in a wet preparation and cultured appropriately. A Wright's stain of epidermal scrapings of cutaneous lesions should be performed if genital herpes is suspected. A therapeutic trial of tetracycline therapy may be indicated for suspected *Chlamydia* infections.
4. Further evaluation of these symptoms may require excretory urography, voiding cystourethrography, retrograde urography, cystoscopy, and other, more specialized tests.
5. Sterile pyuria suggests renal tuberculosis.

## Renal and Ureteral Colic

### Definition

Renal colic, which is most often unilateral, is characterized by a severe crescendo-decrescendo type of pain, which usually radiates from the costovertebral angle toward the hypochondrium. The pain of ureteral colic has similar characteristics but typically radiates around the flank toward the inguinal ligament and into the scrotum or labium major.

## Etiology

Renal colic is usually produced by acute inflammation or bleeding within the kidney with stretching of the renal capsule; it results from conditions such as acute pyelonephritis or an expanding cyst. Ureteral colic is most often associated with the passage of a renal calculus.

## Associated Symptoms

The pain is commonly associated with nausea and vomiting. The presence of chills and fever suggests either a primary or secondary urinary tract infection. Gross hematuria may be seen with the passage of a stone or bleeding from a cyst.

## Physical Examination

The physical examination is usually unremarkable except for the presence of flank tenderness.

## Laboratory Findings

1. Urinalysis. Hematuria as the sole urinary abnormality supports the diagnosis of calculus. The presence of pyuria and bacteriuria suggests infection of the urinary tract.
2. X-ray. Abdominal films may show the presence of an opaque stone. If not, an intravenous pyelogram (IVP) should be performed to reveal calculi not visualized in plain films to determine their location more precisely and to rule out obstruction. An IVP will also show masses and cysts. If the affected kidney is not visualized, delayed films should be taken. When intravenous pyelography is not helpful, renal ultrasound can help rule out obstruction.

---

# Nephrolithiasis

---

## Etiology

1. Calcium oxalate and calcium phosphate stones. Hypercalciuria is the most common cause of such stones. Hypercalciuria (> 150 mg/24 hours) may occur in sarcoidosis, hypervitaminosis D, distal renal tubular acidosis, hyperparathyroidism, idiopathic hypercalciuria, prolonged immobilization, hyperadrenocorticism, and excessive milk intake. Primary and secondary oxalosis results in the formation of calcium oxalate stones. They often follow ileal bypass surgery.
2. Triple phosphate stones. These occur most often in patients who have had frequent urinary tract infections with urea-splitting organisms and who have undergone multiple manipulative procedures.
3. Cystine stones. These are found exclusively in patients with congenital cystinuria.
4. Urate stones. These are usually associated with hyperuricemic states (primary gout, secondary gout, and idiopathic hyperuricemia). However, many patients with uric acid calculi do not have hyperuricemia or increased uric acid excretion.

## Diagnostic Approach

HISTORY AND PHYSICAL EXAMINATION

1. The history should include information concerning the following: the age at which symptoms of stones were first noted; family history of nephrolithiasis; history of

fractures or prolonged immobilization; previous urinary tract infections or manipulations; and the intake of milk, alkali, salt, and vitamins A, D, and C.

2. The physical examination should include investigation for the band keratopathy associated with hypercalcemic states.

LABORATORY PROCEDURES

1. At least two determinations of serum calcium should be performed. In addition, serum levels of phosphorus, alkaline phosphatase, total protein and albumin, uric acid, creatinine, and electrolytes should be obtained.

2. A midstream urine specimen should be collected for culture and sensitivity studies because urinary tract infections are commonly associated with nephrolithiasis.

3. The urinary pH should be determined. A persistently alkaline urine in the presence of hyperchloremic acidosis suggests renal tubular acidosis.

4. Quantitative calcium and uric acid determinations should be performed on two separate 24-hour urine specimens while the patient is on a regular diet with a known calcium intake in order to detect hypercalciuria and increased uric acid excretion. If hypercalciuria is present, an attempt should be made to differentiate between enhanced intestinal absorption of calcium (e.g., as occurs in sarcoidosis and hypervitaminosis D) and increased renal excretion of calcium (e.g., as noted in hyperparathyroidism and idiopathic hypercalciuria). With respect to idiopathic hypercalciuria, both increased intestinal absorption and decreased renal resorption of calcium have been identified as causative mechanisms. Hyperuricemia and increased urinary uric acid excretion favor the formation of uric acid stones as well as calcium oxalate and phosphate calculi.

5. The urine should be examined for the presence of cystine crystals. The diagnosis of cystinuria is based on the demonstration of such crystals in cold acidified urine, a positive nitroprusside test, increased urinary excretion of cystine (> 300 mg/24 hours), and the demonstration of the specific aminoaciduria by urinary chromatography.

6. When urate stones are found, an investigation for primary or secondary causes of hyperuricemia is warranted. However, as noted previously, urate stones may occur in the absence of hyperuricemia or increased uric acid excretion.

7. Pure oxalate stones may occur with primary or secondary oxalosis.

8. Architectural and chemical analyses should be performed on all stones that are passed.

9. Plain films of the abdomen and intravenous pyelograms should be obtained routinely.

---

## Polyuria

### Definition

Polyuria is an excessive output of urine. It may occur in association with many normal or pathologic states. Polyuria per se is not hazardous, provided the lost fluid and solutes are replaced. However, polyuria may become deleterious if such losses are excessive and replacement is inadequate. Hypotension and cardiovascular collapse may then ensue.

### Etiology

1. Polyuria may represent an appropriate physiologic response to osmolar, sodium, or fluid loads, or it may be secondary to diuretic therapy.
   a. Osmolar loads may result in the excretion of isotonic urine. The following are examples of solute loads that may produce osmotic diuresis and polyuria:
      (1) Glycosuria, as in diabetes mellitus.
      (2) Administration of mannitol or urea.
      (3) Hyperalimentation therapy with amino acids or glucose.

**b.** Sodium loads that are accompanied by increased water intake may result in a sodium diuresis and the excretion of isotonic urine. This may occur under the following circumstances:

(1) High dietary intake of sodium (rare).

(2) Administration of excessive quantities of salt and water by intravenous or tube feedings.

(3) Rapid resorption of edema fluid.

**c.** Polyuria may sometimes be the result of compulsive water drinking, so-called psychogenic polydipsia. The condition is usually associated with psychic disturbances. Typically, both the plasma and urine osmolalities are low and there is a lack of responsiveness to vasopressin. Occasionally, dilutional hyponatremia and water intoxication may occur. When plasma osmolality is normal, the diagnosis can be made by a normal response to water deprivation.

2. Polyuria may represent an inappropriate response to a pathologic state.

**a.** Nephrogenic diabetes insipidus. In this condition, there is a urinary concentrating defect that is unresponsive to the antidiuretic hormone (ADH), vasopressin. This impairment in renal concentrating ability may occur in the following conditions:

(1) Renal disease. The inability to concentrate urine adequately may result in obligatory polyuria. The most common causes are listed below.

(a) Chronic renal failure, particularly if associated with interstitial disease.

(b) Recovery from acute renal failure.

(c) Acute pyelonephritis.

(2) Hypercalcemia.

(3) Hypokalemia.

(4) Congenital tubular disorders, usually associated with renal tubular acidosis.

(5) Drug-induced disease (e.g., methoxyflurane anesthesia, lithium carbonate, demeclocycline, potent diuretics).

The diagnosis of nephrogenic diabetes insipidus is based on the following criteria: the occurrence of dilute urine in the presence of normal or increased serum osmolality; an inability to concentrate urine adequately with fluid restriction; and a lack of responsiveness to vasopressin.

**b.** Central diabetes insipidus. This disorder represents a complete or partial defect in the pituitary secretion of ADH, which results in impaired renal concentrating ability and attendant polyuria. The characteristic features are mild serum hyperosmolality, a dilute urine, and responsiveness to vasopressin.

## Diagnostic Approach

1. Rule out administered fluid or solute loads, or both, and psychogenic polydipsia as possible causes of polyuria by the history and by a review of the fluid and electrolyte balance.

2. Determine the urine and serum osmolality.

**a.** If the urine osmolality is elevated above that of the serum, rule out glycosuria.

**b.** If the urine is isosmotic with respect to serum, check for evidence of renal disease, and exclude glycosuria, administered diuretics, and solute loads as possible causes.

3. If the urine is hypotonic compared to serum osmolality, test for renal concentrating ability by restricting the fluid intake.

**a.** If the urine becomes concentrated with fluid restriction, it can be concluded that fluid intake was excessive and that it was either psychogenic or iatrogenic in origin.

**b.** If the ability to concentrate urine is impaired, it can be assumed that the nephron is unable to conserve water adequately, indicating either nephrogenic or true diabetes insipidus. The patient's response to vasopressin should then be determined.

**(1)** If the patient is responsive to vasopressin, the diagnosis is true diabetes insipidus.
**(2)** If the patient is unresponsive to vasopressin, it can be concluded that the patient has some type of renal disease (e.g., postobstructive uropathy, hypokalemic nephropathy, hypercalcemic nephropathy) causing nephrogenic diabetes insipidus.

## Oliguria and Anuria

### Definition

Oliguria is that amount of urine output below which the normal load of metabolic waste products (usually 400–500 ml/24 hours) cannot be excreted. Anuria is arbitrarily defined as a urinary output below 100 ml/24 hours.

### Etiology

1. Prerenal or functional impairment of renal perfusion. The response of the kidneys to renal hypoperfusion is appropriate.
    a. Absolute volume depletion (e.g., shock and dehydration).
    b. Diminished "effective" circulating blood volume without total volume depletion.
        **(1)** Congestive heart failure.
        **(2)** Cirrhosis of the liver.
        **(3)** Nephrotic syndrome.
        **(4)** "Third space" losses (e.g., peritonitis, bowel obstruction).
2. Obstructive uropathy.
    a. Prostatic or urethral obstruction.
    b. Bilateral ureteral obstruction.
3. Vascular disease.
    a. Acute arterial obstruction.
    b. Renal vein obstruction.
4. Renal parenchymal disease.
    a. Diffuse acute glomerular disease (e.g., acute glomerulonephritis, acute vasculitis, disseminated intravascular coagulation).
    b. Acute tubular necrosis (e.g., prolonged prerenal failure, abruptio placentae, nephrotoxins, sepsis, shock, myoglobinuria).
    c. Acute interstitial nephritis.
        **(1)** Hypersensitivity type (e.g., sensitivity to methicillin, ampicillin, nonsteroidal anti-inflammatory drugs, cephalosporins).
        **(2)** Acute urate nephropathy.
        **(3)** Hypercalcemic nephropathy.
    d. Postcontrast media (e.g., multiple myeloma, diabetes mellitus).
    e. Any of the above superimposed on chronic renal failure.
    f. Nonsteroidal anti-inflammatory drugs (NSAIDs).

### Diagnostic Approach

The history, physical examination, and course of the disease are as important as laboratory studies in establishing the diagnosis and in differentiating between renal and extrarenal causes of oliguria and anuria.

HISTORY

1. A history of previous surgery, gastrointestinal bleeding, dehydration, and fluid losses may provide clues to the etiology of acute renal failure.
2. Inquiry should be made concerning the use of potentially nephrotoxic drugs or

combinations of drugs that may act synergistically to cause acute renal failure. Diuretics, the aminoglycosides, and NSAIDs are common offenders.

3. The possible use of drugs capable of causing hypersensitivity interstitial nephritis (e.g., penicillins, NSAIDs, cephalosporins) should be looked into.

4. Because anuria occurs more frequently in obstructive uropathy and the nephritides than in acute tubular necrosis, evidence for the presence of these conditions should be sought.

5. It is necessary to establish evidence of previous renal insufficiency to confirm the diagnosis of acute renal failure superimposed on chronic renal disease.

PHYSICAL EXAMINATION

The most important aspect of the physical examination is the evaluation of the condition of the circulation and the state of hydration. Findings such as poor tissue turgor, orthostatic hypotension, tachycardia, and weight loss support the diagnosis of hypovolemia and prerenal azotemia. On the other hand, edema, distended neck veins, and pulmonary congestion suggest an adequate or increased circulatory volume, as may occur in congestive heart failure or cirrhosis of the liver. Decreased "effective" renal blood flow may nevertheless occur in these conditions.

LABORATORY FINDINGS

1. Urinalysis.
   a. Heavy proteinuria, hematuria, and red blood cell casts suggest primary glomerular disease.
   b. Mild proteinuria, the presence of eosinophils on a Wright's stain, and epithelial cell casts support the diagnosis of hypersensitivity interstitial nephritis.
   c. Trace to mild proteinuria with renal epithelial cells, numerous granular casts, and cellular debris supports the diagnosis of acute tubular necrosis, but may occur in severe prerenal failure.
   d. Myoglobinuria, hemoglobinuria, or urate crystals may be seen in some specific types of acute renal failure.

2. Serum chemistries.
   a. A rising serum creatinine above 2.5 mg/100 ml strongly suggests established renal failure as opposed to prerenal disease.
   b. The BUN-creatinine ratio is usually 10 to 15 : 1 in renal parenchymal disease but is greater than 20 : 1 in prerenal disease.
   c. Hyperchloremic acidosis suggests tubular dysfunction and interstitial disease.

3. Determination of urinary sodium, osmolality, urea, and creatinine.
   a. These procedures are most helpful in differentiating between prerenal (physiologic) oliguria and established acute renal failure. As a rule, with functional oliguria a normal kidney responds to hypoperfusion by retaining salt and water to maintain circulating blood volume. In prerenal failure, urinary sodium is usually less than 10 mEq/liter, urine is concentrated (osmolality > 500 mOsm/kg), and a urine/plasma urea and creatinine ratio greater than 14 : 1 is present. The fractional excretion of sodium is less than 5 percent.
   b. In established acute renal failure, tubular destruction and dysfunction are present. Urinary sodium exceeds 20 mEq/liter, the urine is isosmotic (300 mOsm/kg) and the U/P urea and creatinine ratios are less than 14 : 1. A "prerenal" picture may occur with early acute glomerulonephritis. The fractional excretion of sodium is greater than 10 percent.
   c. Because most diuretics impair tubular function, pretreatment with these drugs causes the appearance of a urine consistent with renal failure although, in actuality, prerenal failure may be present. This may also occur in patients with chronic renal insufficiency.

4. Administration of fluids and diuretics.
   a. A fluid challenge with the administration of 500 to 1000 ml of normal saline

over a 30-minute period to a patient who does not have congestive heart failure or is not fluid overloaded may be helpful in differentiating between prerenal and established renal failure. The occurrence of diuresis favors the latter diagnosis.

    **b.** Should volume expansion fail to induce a diuresis, a diuretic should be administered. Unresponsiveness to a large dose of furosemide (250–500 mg) or mannitol (25 g) supports the diagnosis of established renal failure. On the other hand, a good diuretic response favors the diagnosis of prerenal azotemia. However, adequate diuresis may sometimes occur when established oliguric chronic renal failure reverts to a nonoliguric phase.

**5.** Radiographic diagnosis. Technetium scanning is most helpful in distinguishing vascular occlusion from obstructive uropathy and renal parenchymal disease. Bladder catheterization with a large residual urine suggests bladder outlet obstruction. CT scan, radioisotope scan, or ultrasound can be used to demonstrate the presence of disease in both kidneys and to look for signs of obstruction. Retrograde pyelography should be performed if a question of obstruction still remains after these procedures.

**6.** Serial observations. A definitive diagnosis cannot always be made at the time of initial evaluation of the oliguric patient. Serial measurements of various parameters of renal function, particularly the serum creatinine levels, are extremely valuable in this regard. Rising serum creatinine levels usually establish the diagnosis of acute renal failure.

## Uremia

### Definition

Uremia is a symptom complex found in renal failure. The gastrointestinal, cardiovascular, and central nervous systems are particularly involved. Uremic manifestations are believed to be related to the accumulation of as yet unidentified dialyzable substances in the blood. A uremic individual may also have symptoms and signs related to altered fluid and electrolyte balance. Patients sometimes present with uremic symptoms without any knowledge of antecedent renal disease.

### Clinical Features

A patient with uremia may have some or all of the following manifestations:

**1.** Gastrointestinal symptoms include anorexia, nausea, vomiting, diarrhea, and hiccups. The nausea and vomiting resemble the morning sickness of pregnancy. The patient may awake feeling reasonably well but have nausea and vomiting at the very sight, smell, or taste of food.

**2.** The spectrum of nervous system manifestations is broad. The sensorium may range from mental alertness to coma. Personality changes, irritability, delusions, and hallucinations may occur. Muscle twitching and asterixis are not uncommon. Peripheral neuropathy is sometimes observed.

**3.** Cardiovascular manifestations include fibrinous pericarditis and sometimes cardiac tamponade. Pulmonary edema and circulatory volume overload may occur.

**4.** Other uremic signs include the Kussmaul breathing of metabolic acidosis, increased cutaneous pigmentation, pruritus, anemia, and a uremic breath odor.

**5.** The insidious onset of weakness and anemia may be the only clue to severe renal insufficiency.

**6.** Severe azotemia and elevated serum creatinine levels are a reflection of decreased renal function.

## General Principles

1. In patients with uremia, it is essential, as a first step, to attempt to correct the biochemical abnormalities either by medical means or by dialysis. When uremia is severe, dialysis is the therapy of choice and should be instituted without delay. Diagnostic studies can then be initiated.
2. It is important to differentiate between acute and chronic renal failure or a combination of the two. A special effort should be made to distinguish between reversible and irreversible renal disease. The diagnostic approach to uremia is basically the same as that outlined in the section Oliguria and Anuria.

## Diagnostic Approach

HISTORY

1. A history of hypertension, proteinuria, anemia, hematuria, analgesic abuse, debilitation, and chronic weight loss supports the diagnosis of long-standing renal disease.
2. Recent exposure to nephrotoxins, a major bleeding episode, or hypotensive states are helpful in establishing the diagnosis of acute renal failure.
3. Symptoms of obstructive uropathy (e.g., urinary tract infections, symptoms of prostatism), particularly in the elderly, are helpful in the diagnosis of obstructive uropathy.

PHYSICAL EXAMINATION

1. The state of hydration and the condition of the circulation should be evaluated.
2. Hypertension may occur in either acute or chronic disease.
3. Hypotension commonly accompanies dehydration and volume depletion.
4. A distended urinary bladder suggests outlet obstruction.
5. The physical findings specifically related to uremia are described under Clinical Features.

LABORATORY STUDIES

1. Azotemia, acidosis, anemia, hyperphosphatemia, hyperuricemia, and other biochemical abnormalities may occur in both acute and chronic renal failure.
2. Useful diagnostic modalities are ultrasound and CT scan. The presence of small kidneys implies chronic renal failure. Normal-sized or large kidneys suggest acute disease. However, some patients with chronic disease have normal-sized kidneys.
3. Urinalysis and the other diagnostic tests outlined in the section Oliguria and Anuria are helpful in determining whether the renal failure is due to glomerular, vascular, obstructive, or interstitial disease.
4. A percutaneous renal biopsy is sometimes necessary to establish a definitive diagnosis.

## Nonoliguric Renal Failure

A small number of patients may develop acute renal failure without oliguria following a toxic, ischemic, or other major insult to the kidneys. In some patients with chronic renal insufficiency or partial obstructive uropathy, nonoliguric renal failure may develop insidiously.

Patients with acute nonoliguric renal failure usually run a more benign course than those with oliguria or anuria. On occasion, however, they may develop uremia and require dialysis.

The laboratory abnormalities are similar to those found in oliguric acute renal failure except for the maintenance of a "good urinary output," usually about 1000 ml in 24 hours.

The diagnostic approach is the same for other types of acute renal failure.

---

### Laboratory Abnormalities in Renal Disease: Urinalysis

---

It is not unusual for a patient with renal disease to have no history or physical findings suggestive of renal disease. Many patients are discovered to have kidney disease because of abnormal findings on routine urinalysis. Others are picked up when azotemia or electrolyte abnormalities are found on routine biochemical screening. Of course, many patients have symptoms directly referable to the urinary tract or other symptoms (e.g., edema) that bring up the possibility of a renal abnormality. The two most common urinary abnormalities that suggest renal disease are hematuria and proteinuria. These conditions are discussed separately from other aspects of the urinalysis. The urine should be a clean catch, midstream specimen.

1. Appearance. The appearance of the urine may give a clue to the presence of a renal or systemic abnormality. Cloudiness or turbidity on standing is usually secondary to the precipitation of urates and phosphates and, less commonly, to pyuria. Normal urine is yellow to amber in color. Bile may produce cola-colored urine. Blood, hemoglobin, and myoglobin may impart a red or reddish-brown color to the urine. Urine containing porphyrins changes to a port wine color on standing. The urine may also be discolored by food (e.g., beets) or drugs (e.g., methylene blue, phenolphthalein). A white foam may occur when urine is shaken. Foaming is increased with proteinuria. Yellow foam suggests the presence of bile salts and bile pigments.

2. Concentration. Urine concentration is best determined by recording the osmolality. Urine concentration can be approximated by measuring the specific gravity with a refractometer (preferred method) or a urinometer. A urinometer should be calibrated before use to be sure it reads 1.000 with distilled water. A single determination of osmolality or specific gravity is of limited usefulness unless the results are related to the clinical setting (e.g., the state of hydration). Urine osmolality is of greatest value when compared to serum osmolality in a specific clinical situation (e.g., oliguria).

3. pH. Urine is almost always acid except during the alkaline tide or when there is infection with a urea-splitting organism. The urine is alkaline in renal tubular acidosis. The overall clinical situation must be known for such a measurement to be useful. For example, an alkaline urine in the presence of systemic acidosis suggests a renal acidification defect, whereas an alkaline urine with systemic alkalosis is appropriate.

4. Glucose. Methods that employ glucose oxidase (e.g., dipstick) detect only glucose, whereas other methods detect not only glucose but other reducing substances as well (e.g., salicylates, dextran, urates, antibiotics, pentose sugars), and thus produce false-positive results. When glycosuria is found, it should be determined whether it is secondary to hyperglycemia or renal glycosuria. This is best accomplished with an oral glucose tolerance test, which yields a normal result in renal glycosuria.

5. Other substances. Ketonemia results in a positive finding for acetone in the urine. This occurs most commonly in diabetic ketoacidosis. Ketonuria alone may be found on starvation or fasting and in methanol poisoning.

6. Microscopic examination. Examination of the urinary sediment is essential for the evaluation of renal disease.
   a. Red blood cells. More than 2 RBCs per high-power field (HPF) are significant. Additional workup should proceed as indicated under Hematuria.
   b. White blood cells. More than 4 to 5 WBC/HPF in a well-collected specimen is significant. The patient should be evaluated for urinary tract infection or re-

nal parenchymal inflammation. The presence of eosinophils on a Wright's stain is helpful in diagnosing hypersensitivity interstitial nephritis. When WBCs are found together with vaginal epithelial cells, it can be assumed that the collection technique was poor.

**c.** Tubular epithelial cells are nonspecific findings seen in various types of inflammatory parenchymal disease.

**d.** RBC casts. Such casts are virtually pathognomonic of glomerular inflammation, but they have been reported to occur in acute tubular necrosis.

**e.** WBC casts. These casts are indicative of renal infection (e.g., pyelonephritis).

**f.** Hyaline and granular casts. Such casts may be normal when only 1 to 2/HPF are seen in a concentrated urine. Showers of such casts (20–30/HPF) may be seen in acute renal failure.

**g.** Waxy casts. Waxy casts are nonspecific and may be found in both normal and pathologic urines.

**h.** Mixed cellular casts. Casts of this type generally occur in renal inflammatory disease.

**i.** Crystals. Crystalluria may occur in normal or pathologic urines. Most are not significant. Cystine crystals are abnormal, as are massive precipitations of sulfonamide or uric acid crystals in oliguric patients.

**j.** Tissue fragments. Pieces of the renal papillae are diagnostic of papillary necrosis.

**k.** Bacteria. The presence of bacteria may indicate infection.

---

## Proteinuria

---

### General Principles

1. Proteinuria is often the first and occasionally the only abnormality in patients with renal disease. Proteinuria represents glomerular damage and is often associated with gross or microscopic hematuria.
2. The major protein in the urine in patients with renal disease is albumin. Globulins predominate in certain tubular disorders and plasma cell dyscrasias (e.g., multiple myeloma).
3. Qualitative tests for proteinuria should include either the heat and acetic acid method or sulfosalicylic acid.
4. The measurement of the 24-hour protein excretion is of the utmost importance in the evaluation of any patient with proteinuria.
5. Proteinuria is considered significant when urinary excretion exceeds 150 mg in 24 hours.

### Etiology and Classification

1. Heavy proteinuria. Heavy proteinuria is defined as the excretion of more than 3.5 g of protein in 24 hours. It is most often associated with the nephrotic syndrome. The causes of heavy proteinuria and the nephrotic syndrome are all types of glomerulonephritis; systemic illnesses such as connective tissue disease, diabetes mellitus, and multiple myeloma; amyloidosis; allergic disorders such as bee sting and drug reactions; circulatory conditions such as pericarditis, chronic congestive heart failure, and renal vein thrombosis; infections such as malaria, cytomegalic inclusion disease, typhus, herpes zoster, hepatitis B, bacterial infections; solid tumors; and lymphomas.
2. Moderate proteinuria. Moderate proteinuria is defined as a 24-hour excretion of 1.0 to 3.5 g of protein in 24 hours. The causes of moderate proteinuria are essentially the same as those causing heavy proteinuria.
3. Minimal proteinuria. Minimal proteinuria is defined as the excretion of less than 1.0 g of protein in 24 hours. The causes include mild glomerular disease (pyelonephritis, nephrosclerosis, hypercalcemia, obstructive uropathy, tumor, nephrocalcinosis, acute tubular necrosis, and congestive heart failure), functional

proteinuria, postural proteinuria, and asymptomatic persistent proteinuria. Functional proteinuria is transient proteinuria associated with febrile illness or exercise. Postural proteinuria is proteinuria associated with the upright position. Asymptomatic persistent proteinuria is almost always indicative of renal disease.

## Diagnostic Approach

HISTORY

Because proteinuria may be the result of primary or secondary renal disease, evidence of systemic illness that may involve the kidney should be sought and excluded (e.g., connective tissue disease, diabetes mellitus). A careful drug history should be taken to exclude potentially nephrotoxic agents (e.g., gold salts, nonsteroidal anti-inflammatory drugs).

PHYSICAL EXAMINATION

1. Arterial hypertension may produce minimal to moderate proteinuria. When associated with moderate to heavy proteinuria, primary glomerular disease should be considered. When hypertension and proteinuria begin simultaneously, primary renal disease should be suspected.
2. The combination of proteinuria, hypoproteinemia, and edema is suggestive of the nephrotic syndrome.
3. Arthritis, an erythematous rash, and purpura suggest connective tissue disease.
4. Retinopathy may be seen in systemic hypertension, diabetes, or vasculitis. Diabetic retinopathy is almost always associated with diabetic nephropathy.
5. Peripheral neuropathy may be observed in patients with diabetes or chronic renal failure.

LABORATORY STUDIES

1. Urinalysis. The presence of fatty casts, oval fat bodies, and doubly refractile fat globules suggests the lipiduria of the nephrotic syndrome. Red cell casts are virtually pathognomonic for glomerulonephritis. Glycosuria suggests diabetes mellitus, although renal glycosuria may be present.
2. The 24-hour urinary protein excretion. All patients with proteinuria should have a 24-hour urine collection for total protein. Patients exhibiting minimal to moderate proteinuria should be checked routinely for postural or orthostatic proteinuria. The combined study can be performed as follows: The patient voids at 7 A.M. and discards the urine. All urine thereafter is collected in a single bottle. At 8 P.M. the patient assumes the recumbent position in bed. At 10 P.M. he voids into the same bottle without getting out of bed. At 7 A.M. the next morning, without rising, he voids into another bottle. The urine in the two bottles is the 24-hour urine collection, the second bottle representing the urine voided during recumbency. In patients with postural proteinuria, the total urinary protein excretion usually exceeds 150 mg (but is less than 1 g), but the protein excreted during recumbency should not be greater than 75 mg.
3. Serum and urinary protein electrophoresis should be performed in every patient suspected of having a plasma cell dyscrasia. The presence of light chains in the urine may be the only manifestation of multiple myeloma.
4. Hypercholesterolemia and hypoproteinemia with a decreased albumin fraction are seen in most cases of the nephrotic syndrome.
5. Hyperproteinemia with an increased gamma globulin fraction may occur in multiple myeloma.
6. An abnormal glucose tolerance test and glycosuria may be the only other manifestations of diabetes mellitus in a patient with diabetic nephropathy. Abnormal glucose tolerance, however, may occur in renal failure from any cause.
7. Serologic tests for streptococcal antibodies, $HB_sAg$, connective tissue disease, syphilis, and serum complement (C3) should be performed.

8. Radiologic examinations. Chest films may show the type of circulatory congestion associated with uremia or congestive heart failure. Bone films may reveal the punched-out lesions of multiple myeloma or the changes observed with chronic renal failure. Small kidneys in abdominal films denote chronic renal disease. Intravenous pyelography may reveal obstructive uropathy, polycystic disease, and other abnormalities. Asymmetric size and function on pyelography are seen in renal vein thrombosis. Renal arteriography may be useful in the diagnosis of renovascular hypertension and polyarteritis nodosa.

9. Renal biopsy is indicated when all other studies fail to reveal the etiology of renal disease, when the findings will influence the management of the disease (e.g., systemic lupus erythematosus), and as an aid in determining the prognosis. If performed, the biopsy should be examined by light and electron microscopy as well as by immunofluorescent techniques.

## Hematuria
## (Without Proteinuria)

Hematuria may be gross or microscopic (in excess of 2 RBC/HPF), painful or painless. It may occur with or without proteinuria or the presence of formed elements in the urine. Hematuria may originate anywhere in the urinary tract (i.e., the kidney, ureter, bladder, prostate gland, or urethra). At times, it may reflect a generalized disorder of the clotting mechanism.

Gross hematuria must be differentiated from myoglobinuria, hemoglobinuria, and porphyria. The finding of red cells in the urinary sediment establishes the diagnosis of hematuria. The other conditions are identified by specific laboratory tests. It should be noted that either extremely concentrated or extremely dilute urine may cause lysis of red cells with resultant hemoglobinuria.

Diffuse renal parenchymal disease usually presents with painless smoky or cloudy urine associated with proteinuria and the presence of formed elements in the urine. However, gross hematuria is not a rare occurrence in diffuse renal disease. The approach to this group of patients is discussed in the preceding section, Proteinuria.

In a patient with gross hematuria, the rate and amount of blood loss can be estimated by performing serial urinary hematocrit readings. A hematocrit value of less than 1 percent indicates that the blood loss is slight. Unless blood loss is massive, hematuria does not cause anemia. If anemia is present, other causes, such as chronic renal failure, tuberculosis, neoplasm, and blood dyscrasias, should be considered.

### Etiology

1. Painless hematuria may signify primary renal disease such as tumor, polycystic kidney disease, posttraumatic damage, postexercise hematuria, infection including tuberculosis, or other disease of the urinary tract (e.g., bladder tumor).

2. Painful hematuria is usually caused by nephrolithiasis, renal infarction, or urinary tract infection.

### History

1. A careful menstrual history should be obtained from any woman with a history of blood in the urine to be sure that bleeding is from the urinary tract and not vaginal in origin.

2. Hematuria associated with dysuria, frequency, urgency, and suprapubic pain usually denotes cystitis, but tuberculosis must also be considered.

3. Hematuria with ureteral or renal colic suggests nephrolithiasis or renal infarction.

4. Bleeding at the beginning of urination suggests an origin in the posterior urethra, whereas the source of terminal hematuria is usually the prostate gland or the trigonal area of the bladder.
5. Inquiry concerning the presence of a blood dyscrasia or the use of anticoagulants is warranted in any patient with hematuria. Patients taking anticoagulants who develop hematuria should be investigated because they often turn out to have significant lesions of the urinary tract.
6. A history of increased sexual activity, perineal pain, dysuria, and terminal hematuria suggests prostatitis.
7. A family history of polycystic kidney disease or sickle cell anemia suggests these conditions as possible causes of hematuria.
8. An intensive search for neoplasm is always indicated if all of the foregoing conditions are excluded.

### Physical Examination

1. The presence of petechiae, ecchymoses, lymphadenopathy, or splenomegaly may be indicative of a blood dyscrasia or clotting disorder.
2. A tender, boggy prostate gland suggests prostatitis.
3. Costovertebral angle tenderness and fever suggest renal inflammation.
4. Suprapubic tenderness is commonly associated with bladder inflammation.
5. Bilaterally enlarged kidneys are often found in polycystic disease.
6. A unilateral renal mass suggests neoplasm or cyst.
7. The presence of atrial fibrillation or valvular heart disease suggests renal embolism and infarction as possible causes of hematuria.

### Laboratory Studies

1. Urinalysis may help to differentiate diffuse renal parenchymal disease from disease of the lower urinary tract. Dysuria and bacteriuria suggest infection of the urinary tract. Hematuria and pyuria without bacteriuria suggest the possibility of renal tuberculosis.
2. Blood count. The presence of anemia suggests renal failure or a systemic illness. Polycythemia is sometimes seen with renal cell carcinoma, polycystic disease, isolated renal cysts, uterine leiomyomata, and other conditions.
3. Intravenous pyelogram. Patients with hematuria should have intravenous pyelography before cystoscopy or other urinary tract manipulations are performed. Pyelography is important in the diagnosis of cystic disease, nephrolithiasis, and tumors. It is especially indicated in children in whom renal neoplasms are frequent causes of hematuria.
4. Cystoscopy. Performed after urinalysis and intravenous pyelography, cystoscopy is the best procedure for evaluating the lower urinary tract.
5. Arteriography is helpful in the diagnosis of cysts, tumors, thrombosis, and infarction.
6. Ultrasound is a good method for diagnosing renal cysts and differentiating between cystic and solid tumors. A CT scan may also be helpful.

## Tests of Renal Function

The best clinical guide for evaluating renal function is the creatinine clearance. This test estimates the glomerular filtration rate (GFR). The urea clearance is less reliable. Clearance procedures are particularly useful in detecting early renal function impairment and in following the course of renal disease. However, clearance tests are of little help in determining the cause of kidney disease. The blood urea nitrogen (BUN) and serum creatinine have limited usefulness as indicators of the GFR; the serum creatinine has some advantages over the BUN. In some instances, the two determinations together have some advantage over either test alone (see Serum Creatinine, paragraph **2,** below). Tests for renal concentrating ability are useful in evaluating patients with oliguria. Impaired concentrating ability is an early sign of abnormal renal function in many chronic renal disorders.

## Concentration Tests

1. The normal kidney can produce urine with an osmolality that is 4 to 5 times that of plasma.
2. The most reliable test of the concentrating ability of the kidney is the determination of the osmolality of urine by freezing point depression.
3. To perform a concentration test, examine at hourly intervals freshly voided urine obtained after an overnight fast until the highest urine concentration is obtained. The fast is continued until the test is completed. A specific gravity greater than 1.020 or an osmolality greater than 800 mOsm per kilogram of water is considered normal. In patients with known or suspected azotemia, no attempt should be made to concentrate the urine by dehydrating the patient because it may be hazardous to do so.
4. Factors that affect renal medulla hypertonicity (e.g., high fluid intake prior to the test, diuretics, low-protein diet, sodium restriction) may interfere with the concentration test.
5. Concentration defects may be early findings in essential hypertension, diabetic nephropathy, hypokalemia, hypercalcemia, nephrogenic diabetes insipidus, sickle cell disease, interstitial nephritis, treatment with lithium, and polycystic kidney disease. Renal concentrating ability is also reduced with advancing age.

## Blood Urea Nitrogen

The normal range for blood urea nitrogen (BUN) is 10 to 20 mg/100 ml. The BUN is not a good test for detecting early renal function impairment because the BUN may be normal with as much as a 50 percent reduction in the GFR. Azotemia may be produced not only by renal disease but also by extrarenal disorders, such as dehydration, hypotension, hypovolemia, gastrointestinal hemorrhage, and increased protein intake. When due consideration is given to extrarenal factors, the BUN can be used to follow the course of renal disease. It is not a satisfactory method for evaluating small changes in renal function early in the course of renal failure.

## Serum Creatinine

1. The serum creatinine is a more useful guide to the GFR than is the BUN, but it may not always detect significant changes. The normal serum creatinine level is 0.7 to 1.5 mg/100 ml. Patients with a small muscle mass may have "normal" creatinine levels in spite of significant impairment of renal function.
2. The BUN-serum creatinine ratio is of additional clinical value. Normally, this ratio is 10 to 12 : 1. A high ratio suggests prerenal azotemia, and a low one, decreased protein intake, liver disease, or muscle necrosis. A proportionate rise in both the BUN and the serum creatinine concentrations, with maintenance of the 10 : 1 ratio, suggests renal parenchymal disease.

## Endogenous Creatinine Clearance

1. Clearance is defined as the volume of blood cleared of a substance per unit of time. It is reported in milliliters per minute. The endogenous creatinine clearance is preferred over the urea clearance for estimating the GFR.
2. The creatinine clearance is measured by the formula $C = \dfrac{U \times V}{P}$, in which C is

clearance in milliliters per minute, U is the urine creatinine concentration in milligrams per 100 milliliters, V is urine flow in milliliters per minute, and P is the serum creatinine concentration in milligrams per 100 milliliters.

3. Creatinine clearances are commonly employed to estimate renal function in patients with renal disease. As a rule, the creatinine clearance tends to overestimate the true GFR, especially when the GFR is low. However, serial determinations of creatinine clearance regularly parallel the rise and fall of the actual GFR.

4. A patient in a steady state excretes a constant amount of creatinine in 24 hours. Most men excrete at least 1000 mg of this substance in 24 hours, and women, more than 700 mg in the same period. Omissions in urine collection or sudden changes in renal function are possible causes of reduced excretion of creatinine. Sometimes, a patient with a small muscle mass has a lower than normal total urine creatinine excretion. Whenever the 24-hour urine creatinine excretion is below normal, the test should be repeated. It should also be rechecked if urine creatinine excretion is not comparable to that determined in previous studies.

5. Normal values of the creatinine clearance range from 100 to 150 ml/min in men and 85 to 125 ml/min in women. The GFR declines slowly above the age of 40. By the age of 70, the creatinine clearance may be 50 percent of normal even in the absence of renal disease.

### Urine Electrolytes

There are no "normal" values for the major urinary electrolytes—sodium, potassium, and chloride. The urinary concentration of these electrolytes varies depending on intake (dietary, parenteral, or both), the presence or absence of renal disease, and the responsiveness of the body to such conditions as hypovolemia, hyperosmolality, and hypoosmolality. Isolated urinary electrolyte determinations are of little significance unless a specific problem is being evaluated (e.g., prerenal versus acute renal failure, the syndrome of inappropriate ADH, other hyponatremic states) or when an attempt is being made to alter or maintain the electrolyte tolerance of the patient.

## ELECTROLYTE DISORDERS
S. Robert Contiguglia
Jeffrey L. Mishell
Melvyn H. Klein

### Hypernatremia

#### Definition

Hypernatremia is defined as an abnormally high serum sodium concentration (> 145 mEq/liter). In hypernatremia, the total body sodium content is high with respect to total body water. Hypernatremia is usually due to excessive water loss and rarely to increased total body sodium.

#### Etiology

1. Hypernatremia due to increased body sodium (usually iatrogenic).
   a. Excess solute administration in proportion to water intake.
      (1) Infants inadvertently given preparations with a high sodium content.
      (2) Hyperalimentation by intravenous or nasogastric tube feeding.
   b. Volume depletion (e.g., from diuretics, gastrointestinal losses) and replacement by isotonic or hypertonic solutions.
   c. "Essential" hypernatremia.
2. Hypernatremia due to excessive water loss. This condition is usually averted in the conscious patient because thirst causes the patient to drink until the water

deficit is corrected. Fluids lost from the body are almost always hypotonic with respect to sodium. Thus, hypernatremia may ensue if the fluid losses are not adequately replaced. In the evaluation of hypernatremia due to excessive water loss, both the urine and serum osmolality should be determined.

  **a.** Urine maximally concentrated (hyperosmotic) in response to the hyperosmolar state.
   **(1)** Gastrointestinal losses.
   **(2)** Perspiration.
   **(3)** Hyperpnea.
   **Note:** Elderly persons and patients with renal insufficiency may not be able to concentrate the urine maximally even though the hypernatremia is due to one or more of the preceding causes.

  **b.** Urine not maximally concentrated (isosmotic or hyposmotic) in response to the hyperosmolar state.
   **(1)** Diuretic therapy.
   **(2)** Hypercalcemic nephropathy.
   **(3)** Hypokalemic nephropathy.
   **(4)** Osmotic diuresis.
    **(a)** Diabetes mellitus.
    **(b)** Osmotic diuretics.
   **(5)** Polyuric phase of acute tubular necrosis.
   **(6)** Postobstructive uropathy.
   **(7)** Diabetes insipidus (large urine volume, dilute urine).
    **(a)** True diabetes insipidus (secondary to hypothalamic or pituitary disease)—responsive to vasopressin.
    **(b)** Nephrogenic diabetes insipidus—not responsive to vasopressin.

### Diagnostic Approach

1. Rule out iatrogenic causes of hypernatremia. If iatrogenic causes are excluded, the hypernatremia can only be due to excessive extrarenal or renal fluid losses.
2. Measure the serum and urine osmolality.
  **a.** If the urine is hypertonic (osmolality increased), the fluid was lost by an extrarenal route—the gastrointestinal tract or perspiration.
  **b.** If the urine is isotonic (isosmotic) or hypotonic (hyposmotic), the fluid losses were probably sustained through the kidney. The renal disorders that may be responsible for this type of abnormality are listed in paragraph **2b** above.

---

## Hyponatremia

### Definition

Hyponatremia is defined as an abnormally low serum sodium concentration (< 135 mEq/liter). Because the ionic components of the serum are largely responsible for its osmolality, hyponatremia results in a lowered serum osmolality. The symptoms of hyponatremia are essentially those of reduced serum osmolality. Hyponatremia may occur in a variety of clinical disorders. Because treatment of these conditions may differ markedly, it is always important to determine the cause of hyponatremia. All hyponatremic states, with the exception of hyperlipidemia and hyperglycemia, are associated with low osmolality of the serum and extracellular fluids. In other words, total body sodium is inappropriately low with respect to total body water.

### Etiology and Classification

1. Pseudohyponatremia.
  **a.** Hyperlipidemia. Hyperlipemic states may be associated with spurious hypo-

natremia. The diagnosis is established by finding a high lipid content in the serum and normal serum osmolality.

**b.** Hyperglycemia. Hyperglycemia may induce factitious hyponatremia because every 100 mg/100 ml rise in the serum glucose concentration produces a decline of approximately 3 mEq/liter in the serum sodium level. The diagnosis is based on finding hyponatremia and hyperglycemia together with a normal or elevated serum osmolality.

**2.** Dilutional hyponatremia. This is a state in which an excess of total body sodium and water results in edema or ascites, or both. Serum osmolality is low. Dilutional hyponatremia occurs in congestive heart failure, hepatic cirrhosis, and nephrosis. Increased water intake continued with marked sodium restriction or diuretic therapy, or both, may aggravate any of these conditions.

**3.** Hyponatremia due to sodium depletion. Conditions associated with both sodium and water depletion are characterized by the absence of edema or ascites. Symptoms and signs of extracellular fluid volume depletion, tachycardia, decreased central venous pressure, a high hematocrit reading, and elevated serum total proteins may be noted. The history and urine sodium concentrations are important diagnostically.

   **a.** Decreased urine sodium concentration ($<$ 10 mEq/liter), usually associated with a decreased chloride concentration.

      **(1)** Gastrointestinal losses.

         **(a)** Vomiting or nasogastric suction, or both, commonly associated with hypokalemic alkalosis.

         **(b)** Diarrhea, commonly associated with hypokalemic acidosis.

      **(2)** Excessive perspiration with replacement of water but not sodium losses.

      **(3)** Volume depletion without replacement of lost fluids and electrolytes after diuretic therapy.

   **b.** Increased urine sodium concentration ($>$ 10 mEq/liter). Causes include adrenocortical insufficiency and salt-losing nephropathy. Occasionally, urinary sosodium concentration may be increased and chloride concentration decreased after severe vomiting.

**4.** Hyponatremia due to other causes. The disorders included in this category are not associated with edema or volume depletion.

   **a.** Iatrogenically induced hyponatremia secondary to diuretic therapy and the administration of water.

   **b.** Syndrome of inappropriate secretion of antidiuretic hormone (ADH). This condition may be idiopathic or may be associated with one of the following disorders: diseases of the central nervous system (e.g., strokes, mass lesions, meningitis), pulmonary disease (e.g., tuberculosis, pneumonia, bronchogenic carcinoma), and drugs (chlorpropamide, narcotics, barbiturates, vincristine, antidepressants, and clofibrate).

      **(1)** Criteria for the diagnosis.

         **(a)** Hypotonicity of the body fluids.

         **(b)** Urine osmolality greater than 150 mOsm per kilogram of water.

         **(c)** Normal renal, adrenal, and thyroid function.

         **(d)** Increased urinary excretion of sodium ($>$ 30 mEq/liter) during volume expansion.

         **(e)** Elevated serum concentration of ADH.

         **(f)** Reversal of the syndrome by adequate fluid restriction.

      **(2)** Comment. When a steady state is reached, some of the abnormalities described may not be present.

## Diagnostic Approach

Once the diagnosis of hyponatremia is made, the serum sodium level should be rechecked and the serum osmolality determined.

**1.** If the serum osmolality is normal or high in the presence of confirmed hyponatremia, the possibility of hyperlipidemia or hyperglycemia, or both, should be investigated.

2. If the serum osmolality is low, confirming the diagnosis of true hyponatremia, the status of the extracellular fluid volume should be assessed.
   a. If edema or ascites is present, the hyponatremia is dilutional.
   b. If volume depletion is present, the hyponatremia is due to sodium depletion. The diagnosis is usually revealed by the history and a determination of the urine sodium concentration.
   c. If the extracellular fluid volume appears to be normal, iatrogenic causes of hyponatremia and the syndrome of inappropriate secretion of ADH must be excluded.

# Hyperkalemia
# (Hyperpotassemia)

## Definition

Hyperkalemia is defined as an abnormally high serum potassium concentration ($> 5.5$ mEq/liter).

## Etiology

1. Excessive intake of potassium, especially in renal insufficiency.
2. Increased cellular release of potassium (e.g., acidemia, rhabdomyolysis, succinylcholine therapy, severe muscle disease).
3. Decreased renal excretion of potassium (e.g., oliguric renal failure, potassium-blocking diuretics, interstitial nephritis, Addison's disease, isolated hypoaldosteronism).

## Symptoms and Signs

1. Neuromuscular symptoms and signs predominate; they include weakness, occasionally paralysis, loss of deep tendon reflexes, irritability, and confusion.
2. The following more or less sequential changes may be seen in the electrocardiogram: progressive increase in the amplitude of the T waves; decreased amplitude of the R wave with concomitant increased depth of the S wave, S-T segment depression, and prolongation of the QRS and P-R intervals; continued widening of the QRS and T waves, and their eventual replacement by a sine curve; and finally, ventricular tachyarrhythmia or asystole.

## Diagnostic Approach

The major goal is to find the cause of the hyperkalemia and to correct it if possible. When hyperkalemia is severe ($\geq 7.0$ mEq/liter), diagnostic investigations should be postponed until the life-threatening situation is controlled or corrected.

# Hypokalemia
# (Hypopotassemia)

## Definition

Hypopotassemia is defined as an abnormally low serum potassium concentration ($< 3.5$ mEq/liter).

## Etiology

1. Nonrenal causes.
   a. Decreased potassium intake.

**b.** Gastrointestinal losses of potassium.
   **(1)** Associated with alkalosis and volume depletion.
      **(a)** Gastric suctioning and vomiting.
      **(b)** Villous adenoma.
      **(c)** Neoplasms of the colon.
      **(d)** Chronic laxative abuse.
   **(2)** Associated with acidosis.
      **(a)** Diarrheal states.
      **(b)** Zollinger-Ellison syndrome.
      **(c)** Ureterosigmoidostomy.
**2.** Renal causes.
   **a.** Potassium wasting associated with metabolic acidosis.
      **(1)** Renal tubular acidosis.
      **(2)** Postobstructive uropathy.
      **(3)** Diuretic phase of acute tubular necrosis.
      **(4)** Chronic pyelonephritis.
   **b.** Potassium wasting associated with metabolic alkalosis.
      **(1)** Diuretic therapy (e.g., furosemide, ethacrynic acid, thiazides). Treatment with potent diuretics may cause hypochloremic alkalosis, which is usually associated with volume depletion.
      **(2)** Disorders with increased aldosterone secretion and hypertension (e.g., primary aldosteronism, malignant hypertension, renovascular hypertension, and essential hypertension with vomiting and diarrhea, diuretic therapy, oral contraceptives, steroid therapy).
      **(3)** Disorders with increased aldosterone secretion without hypertension (e.g., salt-losing nephropathy, juxtaglomerular hyperplasia).
      **(4)** Disorders with normal or decreased aldosterone and hypertension (e.g., licorice ingestion, Cushing's syndrome, certain congenital enzyme deficiency syndromes, Liddle's syndrome).

## Symptoms and Signs

1. Most symptoms are nonspecific. They include anorexia, nausea, vomiting, abdominal distention, ileus, weakness, decreased deep reflexes, and a depressed sensorium.
2. The electrocardiographic findings include lowering, flattening, notching, or inversion of the T waves; prominent U waves; depression of the S-T segments; and arrhythmias.
3. Nephrogenic diabetes insipidus, rhabdomyolysis, and aggravation of hepatic coma may also occur.

## Diagnostic Approach

1. Patients with hypokalemia require a thorough investigation to determine whether the potassium loss is the result of renal or extrarenal mechanisms. Extrarenal potassium depletion is easily recognized by the clinical picture and is correctable by appropriate treatment with potassium salts and fluids.
2. To determine whether potassium depletion is renal in origin, the 24-hour urinary excretion of potassium should be measured while the patient is on a regular salt intake. Urinary potassium excretion of less than 20 mEq/24 hours in a hypokalemic individual is excellent evidence against renal potassium wasting. On the other hand, urinary potassium excretion greater than 20 mEq/24 hours, especially if it is more than 60 mEq, is strongly suggestive of renal potassium wasting.
3. The problem of hypokalemia with hypertension is discussed in the section Arterial Hypertension, Chapter 3.
4. In patients with both metabolic alkalosis and potassium wasting, volume depletion may cause the abnormal state to persist. Every effort should be made not

only to ascertain the cause of the metabolic alkalosis but also to determine whether volume depletion is a contributing factor, and if it is, to correct it.

## Hyperphosphatemia

Hyperphosphatemia in the adult is defined as an elevation of serum phosphate levels above normal (3.0–4.5 mg/100 ml). Elevation of serum phosphorus occurs predominantly in acute or chronic renal insufficiency and is aggravated by catabolic stress. Hyperphosphatemia has been reported to occur frequently in lactic acidosis. Large amounts of phosphate administered orally, parenterally, or rectally may cause transient hyperphosphatemia even in the presence of normal renal function. The association of hyperphosphatemia and hypocalcemia has been reported to occur following the administration of large quantities of phosphate, in acute and chronic renal failure, from cytolysis during chemotherapy for neoplastic disease, and in hypoparathyroidism.

## Hypophosphatemia

Hypophosphatemia is defined as a serum phosphate level below 3.0 mg/100 ml. Hypophosphatemia is considered profound when serum phosphorus levels are less than 1.0 mg/100 ml.

The clinical conditions most often associated with hypophosphatemia are alcoholism, diabetic ketoacidosis, the healing phase of severe burns, liver disease, and respiratory or metabolic alkalosis.

### Etiology

1. Decreased intake of phosphate.
2. Impaired absorption of phosphate (e.g., aluminum hydroxide, carbonate antacids).
3. Excessive renal loss of phosphate.
   a. Primary and secondary hyperparathyroidism.
   b. Renal tubular disorders.
   c. Acidosis.
4. Intracellular shift of phosphate.
   a. Carbohydrate loading (e.g., iatrogenic).
   b. Hyperalimentation.
   c. Nutritional recovery syndrome.

### Clinical Features

1. Acute depletion.
   a. Hemolytic anemia.
   b. Rhabdomyolysis.
   c. Increased susceptibility to infection (defective leukocyte function).
   d. Petechiae (defective platelet function).
   e. Metabolic encephalopathy.
2. Chronic depletion.
   a. Anorexia, weakness, bone pain, and pathologic fractures due to osteomalacia.
   b. Increased urinary concentration of calcium, magnesium, and bicarbonate.
   c. Augmented intestinal calcium absorption.
   d. Usually normal serum calcium levels.
   e. Normal or low plasma parathyroid hormone levels.

## Hypermagnesemia

Hypermagnesemia is defined as an elevation of serum levels of magnesium above normal values (1.5–2.4 mEq/liter). Hypermagnesemia occurs almost exclusively in chronic renal insufficiency. It is aggravated by increased intake of magnesium, especially magnesium-containing antacids and laxatives. Symptoms include paresthesias, vasodilatation, mild hypotension, and, at very high levels, decreased tendon reflexes, muscle weakness, and even flaccid paralysis.

## Hypomagnesemia

### Definition

Hypomagnesemia is defined as a decrease in serum levels of magnesium below normal values (1.5–2.4 mEq/liter).

### Etiology

1. Decreased intake of magnesium (e.g., parenteral alimentation, alcoholism).
2. Defective gastrointestinal absorption of magnesium.
   a. Malabsorption syndromes.
   b. Short bowel syndromes.
   c. Intestinal bypass surgery.
   d. Laxative abuse.
   e. Frequent enemas.
   f. Malnutrition.
   g. Isolated magnesium malabsorption.
3. Excessive renal loss of magnesium.
   a. Diuretics.
   b. Ketoacidosis.
   c. Hyperaldosteronism and Bartter's syndrome.
   d. Syndrome of inappropriate ADH secretion.
   e. Hypercalciuria.
   f. Salt-wasting states.
   g. Primary magnesium wasting.
4. Intracellular shift of magnesium (e.g., nutritional recovery).
5. Miscellaneous.
   a. Primary hyperparathyroidism.
   b. Postparathyroidectomy.

### Clinical Features

1. Malnutrition.
2. Cardiac arrhythmias.
3. Muscle weakness.
4. Neurologic dysfunction (e.g., myoclonus, hyperreflexia, positive Trousseau sign, tremor, spasticity).
5. Hypokalemia and hypocalcemia are commonly associated with hypomagnesemia.

## Hyperchloremia and Hypochloremia

Chloride ion is the major extracellular anion. Along with sodium, it is the major contributor to serum osmolality. As a rule, serum chloride levels vary in direct proportion to the serum sodium concentration in hyperosmolar and hypoosmolar states unless there is an acid-base abnormality.

Serum chloride is inversely proportional to serum bicarbonate in most acid-base disorders unless there is anion accumulation (e.g., metabolic acidosis due to diabetic ketoacidosis). This matter is discussed in the next section.

## Hypercalcemia and Hypocalcemia

See Chapter 9.

## BLOOD-GAS AND pH ABNORMALITIES
### N. Balfour Slonim

Abnormalities of blood $O_2$, $CO_2$, and pH are diagnostically revealing as well as clinically significant. If values are extreme or changing rapidly, such abnormal laboratory findings may be of critical importance. These three vital, interrelated blood parameters should not be ignored in any diagnostic situation.

For the purpose of blood-gas and pH determination there is no substitute for *arterial* blood. When reliable information is most needed—in the care of the critically ill patient—blood samples from nonarterial sources are least reliable. Discussion of the anaerobic technique of analysis of arterial blood samples for $O_2$, $CO_2$, and pH is outside the scope of this chapter, but it should be emphasized that all techniques in present use, whether they involve physical or chemical principles, are a challenge to the precision and skill of the analyst; respiratory gas exchange occurs in the pulmonary capillaries in a fraction of a second!

## Pathophysiology

In the interpretation of blood-gas and pH abnormalities, physiologic principles provide the conceptual framework. Hypoxemia always precedes $CO_2$ retention in the course of diffuse bronchopulmonary disease for the following reasons: (1) $CO_2$ is about 20 times as diffusible across the pulmonary alveolocapillary membrane as $O_2$, and (2) the slopes of the $O_2$ and $CO_2$ dissociation curves differ so that regional hyperventilation in ventilation-perfusion mismatching can compensate for regional hypoventilation with respect to $CO_2$ but not with respect to $O_2$.

## Hypoxemia

### Definition

Hypoxemia is an arterial blood $PO_2$ that is less than the normal value of 100 $\pm$ 10 mm Hg for a healthy resting person at sea level. Arterial $PO_2$ decreases with age and is lower at higher altitudes.

### Symptoms and Signs

Hypoxemia is a common clinical occurrence and should be suspected when a patient exhibits tachycardia, cyanosis, dyspnea, restlessness, impaired cerebral function, and polycythemia. Unfortunately, cyanosis does not appear until arterial oxyhemoglobin saturation falls to 83 percent and the arterial $PO_2$ to 48 mm Hg. At least 5 g of deoxygenated hemoglobin per 100 ml of blood must be present in the systemic capillary circulation to produce the color that character-izes cyanosis. Hence, cyanosis is seen at $PO_2$ levels higher than 48 mm Hg in polycythemia and at $PO_2$ levels lower than 48 mm Hg in anemia. Indeed, patients who have chronic severe anemia may die of hypoxemia without cyanosis. Good illumination is required to detect cyanosis, and it may be obscured by skin pig-mentation. Acrocyanosis, as well as other regional cyanosis, may reflect only local conditions and not arterial hypoxemia.

## Etiology

Clinical arterial hypoxemia results from any of four pathophysiologic mecha-nisms, which may occur singly or in combination (Table 7-1).

1. The most common mechanism is ventilation-perfusion ($\dot{V}_A/\dot{Q}_c$) abnormality, or mismatching of the distribution of inspired gas with the distribution of pulmo-nary capillary blood flow. This occurs in acute and chronic diffuse bronchopul-monary diseases:
   a. Chronic bronchitis.
   b. Pulmonary emphysema.
   c. Asthma.
   d. Extensive acute and chronic pneumonias: infectious, chemical, allergic, aspi-ration.
   e. Pulmonary embolism with or without infarction.
   f. Adult respiratory distress syndrome.
   g. Acute severe bronchitis or bronchiolitis.
   h. Pulmonary atelectasis.
   i. Extensive pulmonary tuberculosis.
   j. Pneumoconiosis (e.g., silicosis, asbestosis, coal workers' pneumoconiosis).
   k. Pneumothorax.
   l. Kyphoscoliosis.
   m. Mucoviscidosis or fibrocystic disease.
   n. Fibrothorax.
   o. Extensive pulmonary neoplasm.
   p. Extensive pulmonary granulomata.
   q. Diffuse bronchiectasis.
   r. Primary pulmonary hypertension.
   s. Radiation fibrosis.
   t. Acute anterior poliomyelitis with respiratory paralysis.
   u. Unilateral bronchostenosis.
2. The second most common mechanism is generalized alveolar hypoventilation (not to be confused with the *regional* hypoventilation that occurs in ventilation-per-fusion mismatching) due to one of the following:
   a. Structural thoracic abnormalities (e.g., kyphoscoliosis, chest trauma).
   b. Neuromuscular diseases affecting breathing.
   c. Obesity-hypoventilation (Pickwickian) syndrome.
   d. Sleep-apnea syndrome.
   e. Drugs or toxins decreasing respiratory drive.
3. A less common mechanism of hypoxemia is decreased pulmonary diffusing capac-ity. There are two types:
   a. Decreased alveolocapillary membrane surface area.
      (1) Loss or destruction of lung tissue (e.g., lung resection).
      (2) Compression of lung or restriction of lung expansion (e.g., pneumo-thorax, "vanishing lung" syndrome).
   b. Increased length of the gas diffusion pathway—*alveolocapillary block syn-drome*. This occurs in diffuse parenchymatous bronchopulmonary diseases and certain cardiovascular conditions:
      (1) Acute or chronic diffuse interstitial pneumonitis (e.g., Hamman-Rich syndrome); interstitial pulmonary fibrosis.
      (2) Pulmonary edema.

**Table 7-1.** The four pathophysiologic mechanisms of arterial hypoxemia and patterns of response to oxygen breathing and physical exercise

| Mechanism | Condition* | $PO_2$ Alveolar | $PO_2$ Arterial | $PCO_2$ Alveolar | $PCO_2$ Arterial |
|---|---|---|---|---|---|
| 1. Ventilation-perfusion mismatching | Initial | Normal to high | Low | Normal to low | Low to high |
| | Oxygen | Marked increase | Variable increase | Normal to high | Normal to high |
| | Exercise | Normal to high | Slight increase | Normal to low | Low to high |
| 2. Generalized alveolar hypoventilation | Initial | Low | Low | High | High |
| | Oxygen | Marked increase | Marked increase | Increase | Increase |
| | Exercise | Varies | Varies | Varies | Varies |
| 3. Pulmonary diffusing capacity decrease | Initial | High | Low | Low | Low |
| | Oxygen | Marked increase | Marked increase | Increase | Increase |
| | Exercise | Slight increase | Decrease | Decrease | Decrease |
| 4. Right-to-left shunt | Initial | Normal to high | Low | Normal to low | Normal to low |
| | Oxygen | Marked increase | Slight increase | Increase | Increase |
| | Exercise | Slight increase | Decrease | Slight decrease | Slight increase |

*(1) Initial: spontaneous initial condition; physiologic measurement. (2) Oxygen: effect of breathing 100 percent $O_2$ for 15 minutes; oxygen breathing test. (3) Exercise: effect of physical exercise; exercise test.

**(3)** Pulmonary sarcoidosis.

**(4)** Mitral stenosis with chronic pulmonary vascular congestion.

**(5)** Pulmonary berylliosis.

**(6)** Lymphangitic carcinomatosis.

**(7)** Pulmonary adenomatosis.

**(8)** Alveolar proteinosis.

4. The least common mechanism of hypoxemia is right-to-left cardiac or pulmonary circulatory shunt. Although there are innumerable small shunts that cause venous admixture in ventilation-perfusion mismatching, the term *cardiac* or *pulmonary circulatory shunt* refers to discrete gross anatomic shunts.

   **a.** Congenital right-to-left shunts.

   **b.** Acquired right-to-left shunts.

   **c.** Pulmonary hemangioma.

## Diagnostic Approach

Unfortunately, a given bronchopulmonary disease may produce hypoxemia by more than one of these four mechanisms. Differential diagnosis of the diseases that produce hypoxemia proceeds as follows:

1. Ventilation-perfusion mismatching is established and quantified by the following tests and procedures:

   **a.** Single-breath nitrogen test.

   **b.** Closed-circuit helium equilibration mixing index.

   **c.** Distribution of inhaled radioactively labeled gas (e.g., xenon).

   **d.** Distribution of intravenously injected solution of radioactively labeled gas (e.g., xenon).

   **e.** Lung scan after intravenous injection of radioactively labeled particulates (e.g., radioiodinated macroaggregated serum albumin).

2. Generalized alveolar hypoventilation is established and quantified by the following tests:

   **a.** Spirometry. The minute volume of breathing is less than predicted.

   **b.** Analysis of an alveolar gas sample reveals low $PO_2$ and high $PCO_2$.

3. Decreased pulmonary diffusing capacity is established and quantified by any of several carbon monoxide diffusing capacity tests. Tests of pulmonary diffusing capacity can measure a decrease but cannot distinguish between the conditions listed in paragraphs **3a** and **3b**, above. Unfortunately, the validity of these tests is decreased in patients who have ventilation-perfusion mismatching, generalized alveolar hypoventilation, or both.

4. Right-to-left shunt is established by the following tests and procedures:

   **a.** Chest roentgenography with special views and techniques, as indicated (e.g., tomography).

   **b.** $O_2$ breathing test with analysis of arterial blood sample. A physiologic diagnosis of right-to-left shunt.

   **c.** Angiocardiography. An anatomic diagnosis of the structure and location of a right-to-left shunt.

   **d.** Cardiac catheterization, with calculation of right-to-left shunt flow.

5. Identification of the mechanism of arterial hypoxemia may require the $O_2$ breathing test and an exercise test. Table 7-1 shows the characteristic responses of each of the four pathophysiologic mechanisms of clinical arterial hypoxemia to these two tests.

6. The *alveolar-arterial $PO_2$ difference* [$P(A-a)O_2$] is of diagnostic value in certain clinical situations.

   **a.** To obtain this difference, subtract the measured arterial blood $PO_2$ from the mean alveolar gas $PO_2$, which is calculated using the *alveolar gas equation*. In health, $P(A-a)O_2$ is a function of age. The diagnostic sensitivity of $P(A-a)O_2$ depends on the selection of an appropriate normal range of values for the particular patient.

**b.** $P(A-a)O_2$ is used clinically in the following situations.
   **(1)** The differential diagnosis of acute pulmonary embolism, considering also the arterial blood gases; increased $P(A-a)O_2$, decreased arterial $PCO_2$, and decreased arterial $PO_2$ all favor the diagnosis of acute pulmonary embolism.
   **(2)** To determine the presence or absence of parenchymal lung disease.
   **(3)** To assess arterial hypoxemia in coma, for example, in drug overdose situations, where it is used to distinguish hypoventilation from parenchymal lung disease.

---

## Abnormalities of Blood $PCO_2$

### Definition

The arterial blood $PCO_2$ of a healthy resting man breathing air spontaneously at sea level is $40 \pm 2$ mm Hg. Arterial blood $PCO_2$ is promptly and strongly affected by changes in alveolar ventilation rate. Although arterial $PCO_2$ equals alveolar $PCO_2$ over a wide range of clinical conditions, in moderate to severe ventilation-perfusion mismatching, arterial $PCO_2$ is greater than alveolar $PCO_2$, and hypoxemia is always already present. Although hypoxemia is the only clinically important blood $PO_2$ abnormality, hypocapnia and hypercapnia are both clinically important.

### Hypocapnia

PATHOPHYSIOLOGY

The clinical signs of hypocapnia are always the result of alveolar hyperventilation. Significant physiologic responses are:
1. Slightly decreased systemic arterial blood pressure.
2. Systemic venoconstriction.
3. Cerebral vasoconstriction and decreased cerebral blood flow.
4. Respiratory alkalosis with decreased concentration of ionized calcium in extracellular body fluids.
5. The respiratory alkalosis of chronic hypocapnia induces the kidney to excrete $HCO_3^-$, producing a compensatory metabolic acidosis that corrects the pH abnormality.

SYMPTOMS AND SIGNS

1. Dizziness.
2. Numbness and tingling of hands and feet.
3. Psychomotor impairment.
4. Signs of tetany.
5. Carpopedal spasm.

ETIOLOGY

1. Exposure to high altitudes (physiologic).
2. Normal pregnancy (physiologic).
3. Psychogenic hyperventilation.
   **a.** Hysterical.
   **b.** Voluntary.
4. Passive hyperventilation with mechanically controlled or assisted ventilation.
5. Compensatory alveolar hyperventilation in response to primary metabolic acidosis.
6. Salicylates.
7. Progestogens.
8. Primary central nervous system disease.

9. Severe anemia.
10. Pneumonia, asthma, or pulmonary edema.
11. Gram-negative sepsis.
12. Restrictive lung diseases, such as pulmonary fibrosis.
13. Hepatic failure.

DIAGNOSTIC APPROACH

The cause of hyperventilation is usually readily apparent from the following:
1. History.
2. Physical examination.
3. Mental status and neurologic examination.
4. Routine laboratory workup.
5. The presence of primary metabolic acidosis, shown by low arterial blood pH.
6. Consideration of altitude and ambient pressure.
7. Rarely, cerebrospinal fluid acidosis, stimulating the central chemoreceptors (resulting in hyperventilation and arterial hypocapnia).

## Hypercapnia

PATHOPHYSIOLOGY

1. Responses to *mild hypercapnia:*
   a. Breathing frequency increases.
   b. Tidal volume increases.
   c. Body heat loss increases.
   d. Acute hypercapnia produces respiratory acidosis; chronic respiratory acidosis induces the kidney to retain $HCO_3^-$, producing compensatory metabolic alkalosis.
2. Responses to *moderate hypercapnia:*
   a. Cerebral vasodilation and increased cerebral blood flow.
   b. Intracranial and cerebrospinal fluid pressure increase.
   c. The sympathoadrenomedullary system discharges, but catecholamines are inhibited by the concomitant respiratory acidosis.
   d. Hyperbaric $O_2$ convulsions are inhibited.
3. Responses to *severe hypercapnia:*
   a. Body core temperature decreases.
   b. Narcosis.
   c. Unconsciousness.
   d. Death.

SYMPTOMS AND SIGNS

1. Transient, throbbing headache.
2. Flushed face.
3. Nausea.
4. Sweating.
5. Tachycardia.
6. Palpitation.
7. Insomnia.
8. Somnolence.
9. Tunnel vision.

ETIOLOGY

1. Acute or chronic obstructive bronchopulmonary conditions.
   a. Pulmonary emphysema.
   b. Chronic bronchitis.
   c. Status asthmaticus.

    **d.** Bronchiolitis: infectious or chemical.
    **e.** Mechanical obstruction of trachea or bronchi by water (drowning), blood (hemorrhage), bronchial secretions, or pus.
**2.** Obstruction of the upper respiratory tract.
**3.** Generalized alveolar hypoventilation.
    **a.** Thoracic skeletal conditions, chest wall disease, or chest trauma affecting breathing (e.g., kyphoscoliosis, flail chest, ankylosing spondylitis).
    **b.** Neuromuscular conditions affecting breathing.
        **(1)** Muscular dystrophy.
        **(2)** Myasthenia gravis.
        **(3)** Intoxications (e.g., pesticides, curare, nerve gas).
        **(4)** Acute or chronic infectious diseases (e.g., poliomyelitis, Guillain-Barré syndrome, diphtheria, tetanus).
    **c.** Obesity-hypoventilation (Pickwickian) syndrome.
    **d.** Central nervous system conditions affecting breathing.
        **(1)** Cerebrovascular accident.
        **(2)** Increased intracranial pressure (e.g., intracranial tumor, head trauma).
        **(3)** Meningitis or encephalitis.
        **(4)** Pharmacologic depression of respiratory centers (e.g., barbiturates, morphine, tranquilizers, alcohol).
    **e.** Hypoventilation with mechanical respirator.
    **f.** Extreme abdominal distention or pain, traumatic or postsurgical, interfering with diaphragmatic breathing.
    **g.** Other causes.
        **(1)** Severe hypothyroidism.
        **(2)** Starvation cachexia.
        **(3)** Severe electrolyte disturbance.
        **(4)** Acute intermittent porphyria.
**4.** Restrictive and other bronchopulmonary conditions.
    **a.** Pneumothorax, hemothorax, hydrothorax.
    **b.** Restrictive disease of the pleurae (e.g., fibrosis, calcification).
    **c.** Extensive infiltrative disease or fibrosis of lung parenchyma.
    **d.** Severe pulmonary edema.
**5.** Sleep-apnea syndrome.
**6.** Oxygen therapy for chronic lung failure.

DIAGNOSTIC APPROACH

The precise diagnosis of the disease or condition producing primary hypercapnia is established as follows:
**1.** Arterial hypoxemia is always also present, unless the patient is breathing $O_2$.
**2.** If the simultaneously determined arterial blood pH is low, then respiratory acidosis is either uncompensated or partially compensated by metabolic alkalosis. If the pH is within normal limits, then either (a) respiratory acidosis is completely corrected by compensatory metabolic alkalosis, or, rarely, (b) a primary coexisting metabolic alkalosis may be just sufficient to correct fully the low pH of hypercapnia. The combination of high $PCO_2$ and normal pH indicates chronicity and stability of the inciting etiologic agent.
**3.** If respiratory acidosis is the only primary acid-base disturbance present, differential diagnosis is then made by the following procedures:
    **a.** History.
    **b.** Physical examination.
    **c.** Routine laboratory studies.
    **d.** Chest roentgenography.
    **e.** Electrolyte profile.
    **f.** Pulmonary function tests.
    **g.** Neurologic examination.
    **h.** Special laboratory studies as indicated (e.g., porphyria, hypothyroidism).

## Abnormalities of Blood pH

### Definition

In clinical use, the term "blood pH" means *plasma pH*. The normal arterial blood pH of a healthy resting man at sea level is 7.40 ± 0.05. Deviations of arterial blood pH from this range of normal values result from one or more *primary* acid base disturbances, which induce the pH homeostatic mechanisms to respond with *secondary* pH-compensating processes. Such responses always tend to restore pH toward normal. *Acidemia* means low blood plasma pH, and *alkalemia* means high blood plasma pH.

### Etiology

METABOLIC (NONRESPIRATORY) ACIDOSIS

Metabolic acidosis is the result of acid excess (metabolic overproduction or ingestion of acid), impaired renal excretion of the daily acid load, or loss of body base ($HCO_3^-$). Acid overproduction is often the result of diabetic ketoacidosis. Impaired renal excretion of acid results in retention of nonvolatile acids (acids other than $H_2CO_3$, which is excreted by the lungs as $CO_2$) and uremic acidosis. In ambulatory patients, diarrheal loss of body base stores (base deficit) is the most common cause of hyperchloremic (normal anion gap) metabolic acidosis. The second most common cause of hyperchloremic metabolic acidosis is renal tubular acidosis, which may be primary (hereditary) or secondary (the result of kidney injury from toxic chemical substances or drugs).

Lactic acidosis occurs when, for any reason, metabolic need exceeds the rate of mitochondrial $O_2$ consumption (oxidative metabolism). Under this condition, anaerobic metabolism accelerates and lactic acid accumulates.

Regardless of cause, metabolic acidosis is characterized by decreased plasma pH (acidemia), decreased plasma $HCO_3^-$ concentration, and decreased arterial blood $PCO_2$. The hypocapnia moderates but does not fully correct the acidemia. Severe acidosis may impair myocardial contractility and dilate peripheral arterioles, causing circulatory shock. The symptoms of acidosis—fatigue, anorexia, nausea, vomiting, and dyspnea—may be difficult to distinguish from those of the underlying disorder that produced the acidosis.

1. Hyperchloremic (normal anion gap).
   a. Diarrhea.
   b. Renal tubular acidosis.
   c. Dehydration.
   d. Interstitial renal disease.
   e. Ureterosigmoidostomy.
   f. Carbonic anhydrase inhibitor (e.g., acetazolamide).
   g. Arginine hydrochloride.
   h. Ammonium chloride.
2. Increased undetermined anion (high anion gap).
   a. Diabetic ketoacidosis.
   b. Renal failure with uremic acidosis.
   c. Alcoholic ketoacidosis.
   d. Lactic acidosis (may occur in the clinical setting of shock, sepsis, or cardiac arrest).
   e. Salicylate intoxication.
   f. Methanol intoxication.
   g. Ethylene glycol intoxication.
   h. Paraldehyde intoxication.
   i. Starvation ketoacidosis.
   j. Physical exercise (physiologic).

METABOLIC (NONRESPIRATORY) ALKALOSIS

*Metabolic alkalosis* is an acid-base disturbance characterized by increased plasma $HCO_3^-$ concentration and alkalemia. This disturbance is often partially compensated for by respiratory acidosis. The pH increase results from decreased $H^+$ concentration, increased $HCO_3^-$ concentration, or both.

Metabolic alkalosis may result from either base excess or acid deficit. The clinical causes of metabolic alkalosis include the following:

1. Chloruretic diuretics.
2. Nasogastric suction.
3. Vomiting.
4. Alkali therapy or excessive use of antacids.
5. Mineralocorticosteroid excess.
   **a.** Endogenous (e.g., aldosteronism).
   **b.** Exogenous (e.g., deoxycorticosterone acetate, licorice intoxication).
6. Glucocorticosteroid excess.
   **a.** Endogenous (e.g., hyperadrenocorticism, Cushing's syndrome).
   **b.** Exogenous (e.g., therapy with glucocorticosteroids, ACTH).
7. Severe $K^+$ deficit (usually depletion).
8. $Cl^-$ deficit (usually restriction of $Cl^-$ intake).
9. Intravenous phosphate or sulfate salts in an $Na^+$-depleted patient.

## Diagnostic Approach

Precise diagnosis, and thus proper therapy, of acid-base disorders requires identification of the *primary* inciting—as opposed to *secondary* compensatory—process. Usually one, but sometimes more than one, of the four possible primary acid-base disturbances is found; any primary disturbances and their etiologic agents must be identified and distinguished from any secondary compensatory responses. First, make a clinical assessment of the patient and try to predict what acid-base disorders will be found.

GRAPHIC APPROACH

1. Review the history for potential causes of acid-base disturbance.
2. Review the physical examination for signs of acid-base disturbance.
   **a.** Nasogastric tube.
   **b.** Cyanosis.
   **c.** Evidence of bronchopulmonary disease.
   **d.** Fever.
   **e.** Hypotension.
   **f.** Jaundice.
   **g.** Signs of alkalemic tetany.
3. Review the laboratory values for blood $CO_2$ content and $K^+$ concentration, and calculate the undetermined anion concentration (anion gap) as follows:

Undetermined anion concentration $= [Na^+] - [CO_2] - [Cl^-]$

The value is normally less than 12 to 14 mEq/liter and consists of phosphates, anionic proteins, sulfates, and anions of various organic acids. Slight elevations to 15 or 16 mEq/liter sometimes occur in respiratory alkalosis. Increased undetermined anion concentration indicates metabolic acidosis. However, the converse is not true; metabolic acidosis may be hyperchloremic as in normal anion gap acidosis: diarrhea, renal tubular acidosis (proximal and distal), hyperalimentation acidosis, acetazolamide effect, early renal failure acidosis, and possibly, hyperparathyroidism. Larger undetermined anion gaps are more likely due to increased organic acids. Values greater than 25 mEq/liter occur only in diabetic ketoacidosis; methanol, ethylene glycol, or salicylate intoxication; and lactic acidosis.

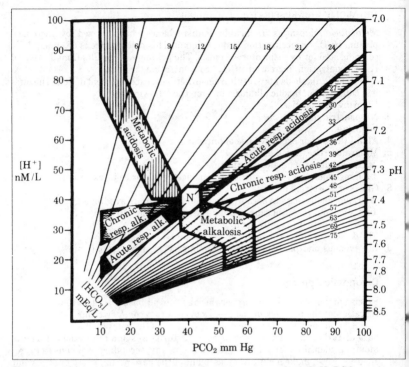

**Fig. 7-1.** Acid-base map showing the usual compensatory range of pH, $PCO_2$, and plasma $HCO_3^-$ concentration in simple acid-base disorders. Values on the vertical axis represent plasma $H^+$ concentration (*left*) in nanomoles/liter, or pH (*right*). Values on the horizontal axis represent $PCO_2$ in mm Hg. Diagonal lines are isopleths for the plasma $HCO_3^-$ concentration in mEq/liter. Clear area in the center of the graph is the range of normal. Note that the metabolic component (plasma $HCO_3^-$ concentration) and the respiratory component (arterial blood $PCO_2$) of the acid-base equation always change in the same direction. (Reprinted by permission from M. Goldberg, et al. Computer-based instruction and diagnosis of acid-base disorders: A systemic approach. *J.A.M.A.* 223:269, 1973. Copyright 1973, American Medical Association.)

Acidosis is usually associated with hyperkalemia unless (a) the acidosis develops in a patient already $K^+$-depleted or (b) the acidosis is due to loss of $KHCO_3$ from the body (e.g., in diarrhea, acetazolamide therapy, or renal tubular acidosis). Alkalosis is usually associated with hypokalemia, except when $K^+$-loading predominates due to increased $K^+$ intake or increased rate of tissue breakdown.

4. Review other laboratory data for acid-base clues.
   a. Polycythemia.
   b. Hyperglycemia.
   c. Elevated BUN.
   d. Elevated $NH_3$.
   e. Decreased pulmonary function.
   f. Positive blood culture.
5. Analyze and interpret pH, $PCO_2$, and $HCO_3^-$ as follows. Plot $PCO_2$ and pH on any of the three available two-dimensional graphs (Fig. 7-1) or on the three-dimensional acid-base surface model of the Henderson-Hasselbalch buffer equa-

tion. Visual inspection of the position of this plotted acid-base point relative to both the isobar $PCO_2 = 40$ (line of pure metabolic disturbance) and the patient's $CO_2$ titration, or blood buffer, curve (line of pure respiratory disturbance) indicates either an apparently (but not necessarily) pure primary respiratory or metabolic disturbance or an obviously mixed disturbance consisting of one or more primary components with or without secondary compensatory responses. Using the other clinical information from paragraphs **1** through **4** above, deduce the nature, sequence, and cause of acid-base events.

TABULAR APPROACH

See Table 7-2.

RULES OF THUMB FOR INTERPRETATION OF ACID-BASE DISORDERS

Rules of thumb provide a useful alternative to the graphic method of interpretation. However, it must be remembered that such rules are linear approximations of nonlinear relationships and assume normal in vivo buffering, including normal hemoglobin concentration (see Table 7-3).

PRINCIPLES OF ACID-BASE INTERPRETATION

1. We live on the brink of acidosis. Failure of either lungs or kidneys precipitates acidosis. Body buffer systems neutralize acid more effectively than they neutralize base. Thus, a base challenge is tolerated more poorly. In health, metabolism of dietary and endogenous protein produces about 1 mEq/kgm/day of acid. However, critical illness may increase the rate of endogenous acid production by a factor of two to three.
2. The *law of electroneutrality* states that in any solution the sum of the anionic ( − ) charges equals the sum of the cationic ( + ) charges. The concept of anion gap, the undetermined anion concentration, is based on the law of electroneutrality.
3. Acid-base disturbances are chemically additive, but their pathophysiologic effects may be multiplicative.
4. $H^+$ concentration is a regulated variable. The pH-compensating response to a primary acid-base disturbance results from the operation of physiologic processes that regulate $H^+$ concentration in extracellular fluid.
5. Because anemia, hypoproteinemia, and decreased muscle mass reduce body buffering capacity, patients who have these conditions are vulnerable to wider pH swings for a given acid-base challenge.
6. Respiratory acid-base changes occur in minutes, whereas metabolic acid-base changes require hours or days.
7. Alveolar ventilation rate is the ultimate regulator of alveolar $PCO_2$. One minute of apnea increases $PCO_2$ about 4 mm Hg.
8. Arterial hypoxemia always precedes $CO_2$ retention in the course of diffuse bronchopulmonary disease.
9. $CO_2$ retention occurs only when the function of both lungs is impaired or when both lungs are diseased. Unilateral pneumonectomy does not result in $CO_2$ retention if the remaining lung is healthy. $CO_2$ retention results from hypoventilation, $\dot{V}/\dot{Q}$ mismatching, or extensive loss of lung tissue.
10. Respiratory compensation for metabolic disturbances is incomplete. The respiratory compensation for metabolic alkalosis is unpredictable.
11. Plasma $Cl^-$ and $HCO_3^-$ concentrations tend to change in opposite directions. In metabolic alkalosis $Cl^-$ falls and $HCO_3^-$ rises, whereas in metabolic acidosis $HCO_3^-$ falls, but $Cl^-$ seldom rises much above normal.
12. A pH rise of 0.1 unit is associated with a corresponding fall in plasma $K^+$ concentration of about 0.5 mEq/liter and a pH fall of 0.1 unit is associated with a plasma $K^+$ rise of the same extent.
13. Acid urine in a patient who is alkalemic is often evidence of hypokalemia or intracellular $K^+$ deficit, or both.

**Table 7-2.** Diagnosis of acid-base disorders

| $PCO_2$ | Low pH | Normal pH | High pH |
|---|---|---|---|
| High | Respiratory acidosis with or without incompletely compensating metabolic alkalosis or coexisting metabolic acidosis | Respiratory acidosis and compensatory metabolic alkalosis | Metabolic alkalosis with coexisting respiratory acidosis or incompletely compensating respiratory acidosis |
| Normal | Metabolic acidosis | Normal | Metabolic alkalosis |
| Low | Metabolic acidosis with coexisting respiratory alkalosis or incompletely compensating respiratory alkalosis | Respiratory alkalosis and compensatory metabolic acidosis | Respiratory alkalosis with or without incompletely compensating metabolic acidosis or coexisting metabolic alkalosis |

**Table 7-3.** Rules of thumb for interpretation of acid-base disorders

| | |
|---|---|
| Metabolic acidosis | Arterial $PCO_2$ decreases by about 1 to 1½ times the decrease of plasma $HCO_3^-$ concentration |
| Metabolic alkalosis | Arterial $PCO_2$ increases by about ½ to 1 times the increase of plasma $HCO_3^-$ concentration |
| Respiratory acidosis | $PCO_2$ above 50 mm Hg suggests a *primary* respiratory disorder |
| Acute | In acute uncompensated respiratory acidosis, plasma $HCO_3^-$ concentration increases but does not exceed 30 mEq/liter. For each mm Hg that $PCO_2$ increases above 40, pH decreases about ¾ of a point below 7.40 in the second decimal place |
| Chronic | In fully compensated respiratory acidosis, for each mm Hg that $PCO_2$ increases above 40, plasma $HCO_3^-$ concentration increases about ⅓ of a mEq/liter and pH decreases about ¼ point below 7.40 in the second decimal place. For each 10 mm Hg increment of arterial $PCO_2$ above 40, plasma $HCO_3^-$ concentration increases by about 4 mEq/liter |
| Respiratory alkalosis | |
| Acute | In primary acute respiratory alkalosis, for each mm Hg that $PCO_2$ decreases below 40, pH increases about 1 point above 7.40 in the second decimal place. For each 10 mm Hg decrement of arterial $PCO_2$, plasma $HCO_3^-$ concentration decreases by about 2.5 mEq/liter but is rarely less than 18 mEq/liter |
| Chronic | Plasma $HCO_3^-$ concentration decreases by at least as much as it does in acute respiratory alkalosis but is rarely less than 15 mEq/liter |

Source: Modified from W. D. Kaehny, Pathogenesis and Management of Respiratory and Mixed Acid Base Disorders. In R. W. Schrier (ed.), *Renal and Electrolyte Disorders*, 2nd ed. Boston: Little, Brown, 1980. P. 170. Used by permission.

## Comments

Rational therapy requires an understanding of the mechanism, nature, extent, and significance of the acid-base abnormality. It is important to identify mixed acid-base abnormalities when present and to distinguish a compensatory change from a coexisting primary disorder. Rational therapy also requires knowledge of the time-course of acid-base changes and often involves prediction of the reversibility of the underlying disorder producing a primary acid-base abnormality.

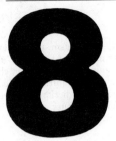

# Musculoskeletal Problems

## CLUBBING
### H. Harold Friedman

### Definition

Clubbing is a condition characterized by bulbous enlargement of the distal phalanges of the fingers and toes. Hypertrophic osteoarthropathy is a more advanced stage of clubbing associated with periosteal proliferation of the long bones, often with arthralgia or joint swelling. Both conditions may occur at any age.

### Clinical Features

1. Clubbing usually occurs first in the thumb and index finger, and later spreads to the other fingers. The earliest evidence of clubbing is thickening and sponginess of the nail bed, manifested by increased ballotability and curvature of the nail in its bed and an increase in the angle made by the nail and the dorsum of the distal phalanx. The normal base angle when viewed from the side (profile view) is 160 degrees. In early clubbing, the base angle is obliterated and becomes 180 degrees or greater. Later there may be warmth and redness and sometimes tenderness of the distal phalanges. Sometimes the patient has a burning sensation in the affected areas, but pain is uncommon. Hypertrophic osteoarthropathy should always be looked for in the presence of clubbing. It may precede the detection of pulmonary neoplastic disease by weeks or months. Clubbing and hypertrophic osteoarthropathy may disappear and reappear synchronously with remission and exacerbations of the underlying disease.
2. When the periosteum of the long bones is involved, there may be pain near the joints as well as redness, warmth, and tenderness.
3. The joints adjacent to long bone involvement may be swollen.
4. Early on the x-rays are normal. Later there is flaring of the ungual process and demineralization. The long bones may reveal periosteal thickening, especially near the joints.

### Differential Diagnosis

Clubbing should be differentiated from (1) exaggerated curving of the nail, a normal variant, particularly in blacks; (2) Heberden's nodes; (3) cysts of the bony phalanges; and (4) infectious processes.

When joint symptoms predominate, confusion with arthritis may occur. If there is superficial warmth, redness, and tenderness in a lower extremity, thrombophlebitis or cellulitis may be considered.

## Associated Conditions

Clubbing and hypertrophic osteoarthropathy are relatively innocuous, but they are important because of their frequent association with significant underlying disease. The hereditary forms are not related to any systemic disorder. The major conditions associated with clubbing and hypertrophic osteoarthropathy are listed below. Their incidence is as follows: pulmonary disease, 75 to 80 percent; cardiovascular abnormalities, 10 to 15 percent; diseases of the gastrointestinal tract, including the liver, 5 to 15 percent; and miscellaneous disorders, 5 to 15 percent.

1. Pulmonary disease.
   a. Bronchogenic carcinoma (rare with metastatic lung tumor).
   b. Pleural neoplasms.
   c. Chronic infections other than tuberculosis (e.g., bronchiectasis, abscess, empyema).
   d. Emphysema with cor pulmonale.
   e. Mediastinal lesions.
2. Cardiac disorders.
   a. Cyanotic congenital heart disease.
   b. Infective endocarditis.
   c. Pulmonary arteriovenous fistula.
3. Chronic liver disease (cirrhosis).
4. Gastrointestinal disorders.
   a. Ulcerative colitis.
   b. Granulomatous colitis.
   c. Regional enteritis.
   d. Neoplasms.
   e. Steatorrhea of unknown cause.
5. Hyperthyroidism.
6. Hemoglobinopathies.
7. Unilateral clubbing is usually due to local vascular disease (e.g., anomalies of the aortic arch, aortic or subclavian aneurysm, pulmonary hypertension with persistent patency of the ductus arteriosus).

## Diagnostic Approach to Bilateral Clubbing

### History

A family history of clubbing and long duration of clubbing without evidence of associated illness suggest that it is of the hereditary type. Specific information related to associated illnesses should be sought in the history: cough, dyspnea, cigarette smoking, cyanosis, fever, jaundice, alcoholism, diarrhea, and tremulousness.

### Physical Examination

Specific points related to associated illness should be sought: wheezes, rales, supraclavicular nodes, murmurs, jaundice, vascular spiders, palmar erythema, enlarged liver, abdominal mass (regional enteritis), thyromegaly, and thyroid eye signs.

## Laboratory Studies

1. CBC.
2. Urinalysis.

3. Chest films.
4. Electrocardiogram.
5. Liver function tests.
6. $T_4$; $T_3$ resin uptake or $T_3$ RIA, or both.
7. Arterial blood gases.
8. Stools for occult blood.
9. Sigmoidoscopy, barium enema, and upper GI and small bowel study if the history suggests gastrointestinal disease or if stools are positive for blood.

## PERIPHERAL JOINT ARTHRITIS

Kenneth P. Glassman
Herbert Kaplan

The diagnostic challenge presented by the patient with pain or swelling in the elbows, knees, or the joints of the hands and feet is considered in this section. Although disorders that affect the peripheral articulations may also involve the shoulders, hips, and spine, these disorders are covered separately. The following abbreviations are used in this chapter:

ANA = antinuclear antibody
ARF = acute rheumatic fever
AS = ankylosing spondylitis
CTD = connective tissue disease(s)
DIP = distal interphalangeal
DNA = deoxyribonucleic acid
ECM = erythema chronicum migrans
ESR = erythrocyte sedimentation rate
$HB_sAg$ = hepatitis B surface antigen
IP = interphalangeal
JRA = juvenile rheumatoid arthritis
MCP = metacarpophalangeal
MCTD = mixed connective tissue disease
MTP = metatarsophalangeal
NSAID = nonsteroidal anti-inflammatory drug(s)
OA = osteoarthritis
PAN = polyarteritis nodosa
PIP = proximal interphalangeal
PMR = polymyalgia rheumatica
RA = rheumatoid arthritis
RF = rheumatoid factor
RNP = ribonucleoprotein
SLE = systemic lupus erythematosus

## Etiology

The more common causes of peripheral joint disease diagnosed in office practice, listed in order of decreasing frequency, are as follows:
1. Osteoarthritis.
2. Bursitis, tendinitis.
3. Connective tissue diseases (rheumatoid arthritis, systemic lupus erythematosus, mixed connective tissue disease, polymyalgia rheumatica, scleroderma, dermatomyositis, polyarteritis nodosa, acute rheumatic fever).
4. Crystalline arthropathies (gout, pseudogout).

5. Rheumatoid variants (ankylosing spondylitis, psoriatic arthritis, Reiter's syndrome, palindromic rheumatism, enteropathic arthropathy, juvenile rheumatoid arthritis).
6. Infectious arthritis (bacterial and viral).
7. Joint trauma.
8. Lyme disease.
9. Miscellaneous disorders (sarcoidosis, hyperparathyroidism, myxedema, chronic active hepatitis, hemophilia, neuropathic arthropathy, pharmacologic arthritis, Behçet's syndrome, Whipple's disease, malignancy, pigmented villonodular synovitis).

# Diagnostic Approach

## History

### MODE OF ONSET

An acute, dramatic onset suggests crystalline arthropathy or infectious arthritis. However, acute rheumatic fever, rheumatoid arthritis, juvenile rheumatoid arthritis, Reiter's syndrome, and psoriatic arthritis may also begin suddenly. The chronic course of osteoarthritis frequently is punctuated by acute exacerbations of painful, swollen, and occasionally warm joints. An acute onset of painful muscles in the proximal upper or lower extremities, or both, suggests PMR, which may be associated with mild synovitis of small joints (see Myalgia, this chapter).

### TRAUMA

1. A history of trauma, recent or remote, may be significant in predisposing to osteoarthritis, tendinitis, or bursitis.
2. Acute gouty or pseudogout arthritis is often triggered by relatively mild trauma to the involved joint and is also a cause of acute arthritis in the first week after a major surgical procedure.

### ANTECEDENT INFECTION

1. A history of an infected skin laceration or any other bacterial focus may be the clue to infectious arthritis.
2. An antecedent streptococcal pharyngitis or scarlet fever should arouse suspicion of acute rheumatic fever.
3. Recent urethritis suggests gonococcal arthritis or Reiter's syndrome. The onset of gonococcal arthritis may also be associated with a menstrual period.
4. Fever and skin rash followed by polyarthritis suggests rubella, infectious mononucleosis, arthritis associated with viral hepatitis, Lyme disease, or juvenile or adult-onset Still's disease.
5. An acute arthritis at the site of a total joint replacement in a patient with recent genitourinary instrumentation or dental cleaning should arouse suspicion of a septic joint.

### DRUGS

1. A history of intravenous drug abuse should suggest the possibility of infectious arthritis.
2. Penicillin, sulfonamides, and horse serum injections are common causes of foreign protein reactions (serum sickness) typified by urticaria and polyarthritis.
3. Antihypertensive drugs, diuretics, and levodopa produce hyperuricemia and are common causes of secondary gout. Chemotherapy agents used in malignant disease may also cause secondary gout.
4. Anticonvulsant drugs, hydralazine, procainamide, isoniazid, and some antibiotics may cause an SLE-like syndrome with polyarthritis.

5. Acute joint swelling in patients taking anticoagulants suggests hemarthrosis. However, hemarthrosis may also occur in patients with hereditary clotting disorders or trauma.

PREVIOUS RESPONSES TO THERAPY

1. A therapeutic response or failure to respond to a specific drug may be of some diagnostic significance.
2. A good result from the administration of colchicine is almost pathognomonic of gout, although a beneficial response has also been reported in sarcoid arthritis, rheumatoid arthritis, and pseudogout.
3. A dramatic response to large doses of salicylates may be obtained in most acute joint inflammations. These drugs are less effective in Reiter's syndrome, crystalline arthropathy, and infectious arthritis.
4. Systemic steroids may alleviate the arthritis of connective tissue disease and gout, but they are less effective in infections, osteoarthritis, Reiter's syndrome, and psoriatic arthritis. They are not indicated in infectious arthritis.
5. The response to drugs with a broad spectrum of anti-inflammatory and analgesic activity is of little or no diagnostic value in either acute or chronic arthritis. A striking response to indomethacin or phenylbutazone in patients with severe lower back pain suggests the presence of ankylosing spondylitis or another seronegative spondyloarthropathy.

FAMILY HISTORY

1. A family history of "arthritis" is generally of little diagnostic significance.
2. A well-documented family history of gout, Heberden's nodes, psoriasis, ankylosing spondylitis, hemoglobinopathy, or abnormal bleeding may be of value.

## Physical Examination

In the physical examination, extraarticular manifestations of rheumatic disorders may provide important clues to specific diagnoses. Some of the more important of these findings are listed below.

1. Mucocutaneous lesions.
   a. Patchy alopecia may be seen in SLE and RA. The hair of the forehead is characteristically short and brittle in SLE.
   b. A combination of painful oral and genital ulcers with iritis suggests Behçet's syndrome. Ulcerative lesions of the penis and scrotum, or of the vulva and vagina, are commonly observed. Pyoderma may be noted.
   c. Painful oral ulcers, balanitis circinata and keratodermia blennorrhagica are features of Reiter's syndrome.
2. Cutaneous lesions.
   a. Erythematous cutaneous lesions, a malar butterfly rash (especially one precipitated by sun exposure), and erythematous lesions of the fingertips should suggest SLE.
   b. Subcutaneous nodules in the olecranon bursa, along the extensor surface of the forearm or along bony protuberances, are almost pathognomonic of RA, but they also are seen, although rarely, in patients with acute rheumatic fever and SLE. Subcutaneous nodules may be indistinguishable from the tophi of gout. Tophi commonly occur in the cartilage of the helix of the ear, the olecranon and patellar bursae, and the tendons.
   c. Indolent ischemic ulcers on the distal portion of the leg occur in RA with Felty's syndrome or vasculitis, and in SLE.
   d. Pyoderma gangrenosum as well as erythema nodosum is often associated with the arthropathy of ulcerative colitis.
   e. The presence of cutaneous psoriasis suggests the possibility of psoriatic arthritis, as do multiple pitted lesions of the nails with or without subungual keratoses and onycholysis.

**f.** Edematous, indurated, and atrophic changes in the skin, fingertip ulcerations, and hyperpigmentation are features of scleroderma.

**g.** Erythema over the knuckles, a dusky erythematous eruption in a "shawl" distribution over the shoulders, a lilac or heliotrope discoloration of the upper eyelids, and diffuse or localized muscle induration should suggest dermatomyositis.

**h.** A small red macule at the site of a tick bite that expands to form a large annular lesion with bright red outer border and partial central clearing may suggest ECM of Lyme disease.

**i.** Sweaty palms with thenar and hypothenar erythema are common in RA.

**j.** A salmon-colored macular, evanescent rash is characteristic of juvenile and adult-onset Still's disease.

**k.** Raynaud's phenomenon on examination or a convincing history of finger blanching suggests scleroderma, RA, or SLE.

3. Ocular lesions.

**a.** Keratoconjunctivitis sicca, xerostomia, nasopharyngeal ulceration, and parotid enlargement are manifestations of Sjögren's syndrome, which may be primary or associated with RA in about half the cases and less commonly with other connective tissue disease.

**b.** Conjunctivitis and iritis occur in Reiter's syndrome, sarcoidosis, AS, JRA, and Behçet's syndrome.

**c.** Retinal cytoid bodies are a manifestation of SLE. Retinal granulomata may be observed in sarcoidosis and tuberculosis.

4. Lymphadenopathy. A nonspecific abnormality, lymphadenopathy is not uncommon in SLE, RA, JRA, sarcoidosis, Lyme disease, and the arthritis seen in lymphomas.

5. Cardiopulmonary abnormalities.

**a.** Wheezing, cough, and shortness of breath may occur as a result of the pulmonary parenchymal disease sometimes found in RA, SLE, scleroderma, polymyositis, polyarteritis nodosa, and sarcoidosis.

**b.** Pleurisy with or without effusion may occur early in RA and SLE.

**c.** Cardiac involvement (pericarditis, heart block) may be a feature of any of the connective tissue diseases, Reiter's syndrome, or Lyme disease.

**d.** Aortic insufficiency may occur in acute rheumatic fever, RA, AS, Reiter's syndrome, and Behçet's syndrome.

**e.** Decreased chest expansion is a feature of ankylosing spondylitis.

6. Hepatosplenomegaly may be found in CTD, sarcoidosis, infections, Lyme disease, and chronic active hepatitis. Splenomegaly is a feature of Felty's syndrome, systemic JRA, and SLE.

7. Neurologic abnormalities.

**a.** Polyneuritis or mononeuritis multiplex may occur in the connective tissue diseases and neuropathic arthropathies.

**b.** Long tract signs and motor weakness may result from cervical cord compression most commonly due to C1-C2 subluxation in RA, ankylosing spondylitis, and less commonly, SLE.

**c.** Peripheral nerve entrapment syndromes may occur in RA, myxedema, and gout.

**d.** Neurologic manifestations of Lyme disease are protean and include cranial neuritis (Bell's palsy), meningitis, motor and sensory radiculoneuritis, chorea, and myelitis.

## Etiology of Peripheral Joint Disease

The mode of onset, clinical course, and pattern of joint involvement provide a convenient basis for classifying the clinical patterns of peripheral joint disease.

Four major categories can be identified: (1) acute polyarthritis, (2) chronic poly-arthritis, (3) acute monarthritis, and (4) chronic monarthritis. It should be recognized that although this classification is useful in the diagnostic approach to joint disease, it is not all-encompassing. Moreover, it should not be implied that all cases can be grouped into these categories. The most common causes of these clinical patterns are listed below.

## Acute Polyarthritis

1. Acute rheumatic fever.
2. Rheumatoid arthritis.
3. Other connective tissue diseases.
4. Seronegative spondyloarthropathies.
5. Infectious arthritis (especially gonococcal).
6. Gout.
7. Pseudogout.
8. Foreign protein reaction (serum sickness).
9. Palindromic rheumatism.
10. Sarcoidosis.

## Chronic Polyarthritis

1. Rheumatoid arthritis.
2. Other connective tissue diseases.
3. Seronegative spondyloarthropathies.
4. Chronic gouty arthritis.
5. Osteoarthritis.
6. Sarcoidosis.
7. Malignancy.

## Acute Monarthritis

1. Gout.
2. Pseudogout.
3. Traumatic joint disease.
4. Infectious arthritis (bacterial, tubercular, fungal).
5. Rheumatoid arthritis.
6. Osteoarthritis.
7. Seronegative spondyloarthropathies.
8. Lyme disesae.
9. Intermittent hydrarthrosis.

## Chronic Monarthritis

1. Infectious arthritis (bacterial, tubercular, fungal).
2. Traumatic arthritis.
3. Osteoarthritis.
4. Gout.
5. Pseudogout.
6. Neuropathic arthropathy.
7. Neoplasms (pigmented villonodular synovitis, osteochondromatosis, synovioma, metastatic).
8. Lyme disease.

## Clinical Features of Peripheral Joint Disease

The clinical manifestations and the pattern of joint involvement may provide useful clues to the diagnosis of arthritis.

### Acute Polyarthritis

1. Acute migratory polyarthritis in children and young adults beginning shortly after a streptococcal infection suggests ARF. Typically, there is swelling, heat, redness, tenderness, pain, and limitation of motion of two or more joints, most commonly the knees, ankles, elbows, wrists, hips, and small joints of the feet. According to the modified Jones criteria, the presence of two major criteria, or one major and two minor criteria, of those listed below, is considered diagnostic of ARF.
   a. Major manifestations.
      (1) Carditis.
         (a) Significant murmurs.
         (b) Cardiomegaly.
         (c) Pericarditis.
      (2) Polyarthritis.
      (3) Chorea.
      (4) Erythema marginatum.
      (5) Subcutaneous nodules.
   b. Minor manifestations.
      (1) Clinical.
         (a) History of previous ARF or evidence of rheumatic heart disease.
         (b) Arthralgias.
         (c) Fever (> 38°C).
      (2) Laboratory.
         (a) Elevated sedimentation rate and positive C-reactive protein test.
         (b) Electrocardiographic changes, chiefly prolongation of the P-R interval.
   c. Supporting evidence of streptococcal infection.
      (1) Laboratory.
         (a) Positive throat culture.
         (b) Positive antibody test (ASO titer).
      (2) Recent scarlet fever.
2. Although RA usually begins insidiously, it may begin as an acute polyarthritis. Favoring RA are the presence of prolonged morning stiffness and symmetric involvement of the small joints of the hands and feet. The need for a hot bath or shower in the morning in order to "get going" is also a helpful diagnostic finding, especially if this information is volunteered by the patient.
3. SLE may present as an acute polyarthritis. The American Rheumatism Association has proposed criteria for making the diagnosis of SLE. The presence, serially or simultaneously, of four or more manifestations strongly supports the diagnosis of SLE and militates against the presence of another CTD. The manifestations are listed in Table 8-1.
4. Seronegative spondyloarthropathies, such as psoriatic arthritis, Reiter's syndrome, and enteropathic arthropathy, may begin as an acute polyarthritis. The distinguishing features are discussed below (see Chronic Polyarthritis).
5. Gonococcal arthritis is usually a febrile illness beginning 1 to 2 weeks after a gonorrheal infection with evidence of a migratory polyarthritis. Eventually, the infection localizes to one or more joints. Signs of joint inflammation and tenosynovitis may be observed. Macular, hemorrhagic, vesicular, or pustular skin lesions are often seen. Culture of the synovial fluid is positive in less than 50 per-

**Table 8-1.** Criteria for the classification of systemic lupus erythematosus*

| Criteria | Definition |
|---|---|
| 1. Malar rash | Fixed erythema, flat or raised, over the malar eminences, tending to spare the nasolabial folds |
| 2. Discoid rash | Erythematosus raised patches with adherent keratotic scaling and follicular plugging; atrophic scarring may occur in older lesions |
| 3. Photosensitivity | Skin rash as a result of unusual reaction to sunlight, by patient history or physician observation |
| 4. Oral ulcers | Oral or nasopharyngeal ulceration, usually painless, observed by a physician |
| 5. Arthritis | Nonerosive arthritis involving 2 or more peripheral joints, characterized by tenderness, swelling, or effusion |
| 6. Serositis | Pleuritis—convincing history of pleuritic pain or rub heard by a physician or evidence of pleural effusion *OR* Pericarditis—documented by ECG or rub or evidence of pericardial effusion |
| 7. Renal disorder | Persistent proteinuria greater than 0.5/day or greater than 3 + if quantitation not performed *OR* Cellular casts—may be red cell, hemoglobin, granular, tubular, or mixed |
| 8. Neurologic disorder | Seizures—in the absence of offending drugs or known metabolic derangements; e.g., uremia, ketoacidosis, or electrolyte imbalance *OR* Psychosis—in the absence of offending drugs or known metabolic derangements, e.g., uremia, ketoacidosis, or electrolyte imbalance |
| 9. Hematologic disorder | Hemolytic anemia—with reticulocytosis *OR* Leukopenia—less than 4,000/μl total on 2 or more occasions *OR* Lymphopenia—less than 1,500/μl on 2 or more occasions *OR* Thrombocytopenia—less than 100,000/μl in the absence of offending drugs |
| 10. Immunologic disorder | Positive LE cell preparation *OR* Anti-DNA: antibody to native DNA in abnormal titer *OR* Anti-Sm: presence of antibody to Sm nuclear antigen *OR* False positive serologic test for syphilis known to be positive for at least 6 months and confirmed by *Treponema pallidum* immobilization or fluorescent treponemal antibody absorption test |
| 11. Antinuclear antibody | An abnormal titer of antinuclear antibody by immunofluorescence or an equivalent assay at any point in time and in the absence of drugs known to be associated with "drug-induced lupus" syndrome |

*The proposed classification is based on 11 criteria. For the purpose of identifying patients in clinical studies, a person shall be said to have systemic lupus erythematosus if any 4 or more of the 11 criteria are present, serially or simultaneously, during any interval of observation.
Source: Reprinted from the Primer on the Rheumatic Diseases, 8th edition. Copyright © 1983. Used by permission of the Arthritis Foundation.

cent of cases and is not necessary for the diagnosis. A good therapeutic response to penicillin but not to salicylates strongly supports the diagnosis in an appropriate clinical setting, even when bacteriologic studies are negative.

6. Infectious arthritis of other origin may present a similar picture. Joint involvement is by local extension or hematogenous spread.

7. Gout and pseudogout may show up in acute polyarticular form, but this is rare. The diagnosis depends on the demonstration of urate or calcium pyrophosphate dihydrate crystals, respectively, in the synovial fluid.

8. Foreign protein reactions, including serum sickness, may look like an acute polyarthritis. Clues to the correct diagnosis are a history of drug or horse serum administration and the presence of urticaria.

9. Palindromic rheumatism is an acute migratory polyarthritis in which the pattern of onset of the inflammation mimics the pattern of resolution.

## Chronic Polyarthritis

1. A progressive, symmetric polyarthritis with fusiform swelling of the joints, muscle atrophy, and, eventually, deformities is characteristic of RA. There is a predilection for involvement of the PIP and MCP joints of the fingers, the MTP joints of the feet, and the toes, wrists, knees, elbows, shoulders, and hips. Stiffness after inactivity, especially in the morning upon arising, is a characteristic symptom. Subcutaneous nodules, when present, are virtually pathognomonic. The outcome of a test for RF is positive in 70 to 80 percent of cases.

2. A chronic rheumatoid arthropathy may occur in other CTD, especially in SLE. Recurrent or persistent small joint inflammation in the absence of deformity or radiographic erosions also suggests SLE. Ankylosis and contractures are uncommon. An overlap syndrome, labeled MCTD, incorporates clinical features of SLE, scleroderma, and polymyositis. The articular manifestations resemble those seen in SLE, with arthritis or arthralgias in over 90 percent of patients. Marked swelling of the hands, particularly the fingers, leads to a sausagelike appearance. Raynaud's phenomenon, a low incidence of renal involvement, and a good response to steroid therapy further characterize this entity.

3. Polyarthritis may occur in the seronegative spondyloarthropathies. In these diseases, joint involvement tends to be asymmetric and progression to deformity is less common than in RA. Interphalangeal synovitis of the toes ("sausage toes") is a feature of Reiter's syndrome, psoriatic arthritis, and the peripheral arthritis of AS. Spondylitis and sacroiliitis are commonly observed in the HLA group of diseases. Tests for RF are usually negative. There is a link between HLA-B27 and the seronegative spondyloarthropathies.

   a. Reiter's disease is characterized by a combination of urethritis, iritis or conjunctivitis, arthritis, and often diarrhea, balanitis, and keratodermia blennorrhagica. Heel pain in a young male should suggest this diagnosis. Spinal involvement similar to that of AS may occur; asymmetric sacroiliac involvement is the rule in Reiter's disease.

   b. Psoriatic arthritis may mimic RA. Involvement of the DIP joints, typical changes in the nails, cutaneous psoriasis, and a positive family history are clues to the diagnosis.

   c. AS with peripheral arthritis is not often mistaken for RA when the spinal involvement dominates the clinical picture, but it may begin with peripheral joint signs.

   d. Enteropathic arthritis (e.g., arthritis associated with regional enteritis and ulcerative colitis) may simulate the polyarthritis of RA. The joint symptoms may precede the gastrointestinal disease.

4. Although chronic gouty arthritis may mimic RA, advanced deforming arthritic changes due to gout are uncommon. A long history of acute episodic arthritis with remissions between attacks can usually be obtained. Hyperuricemia, the demonstration of urate crystals in the synovial fluid, response to colchicine, and biopsy of a gouty tophus have confirmatory value.

5. Osteoarthritis is a polyarticular disease, with symptoms usually related to involvement of the knees, hips, vertebral column, and hands. Heberden's nodes are bony protuberances of the DIP joints of the fingers, often associated with flexion and angulation of the distal phalanges. Local pain, tenderness, and some warmth may be present. Tender, knobby enlargement of the PIP joints (Bouchard's nodes) is not uncommon and may cause confusion with RA. Degenerative changes in the knees are often manifested by pain, joint swelling, crepitus, and deformity. Slight increase in skin temperature over the joint is a common finding. Involvement of the spine and hips is discussed in the sections Painful Hip and Low Back Pain, later in this chapter.

6. The joint swelling present in cases of hypertrophic osteoarthropathy may be mistaken for a polyarthritis of other origin. The presence of clubbing and an association with chronic pulmonary disease, bronchogenic carcinoma, cyanotic congenital heart disease, cirrhosis, or enteropathic disease usually make the diagnosis apparent. The presence of periosteal proliferation on x-ray is confirmatory.

### Acute and Chronic Monarthritis

1. Acute monarticular arthritis in a male involving the MTP joint of the great toe, instep, heel, ankle, knee, wrist, hand, or elbow, with complete recovery between attacks, is virtually pathognomonic of gout. The diagnosis is established by the demonstration of urate crystals in the synovial fluid or a therapeutic response to adequate doses of colchicine. Hyperuricemia is usually but not always present. Tophi are found in advanced cases.

2. Acute monarticular arthritis may also be due to pseudogout (chondrocalcinosis). The diagnosis depends on finding calcium pyrophosphate dihydrate crystals in aspirated synovial fluid and on the presence of calcium deposits in the menisci or the articular cartilages.

3. Trauma frequently affects only one joint. Since the trauma is usually severe, the diagnosis is generally evident from the history.

4. Pyogenic, tuberculous, or gonococcal arthritis is commonly monarticular, and evidence of antecedent or concomitant infection is not difficult to obtain. Cytologic and bacteriologic study of the synovial fluid establishes the etiologic diagnosis.

5. Although several joints are usually affected in osteoarthritis, involvement of a single weight-bearing joint, such as the knee or hip, may dominate the clinical picture. Further details may be found under the heading Chronic Polyarthritis, above, and in the section Painful Hip, later in this chapter.

6. RA and especially JRA may be monarticular at the onset of the disease. Local signs of inflammation are commonly observed. The diagnosis may become apparent only after a prolonged period of observation. Infectious arthritis and other causes of monarthritis must be excluded.

7. Neuropathic arthropathy (Charcot's joint) is characterized by joint hypermobility, effusion, and disproportionately little pain in association with a primary neurologic disorder such as tabes dorsalis, diabetic neuropathy, or syringomyelia.

8. Pigmented villonodular synovitis, synovial chondromatosis, and chondrosarcoma are less common causes of monarthritis.

9. The typical pattern of arthritis in Lyme disease is intermittent mono- or pauciarticular (< four joints) synovitis of large joints, especially the knees. Approximately 10 percent of cases develop chronic arthritis with cartilage damage and erosions.

---

## Diagnostic Procedures in Arthritis

### Synovial Fluid Analysis

Synovial fluid analysis should include the following: white cell count, differential count, crystal identification, gram and acid-fast stains, and culture. The pertinent findings on examination of joint fluid are summarized in Tables 8-2 and 8-3.

**Table 8-2.** Examination of joint fluid

| Measure | Normal | Group I (noninflammatory) | Group II (inflammatory) | Group III (septic) |
|---|---|---|---|---|
| Volume (ml) (knee) | <3.5 | Often >3.5 | Often >3.5 | Often >3.5 |
| Clarity | Transparent | Transparent | Translucent-opaque | Opaque |
| Color | Clear | Yellow | Yellow to opalescent | Yellow to green |
| Viscosity | High | High | Low | Variable |
| WBC (per cu mm) | <200 | 200 to 2000 | 2000 to 100,000 | >100,000* |
| Polymorphonuclear leukocytes (%) | <25% | <25% | 50% or more | 75% or more* |
| Culture | Negative | Negative | Negative | Often positive |

*Lower with infections caused by partially treated or low-virulence organisms.
Source: Reprinted from Primer on the rheumatic diseases, *J.A.M.A.* 224:661, 1973.

**Table 8-3.** Differential diagnosis by joint fluid groups

| Group I (noninflammatory) | Group II (inflammatory) | Group III (septic) | Hemorrhagic |
|---|---|---|---|
| Degenerative joint disease | Rheumatoid arthritis | Bacterial infections | Hemophilia or other hemorrhagic diathesis |
| Trauma* | Acute crystal-induced synovitis (gout and pseudogout) | | Trauma with or without fracture |
| Osteochondritis dissecans | Reiter's syndrome | | Neuropathic arthropathy |
| Osteochromatosis | Ankylosing spondylitis | | Pigmented villonodular synovitis |
| Neuropathic arthropathy* | Psoriatic arthritis | | Synovioma |
| Subsiding or early inflammation | Arthritis accompanying ulcerative colitis and regional enteritis | | Hemangioma and other benign neoplasms |
| Hypertrophic osteoarthropathy† | Rheumatic fever† | | |
| Pigmented villonodular synovitis* | Systemic lupus erythematosus† | | |
| | Progressive systemic sclerosis (scleroderma)† | | |

*May be hemorrhagic
†Groups I or II
Source: Reprinted from Primer on the rheumatic diseases, *J.A.M.A.* 224:661, 1973.

Table 8-4 contains information concerning commonly used laboratory tests in the diagnosis of arthritis.

## Suggested Workup for Acute Arthritis

1. CBC.
2. Urinalysis.
3. ESR (Westergren).
4. Biochemical screening.
5. Test for RF, including titer.
6. ANA, including titer.
7. HB$_s$Ag.
8. HLA-B27, if compatible with spondyloarthritis.
9. Exclusion of infectious process clinically, and if necessary, by cytologic study and culture of synovial fluid.
10. Synovial fluid analysis to rule out crystalline arthropathy when appropriate. Culture of cervix, rectum, throat, and skin lesions when indicated.
11. X-rays of involved and contralateral joints.
12. Chest films to rule out sarcoid arthritis.
13. Electrocardiogram.
14. Antispirochetal (Lyme) antibodies.

## Suggested Workup for Chronic Arthritis

1. CBC.
2. Urinalysis.
3. ESR (Westergren).
4. Biochemical screening.
5. Liver profile.
6. Test for RF, including titer.
7. ANA, including titer.
8. HLA-B27, if compatible with spondyloarthritis.
9. Serologic test for syphilis.
10. Thyroid function tests, if appropriate.
11. X-rays of involved and contralateral joints.
12. Chest films.
13. Electrocardiogram.
14. Synovial fluid analysis.
15. Special procedures, when appropriate.
    a. Immunoglobulins.
    b. Serum complement.
    c. Creatinine clearance.
    d. Coagulation screening.
    e. Esophageal motility studies.
    f. Contrast studies of the gastrointestinal tract.
    g. Biopsy of subcutaneous nodules, tophi, or synovium.
    h. Electromyogram.
    i. Technetium bone scan.
16. Antispirochetal (Lyme) antibodies.

---

# MYALGIA
Kenneth P. Glassman
Herbert Kaplan

## Definition

---

Myalgia is poorly localized aching in a muscle or group of muscles. Although any of the diseases that primarily affect the joints may also cause muscle pain, this

**Table 8-4.** Diagnostic procedures in arthritis

| Test | Purpose | Results and interpretation |
| --- | --- | --- |
| CBC | Routine | Anemia common in RA, connective tissue diseases, rheumatoid variants<br>Leukocytosis in infectious arthritis, juvenile RA, crystalline arthropathy, occasionally RA; eosinophilia rare in RA<br>Leukopenia common in SLE; also occurs in Felty's syndrome |
| ESR (Westergren method) | Routine | Nonspecific sign of inflammatory disease<br>May parallel severity of RA<br>When normal, favors noninflammatory joint disease<br>Strikingly elevated in polymyalgia rheumatica<br>Normal values increase with age |
| Urinalysis | Routine | Proteinuria in nephropathy of SLE, polyarteritis nodosa, scleroderma, gout<br>Pyuria in gonorrhea, Reiter's syndrome<br>Cylindruria and RBC casts in SLE nephritis |
| RF | Diagnosis of RA | Nonspecific test, not absolutely pathognomonic of RA, but is suggestive of the diagnosis when titer exceeds 1 : 80<br>May be positive in 5–10% of normal individuals above the age of 50 years and in 20–30% of cases of SLE. Sometimes positive in connective tissue diseases, rheumatoid variants, and diseases associated with hypergammaglobulinemia |

| Test | Purpose | Comments |
|---|---|---|
| ANA | Diagnosis of SLE, MCTD | ANA more sensitive than LE cell phenomenon but less specific for the diagnosis of SLE. What constitutes a significant titer and the importance of the pattern of ANA varies with different laboratories and the techniques of performing the test<br>ANA rarely if ever absent in SLE but frequently positive in low titer in other CTD and in 5% of "healthy" elderly individuals<br>High titer of speckled ANA seen in MCTD |
| Antibody to RNP | Diagnosis of MCTD | Positive in very high percentage of MCTD<br>May be positive in SLE |
| Antibody to native DNA | Diagnosis of SLE | High titer strongly suggestive of SLE<br>May be positive in some patients with RA |
| HLA-B27 (histocompatibility antigen) | Detection of occult axial arthropathy | Positive in 85–95% of patients with AS and Reiter's syndrome<br>May be positive in enteropathic and psoriatic arthropathy with spinal involvement |
| Anti-DNA | Reflects activity of SLE | Serial determinations of value in monitoring efficacy of therapy in SLE |
| Skin biopsy for immunofluorescence | Diagnosis of SLE | Immunoglobulins at dermal-epidermal junction in sun-protected areas in 50–60% of patients with SLE |
| HB$_s$AG | Detection of hepatitis B infection | Present in arthritis of type B viral hepatitis<br>Positive in some patients with PAN |
| Liver profile | Diagnosis of arthritis associated with liver disease | Abnormal in acute viral hepatitis, chronic active hepatitis, primary biliary cirrhosis, sarcoidosis |
| T$_4$ and T$_3$ resin uptake, TSH | Diagnosis of hypothyroidism | Performed to rule out hypothyroidism, which may produce rheumatoid-like arthropathy and a carpal tunnel syndrome |

**Table 8-4** (continued)

| Test | Purpose | Results and interpretation |
|------|---------|----------------------------|
| CPK, SGOT, aldolase | Diagnosis of polymyositis | One or all elevated in polymyositis<br>CPK often elevated in myopathy of hypothyroidism<br>Enzymes normal in polymyalgia rheumatica and other connective tissue diseases |
| Serum calcium, phosphorus, alkaline phosphatase | Detection of arthritis associated with intrinsic bone disease | Hypercalcemia, hypophosphatemia, and elevated alkaline phosphatase in hyperparathyroidism<br>Hypercalcemia, often present in sarcoidosis, metastatic malignancy<br>Alkaline phosphatase increased in osteomalacia |
| *Borella burgdorferi* antibodies | Detection of infection with the Lyme spirochete | Elevated IgM titers peak 4–6 weeks after infectious IgG titers stay elevated in chronic cases; false positives occur in other autoimmune diseases (SLE, RA) and other spirochetal infections (syphilis, relapsing fever) |

| | | |
|---|---|---|
| Serum protein electrophoresis, immunoglobulins | Detection of hyperglobulinemia and dysproteinemias | Hyperglobulinemia seen in sarcoidosis, enteropathic arthropathy, lymphomas, other malignancies, and advanced stages of some connective tissue diseases<br>Diffuse hypergammaglobulinemia in chronic infection, liver disease, SLE, and RA<br>Monoclonal gammopathy in myeloma, macroglobulinemia, some cases of primary amyloidosis or carcinoma, and some normal elderly persons |
| Serum uric acid | Detection of hyperuricemia | Causes of hyperuricemia<br>Asymptomatic, genetic<br>Gout (primary or secondary)<br>Drugs (e.g., salicylates, diuretics)<br>Hematologic disorders (e.g., polycythemia, leukemia, hemolytic anemias)<br>Renal disease<br>Hypertension<br>Hereditary disorders (e.g., Lesch-Nyhan syndrome)<br>Endocrine disorders |

discussion is limited to patients with muscle pain and minimal or no articular involvement.

---

## Etiology

---

Myalgia may be secondary to rheumatic or nonrheumatic conditions. The causes are listed in order of decreasing frequency within each group.
1. Rheumatic disorders.
    **a.** Fibrositis and psychogenic rheumatism. Both conditions are diagnosed by exclusion. A consideration of whether they are the same condition or separate entities is beyond the scope of this discussion.
    **b.** Tendinitis and peritendinitis.
    **c.** Connective tissue diseases.
    **d.** Ankylosing spondylitis.
    **e.** Polymyalgia rheumatica.
    **f.** Sarcoidosis.
2. Nonrheumatic disorders.
    **a.** Infectious diseases (viremia, bacteremia).
    **b.** Disease of the spinal column (intervertebral disk protrusion, spondylolisthesis, osteoporosis of the spine).
    **c.** Peripheral nerve entrapment syndromes (e.g., carpal tunnel syndrome).
    **d.** Neoplasms, including hypertrophic osteoarthropathy.
    **e.** Endocrine disorders (hypothyroidism, hyperparathyroidism, acromegaly, osteomalacia).
    **f.** Peripheral neuritis, including diabetic neuropathy, pernicious anemia.
    **g.** Drug-induced myalgia.
        **(1)** Steroid-induced pseudorheumatism.
        **(2)** Hypokalemia secondary to diuretics.
        **(3)** SLE syndrome secondary to anticonvulsants, hydralazine, procainamide, isoniazid, antibiotics.
        **(4)** Chloroquine.
    **h.** Reflex sympathetic dystrophy (shoulder-hand syndrome).
    **i.** Alcoholism, acute and chronic.
    **j.** Parkinson's disease.
    **k.** Paget's disease of bone.
    **l.** Postgastrectomy (subtotal).

---

## Clinical Features

---

Table 8-5 lists the clinical features of the most common causes of myalgia. Table 8-6 lists criteria for the classification of fibromyalgia.

---

## Diagnostic Approach

---

### History

1. Mode of onset.
    **a.** An insidious onset and gradual course are typical of most of the etiologic entities. A sudden onset is reported in the majority of patients with polymyalgia rheumatica and those with occult or overt infections.
    **b.** Acute muscle pain, often associated with muscle swelling during the course of an alcoholic bout, is seen in alcoholic myopathy.
2. Area of involvement.
    **a.** The more localized and symmetrical the area of discomfort, the more likely it is that the diagnosis is fibrositis.

    **b.** Specific localization over a tendon is helpful, as in bicipital tendinitis, de Quervain's disease, or the carpal tunnel syndrome.

    **c.** Involvement of the muscles of the neck, the pelvic and pectoral girdles, and the thighs and upper arms occurs in polymyalgia rheumatica. The muscles below the elbows and knees are not affected in this condition.

    **d.** Concomitant arthritis in an adjacent or distant joint suggests one of the connective tissue diseases. However, CTD may be present with myalgia unassociated with articular involvement.

    **e.** Episodic or continuous aching in the low back region or shoulder girdle occurring in a young male, with or without sciatic radiation and improved by activity and NSAID, suggests AS.

    **f.** Pain in the muscles of the pelvic girdle and thighs may occur in Paget's disease.

**3.** A history of use of any of the drugs listed above as etiologic agents suggests drug-induced myalgia.

**4.** Response or lack of response to therapy.

    **a.** Anti-inflammatory drugs (salicylates, steroids, indomethacin, phenylbutazone, and other NSAID) may give some relief in both rheumatic and nonrheumatic conditions. Hence, the response to these agents is of little diagnostic value, although dramatic relief of low back pain with indomethacin or phenylbutazone suggests AS.

    **b.** Failure to respond to anti-inflammatory analgesic treatment should suggest fibrositis psychogenic rheumatism, peripheral neuritis, nerve entrapment, reflex neurovascular dystrophy, endocrinopathy, Parkinson's disease, or nonmuscular causes of pain.

## System Review

In the system review, areas of inquiry specifically applicable to the evaluation of myalgia are listed below.

**1.** Weight loss, malaise, anorexia, and fever suggest neoplasia (with or without associated dermatomyositis), granulomatous disease (sarcoidosis, tuberculosis), infection, or giant cell arteritis.

**2.** The well-known but nonspecific symptoms of hypothyroidism suggest the myopathy associated with this disease.

**3.** Recurrent and severe headaches, especially in the temporal region, a history of tender spots over the scalp, claudication of the jaw, and unilateral or bilateral blurring or loss of vision suggest temporal arteritis associated with polymyalgia rheumatica.

**4.** Neuropsychiatric evaluation during the history-taking process is most important in evaluating a patient with myalgia. Overemphasis by the patient of a "strong family history of arthritis," multitudinous complaints, strong denial of any emotional problems, grimacing, and autopalpation during the teary-eyed recitation of symptoms all may be clues to psychogenic rheumatism.

## Physical Examination

GENERAL EXAMINATION

The abnormalities noted in the section Peripheral Joint Arthritis, earlier in the chapter, should also be sought in evaluating the patient who has myalgia. Abnormalities on the general physical examination that are specifically pertinent to the patient with myalgia are as follows:

**1.** Lethargy, a husky voice, dry skin and hair, edema, and delayed tendon reflex relaxation suggest hypothyroidism. The well-known facies and bone structure of acromegaly should suggest the myopathy associated with this disease.

**2.** The motor, sensory, and reflex changes caused by nerve root compression in the cervical or lumbar area may be observed in patients in whom myalgia is second-

**Table 8-5.** Clinical features of the most common causes of myalgia

| Cause | History | Physical examination | Laboratory data | Course |
|---|---|---|---|---|
| Fibrositis | Symmetrical, reproducible, relatively localized muscular aching with or without morning stiffness; occurs predominantly in females | Reproducible, localized muscle tender points | Negative | Chronic, nonprogressive, nondeforming; must first rule out all other rheumatic diseases |
| Psychogenic rheumatism | Pain described in bizarre terms (tearing; pulsating); role of emotions vigorously denied | Nonreproducible tender points; histrionic reaction to light palpation | Negative | Chronic; psychiatric consultation indicated; refractory to medical management |
| Tendinitis, peritendinitis, capsulitis (especially shoulder) | Acute or insidious onset, often associated with trauma or excessive use of muscle involved | Local tenderness over tendon insertion and contiguous muscle; periarticular tenderness; limited motion common | Negative | Self-limited, although it may result in joint deformity (especially with shoulder involvement) |
| Rheumatoid arthritis | Muscular symptoms may precede articular symptoms; often severe pain and stiffness | Usually significant synovitis in the peripheral joints; subcutaneous nodules; muscle wasting if severe | ESR elevated; RF positive; minimal inflammation on muscle biopsy | Severe muscle symptoms in RA often associated with more ominous course |
| Polymyalgia rheumatica | Typically, elderly female, with relatively acute onset of aching and stiffness of the proximal muscles and pelvic and shoulder girdles | Painful and tender proximal muscles without true weakness; minimal synovitis; possible temporal artery tenderness | Striking elevation of ESR; other tests negative | Dramatic response in 6 hours to steroids; may be a prodrome of RA, other connective tissue disease, or cancer |

| | | | | |
|---|---|---|---|---|
| Dermatomyositis, SLE, scleroderma, MCTD | Usually insidious onset except in dermatomyositis | Abnormal muscle consistency, wasting, weakness; skin induration in SLE and dermatomyositis | Abnormal SGOT, CPK, aldolase in dermatomyositis; positive anti-PM1 in dermatomyositis; positive ANA in SLE; positive RNP in MCTD; soft tissue calcification in scleroderma and dermatomyositis; abnormal esophageal motility may be present in all; muscle biopsy abnormal in dermatomyositis; EMG abnormal | Variable; better prognosis in MCTD |
| Infection | Acute onset associated with overt or occult infection | Fever and signs associated with infection | Leukocytosis, elevated ESR | Improves with treatment of infection |
| Drug-induced | Steroids, diuretics, hydralazine, chloroquine; drug-induced SLE (anticonvulsants, procainamide) | Usually negative although more pulmonary involvement than in primary SLE. Muscle weakness in steroid myopathy | Eosinophilia, hypocalcemia. Positive ANA (antihistone antibodies in drug-induced SLE) | Remission occurs when offending drug is stopped |
| Seronegative spondyloarthropathy (AS, Reiter's Syndrome, psoriatic arthritis) | Chronic low back or neck ache, or both; marked morning stiffness relieved by activity. Buttock and thigh radiation. Chronic myalgia with history of iritis, scaly skin rash, balanitis | Sacroiliac joint tenderness, loss of lumbar lordosis. Peripheral synovitis in 25% | ESR often elevated. HLA-B27+ in 80 to 90% of AS and Reiter's, 70% of psoriasis with spine involvement. Spine and sacroiliac joints may be normal radiographically early in course | Usually good response to indomethacin or phenylbutazone; less striking benefit from other NSAID. Deformity may be less with maintenance physical therapy program |

**Table 8-6.** The American College of Rheumatology 1990 criteria for classification of fibromyalgia*

1. History of widespread pain
   *Definition:* Pain is considered widespread when all the following are present—pain in the left side of the body, pain in the right side of the body, pain above the waist, and pain below the waist. In addition, axial skeletal pain (cervical spine, anterior chest, thoracic spine, or low back) must be present. In this definition, shoulder and buttock pain is considered as pain for each involved side. "Low back" pain is considered lower segment pain
2. Pain in 11 of 18 tender point sites on digital palpation
   *Definition:* On digital palpation, pain must be present in at least 11 of the following 18 tender point sites:
   *Occiput*—bilateral, at the suboccipital muscle insertions
   *Low cervical*—bilateral, at the anterior aspects of the intertransverse spaces at C5–7
   *Trapezius*—bilateral, at the midpoint of the upper border
   *Supraspinatus*—bilateral, at origins, above the scapular spine near the medial border
   *Second rib*—bilateral, at the second costochondral junctions, just lateral to the junctions on upper surfaces
   *Lateral epicondyle*—bilateral, 2 cm distal to the epicondyles
   *Gluteal*—bilateral, in upper outer quadrants of buttocks in anterior fold of muscle
   *Greater trochanter*—bilateral, posterior to the trochanteric prominence
   *Knee*—bilateral, at the medial fat proximal to the joint line
   Digital palpation should be performed with an approximate force of 4 kg
   For a tender point to be considered "positive," the subject must state that the palpation was painful. "Tender" is not to be considered "painful"

---

*For classification purposes, patients will be said to have fibromyalgia if both criteria are satisfied. Widespread pain must have been present for at least 3 months. The presence of a second clinical disorder does not exclude the diagnosis of fibromyalgia.
Source: Reprinted from *Arthritis and rheumatism* 33:160–172, 1990. Used by permission of the American College of Rheumatology.

---

ary to intervertebral disk protrusion. Pain or tingling in the forearm or hand, or both, while tapping over the median nerve at the wrist (Tinel's sign) suggests the carpal tunnel syndrome. Median nerve compression at the wrist may cause aching proximal to the wrist and extending to the shoulder. A masklike facies, a pill-rolling tremor, and rigidity suggest Parkinson's disease.

3. An erythematous, indurated rash over the "shawl" distribution of the shoulders, face, and extremities may be seen in dermatomyositis. Indurated skin is observed in scleroderma. Symptoms and signs of SLE, dermatomyositis, and scleroderma are seen in MCTD.
4. Hepatosplenomegaly, spider angiomata, and clubbed fingers, with or without other physical findings of the alcoholic, suggest alcoholic myopathy.
5. A shiny skin with swollen fingers, atrophic skin, and hyperhidrosis of palms is seen in the shoulder-hand syndrome.
6. Temporal artery thickening or tenderness and bruits over carotid or other peripheral arteries may be found in some cases of polymyalgia rheumatica.

MUSCULOSKELETAL EXAMINATION

Many of the disease entities causing myalgia may show abnormalities of the musculoskeletal system, as described in the section Peripheral Joint Arthritis, earlier in the chapter. Examination of the muscles may reveal various abnormalities.

1. Moderate to exquisite tenderness in many muscle groups without anatomic localization, normal muscle tone, absence of muscle atrophy, and maintenance of a normal range of motion are characteristic of psychogenic rheumatism.

2. Striking proximal muscle stiffness without weakness, normal muscle consistency, and marked periarticular tenderness in the proximal musculature of the shoulder and pectoral girdle in a patient over 55 (female-male ratio 5 : 1) suggest PMR.
3. Proximal muscle weakness, often with induration and muscle tenderness, with or without an associated skin rash, occurs in dermatomyositis.
4. Severe low back pain, with or without percussion tenderness over one or more vertebrae, suggests osteoporosis with possible compression fracture, myeloma, or metastatic bone disease.

## Laboratory Studies

The diagnostic survey outlined in the section Peripheral Joint Arthritis, earlier in the chapter, is applicable to the patient with myalgia.
1. Normal findings on a battery of tests do not rule out organic disease but strongly favor fibrositis or psychogenic rheumatism.
2. An ESR (Westergren) greater than 50 mm/hour with no other abnormality suggests polymyalgia rheumatica.
3. One or more serum enzymes (SGOT, CPK, aldolase) are commonly elevated in dermatomyositis, and the EMG may be abnormal.
4. Decreased thyroid function occurs in hypothyroidism, but the only abnormality may be an elevation of TSH.
5. Hypokalemia is usually diuretic-induced.
6. Hypercalcemia may be associated with the myopathy of hyperparathyroidism, sarcoidosis, myeloma, and metastatic carcinoma.
7. Hyperuricemia is commonly associated with the myopathy of lymphoma, leukemia, sarcoidosis, hyperparathyroidism, and hypothyroidism.
8. The serum alkaline phosphatase level is usually elevated in Paget's disease of the bone, metastatic carcinoma, sarcoidosis, hyperparathyroidism, and osteomalacia.
9. The ANA is likely to be positive in CTD and the drug-induced SLE syndrome. Antihistone antibodies are present in drug-induced SLE.
10. The postprandial blood sugar or glucose tolerance test is abnormal in the occasional patient with diabetes who exhibits diabetic amyotrophy before other abnormalities of this disease are manifested.
11. A characteristic triad of abnormalities is seen in the electromyogram in polymyositis: spontaneous fibrillations with positive, saw-toothed (spike) potentials, complex polyphasic or short-duration potentials on voluntary contraction, and salvos of repetitive high-frequency action potentials.
12. Temporal artery biopsy and arteriograms may be abnormal in polymyalgia rheumatica.
13. Muscle biopsy may show inflammatory changes in polymyositis. Muscle tissue studied with histochemical techniques shows abnormalities in patients with polymyalgia rheumatica and rheumatoid arthritis.

## Radiologic Findings

In a patient with myalgia, the following roentgenographic abnormalities should be sought:
1. Hilar adenopathy or pulmonary parenchymal abnormalities would suggest sarcoidosis, neoplasm, or CTD.
2. Subcutaneous calcifications may be seen in scleroderma and dermatomyositis. Calcification about the shoulder joint is common objective evidence for tendinitis in this area.
3. Subtle changes of sclerosis of the sacroiliac joints, squaring of the vertebrae, and spinal ligamentous calcification occur in ankylosing spondylitis. In the spine, intervertebral disk space narrowing, spondylolisthesis, osteoporosis, and foraminal encroachment secondary to osteoarthritis are capable of causing muscle pain.
4. Radionuclide joint scans may show inflammation before changes are visible in conventional roentgenograms.

# PAINFUL SHOULDER
Robert C. Jacobs

Shoulder pain is the symptom that causes most patients with shoulder disorders to seek medical attention. The pain may arise from the joint structures or the periarticular tissues, or both. It is also important to be aware that the shoulder is a common site of pain referral from cervical, intrathoracic, and diaphragmatic lesions. Contrary to popular belief, nonarticular disorders of the shoulder, not arthritis, cause the vast majority of painful shoulders. Fractures and dislocations are not considered in this discussion.

## Etiology

Omitting fractures and dislocations, approximately 80 to 90 percent of cases of shoulder disability are caused by one of the following conditions: acute and chronic tendinitis and bursitis (often calcific), bicipital tenosynovitis, adhesive capsulitis, and lesions of the musculotendinous cuff. The more common causes of shoulder pain and disability are listed in Table 8-7.

## Clinical Features

### Calcific Tendinitis and Bursitis

Pain, tenderness, and limited motion of the shoulder are characteristic findings in calcific tendinitis. The condition may be acute, subacute, or chronic. On examination, there is tenderness below the tip of the acromion, especially pronounced in acute cases. X-ray films of the shoulder show calcific deposits in the vicinity of the affected tendon.

### Bicipital Tenosynovitis

Bicipital tenosynovitis is a common cause of shoulder pain. The onset is acute or insidious. The pain usually radiates along the course of the bicipital tendon, and muscle tenderness over the tendon in the bicipital groove is characteristic. Shoulder motion is generally limited, particularly in abduction and internal rotation. Yergason's sign (the production of pain on resisted supination of the forearm while the elbow is flexed at 90 degrees) is usually positive. X-ray findings are negative. When the condition is chronic, the shoulder may become "frozen."

### Adhesive Capsulitis

The onset of adhesive capsulitis is acute or insidious. It is often precipitated by trauma or strain but probably has varied causes. In some instances, it represents the end stage of other conditions. The clinical manifestations include localized pain, diffuse periarticular tenderness, and often a profound reduction in shoulder mobility that may eventually result in complete limitation of glenohumeral motion (frozen shoulder). X-ray findings are negative except for demineralization of the humerus in long-standing cases.

### Lesions of the Musculotendinous Cuff

The rotator cuff is able to withstand mild to moderate injury with little effect unless the tendons are already diseased as a result of degenerative changes. The supraspinatus tendon is the one most frequently affected. Partial or complete rupture of this tendon is usually precipitated by a fall with the shoulder ab-

**Table 8-7.** Common causes of shoulder pain

A. Intrinsic lesions
1. Periarticular disorders
   a. Calcific tendinitis
   b. Adhesive capsulitis
   c. Bicipital tendinitis
   d. Lesions of the musculotendinous cuff
2. Articular disorders
   a. Inflammatory lesions
      (1) Connective tissue diseases
      (2) Rheumatoid variants
      (3) Crystalline arthropathies
   b. Osteoarthritis
   c. Neuropathic arthropathy
   d. Traumatic arthritis
   e. Infectious arthritis
   f. Neoplasms
B. Extrinsic lesions
1. Neurologic disorders
   a. Central nervous system (e.g., cervical disks, herpes zoster)
   b. Peripheral nervous system (e.g., neuropathy)
2. Neurovascular syndromes
   a. Thoracic outlet syndromes
      (1) Cervical and first rib syndromes, scalenus anterior syndrome
      (2) Costoclavicular syndrome
      (3) Hyperabduction syndrome
   b. Reflex neurovascular syndromes
      (1) Shoulder-hand syndrome
      (2) Sudeck's atrophy
3. Vascular syndromes
   a. Arterial (e.g., arterial occlusion, Raynaud's phenomenon)
   b. Venous (e.g., venous occlusion, thrombophlebitis)
   c. Lymphatic (e.g., lymphangitis, lymphedema)
4. Psychogenic disorders
5. Viscerogenic disorders (referred pain)
6. Idiopathic disorders (e.g., fibrositic syndromes, myalgias, arthralgias, neuralgias)

---

ducted. The injury is followed by pain, limited motion of the shoulder, and especially, an inability to initiate abduction. Tenderness over the tip of the shoulder and a sulcus at the site of rupture may be noted. Assisted abduction may cause pain when the acromial process impinges on the damaged tendon. Once the arm is elevated to 90 degrees or more, the glenohumeral joint can usually be held in abduction with little or no pain. X-rays may reveal elevation of the humeral head, concavity of the acromial process, and cystic changes in the bone. An arthrogram may demonstrate leakage of dye through the rotator cuff.

## Neurovascular Syndromes

1. **Reflex neurovascular dystrophy (the shoulder-hand syndrome).** The shoulder-hand syndrome is a symptom complex characterized by painful disability of the shoulder in association with painful swelling of the hand. The latter may precede, accompany, or follow the former. Vasomotor disturbances (vasospasm or vasodilatation) are common. The condition may terminate with permanent dystrophic changes and contractures of the hand and fingers. The syndrome may be unilateral or bilateral. Provocative or associated conditions include myocardial infarction, cervical osteoarthritis, trauma, hemiplegia, and other disorders. Approxi-

mately 25 percent of cases are idiopathic. Mottled or diffuse osteoporosis of the humeral head and wrist is a characteristic x-ray finding.
2. Other neurovascular syndromes. The distinctive features of the costoclavicular, hyperabduction, and the scalenus anterior and cervical rib syndromes and their differential diagnosis from the shoulder-hand syndrome are summarized in Table 8-8 (see section The Thoracic Outlet Syndrome, Chapter 10, and p. 41 for additional information).

### Fibromyopathies

See the section Myalgia, earlier in the chapter.

## Diagnostic Approach

### History

1. The history is of little diagnostic assistance. Inquiry should be made concerning previous involvement or the presence of systemic disease.
2. A history of minor trauma or strain is commonly elicited in musculotendinous lesions. Tendon rupture is suggested by a sudden onset of pain and inability to abduct the shoulder precipitated by a fall or a sudden strain in abduction.
3. The diagnosis of a shoulder-hand syndrome should be entertained in patients who have sustained a myocardial infarct, stroke, or trauma to the distal portion of the upper extremity (e.g., Colles' fracture). Cervical radicular syndromes, thoracotomy, and pulmonary disease (e.g., tuberculosis) are also predisposing factors.
4. Analysis of the shoulder pain may be helpful in ruling out pain referred from other localities. Diaphragmatic lesions (e.g., pleurisy) commonly cause pain in the distribution of the trapezius muscle, and disease of the biliary tract, in the right scapular area. Cardiac pain is rarely localized to the shoulder; a retrosternal component is usually present. On the other hand, pain due to intrinsic disease of the shoulder is almost always felt in the deltoid region. Vague, poorly localized pain, unassociated with limited mobility and unaffected by activity, should arouse suspicion of a fibrositic-psychogenic origin.

### Physical Examination

1. Careful examination of all four articulations (glenohumeral, acromioclavicular, scapuloclavicular, and scapulohumeral) is indicated and may help to differentiate between intrinsic and extrinsic disease of the shoulder. The range of motion of the shoulder should be recorded. Localized tenderness suggests tendinitis or a fibrositic syndrome. Diffuse tenderness suggests a more extensive process. A frozen shoulder implies adhesive capsulitis.
2. Signs of joint inflammation and effusion suggest one of the following: crystalline-induced arthropathy, infectious arthritis or a connective tissue disease, tumor, or degenerative change.
3. Popping, snapping, and crepitation on movement are common abnormalities but are nonspecific. Moreover, they may occur in the absence of disease.
4. Limited or painful motion of the neck suggests disease of the cervical spine.
5. Neurovascular abnormalities—shoulder and extremity pain, numbness, paresthesias, swelling of the hand and fingers, and dystrophic changes—suggest a thoracic outlet syndrome or reflex neurovascular dystrophy. The maneuvers employed to diagnose the neurovascular compression syndromes are listed in Table 8-8.

**Table 8-8.** Neurovascular syndromes of the shoulder girdle*

| Syndrome | History | Pulse | Diagnostic test |
|---|---|---|---|
| Costoclavicular syndrome | Symptoms associated with shoulder being forced downward and backward for long periods | Reduced in abnormal shoulder position | Downward and backward bracing of the shoulder reproduces symptoms and signs |
| Hyperabduction syndromes (costoclavicular syndrome) | Hyperabduction in sleep or at work for long periods | Reduced in hyperabduction (also blood pressure and oscillometry) | Hyperabduction; reproduction of symptoms and signs |
| Scalenus anterior, cervical rib, and first rib syndromes | No special postural features | Reduced in resting position or brought on by Adson maneuver | Adson maneuver may reproduce musculoskeletal, neuritic, and vascular signs; tender point at scalenus area |
| Shoulder-hand syndrome (reflex neurovascular dystrophy) | Trauma, intrathoracic disease, or idiopathic; no special postural features | Sometimes reduced | Stellate ganglion block produces transient or prolonged relief |

*Symptoms common to some or all in each disorder: pain of shoulder, and arm or hand, or both; numbness, paresthesias of fingers; swelling of hand(s), fingers; discoloration of hand(s); Raynaud's phenomenon; weakness of hand(s); supraclavicular bruit possible in compression disorders.
Source: Modified from H. H. Friedman, T. G. Argyros, and O. Steinbrocker, Neurovascular syndromes of the shoulder girdle and upper extremity—the compression disorders and the shoulder-hand syndrome, *Postgrad. Med. J.* 35:397, 1959.

## X-Ray Examination

1. All patients with shoulder disability should have roentgenograms of the shoulder taken in both internal and external rotation.
2. Cervical spine films are important in evaluating cervical radicular syndromes associated with shoulder discomfort. Chest films are indicated for the assessment of thoracic outlet and neurovascular syndromes.

## Other Procedures

1. In the presence of effusion, the joint fluid should be aspirated and examined for white cell count, cytologic features, and the presence of crystals. Smears and cultures are indicated when infection is suspected.
2. Plethysmography, nerve conduction studies, and angiography may be useful in evaluating thoracic outlet syndromes.
3. Contrast arthrography is often of material assistance in the diagnosis of rotator cuff tears.
4. MRI may be used to assess the shoulder impingement syndrome, including rotator cuff tears.

## PAINFUL HIP
Joseph C. Tyor

### Definition

This discussion is limited to conditions, exclusive of fractures and dislocations that may cause hip pain in adults.

### Etiology and Clinical Features

1. Intrinsic causes.
   **a.** Periarticular disorders.
      **(1)** Muscle rupture. A history of trauma is usual. Tenderness at the site of rupture, hematoma formation, and deformity of the muscle are usually noted. Some degree of limitation of the hip may be present.
      **(2)** Bursitis.
         **(a)** Trochanteric bursitis commonly causes pain in the thigh and along the posterolateral region of the hip. Direct manual pressure over the greater trochanter usually reproduces the pain. Pain may be noted on external rotation of the hip.
         **(b)** Ischiatic bursitis causes pain and tenderness over the ischial tuberosities. Straight leg raising may be painful and limited.
         **(c)** Iliopectineal bursitis is associated with tenderness over the superior and anterior aspect of the joint capsule, under the psoas muscle and in Scarpa's triangle. Hip extension may be limited.
         **(d)** Obturator bursitis causes painful internal rotation of the hip.
   **b.** Articular disorders.
      **(1)** Connective tissue diseases. Rheumatoid arthritis, scleroderma, polymyositis, systemic lupus erythematosus, and polyarteritis nodosa rarely cause involvement of the hip joint alone. Usually, other joints are also affected.
      **(2)** Rheumatoid variants. Ankylosing spondylitis, Reiter's syndrome, enteropathic arthropathy, and psoriasis may involve the hip joints and lead to permanent articular damage. Usually, joint involvement is not limited to the hip.
      **(3)** Crystalline arthropathies.
         **(a)** Gouty arthritis of the hip is quite rare.
         **(b)** Pseudogout may cause acute arthritis of the hip. The presence of crystals of calcium pyrophosphate in the joint fluid is diagnostic.
      **(4)** Neuropathic arthropathy. Neuropathic arthropathy due to tabes dorsalis, diabetic neuropathy, or other neurologic disorders may affect the hip. It is characterized by effusion, undue mobility and instability of the hip, and disproportionately little pain. Some authorities have suggested that neuropathic hip disease may also result from repeated intraarticular injections of steroids.
      **(5)** Osteoarthritis of the hip. Degenerative arthritis of the hip is usually a disease of older individuals, more common in males, and more often unilateral than bilateral. It may be primary or secondary to long-standing mechanical malalignment of the hip due to congenital dislocation of the hip, Calvé-Perthes disease, slipped capital femoral epiphysis, or trauma (leg fracture, dislocation). The onset is insidious. The chief symptoms are pain, stiffness, and a limp on walking. The pain is usually located in the groin but may be felt along the medial aspect of the thigh. It is commonly referred to the buttock or knee. Initially, the pain is present on standing or walking and relieved by rest. Over a period of time, however, the pain tends to persist in the sitting position or recumbency. Backache from

mechanical strain is a common accompaniment. On physical examination, the lower extremity is often found to be everted, with the hip in a flexed and adducted position. Hip motion is limited in all directions, especially on internal rotation and adduction.

**(6)** Tumors of the hip. Tumors of the hip, including benign cysts, giant cell tumors, osteogenic or synovial sarcomas, and metastatic carcinomas are uncommon causes of the hip pain.

**(7)** Infectious arthritis.

    **(a)** Septic arthritis is usually hematogenous in origin and due to staphylococci, streptococci, or, less commonly, other organisms. Fever and other systemic symptoms are present. Pain may be located in the hip but is commonly referred to the knee. The thigh is flexed, adducted, and internally rotated. Motion is markedly limited. Local signs of inflammation and bulging of the joint capsule are noted commonly. Joint aspiration is essential for early diagnosis and proper treatment, because x-ray signs may not appear for several days. The synovial fluid should be cultured and cytologic studies done.

    **(b)** Tuberculosis of the hip joint is usually associated with pulmonary or visceral tuberculosis. It is more common in adolescents than in adults. A history of preceding trauma is often obtained. The onset is insidious. Nocturnal and rest pain are common. Pain in the knee and thigh, a limp, muscle spasm, fullness in the groin, tenderness over the hip, and limited motion of the hip are usually noted. The diagnosis should be suspected in any tuberculous individual with chronic monarticular arthritis involving the hip. Confirmation by culture of the joint fluid or biopsy is indicated.

**(8)** Aseptic necrosis of the femoral head. Aseptic or avascular necrosis of the femoral head refers to the changes that occur in the bone after interruption of its blood supply by trauma or disease. Avascular necrosis may occur in the osteochondroses, following fracture of the neck of the femur or dislocation of the hip, in sickle cell anemia or other hemoglobinopathies, or in caisson disease and other conditions. The condition is painful. The diagnosis is made radiologically.

**(9)** Bleeding disorders. Hemarthrosis occurs in the vast majority of patients with hemophilia and may lead to permanent joint drainage and deformity.

**2.** Extrinsic causes. Pain may be referred to the hip in degenerative disease of the lumbar spine, pelvic disease, and vascular insufficiency in the lower extremities. Pain in the hip is not commonly of psychogenic origin.

## Diagnostic Approach

**1.** In the history, the type of onset and course of the disease may be of some help. Trauma may itself result in hip pain or may predispose to subsequent development of osteoarthritic changes. A history of conditions such as congenital dislocation of the hip, slipped capital femoral epiphysis, and Calvé-Perthes disease may be important in revealing the underlying cause in osteoarthritis of the hip.

**2.** The location of the pain, its relationship to weight-bearing or walking, and its constancy may provide clues to the severity of the hip joint involvement. Pain at rest and nocturnal pain suggest inflammatory or neoplastic disease.

**3.** Evidence of systemic disease suggests that hip involvement may be secondary to the primary disorder. Infection, tuberculosis, connective tissue disease, and the rheumatoid variants should be ruled out. Usually this can be accomplished on clinical grounds alone.

**4.** Examination of the hip joint should include observation for the presence of an abnormal gait, limp, or deformity. Palpation of the joint and periarticular structures may help to localize the source of difficulty. The range of motion of the hip and the length of the extremity should be measured.

5. Routine laboratory studies should include CBC, urinalysis, and sedimentation rate. In the presence of effusion, the synovial fluid should be aspirated. When an infectious etiologic agent is under consideration, appropriate cultures and cytologic studies are indicated. Examination for urate and calcium pyrophosphate crystals should be done if crystalline arthropathy is suspected.

6. X-ray examination is essential for the proper evaluation of hip pain. An AP roentgenogram of the pelvis, including both hips, and a lateral view of the hip should be taken. Salient features of the more common abnormalities causing hip pain are listed below.

   a. Rheumatoid arthritis and the rheumatoid variants. Early, there is juxtaarticular demineralization of the bone, which is followed by narrowing of the joint space, the appearance of marginal erosions, pseudocyst formation, and eventually bony ankylosis. Protrusio acetabuli may occur occasionally in rheumatoid arthritis.

   b. Osteoarthritis. Reduction of the joint space without osteoporosis is an early finding. Later, spur formation is found at the acetabular margins and around the head of the femur. Sclerosis of the subchondral bone and cyst formation eventually appear. The head of the femur tends to drift laterally and become flattened.

   c. Pseudogout. Roentgenograms show calcification of the articular cartilage and acetabular labra. The calcification is indistinguishable from that produced by degenerative joint disease.

   d. Neuropathic arthropathy. The radiologic picture is that of degenerative arthritis "gone wild," with acetabular erosions, irregularity of the joint space, marked osteophyte formation, bone destruction, the presence of fragmented bone in the joint space, and ossification of the soft tissues.

   e. Infectious arthritis. In septic arthritis, the earliest finding is narrowing of the joint space. Later, destruction of the articular margin and adjacent bone occurs. Eventually, hypertrophic changes and bony ankylosis may occur. Tuberculous arthritis may show little change early in the course of the disease. Later, demineralization without narrowing of the joint space appears. This is followed by destructive changes at the joint margins and contiguous bone. Joint destruction may eventually become quite extensive. Sinus tract formation is often present in advanced cases.

   f. Avascular necrosis of the femoral head. Initially there is separation of the subchondral bone from the articular margin and apparent condensation of the separated fragment within the femoral head, leaving a crescentic lucent area between the two. Over a period of time, intermingled areas of increased and decreased bone density are formed.

7. Suspected avascular necrosis is the main indication for MRI of the hip.

## PAINFUL KNEE
### Arnold Heller

Knee pain is a common complaint in office practice. The etiologic diagnosis is often elusive and imprecise. It is frequently difficult to determine whether the cause is primarily intraarticular or periarticular in origin.

## Etiology and Clinical Features

### Intrinsic Causes

PERIARTICULAR DISORDERS

1. Musculotendinous pain. A history of overt or occult trauma is usual. Knee injuries account for 40 percent of the overuse injuries seen in runners. The most com-

mon form is a musculotendinous patellofemoral pain syndrome resulting from stress or strain of the fibers that stabilize the patella. The causative factors fall into three main categories: training or competition errors, anatomic factors (leg length discrepancy, quadriceps insufficiency, and axial or patellar malalignment), and improper footwear.

Local tenderness at the superior or inferior pole of the patella is common. Tenderness at the insertional sites of the hamstrings at the head of the fibula or posteromedial proximal tibia may be found. Excessively tight hamstrings in children and adults can cause vague knee and calf pain with inability of the patient to take a full stride in running. Tenderness at the lateral compartment of the knee can occur with popliteus tendinitis. Occasionally the strain may be so severe that rupture of the quadriceps from the patella occurs. A palpable defect with incomplete active extension occurs. Rupture of the patellar tendon from the patella more commonly affects the younger athlete.

2. Bursitis and tendinitis.
   **a.** Pes anserinus bursitis commonly causes pain and tendinitis at the proximal anteromedial aspect of the tibial metaphysis. Direct local pressure with active or passive external rotation of the tibia on the femur usually reproduces the pain. Resisting forced active internal rotation may also reproduce the pain.
   **b.** Infrapatellar bursitis causes pain, tenderness, and swelling in the patellar tendon. The tendon itself may be enlarged or the infrapatellar fat pad may seem larger on one side. Knee effusion is usually absent.
   **c.** Prepatellar bursitis is usually associated with a painless effusion in the anterior prepatellar region between the skin and the patella (housemaid's knee). If this region is hot and painful, a pyogenic bursitis must be suspected.
   **d.** Tensor fascia lata tendinitis is associated with tenderness over the distal anterolateral aspect of the proximal tibia, often extending to the insertion site at the tibia (Gerdy's tubercle). Localized pain at the lateral femoral condyle may occur. Pain is noted lateral to the knee on resisting external rotation of the tibia on the femur and also on active abduction of the hip.
   **e.** Osgood-Schlatter disease is a disorder of heterotopic bone formation in an area of tendinitis involving the portion of the proximal tibial epiphysis that forms the patellar tendon attachment to the tibial tubercle. It is characterized by swelling and pain that is made worse by strenuous running or jumping activities and relieved by rest. It occurs in the 10- to 15-year-old age group. It is a self-limiting condition with cessation of symptoms occurring when fusion of the proximal tibial epiphysis takes place. Fragmentation of the tibial tubercle can occur normally with the formation of more than one ossification center. This is not necessarily associated with Osgood-Schlatter disease.

INTRAARTICULAR DISORDERS

1. Inflammatory disorders.
   **a.** Connective tissue diseases. The knee joint is commonly affected in rheumatoid arthritis. Bilateral involvement is common. Monarticular arthritis is more common in juvenile rheumatoid arthritis. Scleroderma, polymyositis, systemic lupus erythematosus, and polyarteritis nodosa rarely cause involvement of the knee joint alone.
   **b.** Axial arthropathies. Ankylosing spondylitis, Reiter's syndrome, enteropathic arthropathies, and psoriatic arthritis can cause monarticular involvement of the knee joint.
   **c.** Crystalline arthropathies.
      **(1)** Pseudogout is a common cause of inflammatory arthritis of the knee, especially when superimposed upon preexisting degenerative arthritis. The presence of calcium pyrophosphate crystals in the synovial fluid is diagnostic. A warm, swollen knee joint is a common finding and must be differentiated from pyogenic arthritis.
      **(2)** Acute primary gouty arthritis of the knee does occasionally occur. Secondary gouty arthritis is the more common cause of inflammatory urate synovitis of the knee.

**d.** Pyogenic arthritis is usually hematogenous in origin and most commonly due to staphylococci. The knee is the joint most likely to be infected by nongonococcal organisms. Gram-negative organisms such as *E. coli, Proteus,* and *Hemophilus influenzae* account for most of the remaining cases. Pyogenic arthritis is characterized by an acute onset of a hot, red, swollen knee. Fever and general malaise may be present. Painful restriction of motion is present. The classic signs of inflammation may be modified or absent in the patient who cannot mount a strong immune defense. Gram-negative organisms are more typically responsible in this type of patient. An indolent infection may be present for months and mistaken for nonpyogenic inflammatory arthritis or recurrent crystalline synovitis. Gonococcal arthritis is unusual as an isolated cause of monarticular arthritis of the knee. Joint aspiration is essential for prompt diagnosis and treatment. Radiographic abnormalities may not appear for 7 to 10 days. Cartilage destruction can begin within 24 hours.

**2.** Noninflammatory disorders.

**a.** Degenerative arthritis of the knee is usually a disease of older individuals, more often unilateral than bilateral. Medial compartment deterioration associated with varus deformity is more common than lateral compartment deterioration with valgus deformity. Both can cause loss of full extension and flexion. Degenerative arthritis may be secondary to occult traumatic disorders and mechanical malalignment. Degenerative arthritis develops slowly over many years. The chief symptoms are pain, stiffness, and weight-bearing discomfort. A limp may be present. The pain may be localized or involve the entire joint. In tibiofemoral compartmental arthritis, a bowleg (varus) or knock-knee (valgus) deformity may develop, depending on which side is more severely involved. The pain is usually relieved by rest. Crepitation or grating can be palpated on flexion-extension maneuvers and aggravated by rotation of the tibia on the femur, both in internal and external rotation, stressing the individual compartment with these maneuvers (McMurray maneuver). If effusion is present, it is usually of a cool type unless an acute calcium pyrophosphate synovitis is present.

**b.** Patellofemoral arthritis. Symptomatic chondromalacia or patellofemoral arthritis is characterized by aching, crepitation, or patellofemoral stiffness that is aggravated by stairwalking, squatting, and sustained running. It may cause stiffness and aching following prolonged driving or sitting. It is less severe when walking on level ground. Painless, cool effusions may occur. Cartilage fibrillation present on the medial facet of the patella is thought to be nonprogressive. Lesions involving the lateral side of the patella are more likely to be symptomatic and progressive. Patellofemoral crepitation on flexion or extension is present in many asymptomatic adults. Skyline patellar radiographic views are necessary to define clearly the severity of degeneration at the patellofemoral joint.

**c.** Meniscus injuries. The most common meniscal injury is a tear. The usual history is that of an acute injury involving rotational stress of the flexed knee. Joint line tenderness and blockage of motion appear to be the most reliable physical signs. Knee effusion may be present. Rotatory stress tests to determine the side of the lesion are not totally reliable. Radiograms should be obtained to rule out other causes of knee pain and mechanical locking. True locking may also be caused by loose bodies.

**d.** Acute ligamentous injuries are characterized by acute trauma associated with painful restriction of motion, effusion, and instability. A thorough history and physical examination are essential. The anterior cruciate ligament may rupture in a noncontact situation due to external rotation of the femur on a fixed tibia. The patient often states that he heard and felt a pop in his knee and may complain of posterolateral knee pain, which represents the rupture of the anterior cruciate ligament at the femur. This may be mistaken for a strain of the lateral head of the gastrocnemius muscle. The most important finding on physical examination during the first 24 hours is a large tense effusion which on aspiration is grossly bloody. Anterior cruciate ligament tears are the most common cause of tense hemarthroses (75 percent). Acute lateral dislocations of the patella and osteochondral fractures are less common. An isolated tear of the meniscus seldom produces a tense hemarthrosis. A first- or second-degree sprain (incomplete tears) of the medial collateral ligament does not lead to a tense hemarthrosis unless the athlete continues to play and aggravates the injury. Third-degree tears (complete) of the medial or lateral collateral ligament may not be accompanied by a tense hemarthrosis, because blood escapes into the soft tissues. The most reliable clinical indicator of anterior cruciate ligament injury is the anterior drawer test performed with the knee held in 20 to 30 degrees of flexion (Lachman's test). If hamstring spasm is present, this test may be negated. Examination under general anesthesia may be necessary with arthroscopy. Stress tests in valgus and varus of the collateral ligaments should be done in 30 degrees of flexion. Ruptures of the posterior cruciate ligament with instability can be perceived by flexing the knee to 90 degrees and appreciating a posterior sag of the tibia on the femur.

**e.** Patellar dislocation and malalignment syndromes. Acute lateral dislocations or subluxations are associated with a history of an acutely painful episode with medial parapatellar tenderness and decreased range of motion, with rather acute apprehension on gentle lateral motion of the patella. Swelling may not be present. Radiograms in patients with recurrent lateral dislocations of the patella may demonstrate loose bodies or avulsion fragments along the medial border of the patella. Pseudolocking or giving way may be reported as occurring in the extended position (not in the flexed position of true locking that occurs with a displaced meniscus). Medial joint line tenderness due to patellar retinacular injury may lead to erroneous diagnosis of meniscal injury.

**f.** Fractures. A history of trauma followed by pain, local tenderness with or without deformity, or effusion may be present. Radiographic studies are imperative for establishing the diagnosis. Radiograms may not reveal the fracture for a period of several weeks. A detailed discussion of fractures is beyond the scope of this text.

**g.** Neuropathic arthropathy. Neuropathic arthropathy due to tabes dorsalis, diabetic neuropathy, or other neurologic disorders may affect the knee. It is characterized by effusion, relatively painless mobility, and instability of the knee, with disproportionately little pain relative to the degree of destruction visualized radiographically.

**h.** Osteochondritis dissecans is a disorder most commonly of the medial femoral condyle of the knee and less commonly of the lateral femoral condyle or the patella. In a child, the symptoms are usually intermittent, nonspecific, and present over a long period of time. There are no special physical findings that allow the diagnosis to be made easily. The tunnel and lateral radiographic views are essential to diagnosis. Both knees should be radiographed because as many as 30 percent of patients have been reported to have bilateral involvement. In the adult, spontaneous osteonecrosis is a similar condition that develops in the juxtaarticular region of the medial femoral condyle and often leads to rapid degeneration of the medial compartment of the knee.

**i.** Bleeding disorders. Hemarthrosis involving the knee joint occurs in patients with hemophilia and may lead to severe destruction of articular cartilage with instability and deformity.

**j.** Tumors of the knee. Benign tumors, including benign cysts, giant cell tumors, osteosarcomas or synovial sarcomas, and metastatic carcinomas, are uncommon causes of knee pain.

**k.** Tuberculosis of the knee, primarily an osseous disease seen in adults, spreads secondarily to the adjacent joint. Destruction of cartilage occurs rather late in the course of the disease. A caseating, granulomatous synovitis is produced.

## Extrinsic Causes

Pain may be referred to the knee in degenerative diseases of the lumbar spine, especially anteriorly in the distribution of the femoral nerve and medially in the distribution of the obturator nerve along the inner thigh. Vascular insufficiency and pelvic disorders may be causes of referred pain to the knee. Disorders of the hip joint commonly radiate to the inner aspect of the knee.

---

# Diagnostic Approach

---

## Initial Evaluation

1. The initial investigation of every patient with knee pain should include a complete history and physical examination. The type of onset and course of the pain may be of some help. Trauma itself may result in knee pain or may predispose to subsequent development of degenerative arthritic changes. A prior history of traumatic effusion following twisting injuries may be important. If a warm effusion is present, one should seek an obvious source of recent or concurrent infection.

2. Evidence of systemic disease, especially if associated with polyarthritis and symmetric joint involvement, suggests inflammatory arthritis due to connective tissue disease.

3. The location of the pain in relationship to transfer activities, weight bearing, walking, and more strenuous activities such as running may provide clues to the severity and location of the involvement. Nocturnal pain and pain at rest suggest the possibility of inflammatory or neoplastic disease.

4. Examination of the knee joint should include observation, auscultation, palpation, and measurements of the range of motion. This should be done with the patient supine, sitting, standing, and ambulating. Thigh and calf circumferences should be measured equidistant from a joint line reference to reveal disuse atrophy. Palpation of the joint during various movements and rotatory stress tests may be helpful in localizing the diseased area. Measurements of the alignment angle of the patella during the excursions of flexion and extension are helpful in ruling out painful subluxation of the patella.

5. When pyogenic arthritis is suspected, the joint should be aspirated. Synovial fluid should be submitted for cell count and differential, Gram stain, and aerobic and anaerobic culture and sensitivity. Examination for urate and calcium pyrophosphate crystals under polarized light microscopy should be done. In an infected joint, the white count is unlikely to be under 25,000 per cubic millimeter. Blood cultures should be done if hematogenous pyogenic arthritis is suspected.

6. Radiographic examinations are essential for the proper evaluation of knee pain. Comparative, symmetric, AP, lateral tunnel, oblique, and skyline patellar views may be of great value. Weight-bearing AP radiograms are essential to assess fully the articular cartilage space narrowing that is present with early degenerative arthritis. Single leg weight-bearing and manual stress techniques in varus and valgus sometimes may be indicated to evaluate further medial and lateral compartmental narrowing, degeneration, and stability.

7. Knee arthrography is a safe procedure that may provide a definitive diagnosis; it is especially helpful in peripheral, midbody, and posterior horn tears in the medial meniscus. It is less accurate in evaluating the lateral meniscus. Arthrography and arthroscopy are complementary procedures in the evaluation of meniscal lesions. Arthrography is also useful in extrameniscal lesions, such as popliteal cysts. Flexing the knee 90 degrees may significantly improve accuracy of diagnosis of a popliteal (Baker's) cyst. Tears of the medial collateral ligament can be evaluated arthrographically within 48 hours of the injury. Tears of the deep fibers of the medial ligament attached to the joint capsule allow contrast material to escape from the joint.

If the articular cartilage overlying a lesion of osteochondritis dissecans is present, it is likely to be stable. If air or contrast media surround the fragment, it is likely to be a loose body.

Irregularities, thinning, or loss of articular cartilage to subchondral bone is seen in various stages of degenerative arthritis. Fraying and irregularity of the meniscus often accompany this condition.

8. An experienced arthroscopist can examine the interior of a knee joint and derive as much or more information about the state of the joint as can be gained from arthrotomy or arthrography alone. This can be done without risking the morbidity often associated with arthrotomy. The condition of the synovial lining, articular cartilage, menisci, synovial-covered fat pads, and cruciate ligaments can be assessed. Loose bodies can be visualized and the functional status of the patellofemoral joint can be determined. Degenerative changes in the patellofemoral joint with or without lateral patellar subluxation can be appreciated. Suprapatellar plicae (congenital folds), which may cause symptoms of internal derangement, can be demonstrated. Knee arthroscopy has been useful in the evaluation of adhesive capsulitis, rheumatoid arthritis, foreign bodies, pigmented villonodular synovitis, and synovial tumors.

9. A bone scan is unnecessary for making a diagnosis in most cases. It can, however, aid in establishing cases of early osteomyelitis before bone changes are present and revealing early cases of "spontaneous" osteonecrosis of the tibia before the appearance of a radiolucent area. Radionuclide scintigraphy in osteoarthritis reveals low values on both sides of the joint (tibial-femoral), whereas in osteonecrosis, high values are found on the femoral side of the joint.

10. Magnetic resonance imaging (MRI) of the knee has some advantages when compared with other modalities used to evaluate meniscal and ligamentous injuries. MRI is painless and noninvasive and does not subject the patient to ionizing radiation. The soft tissues of the knee can be directly visualized with excellent tissue differentiation and high spatial resolution. It is not affected by the presence of a joint effusion, thus making examination of a painful, swollen knee possible.

Potential pitfalls in the interpretation of an MRI can be caused by volume-averaging artifacts due to the concavity of the outer margin of the meniscus and by structures with low signal intensity: the lateral inferior geniculate artery, veins, the transverse ligament, and the popliteus tendon. MRI is very sensitive to intrameniscal degeneration, but it does not replace arthroscopy for diagnostic accuracy.

## LOW BACK PAIN
Charley J. Smyth

Low back pain is one of the most common complaints and causes of disability in persons seen in office practice. It is estimated that 80 percent of the population will experience lower back pain at some time in their lives. The incidence of this condition increases with age, reaching 50 percent in persons over 60 years of age. Despite the frequency with which low back complaints occur, the etiologic diagnosis is often elusive and imprecise. However, with the use of computed tomography (CT scans) and MRI, major advances have been made in the diagnosis of a wide variety of degenerative conditions that can cause low back pain. Sometimes it is impossible to determine whether the cause is primarily musculoskeletal, neurologic, or visceral. In this discussion, primary consideration will be given to musculoskeletal causes of low back pain.

## Etiology

The more common causes of pain in the low back region are as follows:
1. Low back strain. Low back strain may be acute, subacute, or chronic. Conditions

that predispose to strain include postural defects, disk degeneration, osteoarthritis, spondylolisthesis, and repeated trauma.

   **a.** Acute low back strain usually follows injury, the severity of which may be variable. The clinical picture is one of trauma followed by diffuse low back pain accompanied by muscle spasm, tenderness, and limited, painful motion of the back. The course is usually of relatively short duration.

   **b.** Subacute or chronic low back strain is probably the most common disorder causing low back pain. A history of antecedent injury is often absent. The course is chronic, but it may be punctuated by repeated acute exacerbations. Usually there is stiffness and some degree of painful motion of the back. Limitation of motion may or may not be present. Tenderness to palpation or percussion is common. Neurologic findings are negative, although pain may be referred in dermatomal distribution.

**2.** Herniated intervertebral disk is a common cause of low back pain. The L4-L5 and L5-S1 disks are most frequently affected. The L3-L4 disk is involved less frequently, and the other lumbar disks, rarely. More than one disk may herniate in the same patient. If the herniation does not rupture through the longitudinal ligament, the phenomenon is called protrusion; if it does, the term *extrusion* is appropriate. In either case, the nerve root or roots may be displaced and compressed. Herniation of the L5-S1 disk causes compression of the S1 nerve root; L4-L5 herniation causes L5 compression; and L3-L4 herniation, L4 compression. Degenerative changes in the disks predispose to herniation. Disk trouble often begins with a popping or snapping sensation in the back followed by low back pain. Although the initial episode may subside, there is a tendency for recurrence. During the attack, the pain is likely to be severe and incapacitating. After a period of time, the pain usually begins to radiate in sciatic distribution. On examination, one observes the patient's difficulty in standing and walking. A list to the side opposite the pain is common. Tenderness of the musculature on the affected side is often marked. The straight leg raising, sitting knee extension, and popliteal compression findings are usually positive. Neurologic changes are variable. Compression of S1 is suggested by a decreased or absent ankle jerk, hypoesthesia of the lateral foot and sole, and weakness of the calf muscles. Compression of L5 is commonly manifested by sensory loss in the lateral leg and in the dorsomesial aspects of the foot, and by weakness of the toe extensors. Compression of L4 usually results in a decreased or absent knee jerk, hypoesthesia of the medial aspect of the leg, and weakness of the knee extensors.

**3.** Osteoarthritis. Osteoarthritic changes are the results of degenerative changes in the disks, vertebral bodies, and apophyseal joints. The clinical picture is similar to that of chronic low back strain. However, degenerative changes in the disks may occasionally lead to herniation with attendant nerve root compression and radicular pain. In some instances, however, radicular pain may be simulated by pain referred along dermatomes related to specific areas of spinal involvement. The radiologic features are discussed later in the section (p. 325). Although osteoarthritis is usually a primary disorder, its occurrence may be secondary to trauma, neuropathic disorders, steroid therapy, epiphyseal dysplasia, Wilson's disease, ochronosis, infections, vertebral osteochondritis, or chondrocalcinosis. Degenerative disease of the discs and osteoarthritis of the apophyseal joints usually occur together and are called spondylosis. Such degenerative changes are frequently seen in older individuals. The correlation between their presence and back pain is poor. Radiologic identification of such changes does not mean that they are necessarily the source of the symptoms.

**4.** Lumbosacral facet syndrome. This condition produces symptoms similar to those of a root entrapment syndrome involving the fifth lumbar nerve root, but it does not produce the objective findings of such entrapment. A careful history can also bring out differences between the two symptomatically. The facet syndrome appears to result from a stretch injury to either the capsule of the lumbosacral facet joint or the articular branch of the dorsal primary ramus of the L-5 nerve root, which transmits pain sensation from the joint. The perception of pain in the ipsilateral L-5 sensory distribution, to a variable extent, represents a referred pain syndrome. Localized tenderness is found over the affected articulation. Manipulation of the spine may be successful in relieving the disorder.

5. Lumbar claudication syndrome secondary to spinal stenosis. The symptoms consist of bilateral lower extremity nonradicular pain, paresthesias, coldness, and weakness in varying combinations. Unilateral symptomatology may occur but is unusual. The symptoms are precipitated and aggravated by walking or standing, but they are relieved promptly (within 2 to 5 minutes) by sitting or bending forward at the waist. Spinal stenosis may be due to a developmental or acquired abnormality. Possible causes include spondylolisthesis, spondylosis, postsurgical scarring, Paget's disease, and fluorosis. In extreme cases, the cauda equina syndrome may occur, with attendant bladder and bowel dysfunction. Ordinarily, no neurologic deficit is present. The lower extremity pulses are normal, thus excluding a peripheral vascular disease as the cause of claudication. The diagnosis is established by myelography or MRI.

6. Cauda equina syndrome. This disorder is due to an obstruction of the spinal canal that results in the loss of all neurologic function below the level of the lesion. Bladder and bowel dysfunction are cardinal features. Prompt recognition of this condition is essential because it represents a surgical emergency.

7. Other causes.

   a. Ankylosing spondylitis. Ankylosing spondylitis is a common cause of low back pain, especially in young men. The disease usually begins in the sacroiliac joints and spreads cephalad. Typically, there is continuous low back pain, often with radiation to the buttocks and thighs, accompanied by stiffness, muscle spasm, limitation of motion, and tenderness to palpation. With thoracic involvement and attendant inflammation of the costovertebral joints, root pains and decreased chest expansion become manifest. Spread to the cervical spine produces limitation of motion of the neck. When the disease is advanced, there is loss of the lumbar lordotic curve, dorsal kyphosis, and protrusion of the head and neck. The shoulders and hips are commonly diseased, and arthritis of the peripheral joints is not unusual. Iritis and spondylitic heart disease occur in some patients. The radiologic abnormalities described later in the section are characteristic.

   b. Other connective tissue diseases. Diseases such as Reiter's syndrome, ulcerative colitis, regional enteritis, Whipple's disease, psoriasis, and juvenile rheumatoid arthritis may affect the spine and produce sacroiliac arthritis. The radiographic changes in the sacroiliac joints in these conditions are indistinguishable from those seen in ankylosing spondylitis. The differential diagnosis of these disorders is based on the more characteristic extraarticular and systemic manifestations of each disease.

   c. Osteoporosis. Osteoporosis of any origin is another cause of back pain, especially in the elderly, in whom senile or postmenopausal osteoporosis is common. Osteoporotic vertebrae are susceptible to pathologic fracture. The diagnosis is made by x-ray study, but additional laboratory studies are needed to differentiate between the various causes.

   d. Fractures. The relationship between trauma and fracture is usually obvious. The diagnosis is established by physical examination and roentgenographic findings. In pathologic fractures, the relationship to trauma is less evident. Aside from osteoporosis, pathologic fractures are most frequently caused by metastatic carcinoma (usually arising in the breast, kidney, lung, or thyroid gland), multiple myeloma, tuberculosis, eosinophilic granuloma, and other conditions.

   e. Infections. Back pain may occur as a symptom of such systemic infections as viral diseases. Meningitis may, of course, cause backache, but it is usually easily distinguished by the presence of nuchal rigidity, a positive Kernig's sign, and spinal fluid abnormalities. Nontuberculous as well as tuberculous infections may cause backache by direct involvement of the spine and its associated structures. Herpes zoster involving the lumbar nerve roots may present a diagnostic problem until the characteristic rash appears.

   f. Psychogenic rheumatism. Back pain is a common feature of psychogenic rheumatism. The diagnosis should be suspected in neurotic individuals with multitudinous complaints in whom the symptoms fail to fit any anatomic pattern of disease and in whom there is a discrepancy between the multiplicity of symptoms and the paucity of objective findings. Laboratory findings are normal. The diagnosis should be approached with caution because the neurotic individual may have organic disease.

**g.** Fibrositis. A cause of backache, this is the "lumbago" of a generation ago. The characteristic symptoms are pain and muscle stiffness aggravated by tension, fatigue, immobilization, and chilling, and relieved by heat and physical activity. Although the pain is diffuse, one or more "trigger" points may be found on palpation. Laboratory findings are normal. Patients with the fibrositis syndrome should be reexamined frequently to rule out underlying disease.

## Diagnostic Approach

### Initial Evaluation

The preliminary investigation of every patient with low back pain should include a complete history and physical examination with special attention to the back, CBC, sedimentation rate, urinalysis, and x-rays of the lumbosacral spine (AP and lateral views usually suffice, but oblique and special views may be needed to delineate specific pathologic processes more clearly).

HISTORY

1. A history of back pain initiated by injury or strain suggests low back strain, herniated disk, or fracture. Absence of trauma does not exclude these diagnostic possibilities.
2. Occupational and recreational activities that may be related to back pain should be investigated. An effort should be made, when trauma is involved, to learn whether compensation insurance or legal questions are pending.
3. Diagnostic clues to rheumatoid disorders and other systemic disease may be obtained from the general history and system review (see the section Peripheral Joint Arthritis, earlier in the chapter).
4. The pain should be analyzed with respect to its chronology, its character, and the response to previous treatment. The severity of the pain, its localization, radiation, and duration, and the effects of aggravating (cough, sneezing, straining) and alleviating (rest, exercise, activity, drugs) factors should be determined.
   **a.** Low back pain with sciatica is caused most commonly by herniation of a nucleus pulposus. The pain is characteristically aggravated by cough, sneezing, straining, bending, or lifting.
   **b.** In the elderly, lumbar nerve root irritation may be caused not only by osteoarthritis but also by collapse of a vertebral body due to osteoporosis, metastatic carcinoma, or infection.
   **c.** Continuous, severe back pain that is worse at night and is not relieved by ordinary analgesics should arouse suspicion of metastatic carcinoma, multiple myeloma, lymphomas, and abdominal or retroperitoneal malignancy.
   **d.** In young men, continuous, aching low back pain with radiation to the buttocks and thighs or low back pain in sciatic distribution should suggest ankylosing spondylitis.
   **e.** Retroperitoneal or abdominal malignancy should always be considered in individuals with intractable low back pain associated with constitutional symptoms of fatigue, anorexia, and weight loss.
   **f.** A history of back or leg pain, lower extremity weakness, and unsteady gait should suggest disease of the cervical rather than the lumbar spine. Such a history is suggestive of spinal cord compression either by osteoarthritic changes or by posterior dislocation of the odontoid process caused by rheumatoid arthritis.

PHYSICAL EXAMINATION

1. The examination of every patient with backache should include abdominal, pelvic, and rectal examinations, to exclude visceral causes of low back pain. Examination of the hip is also warranted to exclude hip joint involvement (e.g., in ankylosing spondylitis) or hip joint disease causing backache (e.g., osteoarthritis of the hip).

2. The physical examination of the back involves inspection, palpation, determination of the range of motion of the spine, and observation of the gait. The presence or absence of pain during movement should also be noted.

   a. A mechanical cause of low back pain is suggested by poor posture, scoliosis, kyphosis, and obesity. A sharp, angular deformity in the dorsal or lumbar area may suggest tuberculosis. The appearance of the patient with ankylosing spondylitis is characteristic.

   b. Reduction of chest expansion suggests ankylosing spondylitis.

   c. Loss of lumbar lordosis, with muscle spasm and tenderness, is a sign pointing to ankylosing spondylitis, spondylolisthesis, or other congenital lesions with secondary degenerative changes.

   d. Tenderness over the sacroiliac joints is, when supported by a positive iliac compression test, a sensitive indicator of the sacroiliitis found in ankylosing spondylitis and other rheumatoid variants.

   e. Restricted motion of the spine and muscle spasm are nonspecific abnormalities found in many low back disorders.

   f. Localized lumbar spine pain associated with tenderness and muscle spasm suggests involvement of a vertebra or its processes by fracture, tumor, or infection.

   g. The presence of tender or "trigger" points without other abnormalities is suggestive of fibrositis. Disappearance of this pain following local injection of procaine or lidocaine into the tender spot is both diagnostic and therapeutic. However, underlying disease or psychogenic rheumatism is not ruled out by this maneuver. Psychogenic pain is suggested by the presence of cutaneous hyperesthesia at the tender point. It is demonstrable when pain is elicited by lifting and gently pinching a fold of skin over the affected side. Further presumptive confirmation is secured when relief of pain is obtained by the intracutaneous, rather than the intramuscular, injection of the local anesthetic.

3. Special tests are useful in assessing specific problems. Straight leg raising, allowing for tightness of the hamstrings, is a valuable but not infallible indicator of nerve root compression. The sitting knee extension and popliteal compression tests confirm nerve root compression when results are positive. The Patrick's test yields a positive result in hip joint disease. A positive jugular compression test (Naffziger) result is indicative of spinal cord or nerve root involvement.

4. A neurologic examination including tests for reflex, sensory, and motor functions should be done routinely. It is essential for the diagnosis of nerve root compression or lesions of the spinal cord. The findings in L4, L5, and S1 nerve root compression by herniated disks are listed earlier in the section (p. 322).

PSYCHOLOGIC EVALUATION

It is necessary to recognize and evaluate emotional factors in patients presenting with low back pain. Nonorganic physical signs include superficial or nonanatomic distribution of tenderness, distracted straight leg raising, overreaction during the examination, ill-defined weakness, and sensory changes in stocking distribution in the lower extremity.

RADIOLOGIC EXAMINATION

Although different pathologic conditions may cause similar clinical pictures, the radiologic findings are often specific or sufficiently characteristic to establish a diagnosis. Reference will be made to the more common diseases whose skeletal lesions have distinctive roentgenographic appearances in plain radiographs.

Degenerative changes of the lumbar spine from osteoarthritis or structural defects such as congenital malformations, trauma, surgery, spinal misalignment, and herniated disks may be demonstrated by CT scans. The interspaces and facet articulations can be visualized and degenerative changes related to the spinal canal and neural foramina identified. Moreover, soft tissue changes such as ligamentous hypertrophy, lateral spinal stenosis, and herniated disk fragments can be visualized.

MRI is often preferred to CT in disk disease and metastases, but a CT myelogram is equivalent to MRI.

1. Generalized osteoporosis of the spine is a common but nonspecific radiologic abnormality. Partial or complete collapse of one or more vertebral bodies may be an associated finding. Osteoporosis has many possible causes.

2. Osteoarthritis of the lumbar spine is manifested radiologically primarily by disk narrowing and spurring, which is most often located anteriorly. Anterior spurs rarely have clinical significance. Changes in the apophyseal joints consist of narrowing of the joint spaces, spur formation, and bony sclerosis. It should be emphasized that the presence of x-ray findings of osteoarthritis does not necessarily imply that symptomatology is related to these changes.

3. Sacroiliac arthritis is a characteristic feature of ankylosing spondylitis and the other rheumatoid variants. The sacroiliitis is manifested early by irregularity and blurring of the joint margins; later, by sclerosis of the adjacent bone; and eventually, in some cases, by bony ankylosis. The sacroiliac changes in these diseases are radiologically indistinguishable. Osteitis condensans ilii may mimic sacroiliitis by the presence of sclerosis of the iliac bone adjacent to the sacroiliac joints. The joints themselves, however, are uninvolved. Osteoarthritic sacroiliac disease is differentiated by the absence of destructive changes and the presence of sclerosis of subchondral bone with marginal spur formation.

4. Spinal ankylosis may be seen in several disorders:
   a. In ankylosing spondylitis, the vertebrae have a "squared" appearance in lateral views. Other typical radiologic findings include paravertebral ossifications leading eventually to a "bamboo spine"; apophyseal narrowing, sclerosis, and fusion; loss of lumbar lordosis; and occasional destruction of a disk and its adjacent vertebra with pseudoarthrosis formation.
   b. Senile ankylosing hyperostosis is a condition seen in elderly patients, characterized by irregular ossification of the anterior longitudinal ligament. The hyperostosis produces typical "candle-flame" shadows along the anterior aspect of the vertebral bodies.
   c. Paravertebral ossifications bridging adjacent vertebral bodies, limited to one or a few areas, may be seen following trauma or infection, and in psoriatic arthropathy and Reiter's syndrome.

5. Destruction of vertebral bodies may be seen with infection (e.g., tuberculosis, pyogenic organism), neoplasm, and neuropathic disorders.

6. Paget's disease (osteitis deformans) is characterized by a mottled increase in bone density, coarse trabeculation, and at times, fractures.

7. Spondylolysis is a unilateral or bilateral congenital vertebral arch that can be detected only by radiologic studies. Spondylolisthesis is the anterior displacement of a vertebra on the one below, found in some cases of bilateral spondylolysis.

8. Disk rupture may show disk narrowing or no abnormality. When the condition is of long standing, secondary osteoarthritic changes occur. Conclusive x-ray diagnosis depends on myelography or diskography.

9. Computed tomography (CT). This noninvasive method has replaced many other radiologic techniques and is used extensively. The reliability of CT scanning in detecting herniated disks appears to exceed 95 percent. Spinal stenosis due to thickening of the ligamentum flavum, osteophytic entrapment from the facets, and the obliteration of epidural fat can be visualized.

10. Magnetic resonance imaging (MRI) is a rapidly evolving, noninvasive diagnostic imaging technique that has promise as a useful instrument in evaluating patients with low back pain.

## Histocompatibility Antigen Test—HLA-B27

It is now well established that a positive blood test with histocompatibility antigen HLA-B27 has a striking association with ankylosing spondylitis. This test is also positive in a high percentage of patients with Reiter's disease and juvenile ankylosing spondylitis. It is also frequently positive in patients with spondylitis associated with inflammatory bowel disease and psoriatic spondyloarthritis. In patients with unexplained backache, this test may provide a clue to the diagnosis.

## Subsequent Evaluation

1. Usually the diagnosis of broad categories of disease can be established on the basis of the initial examination. Thus, a history of trauma followed by backache with characteristic symptomatology is diagnostic of low back strain. No further workup is indicated, and therapy should be instituted. Failure to respond to conservative management may or may not suggest the need for further investigation. The diagnosis of chronic low back strain is really nonspecific because the clinical picture may be caused by recurrent minitrauma, osteoarthritis, or fibrositis. Again, no further workup is necessary unless there is poor response to treatment or unusual features develop that suggest the original diagnosis was in error.
2. Myelography may be indicated for the precise diagnosis of disk herniations. It may also be helpful in differentiating disk herniations from tumors or other obstructive lesions. Myelography is customarily performed only when conservative therapy fails, when the diagnosis is uncertain, or preoperatively to confirm the presence and site of disk herniations. Electromyography and diskography have more limited applications in the diagnosis of herniated disks.
3. A radiologic survey of other bones and joints may be indicated when osteoporosis, metabolic bone disease, malignancy, connective tissue diseases, or rheumatoid variants are suspected.
4. Bone scans using technetium pertechnetate ($^{99m}$Tc) can be used to demonstrate bone infections and tumors, as well as to detect sacroiliitis with greater frequency than conventional radiologic methods. The amount of uptake of this isotope reflects the blood flow to the involved joint.
5. Additional laboratory tests may be advisable under certain circumstances.
   a. Serum calcium, phosphorus, and alkaline phosphatase, in suspected hyperparathyroidism, malignancy, osteoporosis, and Paget's disease.
   b. Serum uric acid, which is elevated in gout, lymphomas, and leukemia.
   c. Serum protein electrophoresis and immunoglobulins, which may be useful in the diagnosis of multiple myeloma, lymphomas, and connective tissue diseases.
   d. Spinal fluid examination, for the diagnosis of disease of the central nervous system and spinal cord.
6. Systemic or visceral disorders with low back pain (e.g., enteropathic arthropathy) may require barium studies of the gastrointestinal tract or other diagnostic measures (e.g., lymph node biopsy), as suggested by the symptoms and physical findings.
7. In patients with persistent, intractable low back pain of unknown cause, bone marrow biopsy and radioisotope scanning of the skeleton may reveal the presence of malignancy or other conditions undetectable by conventional examinations. Table 8-9 lists the differential diagnosis of a few of the important low back pain syndromes.
   These syndromes are not mutually exclusive. Thus, more than one disorder may be found in the same patient. The symptoms of the syndromes, although typical, are not found in all patients. Hence, clinical judgment is essential to adequately assess the symptomatology. A brief clinical examination is highly reliable for diagnosis and can be performed even when time is limited.

**Table 8-9.** Differential diagnosis of selected lower back pain syndromes

| Clinical features | Lumbar root entrapment syndromes | Lumbosacral facet syndrome | Lumbar claudication syndrome due to spinal stenosis |
|---|---|---|---|
| Pain | Painful radicular paresthesias conforming to one or two dermatomes (unilateral more common than bilateral) <br><br> Pain less when sitting than standing, and usually least when lying down. With a free fragment of nucleus pulposus, back pain may clear entirely, but no relief results from recumbency | Painful radicular paresthesias involving part of the L-5 dermatome (unilateral more than bilateral) <br><br> Pain less when standing than sitting, but unable to maintain any position for a long period of time including recumbency. A "restless" type of pain, and patients often resort to movement to obtain relief | Bilateral lower extremity paresthesias, including numbness, involving two or more dermatomes (unilateral unusual) <br><br> Pain or painful numbness clears promptly (within 2 to 5 minutes) when sitting down or bending forward at the waist. Pain precipitated and aggravated by walking or standing. |
| Onset and course | Onset is often insidious, but commonly follows major load-bearing injury to the lumbar spine | Onset almost always can be pinpointed and results from a combination of flexion and twisting of the low back region | Onset insidious, course progressive; claudication occurs at progressively shorter distances; length of time that can be tolerated in standing position decreases |
| Cauda equina syndrome | Rare | Never | Occurs ultimately, but usually only after the claudication becomes severe |

| Physical findings | **S-1 root**<br>Mechanical: SLR and LS positive<br>Reflex: Decreased or absent ankle jerk.<br>Motor: Decreased strength of gastrocnemius<br>Sensory: Decreased sensation on lateral aspect of foot<br><br>**L-5 root**<br>Mechanical: SLR and LS positive<br>Reflex: No deficit<br>Motor: Decreased strength of extensor hallucis longus, peronei, and tibialis anticus<br>Sensory: Decreased sensation on dorsum of foot<br><br>**L-4 root**<br>Mechanical: SLR or femoral stretch test may be positive, but negative tests do not exclude L-4 involvement<br>Reflex: Decreased or absent knee jerk<br>Motor: Decreased strength of quadriceps<br>Sensory: Decreased anterior thigh and medial aspect of leg | Mechanical:<br>1. Focal tenderness over lumbosacral facet joint<br>2. Pain referred to this joint by the ipsilateral knee-chest position<br>3. Although SLR may be positive at the same degree of hip flexion produced by the knee-chest position, the LS should be negative<br>Reflex: No deficit<br>Motor: No deficit<br>Sensory: No deficit | Mechanical:<br>1. SLR is negative<br>2. LS is negative in the knee-chest position<br>Reflex: No deficit<br>Motor: No deficit<br>Sensory: No deficit<br>Reflex, motor, and sensory changes occur if the cauda equina syndrome is present |

SLR = straight leg raising; LS = Lasègue's sign
Courtesy of Henry G. Fieger, Jr.

## NECK PAIN AND SELECTED CERVICAL SYNDROMES
Walter G. Briney

The human cervical spine is quite susceptible to disease and trauma in that it is interposed between the head and the relatively immobile thoracic spine. The cervical spine offers little protection to the vital structures it encloses—including the lower medulla oblongata, spinal cord, vertebral and spinal arteries, and spinal and sympathetic nerves. For effective use of the senses of sight and hearing, the neck must have a wide range of motion. About 85 percent of this movement occurs at the atlas-axis-skull complex. In addition to the marked mobility of the cervical spine, 32 cervical joints with synovial lining are present and can be involved in inflammatory processes.

## Etiology and Clinical Features of Neck Pain

1. Acute neck pain. This usually results from a relatively sudden insult to the cervical spine and the structures it encloses.
   a. Cervical muscle strain. A history of trauma, such as flexion-extension (whiplash) neck injury, is usually present.
   b. Cervical disk herniation with nerve root compression. This is relatively uncommon. It is attended by severe neck pain with voluntary immobilization of the neck (see the section Cervical Radiculopathies, Chapter 10).
   c. Osteomyelitis. This disease is usually due to *Staphylococcus aureus* and is seen in patients with underlying diseases that make them more susceptible to infection and with the use of corticosteroids or immunosuppressive drugs. Patients with AIDS and IV drug abusers are candidates for opportunistic infections, and appropriate cultures are indicated.
   d. Osteoporosis and vertebral collapse. These conditions occur less commonly in the cervical than in the dorsal and lumbar regions.
   e. Pathologic fracture (tumor).
   f. Meningitis. Neck pain, occipital headache, marked nuchal rigidity, altered sensorium, and fever usually occur.
   g. Subarachnoid hemorrhage. The symptoms may be similar to those produced by meningitis. The onset is usually acute and the headache severe. Change in sensorium may be rapid.
2. Chronic neck pain.
   a. Osteoarthritis (see the section Low Back Pain in this chapter).
   b. Cervical disk herniation (see the section Cervical Radiculopathies, Chapter 10).
   c. Ankylosing spondylitis (see the section Low Back Pain in this chapter).
   d. Chronic infection in the vertebrae and disks. Tuberculosis and fungus disease should be considered diagnostic possibilities.
   e. Metastatic tumor.
   f. Fibrositis, psychogenic rheumatism, and chronic anxiety. These conditions are common causes of neck, upper back, and shoulder pain. They are seen frequently in those who work in a sitting position, especially if they are emotionally labile and unhappy with their life situations. Fibrositis and psychogenic rheumatism are discussed elsewhere in this chapter and in the section Anxiety in Chapter 1.
   g. Rheumatoid arthritis of the cervical spine. This disease is usually associated with evidence of extensive rheumatoid arthritis elsewhere. Subluxation of C1-C2 is the most serious complication of rheumatoid arthritis and can be life-threatening. High neck and occipital pain occur and may be aggravated by coughing or sudden movements. Paresthesias in the arms, electric shock sen-

sations down the back, **paresthesias in the legs,** spastic paraplegia or quadriplegia, urinary retention, **loss of bladder control,** and loss of deep tendon reflexes may be seen. **Vertebral artery compression and "drop" attacks have** also been reported.

## Cervical Syndromes Not Associated with Pain

1. Vertebral artery compression. **Osteophytes from the** intervertebral disk or zygapophyseal joints are **common causes. Posterior** subluxation of vertebrae with a scissoring action may also **cause this condition. Turning** the head to the opposite side or extension **of the neck while looking upward** may decrease vertebral blood flow, causing dizziness, **unsteadiness of gait,** paresthesias of the lips or face, visual disturbances, and **"drop" attacks.**
2. Cervical spondylosis. **Osteophytes from the disks and** zygapophyseal joints may compress the spinal cord. **Hypertrophy of the ligamentum** flavum is a frequently associated finding. A **spastic, ataxic gait,** loss of bladder and bowel control, and other neurologic abnormalities **may result. Extension** of the neck may aggravate the clinical findings.

## Diagnostic Approach

1. Examination of the cervical spine. **Scoliosis and kyphosis are easily recognized.** Palpation may reveal local **areas of tenderness,** and crepitus may be found with rotation. Motion should be **observed with forward flexion, backward extension,** rotation to the left and **right, and lateral bending of the** head to the left and right. Spasm may also be palpable, **particularly over the trapezius muscles.**
2. Radiographic studies.
   a. Cervical spine x-rays **should be obtained with oblique,** lateral flexion and extension and open mouth views. **Straightening of the** spine may be seen. The oblique views can **demonstrate osteophyte encroachment on the** intervertebral foramina. Flexion views **should be examined for the possible C1-C2 sub-** luxation of rheumatoid involvement **of the spine.** Narrowed intervertebral disks, hypertrophic spurring, **and cervical instability may be present.** Osteoporosis and vertebral **collapse can be delineated.** The destructive lesions of tumor or infection **may be identified.** If ankylosing spondylitis is suspected, x-rays of the pelvis **should be obtained for examination of the sacroiliac joints.**
   b. Tomograms are extremely **helpful in outlining structures that are not well** visualized on routine **radiographic studies.**
   c. Bone scans should be **ordered in all cases of obscure** neck pain and are especially helpful for metastatic **tumor and osteomyelitis.**
   d. Computerized tomography (CT scanning) with or **without myelographic dye** may be indicated when **there is physical or other x-ray evidence of a mass** lesion (e.g., tumor, **herniated disk, hypertrophic spurring).** The use of the iodinated dye is an invasive **procedure, and neurological consultation is rec-** ommended before proceeding to this. **In addition, sagittal, coronal, or oblique** views cannot be directly **acquired. Magnetic resonance imaging, although** very costly, may be a **good choice before myelography is performed.**
   e. Magnetic resonance imaging is noninvasive and affords no radiation exposure. The bony **architecture of the cervical spine,** structure of the cord, and surrounding structures **are all visualized with** excellent detail. Sagittal, oblique, and axial images **may be obtained.** MRI is applicable in the evaluation of degenerative **disk disease, infection,** trauma, and neoplasia involving osseous structures, **soft tissue, and the cord.**
3. Lumbar puncture.
   a. Examination of the spinal fluid **may be done at the time of myelography. If**

increased intracranial pressure is suspected, as may occur with subarachnoid hemorrhage, a small needle should be used and only a small amount of fluid withdrawn.

   **b.** Diagnostic tests.

   **(1)** Cell count and differential count. The presence of red blood cells suggests subarachnoid bleeding. Increased numbers (several thousand or more) of granulocytes indicate bacterial meningitis.

   **(2)** A low spinal fluid glucose with a normal blood glucose value suggests bacterial infection.

   **(3)** Modest elevation of the spinal fluid protein is frequently seen with cervical disk disease.

   **(4)** Gram stains, India ink preparations, and cultures should be done if infection is suspected.

**4.** Electromyography of the upper extremities may be helpful in demonstrating nerve root compression in cervical disk disease. Electromyography of the lower extremities is helpful occasionally in cervical spondylosis with spinal cord compression.

**5.** Additional laboratory tests may be of benefit (see the section Low Back Pain):

   **a.** Elevation of the sedimentation rate may indicate infection or inflammatory arthritis.

   **b.** If ankylosing spondylitis is suspected, obtain an HLA-B27 test, which is positive in about 95 percent of cases. The test is also frequently positive in spondylitis due to other causes (see HLA-B27 under Low Back Pain in the preceding section).

**6.** Needle biopsy under fluoroscopic control. This procedure is seldom carried out in disease of the cervical spine because of the risk of damage to adjacent structures. However, it may occasionally be valuable in detecting tumors or infection.

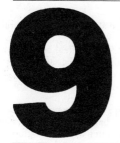

# Endocrine and Metabolic Problems

## HYPERGLYCEMIA
Walter A. Huttner

### Definition

Hyperglycemia is the presence of elevated blood glucose levels in fasting or post-prandial specimens.

The criteria listed below for the diagnosis of normal glucose levels, diabetes mellitus, impaired glucose, and gestational diabetes are based on those recommended by the National Diabetes Data Group and published in *Diabetes* 28:1049, 1979. (Reproduced with permission from the American Diabetes Association, Inc.)

### Blood Glucose Determinations

1. Glucose determinations performed on plasma or serum are preferable to those performed on whole blood. Plasma or serum methods are not dependent on the hematocrit value and are more suitable for use in autoanalyzers. Plasma and serum glucose levels, which are about equal, are approximately 15 percent higher than those obtained from whole blood.
2. Venous blood is customarily used for glucose determinations, although capillary blood may be more convenient in children. In the fasting state, venous and capillary glucose levels are comparable, but the values tend to be higher in capillary than in venous blood for at least 2 hours after eating.
3. Glucose determinations by true glucose methods (e.g., glucose oxidase) are preferred because their use avoids the spuriously elevated values produced by hemolysis, uremia, or other sugars such as fructose or galactose.
4. Home glucose monitoring is performed on capillary whole blood. This has become an important aspect of glucose control in diabetes. The determinations are performed by various monitoring devices.

### The Oral Glucose Tolerance Test

1. Prior to the test, the patient should be on a diet containing at least 150 g of carbohydrate per day for 3 days. Standardized conditions should prevail so that they may be reproduced if desired. The test should be given only to patients who are otherwise healthy, ambulatory, and free from any complicating acute or chronic illness that might impair carbohydrate tolerance. They should not be taking drugs that elevate blood glucose or interfere with the laboratory determination of glucose.
2. The oral glucose tolerance test (OGTT) should be performed in the morning after a fast of at least 10 hours but no more than 16 hours, although water is permitted

during this period. The patient should be seated and should not smoke throughout the test.

3. The dose of glucose administered should be 75 g (1.75 g/kg ideal body weight)—100 g when testing for gestational diabetes. After a fasting blood sample is drawn, glucose is administered in a flavored drink. Zero time is the beginning of the drink. Blood samples are customarily drawn after ½ hour, 1 hour, 2 hours, and 3 hours.

4. The standard OGTT is a 3-hour procedure. If reactive hypoglycemia is suspected, the test should be suspended until the glucose levels begin to rise. Urinary sugar determinations are no longer considered significant, but a qualitative glucose determination on the total urine collection during the test period may be worthwhile.

### Criteria for Normal Glucose Tolerance in Nonpregnant Adults

1. Fasting values:
   a. Venous plasma < 115 mg/100 ml.
   b. Venous whole blood < 100 mg/100 ml.
   c. Capillary whole blood < 100 mg/100 ml.
2. Values between ½ hour and 1½ hours:
   a. Venous plasma < 200 mg/100 ml.
   b. Venous whole blood < 180 mg/100 ml.
   c. Capillary whole blood < 200 mg/100 ml.
3. Two-hour values:
   a. Venous plasma < 140 mg/100 ml.
   b. Venous whole blood < 120 mg/100 ml.
   c. Capillary whole blood < 140 mg/100 ml.
4. Glucose values above these concentrations but below the levels found in diabetes or impaired glucose tolerance should be considered nondiagnostic for these conditions.

### Criteria for Normal Glucose Tolerance in Children

1. Fasting values:
   a. Venous plasma < 130 mg/100 ml.
   b. Venous whole blood < 115 mg/100 ml.
   c. Capillary whole blood < 115 mg/100 ml.
2. Two-hour values:
   a. Venous plasma < 140 mg/100 ml.
   b. Venous whole blood < 120 mg/100 ml.
   c. Capillary whole blood < 140 mg/ml.

### Criteria for the Diagnosis of Diabetes Mellitus

NONPREGNANT ADULTS

Any one of the following criteria is considered diagnostic of diabetes.

1. The presence of classic symptoms of diabetes such as polyuria, polydipsia, rapid weight loss, and ketonuria, associated with gross elevation of blood glucose concentrations.
2. Elevated fasting glucose concentrations on more than one occasion.
   a. Venous plasma ≥ 140 mg/100 ml.
   b. Venous whole blood ≥ 120 mg/100 ml.
   c. Capillary whole blood ≥ 120 mg/100 ml.
   If the fasting glucose values meet these criteria, *an OGTT is not required.*
3. Fasting glucose concentrations that are below those diagnostic of diabetes and that are associated with elevation of *both* the 2-hour sample and another sample

drawn during the time between the administration of glucose and the 2-hour specimen.

  **a.** Venous plasma ≥ 250 mg/100 ml.
  **b.** Venous whole blood ≥ 180 mg/100 ml.
  **c.** Capillary whole blood ≥ 200 mg/100 ml.

CHILDREN

1. The presence of classic symptoms of diabetes together with a random plasma glucose above 200 mg/100 ml or the criteria listed in paragraph 2 below. In asymptomatic individuals, both an elevated fasting glucose and an elevated glucose concentration on more than one occasion during the OGTT.
2. Both the 2-hour specimen and another sample drawn between the administration of the glucose dose (1.75 g/kg ideal body weight [maximum 75 mg]) and the 2-hour sample.
3. Criteria for elevated fasting, 2-hour, and intervening values are the same as those listed for nonpregnant adults.

GESTATIONAL DIABETES

1. Screening test
  **a.** The test should be administered between the twenty-fourth and twenty-eighth weeks of pregnancy to women who have not previously been identified as having glucose intolerance.
  **b.** 50 g of glucose is administered orally without regard to the time of day or the time of the previous meal.
  **c.** A plasma glucose level taken 1 hour later equal to or greater than 140 mg/100 ml indicates the need for a conventional glucose tolerance test.
2. Diagnostic test
  **a.** Prior to the test, the patient should be on an unrestricted diet containing at least 150 g of carbohydrate per day for 3 days.
  **b.** The test should be performed after an overnight fast of 8 to 14 hours.
  **c.** Venous plasma glucose determinations should be performed in the fasting state and at 1 hour, 2 hours, and 3 hours after the administration of 100 g of glucose. The patient should remain seated and not smoke during the test.
  **d.** Two or more of the following plasma glucose levels must be met or exceeded for a positive diagnosis: fasting, 105 mg/100 ml; 1 hour, 190 mg/100 ml; 2 hours, 165 mg/100 ml; 3 hours, 145 mg/100 ml.

## Criteria for Impaired Glucose Tolerance

In adults, three criteria must be met: (1) The fasting glucose concentration must be below the value that is diagnostic of diabetes; (2) the glucose concentration 2 hours after glucose administration must be between normal and diabetic values; and (3) a value between the ½-hour and 2-hour samples must be unequivocally elevated.

In children, two criteria must be fulfilled: (1) The fasting glucose concentration must be below diabetic levels, and (2) the glucose concentration 2 hours after the oral glucose challenge must be elevated to between normal and diabetic values.

## Miscellaneous Considerations

### The Effects of Age on the Oral Glucose Tolerance Test

Glucose tolerance appears to decrease with age. Approximately 50 percent of patients over the age of 60 years have abnormal glucose tolerance test results, but only a minority of these individuals eventually develop frank diabetes mellitus. An approximately equal number will be normal on retesting. Because of impaired glucose tolerance with aging, some authorities add 10 mg/100 ml to each of the maximum normal values (whole blood glucose) for each decade above the age of 50 years. Other authorities feel that with adequate dietary preparation, the effect of age on the OGTT is insignificant. Still other investigators feel that a 3-hour whole blood value of 110 mg/100 ml or greater is the most reliable criterion for the diagnosis of diabetes in the elderly.

### Nondiabetic Causes of Abnormal Glucose Tolerance

1. Fasting hyperglycemia, otherwise unexplained, is virtually diagnostic of diabetes mellitus, especially in a patient with a family history of diabetes. The same holds true for an OGTT that is clearly abnormal. However, the final decision depends on the exclusion of nondiabetic causes of impaired glucose tolerance.
2. The major nondiabetic causes of an abnormal OGTT are as follows:
   a. Inadequate dietary preparation.
   b. Hepatocellular disease.
   c. Chronic disease and prolonged physical inactivity (bed rest).
   d. Malnutrition and starvation.
   e. Potassium depletion due to diuretics, primary aldosteronism, renal disease, or alcoholism.
   f. Stress secondary to strokes, myocardial infarction, surgery, and febrile illnesses.
   g. Endocrinopathies, such as acromegaly, Cushing's syndrome or disease, adrenocortical hyperfunction, prolonged steroid therapy, islet cell tumors (insulinomas, glucagonomas), pheochromocytoma, and thyrotoxicosis.
   h. Chronic renal disease and uremia.
   i. Alimentary hyperglycemia following gastric surgery.
   j. Drugs (e.g., steroids, diuretics, oral contraceptives, nicotinic acid).
3. An abnormal OGTT found in any of the above-mentioned conditions should be considered nondiabetic until proved otherwise, provided the fasting blood sugar is normal. Patients with these disorders should be retested with an oral OGTT after recovery has taken place and normal physical activity has been resumed. Adequate dietary preparation prior to the test is most important. The intravenous OGTT is helpful in differentiating between alimentary hyperglycemia and diabetes mellitus.

### Effect of Drugs on the Oral Glucose Tolerance Test

Drugs may raise or lower blood sugar values. Drugs that can affect glucose tolerance include steroids, some oral contraceptives, diuretics, nicotinic acid, salicylates administered in large doses, alcohol, propranolol, and monamine oxidase inhibitors. As a general rule, a normal OGTT found in patients on any of these medications can be considered valid.

### Diagnosis of Diabetes in the Presence of Conditions That May Impair Glucose Tolerance

There are six conditions, listed below, in which, although the fasting blood sugar is normal, the OGTT is abnormal. It is often difficult and sometimes impossible to determine whether the glucose intolerance is a reflection of the underlying disorder or is the result of coexisting diabetes mellitus.

1. Obesity. An abnormal OGTT in an obese individual should be considered prima facie evidence of diabetes and treated accordingly.
2. Pregnancy. The criteria for the diagnosis of gestational diabetes are listed above (see p. 335).
3. Hyperlipoproteinemia. Familial hyperlipoproteinemia, including types III, IV, and V in the Frederickson classification, is often associated with abnormal glucose tolerance. Until more is known, patients with hyperlipoproteinemia and glucose intolerance should be treated the same as other diabetics with standard regimens including weight reduction and carbohydrate restriction.
4. Degenerative vascular disease. Strokes, intracerebral hemorrhages, and heart attacks are commonly associated with transitory hyperglycemia. Unless the diagnosis of diabetes is unequivocal, a final decision as to whether or not such patients are diabetic should be postponed until complete recovery has taken place and normal physical activity has been resumed.
5. Chronic liver disease. Hepatocellular disease may produce an abnormal OGTT, but fasting hyperglycemia is a rare occurrence. Usually, the glucose intolerance disappears when the liver function returns to normal. There is no available test that distinguishes between hepatic and diabetic glucose tolerance curves.
6. Gout and hyperuricemia. A much higher incidence of glucose tolerance abnormality is found in gouty and hyperuricemic individuals than in the general population. The usual criteria for the diagnosis of diabetes are applicable.

## Intravenous Glucose Tolerance Test

The intravenous GTT is primarily a research tool. It has no demonstrable clinical advantage over the oral test. Its major usefulness is in differentiating between diabetes and alimentary hyperglycemia secondary to gastric surgery.

## HYPOGLYCEMIA
Walter A. Huttner

### Definition

Hypoglycemia is a symptom complex associated with abnormally low blood glucose levels. Plasma glucose values below 50 mg/100 ml are usually diagnostic of hypoglycemia in the presence of typical symptoms. For blood glucose determinations and the preparation and precautions in performing the oral glucose tolerance test, see the preceding section Hyperglycemia. For the diagnosis of hypoglycemic states, the standard 3-hour oral GTT is extended to a 5-hour period.

### Symptoms

The occurrence of hypoglycemic symptoms is related to both the rapidity and the severity of the decline in the blood glucose level. Symptoms that accompany a rapid fall in the concentration of blood glucose include a sensation of "not feeling well," shakiness, sweating, palpitation, restlessness, anxiety, hunger, nausea, and vomiting. Loss of consciousness and even coma may occur. These symptoms, which are largely due to catecholamine release, are alleviated promptly by correction of the hypoglycemia. The symptoms are usually different when the fall in glucose levels is slow and prolonged or severe. Neuroglycopenic symptoms, such as headache, restlessness, reduction in spontaneous conversation and activity, mental confusion, prolonged sleep, stupor, coma, and hypothermia or fever, may occur. Sensory and motor disturbances and bizarre behavior may also be noted.

# Etiology

The causes of hypoglycemia can be divided into three major groups: reactive, fasting, and factitious hypoglycemia. The two types of hypoglycemia found most commonly in practice are reactive functional hypoglycemia and reactive hypoglycemia secondary to diabetes mellitus. The distinction between fasting and reactive hypoglycemia is important clinically because fasting hypoglycemia is not a feature of either reactive functional hypoglycemia or reactive hypoglycemia secondary to diabetes mellitus.

1. Reactive hypoglycemia.
   a. Reactive functional hypoglycemia. Reactive functional hypoglycemia is the most common cause of hypoglycemia in adults. This disorder, which seems to be unusually common in individuals with emotional problems, is characterized by transient postprandial hypoglycemia that occurs 2 to 4 hours after the ingestion of food containing carbohydrate. The symptoms are predominantly those of hyperepinephrinemia, brought about by the rapid decline in the blood sugar concentration. The symptoms usually subside spontaneously within half an hour after their onset. Reactive functional hypoglycemia does not predispose to the subsequent development of diabetes.
   b. Reactive hypoglycemia secondary to diabetes mellitus. Reactive hypoglycemia secondary to mild diabetes mellitus is the second most common type of hypoglycemia found in adults. Low blood sugar values accompanied by symptoms of hyperepinephrinemia typically occur 3 to 5 hours after meals. A family history of diabetes is commonly obtained.
   c. Alimentary hypoglycemia. Alimentary hypoglycemia is found in approximately 5 to 10 percent of patients who have had partial to complete gastrectomies or gastroenterostomies. However, it sometimes occurs in individuals who have not had gastric surgery. The rapid gastric emptying time leads, sequentially, to accelerated absorption of glucose, hyperglycemia, and hypoglycemia. Symptoms usually occur 1½ to 3 hours after meals, corresponding to the time when blood glucose levels are low.
   d. Hereditary fructose intolerance. Patients with familial fructose intolerance may have postprandial reactive hypoglycemia following the ingestion of fructose-containing foods. Since the disease occurs primarily in children and is seldom found in adults, it is not discussed here. The diagnosis is established by the use of an oral fructose tolerance test.
2. Fasting hypoglycemia.
   a. Pancreatic islet cell disease. The symptoms of hypoglycemia due to islet cell tumors (insulinomas) are produced by the excessive secretion of insulin. Approximately 85 percent of these tumors are benign and 15 percent malignant. They occur most frequently between the ages of 35 and 55 years. Insulinomas may be solitary or multiple and may be either macroscopic or microscopic in size. Multiple islet cell tumors are sometimes associated with multiple endocrine adenomatosis and peptic ulceration (Zollinger-Ellison syndrome). Hypoglycemic symptoms usually develop insidiously, but with the passage of time hypoglycemic episodes tend to increase in frequency and severity. Most attacks occur in the early morning or later afternoon hours. They are often precipitated by fasting and physical activity. Neuroglycopenic symptoms predominate over those caused by epinephrine release. Whipple's triad, consisting of symptoms of hypoglycemia, low blood sugar levels, and relief with administration of glucose, is suggestive of organic hypoglycemia but is not specific for hyperinsulinism due to islet cell disease.
   b. Glucagon deficiency. This is an extremely rare cause of hypoglycemia. The failure of plasma glucose and glucagon to rise following an arginine infusion is diagnostic of this condition.
   c. Extrapancreatic tumors. Severe fasting hypoglycemia may occur in the presence of such tumors as mesotheliomas, fibromas, fibrosarcomas, or leiomyosarcomas, particularly when they are large. The neoplasms are usually found

in the pelvis, retroperitoneum, or thorax. The diagnosis is usually based on the association of hypoglycemia with easily identified abdominal or thoracic masses.

d. **Liver disease.** Glycogen storage disease and galactosemia are examples of congenital anomalies that may be associated with hypoglycemia. Hypoglycemia may also occur in severe, diffuse liver disease (e.g., fulminating hepatitis, hepatic necrosis due to toxic agents, cholangitis, cirrhosis) and in some patients with hepatomas.

e. **Leucine sensitivity.** Leucine-induced hypoglycemia is an extremely rare disorder in adults but is a not uncommon cause of fasting hypoglycemia in children below the age of 4 years. The administration of leucine may produce hypoglycemia in patients with islet cell tumors or in those on sulfonylureas.

f. **Alcohol-induced hypoglycemia.** Ethanol-induced hypoglycemia occurs most frequently in alcoholics who are eating little or no food. Occasionally, following a 2- to 3-day fast, the ingestion of alcohol may produce hypoglycemia in a young, healthy person. Patients with hypopituitarism or adrenocortical insufficiency exhibit increased sensitivity to the hypoglycemic effects of alcohol. Ethanol-induced hypoglycemia is promptly corrected by the administration of glucose.

g. **Malnutrition.** Hypoglycemia is relatively common in children with kwashiorkor, but in adults, even severe protein depletion and malnutrition rarely lead to hypoglycemia.

h. **Endocrine disorders.** Fasting hypoglycemia may occur in patients with hypopituitarism or Addison's disease, but it is a relatively uncommon finding in these disorders. The endocrine cause of the hypoglycemia is usually apparent from the clinical picture.

3. **Factitious hypoglycemia.** Hypoglycemia may be induced by ingestion of salicylates in large amounts, monoamine oxidase inhibitors, barbiturates, and other drugs. It may be precipitated in diabetics receiving insulin, when the dose of insulin is too high, when physical activity is excessive, or when food intake is inadequate or delayed. Sulfonylureas may induce hypoglycemia, especially in the presence of renal failure or the use of alcoholic beverages. Insulin has sometimes been used by medical personnel, diabetics, and the relatives of patients, with malingering, suicidal, or homicidal intent. However, insulin overdose is most commonly accidental.

## Diagnostic Approach to Reactive Hypoglycemia

1. A 5-hour oral GTT is the mainstay of the diagnostic approach to suspected reactive hypoglycemia.

   a. In **reactive functional hypoglycemia,** the fasting blood sugar level is normal. The curve is not remarkable except for the occurrence of abnormally low plasma glucose values (50 mg/100 ml or less) between the second and fourth hours of the test.

   b. In **reactive hypoglycemia secondary to mild diabetes mellitus,** the glucose tolerance curve generally shows a normal or slightly elevated fasting blood sugar level, hyperglycemia at the peak value and at 2 hours, and low plasma glucose levels (50 mg/100 ml or less) during the third to fifth hours.

   c. In **alimentary hypoglycemia,** the oral GTT reveals a normal fasting glucose level, peak hyperglycemia at ½ to 1 hour, normal glucose concentration at 2 hours, and hypoglycemia shortly thereafter.

2. Because the intravenous GTT is normal in alimentary hypoglycemia but abnormal in diabetes mellitus, it is useful in differentiating between the two.

3. Once an oral GTT has been performed, when fasting hypoglycemia has to be ruled out, the procedures outlined below (Diagnostic Approach to Fasting Hypoglycemia) should be followed.

4. The most effective method for documenting true hypoglycemia is to teach the

patient to perform self glucose monitoring. Using this procedure, the patient can determine the glucose levels during attacks and bring these to the attention of the physician.

## Diagnostic Approach to Fasting Hypoglycemia

In addition to the oral 5-hour GTT, the following procedures are recommended in the evaluation of patients with suspected fasting hypoglycemia:

1. Determine, on at least two or three occasions, the plasma glucose and insulin levels after an overnight fast. Plasma glucose values of 50 mg/100 ml or less together with plasma insulin levels exceeding 40 μU/ml occurring in association with hypoglycemia symptoms are considered virtually diagnostic of insulinoma.

2. If the plasma glucose and insulin levels are not diagnostic, the overnight fast should be prolonged for 4 hours and the plasma glucose and insulin determinations repeated. If the results still prove to be inconclusive, the fast should be extended for an additional 48 to 72 hours, with only black coffee permitted. During this time, multiple plasma glucose determinations should be obtained. These are usually done at 6-hour intervals or whenever symptoms appear. As soon as low glucose levels and symptoms of hypoglycemia are induced, the test is terminated. Otherwise, at the conclusion of the 3-day period, the patient is exercised and a blood sample is drawn thereafter.

3. In patients with islet cell tumors, the plasma glucose concentration normally falls below 50 mg/100 ml at some time during the fast. Hypoglycemia of this severity is uncommon in patients who do not have disease of the islet cells. Exercise is a valuable adjunct in the evaluation of hypoglycemia because it produces a further drop in plasma glucose concentration in patients with insulinomas or other conditions associated with fasting hypoglycemia and a rise in plasma glucose levels in patients with reactive hypoglycemia.

4. The measurement of plasma insulin levels in conjunction with plasma glucose concentrations is extremely valuable in the diagnosis of islet cell disease. Elevated plasma levels in connection with low fasting plasma glucose levels confirm the diagnosis of insulinoma. However, not all patients with islet cell tumors show fasting hyperinsulinemia. Moreover, normal fasting plasma insulin levels not only do not exclude the diagnosis but may actually support it if they occur in association with low plasma glucose concentrations. During the fast, a fall of plasma glucose to hypoglycemic levels while the plasma insulin remains unchanged or rises is also a significant finding. High fasting plasma insulin levels are not always pathognomonic of insulinoma because they may sometimes occur in obese persons without fasting hyperglycemia, in children with idiopathic hypoglycemia, and, rarely, in patients with nonpancreatic neoplasms. It has also been reported that assay of fasting plasma proinsulin levels may be helpful in the diagnosis of islet cell disease, particularly when fasting plasma insulin levels are not elevated.

5. Tests that induce the secretion of insulin are useful in confirming the diagnosis of islet cell tumors and in the differential diagnosis of hypoglycemia. The procedures used most commonly are the intravenous tolbutamide, leucine, and glucagon tests, in which serial determinations of plasma glucose and insulin are performed following the administration of the test substance. Details of the test procedures and information concerning their interpretation can be found in standard textbooks. These provocative tests for insulin secretion are abnormal in a high percentage of patients with insulinomas. However, false-positive and false-negative results may occur with any of them. All three tests should be employed in suspected islet cell disease because an abnormal response may be obtained with one test but not with another. False-positive results may occur with the tolbutamide test in patients with nonpancreatic causes of hypoglycemia, uremia, or malnutrition, but not in patients with reactive hypoglycemia. With the leucine

test, false-positive results may occur in individuals on the sulfonylureas. In children, the leucine test does not differentiate between insulinoma and the so-called idiopathic hypoglycemia of children. It is the writer's opinion that the glucagon test may prove to be the most reliable provocative test for insulin secretion.

6. Once the diagnosis of islet cell tumor is made on the basis of the foregoing tests, an abdominal CT scan should be performed to help localize the tumor. It is often positive if the islet cell tumor is of significant size. Sometimes, MRI may more clearly delineate the soft tissue mass. A CT scan of the head and serum calcium and phosphorus determinations are indicated to rule out multiple endocrine adenomatosis. If carcinoma is suspected, a liver scan should be done to rule out metastatic disease.

7. Extrapancreatic neoplasms merit consideration as possible causes of hypoglycemia after islet cell tumor has been ruled out, particularly in elderly individuals. Radiologic examinations such as chest and abdominal films, intravenous pyelography, contrast studies of the gastrointestinal tract, CT scan, and MRI are useful diagnostic studies for this purpose.

8. If glucagon deficiency is suspected, an arginine test should be performed. The failure of plasma glucagon and glucose to rise following the administration of arginine by infusion is diagnostic of glucagon deficiency.

9. If pituitary and adrenal hypofunction are suspected causes of hypoglycemia, appropriate laboratory studies to confirm the diagnosis are indicated.

10. The relationship of diffuse liver disease to hypoglycemia is usually apparent from the clinical picture. Liver function tests show abnormalities. Hepatic hypoglycemia is easily corrected by the administration of glucose. Glucagon should be avoided because it may fail to cause hyperglycemia in the presence of severely impaired glyconeogenic reserve.

11. The diagnosis of alcohol hypoglycemia is supported by a fall in plasma glucose levels following an infusion of ethanol.

12. When factitious hypoglycemia due to malingering is suspected, the following procedures merit consideration:

    a. Serum insulin antibody levels. The presence of such antibodies is proof of the administration of insulin.

    b. Sulfonylurea blood levels.

    c. Examination of the urine for tolbutamide excretion products.

    d. Leucine sensitivity test, which produces elevated insulin levels in patients with hypoglycemia due to sulfonylurea compounds.

    e. In patients with hypoglycemia and hyperinsulinism, measurement of the serum C-peptide level can determine whether the insulin in the circulation is endogenously secreted or administered exogenously. If the C-peptide level is low in the presence of high concentrations of circulating insulin, it can be assumed that the insulin is exogenous in origin. On the other hand, if the C-peptide levels are elevated, the implication is that the insulin is secreted endogenously, possibly by an insulinoma.

13. Many investigators rely heavily on encephalographic changes for the diagnosis of questionable cases of hypoglycemia. The disappearance of alpha waves when blood sugar values are low and their reappearance after correction of the hypoglycemia are regarded as specific evidence, provided hyperventilation and severe anoxia are ruled out. The test is considered to be especially valuable in the diagnosis of organic hypoglycemia.

## FAILURE TO MATURE

Janet E. Schemmel

## Definition and Etiology

Failure to mature or the failure to develop secondary sex characteristics is a relatively common disorder. It is frequently, but not always, associated with delayed growth. The condition has many causes. This discussion is limited to males; th problem as related to females is considered in the following section, Amenorrhea The age of presentation varies, often depending on the family history and th patient's identification with his peers. Usually, the patient is seen between th ages of 12 and 17 years; within the last decade, at a slightly younger age The various abnormalities that can occur are listed below.

1. Failure to mature, with growth retardation or failure.
   a. Delayed puberty (constitutional retardation)—most common; commonly fa milial; cause unknown.
   b. Pituitary-hypothalamic disease.
      (1) Idiopathic hypopituitarism (with isolated or multiple tropic hormon losses).
      (2) Pituitary tumor, nonsecreting, with multiple tropic hormone losses.
      (3) Pituitary tumor, secreting, as in Cushing's disease.
      (4) Suprasellar or parasellar tumor.
      (5) Infiltrative disease of the hypothalamus (e.g., sarcoidosis).
      (6) Vascular abnormalities (e.g., internal carotid aneurysm).
   c. Hypothyroidism, juvenile, with or without goiter.
   d. Chronic systemic disease (e.g., congenital heart disease, pulmonary disease steroid treatment for asthmatic and dermatologic patients, chronic renal dis ease).
   e. Cushing's syndrome.
   f. Cryptorchidism.
   g. Testicular failure.
      (1) Infection.
      (2) Trauma.
   h. Anorchism and testicular dysgenesis.
2. Failure to mature, without growth retardation.
   a. Hypogonadotropic hypogonadism, including isolated LRH deficiency (Kal mann's syndrome).
   b. Klinefelter's syndrome and associated syndromes.
3. Delayed puberty secondary to other disease states and syndromes (e.g., myotoni dystrophica, and the obesity, mental retardation, and polydactylism or synda tylism seen in the Laurence-Moon-Biedl syndrome). Deprivational dwarfism i beyond the scope of this text.

## Symptoms

Multiple symptoms may occur. They are usually related to the underlying caus and to the state of growth of the patient.

1. Failure to mature with growth retardation.
   a. Immature genitalia.
   b. Lack of beard.
   c. Delay in growth.
   d. Considered younger than chronologic age by peers and adults.
   e. Immature voice.
   f. In patients with pituitary or hypothalamic disorders (or both), additiona symptoms may be present: (1) headaches, (2) visual complaints, (3) polydipsi and polyuria, (4) easy fatigability or episodic weakness, or both, and (5) fai ure to tan.
   g. In addition to the general symptoms, patients with hypothyroidism may hav (1) somnolence, (2) poor concentration, (3) cold intolerance, (4) constipatio and obstipation, (5) mass in neck, (6) hearing defects, and (7) joint pain, e: pecially hip pain.
   h. Patients with systemic disease frequently have symptoms of their underlyin disease. Cushing's disease or syndrome, uncommon at this age, is discusse in the sections Amenorrhea and Obesity, later in the chapter.

2. Failure to mature without growth retardation. Patients without growth retardation may have few complaints except those of delayed maturity. Patients with hypogonadotropic hypogonadism (Kallmann's syndrome) may complain of inability to smell.

## Signs

### Failure to Mature with Growth Retardation

1. Below height and weight for chronologic age.
2. Immature facies for chronologic age.
3. Immature voice and larynx for chronologic age.
4. Paucity or absence of axillary or pubic hair.
5. Absence of any pubertal breast tenderness or tissue.
6. Span and upper and lower segment heights that are compatible with normal prepubertal dimensions, although occasionally a eunuchoidal habitus may be seen.
7. Tanning may be absent, or the skin may be pale, yellowish, or dry.
8. Blood pressure may be variable, depending on the underlying disease.
9. Genitalia are prepubertal, compatible with the patient's somatic age; the testes may be inguinal or impalpable.
10. In patients with pituitary disorders, additional findings may be noted:
    a. Changing visual acuity and visual field defects.
    b. Cranial bruit.
    c. Pale, yellowish, or dry skin when multiple tropic hormones are lost.
11. Patients with chronic disease frequently demonstrate findings of the underlying disease (e.g., hepatosplenomegaly). The findings in Cushing's disease and syndrome are discussed in the sections Amenorrhea and Obesity, later in the chapter.

### Failure to Mature Without Growth Retardation

1. Normal height or taller than predicted on the basis of the family height history.
2. Commonly, increased span, with the lower segment height greater than the upper segment height.
3. Absent or small scrotal testes and a small phallus.
4. Gynecomastia.
5. Sparsity or absence of the beard and axillary and pubic hair.
6. Obesity (not uncommon).
7. Hyposmia or anosmia, which may be present in hypothalamic hypogonadotropic hypogonadism (Kallmann's syndrome).

## Diagnostic Approach

### Initial Evaluation

Initial studies should be carried out to help clarify the diagnosis, to determine the need for further investigation, and to determine proper treatment. These studies should include the following tests:

1. Hemoglobin and hematocrit values.
2. WBC and differential counts.
3. Platelet count.
4. Sedimentation rate.
5. TSH; free $T_3$ or $T_4$; $T_3$ RIA.
6. Biochemical profile.
7. Serum calcium, phosphorus, and alkaline phosphatase.
8. Plasma FSH, LH, and testosterone; growth hormone; somatomedine.
9. Buccal smear for chromatin pattern.
10. X-rays: chest, skull, and AP; hands and wrists, for bone age.

11. 24-hour urine collection for 17-ketogenic steroids or 17-hydroxycorticoids and creatinine. Alternatively, a 7:00 A.M. serum cortisol and plasma ACTH.

Patients with idiopathic delayed puberty usually have normal findings except for a delayed bone age that correlates with height, facial maturity, and genital development. Plasma gonadotropins may be low or absent. The span is usually prepubertal, occasionally eunuchoidal. A family history of delayed puberty with good response to therapy supports this diagnosis.

In contrast, patients with pituitary disease may demonstrate the following findings: low or absent growth hormone; normal or low-normal thyroid function, reduced 17-ketogenic steroids or 17-hydroxycorticoids, and 17-ketosteroids; low cortisol and ACTH levels, and reduced gonadotropins. Skull x-rays are usually abnormal if a pituitary tumor is present. Enlargement of the sella turcica, with or without intracranial calcification, is a common finding. In idiopathic hypopituitarism, the sella turcica is usually normal. The BUN and plasma glucose are frequently low. The serum phosphorus and alkaline phosphatase are reduced. Slight anemia may be present. Bone age is delayed. The body proportions and span are prepubertal.

## Subsequent Evaluation

Further evaluation should include the following tests to determine tropic hormone losses:

1. Measurement of ACTH, cortisol, and compound S or measurement of 17-ketogenic steroids or 17-hydroxycorticoids before and after metyrapone administration.
2. Plasma TSH. TRH infusion with measurement of TSH may be indicated to separate hypothalamic from pituitary disease.
3. Growth hormone. A number of tests are used to evaluate growth hormone deficiency. These include the following:
   a. Growth hormone drawn 2 hours after the patient goes to sleep.
   b. Growth hormone measurement after 15 minutes of exercise.
   c. Pharmacologic tests.
      (1) Clonidine (ambulatory setting).
      (2) L-dopa (ambulatory setting).
      (3) Insulin tolerance test. This test should be done in the hospital observation unit with the physician in attendance. A rise to 7 ng/ml is probably a normal growth hormone level. After provocative testing, multiple tests may be necessary, since more than 20 percent of normal children may show no response after one pharmacologic test.
      (4) Somatomedin C. A normal somatomedin C level suggests the absence of growth hormone deficiency. Unfortunately, somatomedin levels may be normal in a small percentage of patients with growth hormone deficiency. For details about performing these tests, see the section Amenorrhea, later in this chapter.

      Growth hormone is elevated in Levi-Lorain–type dwarfism. Somatomedin C levels are usually low.
4. Further radiologic investigation, including cranial CT scan, or MRI.

If the diagnosis of primary hypothyroidism is established, tests for thyroid antibodies are indicated; a positive result suggests Hashimoto's struma. If a goiter is present or hearing is abnormal, other members of the family should be examined for familial goiter. A perchlorate test may be indicated in the presence of a goiter when the RAI uptake is elevated (see section Thyroid Enlargement, later in the chapter). Other tests to determine thyroxin-synthesizing defects are not yet available. It should be remembered that patients with juvenile hypothyroidism frequently have normal to accelerated puberty in the presence of delayed growth.

Ordinarily, the history, physical findings, and initial laboratory tests suggest the presence of an underlying chronic disease as the cause of the patient's failure to mature. Electrocardiogram, pulmonary function tests, liver function tests, long bone x-rays, skin tests, urinary electrolyte excretion, and other tests should be carried out when applicable. Serial growth hormone measurements before and after provocative testing may be necessary to prove growth hormone deficiency. At present, growth response to growth hormone administration may be the only conclusive way to diagnose growth hormone deficiency.

Hypogonadotropic hypogonadism may occur as an isolated abnormality or in association with other conditions, such as palatal abnormalities and anosmia. The initial workup usually discloses a eunuchoidal or normal habitus, prepubertal scrotal testes, negative plasma gonadotropins, and delayed bone age. Further investigation for tropic hormone losses should be undertaken to ensure that the defect is isolated. These should include the following:

1. Metyrapone test (see p. 359) with measurement of acetylcortisol and compound S 17-ketogenic steroids or 17-hydroxycorticoids before and after administration of the drug.
2. Growth hormone measurements before and after the oral administration of L-dopa, and arginine infusion or insulin-induced hypoglycemia, or both.
3. TSH. TRH infusion with measurement of TSH may be indicated.
4. Careful testing of the sense of smell.

Testicular biopsy is not necessary. Follow-up study may be indicated in selected patients because tropic hormone losses theoretically may occur at a later date.

More common than hypogonadotropic hypogonadism is Klinefelter's syndrome (and its variants). These patients frequently are eunuchoidal and usually have small testes. Gynecomastia may be present. The buccal smear may be positive, bone age is delayed, and plasma gonadotropins are elevated. A karyotype determination is indicated.

5. Growth hormone releasing factor is not yet available for clinical use.

---

## AMENORRHEA
### Janet E. Schemmel

---

### Definition

---

Amenorrhea is the failure of menstruation to occur in a female of menstrual age. It is considered primary if menstruation has never occurred, and secondary if menses have ceased in a woman who has menstruated previously. The normal menarche is variable but generally occurs between 12 and 15 years of age in this country. A somewhat wider age range of 9 to 17 years has been reported for other countries. In recent years, the age of onset of menstruation appears to be lower than formerly.

---

### Primary Amenorrhea

---

#### Etiology

The causes of primary amenorrhea are many and varied. Occasionally, the past or family history provides clues to the diagnosis, particularly in the presence of chronic disease or a familial disorder. Primary amenorrhea is commonly associated with delayed growth. The most frequent causes are listed below.

1. Delayed puberty of unknown cause.
2. Ovarian dysgenesis (agenesis, dysplasia).
3. Pituitary-hypothalamic disease, associated with idiopathic onset, tumors, infiltrative disease, vascular anomalies.
4. Testicular feminization syndrome.
5. Cushing's syndrome or disease occurring at puberty.
6. Juvenile hypothyroidism.

7. Systemic disease (e.g., chronic renal disease, cystic fibrosis, congenital heart disease).
8. Cervical or uterine abnormalities.
9. Other endocrine disorders, including congenital or acquired adrenal hyperplasia, pseudohermaphroditism, true hermaphroditism, and ambiguous sexual differentiation.

## Symptoms

1. Delayed puberty of unknown cause and ovarian dysgenesis are probably the two most common causes of primary amenorrhea. Delayed growth usually accompanies these conditions. Patients with systemic disease and Cushing's syndrome or disease may also have retardation in growth.
2. The usual symptoms encountered in patients with primary amenorrhea are (a) amenorrhea, in association with absent or delayed development of breast tissue and absence or paucity of pubic and axillary hair, (b) retardation in growth, and (c) a younger appearance than expected for the patient's chronologic age.
3. When primary amenorrhea is due to pituitary-hypothalamic disorders, additional symptoms related to its underlying cause or to the loss of specific tropic hormones may occur, such as (a) headaches, (b) visual disturbances, (c) polydipsia, (d) polyuria, (e) easy fatigability or episodic weakness, or both, and (f) failure of the skin to tan.
4. Patients with hypogonadotropic hypogonadism and testicular feminization may complain only of amenorrhea.
5. The symptoms found in young patients with Cushing's syndrome or disease are similar to those encountered in adults. The usual symptoms are (a) obesity that is not due to excessive food intake and that is chiefly truncal in distribution, (b) easy fatigability and weakness, (c) irritability and difficulty in concentrating, (d) skin problems such as acne and easy bruisability, and (e) growth retardation.
6. Patients with underlying chronic disease frequently have symptoms related to the basic disorder. Delayed growth often coexists.
7. Patients with congenital adrenal hyperplasia due to a 21-hydroxylase defect are usually diagnosed shortly after birth because of the presence of pseudohermaphroditism or adrenal insufficiency, or both. However, when acquired, this rare anomaly may manifest itself primarily with amenorrhea and, sometimes, with mild hirsutism but without any delay in growth. Other rare causes of congenital adrenal hyperplasia are the 11-hydroxylase and 17-hydroxylase deficiencies, both of which may be associated with systemic hypertension. However, significant growth problems are not encountered in these disorders.
8. Patients with ambiguous sexual differentiation may have few symptoms other than amenorrhea and delayed growth.

## Physical Findings

PRIMARY AMENORRHEA WITH ASSOCIATED GROWTH RETARDATION

1. Delayed height and weight for the chronologic age.
2. Immature facies for the chronologic age.
3. Immature voice and larynx for the chronologic age.
4. Paucity or absence of axillary and pubic hair.
5. Minimal or absent breast development.
6. An arm span and upper and lower segment heights that are more compatible with normal prepubertal than with postpubertal dimensions.
7. Normotension, but occasionally systolic hypertension.
8. Skin changes, consisting of absence of tanning or a dry skin that is pale and yellowish.
9. Abnormalities that are suggestive of ovarian dysgenesis: strabismus, webbing of the neck, increased carrying angle of the arms, pedal edema, pes cavus, shortened metacarpals, and a high-arched palate.

**10.** External genitalia that are normal but prepubertal in appearance.
**11.** Findings suggestive of chronic underlying disease, such as chest deformities, heart murmurs, and hepatomegaly.
**12.** Diminished visual acuity, visual field defects, cranial bruits, and a pale yellow or dry skin in some patients with pituitary disorders.

PRIMARY AMENORRHEA WITHOUT ASSOCIATED GROWTH RETARDATION

This group of patients includes those with sexual ambiguity, some cases of ovarian dysgenesis, the testicular feminization syndrome, hypogonadotropic hypogonadism (including Kallmann's syndrome), some patients with congenital (11-hydroxylase or 17-hydroxylase deficiency) or acquired (21-hydroxylase deficiency) adrenal hyperplasia, and some patients with chronic systemic illness. Cases with these disorders may show the following features:

**1.** Immature but otherwise normal facies for the chronologic age.
**2.** Immature voice and larynx for the chronologic age, although the larynx is sometimes enlarged and the voice low-pitched.
**3.** Paucity or absence of axillary and pubic hair except in patients with acquired adrenal hyperplasia, who may show hirsutism.
**4.** Variable breast development—minimal to absent, or normal in the testicular feminization syndrome.
**5.** Normal arm span and upper and lower segment heights, or greater than normal arm span and lower segment height.
**6.** External genitalia showing normal prepubertal development, clitoral hypertrophy, ambiguity, a vaginal dimple, or urethral abnormalities.
**7.** Absent uterus (Rokitansky syndrome).
**8.** Anosmia (Kallmann's syndrome).

---

## Diagnostic Approach

### Initial Workup

**1.** Careful measurement of the arm span, total height, and upper and lower segment heights.
**2.** Skull films to determine the size of the sella turcica and to search for other abnormalities (e.g., intracranial calcification).
**3.** AP x-rays of the wrists and hands to evaluate bone age.
**4.** Chest films to detect bony abnormalities and to determine the heart size.
**5.** Buccal smear for the chromatin pattern.
**6.** TSH; free $T_4$ or $T_3$; $T_3$ RIA.
**7.** A 24-hour urine collection for 17-ketogenic steroids or 17-hydroxycorticoids, 17-ketosteroids, and creatinine.
**8.** Serum electrolytes, BUN, creatinine, calcium, phosphorus, and alkaline phosphatase (biochemical profile).
**9.** Plasma FSH and LH determinations.
**10.** Fasting serum growth hormone, somatomedin C, and prolactin determinations.
**11.** Pelvic examination. Rectal examination may be substituted if necessary.

Patients with primary amenorrhea due to delayed puberty, ovarian dysgenesis, pituitary-hypothalamic disease, or hypothyroidism show evidence of delayed bone maturation. The arm span and the upper and lower segment heights are prepubertal in character. Normal skull films virtually exclude pituitary tumors. Buccal smears are negative in many cases of ovarian dysgenesis. Thyroid function studies may be normal in each of these conditions. However, they may be borderline or low in pituitary disorders and, occasionally, in ovarian dysgenesis. TSH is always elevated in hypothyroidism. Plasma FSH and LH are absent or low in hypopituitarism and delayed puberty but are elevated in patients with ovarian dysgenesis. The serum electrolyte, BUN, creatinine levels, and biochemical profile are normal unless a systemic disease or hypothyroidism is present. The BUN may be less than 10 mg/100 ml in patients with pituitary disease. It may be slightly elevated in some patients with hypothyroidism. The serum calcium i usually normal unless chronic disease is present. Elevated serum phosphorus an alkaline phosphatase values suggest that body growth is occurring. Such a find ing is helpful because the results of growth hormone assays often are not reporte until several weeks after specimens were collected and submitted for analysis On pelvic examination, the genitalia are usually prepubertal in size, but th uterus may be absent or impalpable in ovarian dysgenesis. Uterine or vagina anomalies may be present.

## Subsequent Workup in Primary Amenorrhea with Delayed Growth

The diagnosis of delayed puberty is suggested when the biochemical profile serum electrolytes, BUN and creatinine, growth hormone assay, thyroid functio tests, and excretion of 17-ketogenic steroids and 17-ketosteroids are normal, th buccal smear is positive, plasma FSH and LH are low, bone maturation is re tarded, and serum phosphorus and alkaline phosphatase are elevated.

Ovarian dysgenesis should be suspected if the skull films are negative, th fasting growth hormone level is normal, buccal smears are negative, bone age i delayed, and plasma FSH and LH are elevated. The karyotype should be deter mined; usually it is XO, but a mosaic pattern may occur with or without othe obvious extragenital abnormalities. Because diabetes mellitus is common in ovar ian dysgenesis, serial plasma glucose determinations should be performed on a patients with this disorder. Thyroid antibodies are commonly present in patient with this anomaly.

A pituitary tumor should be suspected when skull films reveal an abnormalit of the sella turcica or show suprasellar calcification. Confirmatory findings c hypopituitarism include delayed bone growth, low or absent plasma FSH and LH absent growth hormone, low or normal thyroid function, positive buccal smear normal or low BUN, and a normal or reduced serum alkaline phosphatase an phosphorus. To establish the diagnosis of pituitary hypofunction, additional stud ies are indicated:

1. Plasma TSH before and after the administration of TRH to differentiate pituitar from hypothalamic disease.
2. Metyrapone test (see p. 359).
3. Growth hormone stimulation tests.
   a. Clonidine. After an overnight fast, 4 μg/kg clonidine is administered b mouth. Growth hormone is measured before and 60 and 90 minutes afte ingestion.
   b. L-Dopa. After an overnight fast, 125–250 mg L-dopa is administered. Growt hormone is measured before and 60 and 90 minutes after ingestion. Proprar olol given on 2 consecutive days prior to the test improves the response. Nau sea limits the usefulness of this test.
   c. Insulin tolerance test to measure the release of growth hormone and plasm cortisol with insulin-induced hypoglycemia. Prior to the test, a fasting bloo sample is drawn for glucose determination, growth hormone assay, an plasma cortisol. Regular insulin is then injected intravenously in a dose c 0.05 to 0.10 units/kg of body weight. Blood samples are collected at 15, 30, 4! and 60 minutes after the injection for glucose determinations. Samples at 3 and 60 minutes are also used for growth hormone assay and plasma cortiso Normally, insulin-induced hypoglycemia causes a rise in growth hormone lev els to at least 20 ng at 60 minutes and a threefold rise in the plasma cortis level. Because the insulin tolerance test is a potentially dangerous procedur a physician should be in attendance at all times.
   d. Arginine infusion test. Arginine is not readily available.
      The test is done as follows: A growth hormone level is obtained, followin which 30 g of arginine diluted in 100 ml of sterile water is infused over a 3( minute period. In children, the dose of arginine is 0.5 mg/kg of body weigh up to a maximum of 30 g. The growth hormone level is measured at 30-minut

intervals for a period of 2 hours after the completion of the infusion. The plasma growth hormone level should rise at least 7 ng/ml. This test is sometimes combined with intravenous insulin.

Response to both arginine and L-dopa does not occur invariably. Failure of the growth hormone levels to rise has been observed in over 25 percent of adults above the age of 50 years.

Somatomedin C levels, if measured, may parallel the growth hormone levels. Growth hormone releasing factor is not yet available for clinical use.

3. Plasma FSH and LH. Measurements before and after LRH administration may be indicated.
4. Visual acuity and visual field tests.
5. Radiologic studies, such as sellar tomography, cranial CT scan or MRI, and arteriography, depending on the circumstances.
6. Patients with suspected hypothyroidism should have a TSH assay and thyroid antibody determinations.
7. Patients with Cushing's syndrome or disease show elevated 17-ketogenic steroids or 17-hydroxycorticoids on initial workup.

   Further investigation should include urinary steroid excretions before and after the administration of dexamethasone, metyrapone, or ACTH (see the section Obesity, later in the chapter). Plasma cortisol and ACTH may be useful.
8. Patients with chronic systemic disease may show abnormalities in the initial workup that are primarily related to the underlying disorder. Usually, bone maturation is delayed and plasma FSH and LH may be lower than expected for the chronologic age. Additional studies to elucidate the diagnosis are advisable.

## Subsequent Workup in Primary Amenorrhea Without Delayed Growth

1. Patients with suspected hypogonadotropic hypogonadism should have workups similar to those performed on patients with hypopituitarism since other tropic hormones may be deficient either initially or at a later date. Those with anosmia have luteinizing hormone deficiency. Luteinizing releasing hormone administration in these individuals is followed by a rise in LH.
2. Patients with the testicular feminization syndrome have normal breast development together with abnormalities of the external genitalia, negative buccal smears, and usually normal excretion of testosterone, 17-ketogenic steroids, and 17-ketosteroids. A karyotype should be obtained in patients with this syndrome. Also, because the mode of inheritance is consistent with either an X-linked recessive or a sex-limited autosomal dominant trait, other members of the family should be studied.
3. The diagnosis of ambiguous sexual differentiation is suggested by abnormality of the external genitalia and pelvic examination findings. In such cases, even if the buccal smear is positive, karyotype should be made. Intravenous pyelography, cystography, vaginography, and urethroscopy are indicated to further elucidate the renal and uterovaginal abnormalities commonly seen in true hermaphroditism or pseudohermaphroditism. Pelvic ultrasound and CT scan are helpful as screening studies.
4. Patients with the common type of congenital adrenal hyperplasia (21-hydroxylase deficiency) rarely have amenorrhea because they are usually diagnosed at a much earlier age. The acquired form of the disease may occur without any associated abnormality of growth. The urinary excretion of pregnanetriol is elevated in these patients with increased excretion of 17-ketogenic steroids. Elevation of the plasma 17-hydroxyprogesterone level is confirmatory.
5. Congenital adrenal hyperplasia due to 11-hydroxylase deficiency is a rare cause of amenorrhea. This syndrome is associated with excessive production of 11-desoxycorticosterone and ultimately with the development of hypertension. The external genitalia are abnormal. The urinary excretion of aldosterone and 17-hydroxycorticoids is reduced.
6. Another variant of congenital adrenal hyperplasia, the 17-hydroxylase deficiency

syndrome, is also associated with amenorrhea and hypertension. The external genitalia are underdeveloped. The urinary excretion of corticosterone and desoxy-corticosterone is elevated, and that of aldosterone and 17-hydroxycorticoids is reduced.

7. Pelvic exploration may be indicated in ambiguous sexual differentiation once congenital or acquired adrenal hyperplasia has been ruled out by appropriate testing.

---

## Secondary Amenorrhea

---

Patients with secondary amenorrhea may have an abrupt cessation of menses, or the amenorrhea may be preceded by a period of oligomenorrhea. Investigation is usually warranted after 4 to 6 menstrual periods have been missed. Pregnancy is an obvious cause and should be excluded before proceeding with further investigations.

### Etiology

1. Polycystic ovary syndrome—probably the most common cause in patients in their teens or early twenties.
2. Pituitary-hypothalamic disease.
   a. Tumors.
      (1) Pituitary, nonsecretory.
      (2) Pituitary, secretory.
         (a) Acromegaly.
         (b) Prolactin-secreting.
         (c) Cushing's disease.
      (3) Suprasellar, parasellar and, rarely, intrasellar.
   b. Hypopituitarism.
      (1) Idiopathic (Simmonds' disease).
      (2) Infarction (Sheehan's syndrome).
   c. Infiltrative disease (e.g., sarcoidosis).
   d. Internal carotid aneurysm and other vascular anomalies.
   e. Prolactin secretion in the absence of radiologic evidence of tumor (idiopathic and drug-induced).
   f. Postpubertal hypogonadotropic hypogonadism.
   g. Cushing's disease.
   h. Empty sella syndrome.
3. Adrenal disease.
   a. Cushing's syndrome.
      (1) Tumor.
      (2) Carcinoma.
   b. Adrenal tumors with virilization.
   c. Addison's disease.
4. Ovarian disease.
   a. Ovarian failure.
      (1) Premature menopause (before the age of 40 years), usually idiopathic.
      (2) Acquired anatomic lesions, including tumors, carcinoma, and infection.
      (3) Normal menopause.
   b. Ovarian tumors.
5. Chronic systemic disease (e.g., kidney, liver, lung).
6. Anorexia nervosa or bulimia, or both.
7. Drug-induced: contraceptives, spironolactone.
8. Intrauterine adhesions (Asherman's syndrome).
9. Idiopathic, including exercise-induced.

## Symptoms

The symptoms in secondary amenorrhea are quite variable. The more common ones are listed below:

1. Amenorrhea, either abrupt in onset or preceded by a period of oligomenorrhea. Galactorrhea may or may not be present.
2. Changes in body weight.
   a. Weight loss, which may be marked, occurs in anorexia nervosa, panhypopituitarism, Addison's disease, some tumors and carcinomas, and idiopathic amenorrhea.
   b. Weight gain may be noted in patients with polycystic ovaries, Cushing's syndrome or disease, adrenal and ovarian tumors, acromegaly, prolactin-secreting tumors, and idiopathic amenorrhea.
3. Weakness and fatigability, which are most prominent in Cushing's disease, panhypopituitarism, Addison's disease, ovarian and adrenal malignancies, and chronic systemic illness.
4. A variety of specific or nonspecific symptoms related to the cause of the amenorrhea. Thus, symptoms of hypopituitarism, hyperadrenocorticism, adrenal insufficiency, or hypothyroidism may be reported by the patient.
5. Increase in body and facial hair noted by patients with polycystic ovaries.
6. Hot flushes in ovarian failure.

## Physical Findings

There are no physical signs that are specifically related to secondary amenorrhea. The findings, if any, are those of the primary disorder.

## Diagnostic Approach

CLINICAL FEATURES

1. Weight loss without skin changes suggests anorexia nervosa, acquired anatomic lesions, systemic disease, infiltrative hypothalamic lesions.
2. Weight loss in a patient with a pale, thin, sallow, yellowish skin suggests possible hypopituitarism.
3. Weight loss with hyperpigmentation and increased numbers of freckles and moles is commonly seen in Addison's disease.
4. Weight gain, with or without skin changes, may be observed in acromegalic patients, many of whom have increased numbers of papillomata and moles as well as a slight increase in body hair.
5. Weight gain, in association with plethora, acne, and striae, is common in Cushing's syndrome or disease.
6. Weight gain, in association with lactation, suggests a prolactin-secreting tumor and hypothyroidism.
7. The association of obesity with mild hirsutism is often noted in patients with the polycystic ovary syndrome.
8. Hirsutism of mild to severe degree may accompany ovarian or adrenal disease.
9. Patients with postpubertal hypogonadism and premature ovarian failure rarely demonstrate any significant change in body weight.
10. A history of excessive exercise may clarify the cause.

INITIAL WORKUP

The following preliminary studies are recommended in the workup of patients with secondary amenorrhea:

1. CBC and platelet count.
2. Sedimentation rate.
3. Chest and skull films.
4. Plasma FSH, LH, and prolactin.

5. Urinary 17-ketogenic steroids or 17-hydroxycorticoids; 17-ketosteroids; and creatinine.
6. TSH; free $T_4$; or thyroid profile.
7. Careful pelvic examination to establish the size of the uterus and ovaries and to detect the presence of infection or masses. (A single index of maturation is usually not helpful.)

SUBSEQUENT WORKUP

1. If the skull films are abnormal, additional studies, cranial CT scan or MRI, and arteriography may be indicated.
2. If acromegaly is suspected, appropriate bone x-rays should be done. A glucose tolerance test, including simultaneous determinations of the glucose and growth hormone levels, should also be performed.
3. Pituitary function studies are indicated in the presence of lactation. If the prolactin level is elevated, a pituitary tumor may be suspected. When the prolactin level is 200 ng/ml or greater, a pituitary tumor is likely in the absence of drug therapy. Lower levels of prolactin may sometimes occur in the presence of a pituitary tumor and in primary hypothyroidism.
4. Appropriate diagnostic studies are warranted whenever systemic disease is suspected.
5. Elevated plasma FSH and LH are indicative of primary ovarian failure.
6. Plasma FSH may be absent or low in prolactin-secreting tumors, hypopituitarism, massive obesity, and anorexia nervosa. Plasma FSH is usually normal in Cushing's disease or syndrome, polycystic ovary disease, and adrenal and ovarian tumors. Plasma FSH and LH may be variable in acromegaly. Plasma LH is frequently elevated in polycystic ovary disease to > 20 mIU/ml. An LH/FSH ratio of > 2.5 supports the diagnosis of polycystic ovary disease. If this disease is considered a possibility, testosterone should be measured. Measurement of LH before and after LRH administration may be useful in the appropriate patient.
7. Further evaluation of pituitary function is indicated in all patients with absent plasma FSH and LH to determine whether other tropic hormone deficiencies exist.
8. Additional studies for the diagnosis of Cushing's disease or syndrome, polycystic ovaries, and suspected ovarian or adrenal tumors are discussed in the sections Obesity and Adrenocortical Hyperfunction later in the chapter. Pelvic ultrasonography may be useful in suspected ovarian disease.
9. The response to progestational agents is often of some help diagnostically. The occurrence of withdrawal bleeding following the administration of medroxyprogesterone acetate (10 mg/day for 4 days) is indicative of previous endometrial stimulation by endogenous estrogen. Failure of such bleeding to occur suggests either estrogen deficiency or a lack of endometrial responsiveness.
10. Estradiol levels are useful in those patients who fail to respond to progesterone and in others to confirm estrogen deficiency.
11. Psychiatric evaluation is indicated in patients with massive obesity or anorexia nervosa.
12. Pelvic ultrasound is useful in establishing the size of the ovaries and uterus.

# ADRENOCORTICAL HYPERFUNCTION
## Janet E. Schemmel

Excessive production of adrenocortical hormones produces distinctive clinical syndromes. The recognized syndromes include Cushing's syndrome, caused by hypercortisolemia; virilization of women and children, related to excessive secretion of 17-ketosteroids or testosterone or both; feminization of men or children, due to the overproduction of estrogen; and hypertension with hypokalemia, which results from increased secretion of aldosterone. Aldosteronism is discussed in the section Arterial Hypertension (see Chapter 3). The virilization and feminization syndromes are beyond the scope of this text. This section will be confined to a discussion of the syndrome of glucocorticoid excess.

## Cushing's Syndrome

### Etiology

1. ACTH-dependent hyperadrenocorticism.
   a. Cushing's disease. This condition is most probably due to hypothalamic dysfunction. Excessive secretion of pituitary ACTH leads to adrenocortical hyperplasia and hypercortisolemia. Pituitary tumors are responsible for most cases.
   b. Nonpituitary tumors (the ectopic ACTH syndrome). An ACTH-like peptide is secreted and leads to adrenocortical hyperplasia and hypercortisolemia. The most common causes are oat cell carcinoma of the lung, pancreatic carcinoma, thymoma, and bronchial adenoma. Other tumors may also cause the syndrome.
2. ACTH-independent hyperadrenocorticism.
   a. Iatrogenic. This is the most common cause of Cushing's syndrome. It is the result of the prolonged and often excessive administration of cortisol, cortisone, or their derivatives.
   b. Adrenal adenomas. There is autonomous secretion of excessive quantities of cortisol with suppression of ACTH production.
   c. Adrenal carcinoma. Autonomous hypersecretion of cortisol and other steroids occurs. ACTH secretion is suppressed.

### Clinical Manifestations

Most of the more common clinical features are listed below.
1. Truncal obesity.
2. Moon facies.
3. Plethora.
4. Increased fragility of the skin with ecchymoses and striae.
5. Muscle atrophy.
6. Easy fatigability and weakness.
7. Mild acne.
8. Hirsutism (virilization suggests adrenal carcinoma).
9. Amenorrhea.
10. Nephrolithiasis.
11. Hypertension.
12. Leukocytosis with lymphopenia and eosinopenia; erythrocytosis.
13. Glucose intolerance.
14. Osteoporosis.
   Patients with the ectopic ACTH syndrome ordinarily have few of the manifestations outlined above. Weight loss rather than weight gain is the rule. Weakness, fatigability, and muscle atrophy are usually profound. Anemia and hypokalemia occur commonly. Cutaneous pigmentation is often pronounced.

### Diagnosis

Confirmation of the clinical diagnosis of Cushing's syndrome is based on the following criteria:
1. Increased urinary excretion of free cortisol or its metabolites, measured as 17-hydroxycorticosteroids (17-OHS) or 17-ketogenic steroids (17-KGS), or both.

2. Loss of the normal diurnal variation in plasma cortisol levels; both the A.M. and P.M. values are usually elevated.
3. Failure of cortisol secretion to be suppressed by low-dose dexamethasone testing.

### Etiologic Diagnosis of Cushing's Syndrome

Once the diagnosis of Cushing's syndrome is established, its etiology must be determined. For this purpose, a variety of laboratory tests and diagnostic procedures are employed. These are outlined in Table 9-1 and summarized below.
1. Iatrogenic hyperadrenocorticism is usually evidenced by a history of prolonged, excessive administration of corticosteroids.
2. Measurement of plasma ACTH levels may distinguish between the ectopic ACTH syndrome, in which the levels are usually high, and adrenocortical tumors, in which the levels are low. The ACTH levels may be normal or increased in Cushing's disease. Chromatography of ACTH, if available, may demonstrate "big ACTH" in the ectopic ACTH syndrome.
3. Cortisol levels not only show a loss of the normal diurnal variation but are elevated as well.
4. Low- and high-dose dexamethasone suppression tests are valuable aids to diagnosis.
   a. In normal and obese individuals, cortisol levels are suppressed with low dosage of dexamethasone.
   b. High-dose testing ordinarily suppresses cortisol levels in patients with Cushing's disease.
   c. Cortisol levels usually are not suppressed with high dosage of dexamethasone in patients with the ectopic ACTH syndrome or adrenocortical adenoma and carcinoma.
5. Metyrapone testing is useful in differentiating adrenal tumors from adrenal hyperplasia. The response to metyrapone is impaired in adrenal tumors but is normal in adrenal hyperplasia.
6. Exogenous ACTH stimulation may cause an exaggerated response in adrenal hyperplasia, a variable response in adenomas, and no response in adrenal carcinoma.

### Diagnostic Approach

A gamut of procedures is available for the investigation of Cushing's syndrome. Not all of the tests are indicated in every case. Selectivity in the choice of diagnostic procedures depends on the circumstances and the judgment of the physician. Repetition of some tests may be necessary.
1. As a first step, it is necessary to confirm the clinical diagnosis by the laboratory tests outlined above under the heading Diagnosis.
2. Once the diagnosis is confirmed, the cause can usually be ascertained by use of the following tests, as dictated by the circumstances (Table 9-1):
   a. Plasma cortisol and ACTH levels.
   b. Response to suppression by dexamethasone testing.
   c. Response to metyrapone testing.
   d. Response to ACTH stimulation.
3. Routine studies are advisable to evaluate the systemic effects of hypercortisolemia.
   a. CBC and platelet count.
   b. Urinalysis.
   c. Biochemical screening.
   d. Serum electrolytes.
   e. Glucose tolerance test or random postprandial glucose determinations.
   f. Radiologic studies.

**Table 9-1.** Etiologic diagnosis of Cushing's syndrome by evaluation of pituitary-adrenocortical function

| Test | Normal | Cushing's disease Hypothalamic | Pituitary tumor | Ectopic ACTH syndrome | Adrenal adenoma | Adrenal carcinoma | Iatrogenic |
|---|---|---|---|---|---|---|---|
| Plasma Cortisol level | N | | I | I | I | I | Variable; depends on method and steroid used |
| Diurnal cortisol | Higher in A.M. than P.M. | | None | None | None | None | Not applicable |
| Plasma ACTH | N | N or I | N or I | N or I* | D | D | D |
| Urinary excretion control | | | | | | | |
| 17-OHS, 17-KGS, free cortisol | N | | I | I | I | I | Variable; depends on steroid used |
| 17-KS | N | | I | I | L | Usually markedly I | Variable; depends on steroid used; usually D |
| Response to high-dose dexamethasone | S | | S | NS | Usually NS | NS | S |
| Response to metyrapone | N | | N to IR | D to NR | NR | NR | NR |
| Response to ACTH stimulation | N | | N to IR | N to slightly IR | D | Usually NR | Variable or slightly IR |

N = normal, I = increased, D = decreased, IR = increased response, NR = no response, S = suppression, NS = no suppression, L = low.
*Inferior petrosal sinus sampling of ACTH, if available, differentiates ectopic ACTH syndrome from pituitary tumor.

        **(1)** Skull films.
        **(2)** Chest films.
        **(3)** X-rays of the lumbar spine.
        **(4)** Intravenous pyelography with nephrotomography for nephrolithiasis and detection of adrenal enlargement.
    **g.** Electrocardiogram.
  **4.** Special procedures if a pituitary tumor is suspected.
    **a.** Visual fields.
    **b.** Pituitary MRI.
  **5.** If adrenal disease is believed to be responsible for the syndrome, the following procedures merit consideration:
    **a.** CT scanning.
    **b.** Arteriography to help differentiate between adrenal hyperplasia and tumor.
    **c.** Isotope scanning of the adrenals with $^{131}$I-19-iodocholesterol to assist in the differential diagnosis of hyperplasia, adenoma, and carcinoma.
  **6.** Inferior petrosal sinus sampling. Although this technique is not widely available, petrosal sinus and peripheral measurement of ACTH before and after administration of corticotrophin-releasing factor clarifies the diagnosis of pituitary as opposed to ectopic ACTH syndrome. Further, this study frequently can localize the pituitary tumor to the right or left side of the pituitary gland, which is especially useful since the MRI is often normal.
  **7.** Determination of the primary site and extent of the neoplasm in the ectopic ACTH syndrome (e.g., lung tomography).

---

## ADRENOCORTICAL HYPOFUNCTION (INSUFFICIENCY)
### Janet E. Schemmel

---

### Definition and Etiology

Adrenocortical insufficiency is a symptom complex that results from deficiency of adrenocortical hormones. It may be primary, as in Addison's disease, or secondary, as in hypopituitarism. The onset may be acute or insidious.

**1.** Primary adrenocortical insufficiency. The term *Addison's disease* refers to primary adrenocortical insufficiency. The course of the disease may be chronic or acute, or an acute phase may be superimposed on a chronic state. Primary atrophy (idiopathic adrenal insufficiency), tuberculosis, and fungal infections are common causes. Adrenal hemorrhage (due to anticoagulants or idiopathic in origin), AIDS, surgical removal of the adrenal glands, drugs (e.g., OP-DDD, aminoglutethimide), congenital adrenal hypoplasia, congenital adrenal hyperplasia, and metastatic carcinoma may also produce primary adrenocortical insufficiency. In present-day medical practice, adrenal suppression from prolonged steroid therapy is probably the most commonly diagnosed cause.

    Idiopathic adrenal insufficiency may be associated with a multiplicity of other diseases including diabetes mellitus, Hashimoto's thyroiditis, thyrotoxicosis (Graves' disease), mucocutaneous candidiasis, hypoparathyroidism, primary ovarian failure, and pernicious anemia. An autoimmune mechanism has been postulated. Polyglandular autoimmune syndromes, Type I and Type II (PGA I and PGA II, respectively), are associated with adrenal insufficiency and may be familial.

**2.** Secondary adrenocortical insufficiency. Adrenocortical insufficiency may also be secondary to hypopituitarism from pituitary or hypothalamic disease. Destruction of pituitary or hypothalamic tissue may be caused by infarction, granulomatous disease (e.g., sarcoidosis, tuberculosis), chromophobe adenoma, suprasellar meningioma, craniopharyngioma, or aneurysm.

## Symptoms

The onset of adrenocortical insufficiency is usually insidious but it can be acute. The spectrum of symptoms in both primary and secondary adrenocortical insufficiency is variable. The following symptoms may be described by the patient: (1) asthenia, weakness, and lethargy, (2) weight loss, (3) easy fatigability, especially in the afternoon, (4) dizziness and syncope, (5) anorexia, nausea, vomiting, and diarrhea, (6) nervousness, irritability, and apathy, and (7) nonspecific complaints such as myalgias, loss of libido, or heat and cold intolerance.

### Primary Adrenocortical Insufficiency

Any of the aforementioned symptoms can occur in primary adrenal disease, but chronic weakness, fatigue, weight loss, and gastrointestinal symptoms are the most frequent complaints. Changes in the color of the skin or increased numbers of moles and freckles are sometimes noted by the patient or his friends. Salt craving and increased salt intake are also common symptoms.

If the patient has PGA I or PGA II, other conditions may be associated. PGA I patients may have mucocutaneous candidiasis and those with PGA II, autoimmune thyroid disease and diabetes mellitus. Further discussion is beyond the scope of this text.

### Secondary Adrenocortical Insufficiency

In addition to many of the symptoms noted above, patients with hypopituitarism may have local symptoms related to its underlying cause and systemic symptoms resulting from specific tropic hormone deficiencies, as follows: (1) impairment of vision or visual field defects, (2) headaches (frontal, vertical, temporoparietal, or varying combinations of these locations), (3) failure to tan after exposure to sunlight, (4) mental confusion and somnolence, (5) loss of libido, amenorrhea, or impotence, (6) loss of body hair and decreased beard growth, (7) growth failure in children, and (8) polydipsia and polyuria. Salt craving does not occur.

### Acute Adrenocortical Insufficiency

Adrenal crisis is characterized by headaches, malaise, restlessness, vomiting, abdominal pain, hyperpyrexia, and shock, which may progress to coma and death. Acute adrenal insufficiency may occur under the following circumstances: (1) failure of the patient with adrenocortical insufficiency to take the prescribed replacement therapy; (2) following acute illness, stress, anesthesia, or surgery in patients with decreased adrenocortical reserve; (3) failure to increase the dosage of steroids in patients with Addison's disease complicated by acute disease or other stressful situations; (4) abrupt withdrawal of adrenocortical hormones in steroid-treated individuals; (5) following injury to the adrenals by trauma, thrombosis, or hemorrhage; (6) after bilateral adrenalectomy; and (7) overwhelming sepsis, with or without hemorrhagic phenomena.

## Physical Findings

### Primary Adrenocortical Insufficiency

The physical findings may be normal, but patients with symptoms of weakness, lethargy, and weight loss usually exhibit changes in the pigmentation of the skin. Sometimes this is the only abnormality detectable on examination. The skin changes observed include hyperpigmentation or tanning of both the exposed and unexposed parts of the body (especially prominent over pressure areas), increased numbers of freckles, and sometimes vitiligo. Brownish-blue discoloration of the lips and gums and other mucous membranes may be present. The blood pressure may be normal, although postural hypotension is more common. The heart size is often reduced. Manifestations of PGA I or II may be present.

### Secondary Adrenocortical Insufficiency

The physical findings may be normal, although the examination may provide evidence suggestive not only of adrenocortical insufficiency but also of hypothyroidism and hypogonadism. Changes in visual acuity or visual field defects may be demonstrable. In the preadolescent age group, growth failure and delayed puberty are frequent findings. The skin of the exposed portions of the body may be pale.

---

## Diagnostic Approach

---

### Primary Adrenocortical Insufficiency

1. A simple procedure called the rapid ACTH test or Cortrosyn (tetracosactrin) test is useful for initial screening. The plasma cortisol level is determined from a blood sample drawn between 7 A.M. and 9 A.M. Cortrosyn (0.25 mg) is then injected intramuscularly. Plasma cortisol levels are then obtained 30 and 45 minutes after the injection. In normal subjects, plasma cortisol levels rise by at least 7 μg/100 ml in 30 minutes or the total value exceeds 18 μg/100 ml. Usually there is at least a twofold rise above the control value to 20 μg/100 ml or above. The plasma cortisol value at 45 minutes should approximate that in the 30-minute sample. A normal response excludes primary adrenocortical failure.
2. If the Cortrosyn test elicits an abnormal response, additional tests may be performed.
   a. CBC and urinalysis.
   b. Serum electrolytes.
   c. BUN.
   d. Skin tests for tuberculosis and fungal diseases.
   e. Chest films, which may show a small heart.
   f. A KUB film to demonstrate adrenal calcification, which suggests tuberculosis or fungal disease. Idiopathic adrenal insufficiency is associated with small adrenal glands on CT scanning of the adrenals. Enlarged glands are consistent with metastatic or granulomatous disease.
   g. Skull films to exclude pituitary lesions.
   h. Serum calcium and phosphorus.
   i. Liver profile.
   j. Antithyroglobulin antibodies, which if present suggest an autoimmune basis for the adrenal disease.
   k. $T_4$; $T_3$ resin uptake or $T_3$ RIA, or both; TSH.
   l. Adrenal antibodies.
3. The most specific and sensitive test for adrenocortical insufficiency is the intravenous ACTH test. On the day before the test, a 24-hour urine collection is made, and the quantities of 17-ketogenic steroids or 17-hydroxycorticoids and creatinine excreted are determined. Subsequently, on three consecutive days, 25 units of ACTH in 1000 ml of 5% dextrose in normal or 0.45 normal saline are infused intravenously over a period of exactly 8 hours. Daily 24-hour urine specimens are collected for 17-ketogenic steroids or 17-hydroxycorticoids and creatinine. A rise in steroid excretion of less than 100 percent of the control value is diagnostic of adrenocortical insufficiency. Normally, a threefold or greater excretion occurs on the first day of the test, with a further increase on the second day and maximum excretion on the third day. The urinary creatinine determinations are made to check on the reliability of the urine collections.

   An equally specific and shorter test for adrenocortical insufficiency is the 48-

hour ACTH test. Cortrosyn in a dose of 0.5 mg dissolved in glucose and water is infused every 12 hours for a continuous 48-hour period, during which time urines are collected for 17-ketogenic steroids or 17-hydroxysteroids and creatinine, as in the 3-day ACTH test. Normally there is at least a twofold increase in the baseline values following the 2-day infusion. Depot Cortrosyn is not yet available.

4. If PGA I or II is suspected, additional studies may be necessary. HLA typing may be indicated.
5. ACTH levels are markedly elevated.
6. Plasma renin levels are considerably elevated and aldosterone levels are usually markedly decreased, if aldosterone deficiency coexists with hydrocortisone deficiency.

## Secondary Adrenocortical Insufficiency

1. Patients with secondary adrenocortical insufficiency generally require a more extensive workup than those with primary disease, not only for the purpose of determining the cause but also to ascertain which tropic hormones are deficient.
2. The tests listed below are recommended for this type of comprehensive survey.
   a. CBC and urinalysis.
   b. Serum electrolytes.
   c. BUN.
   d. Skull films.
   e. Chest films.
   f. Visual acuity, including visual fields, if appropriate.
   g. $T_4$; $T_3$ resin uptake or $T_3$ RIA, or both.
   h. TSH by RIA. If the TSH is low, TRH infusion with measurement of TSH both before and after the infusion should be carried out to detect pituitary or hypothalamic dysfunction.
   i. Fasting serum growth hormone and prolactin determination.
   j. Insulin tolerance test with growth hormone determinations. The L-dopa or arginine infusion test may be substituted in selected cases.
   k. Plasma FSH, LH, testosterone, and plasma estradiol in selected cases. LHRF (luteinizing hormone releasing factor) can facilitate the investigation of patients with low FSH and LH values. A 100 μg bolus of synthetic LHRF is given intravenously with blood samples collected before, and at 20 and 60 minutes after, the injection. Normally there is at least a threefold rise in FSH and LH above the baseline levels. If the 20-minute or 60-minute values for both FSH and LH are above normal, the response is regarded as exaggerated. When the 60-minute levels are the same as or greater than those found at the 20-minute interval, the response is considered to be delayed. A delayed response in the FSH level is seen in most normal women. The LHRF infusion test can also be performed with blood samples taken 20 and 30 minutes after the injection.
   l. Metyrapone test. This test is carried out by collecting 24-hour urine specimens for 17-ketogenic steroids or 17-hydroxycorticoids and creatinine on the day before and the day following the administration of metyrapone. The drug is given orally in a dosage of 750 mg every 4 hours for six doses. A normal response is characterized by an increase of 2.8 times or greater in steroid excretion on the day after the test compared to the control value.
      The metyrapone test can also be carried out as an overnight procedure. Plasma cortisol, 11-deoxycortisol, and/or ACTH levels are measured at 8:00 A.M. on the day before the test. At midnight, 2 g of metyrapone is administered. At 8:00 A.M. the following morning, plasma cortisol, 11-deoxycortisol, and/or ACTH levels are determined. A normal response is a rise in the 11-deoxycortisol level above 10 μg/100 ml.
   m. Plasma ACTH.
   n. Vasopressin assay. Measurements of vasopressin are now commercially available. The determination is best made after a period of water deprivation. Va-

sopressin acts on the pituitary gland as a corticotropin-releasing hormone. Measurement of plasma cortisol levels following the administration of vasopressin has been used to differentiate between pituitary and hypothalamic disease. This test has not achieved wide popularity at present. Corticotropin releasing factor (CRF) is investigational.

3. If skull x-rays show a pituitary tumor or abnormality of the sella turcica, then MRI of the pituitary gland is indicated.

4. If surgical intervention is necessary before the appropriate laboratory studies can be completed, blood samples should be drawn for the following tests: CBC; urinalysis; electrolytes; BUN; creatinine; $T_4$; $T_3$ resin uptake or $T_3$ RIA, or both; plasma TSH; plasma cortisol; fasting growth hormone; plasma FSH and LH; ACTH; prolactin; and testosterone.

## OBESITY
Janet E. Schemmel

### Definition

Obesity may be defined as an excess quantity of body fat. The diagnosis of obesity is usually based on statistics given in life insurance tables. A patient is considered overweight if his weight is 20 pounds greater than the norm established for his age, sex, height, and body build. However, the tables should be considered only as an approximate clinical guide. More precisely, obesity may be defined by a body mass index of more than 30 (weight in kg ÷ by height in square meters). This value correlates well with skin fold measurements of > 30 mm in women and > 23 mm in men. Fat normally constitutes 15 to 20 percent of the total body weight. The degree and interpretation of obesity relate to cultural values.

### Etiology

Obesity is most commonly due to overeating, but it may be associated with the conditions listed below. Although this list is not all-inclusive, it encompasses the more common and several unusual syndromes reported.

1. Diabetes.
2. Pregnancy.
3. Use of contraceptives.
4. Genetic influences (probably more environmental than genetic).
5. Hypothalamic injuries or abnormalities (e.g., Prader-Willi syndrome).
6. Hyperlipemic states.
7. Miscellaneous diseases.
   a. Cushing's syndrome or disease.
   b. Acromegaly.
   c. Islet cell tumor.
   d. Hypothyroidism.
   e. Polycystic ovary syndrome.
   f. Laurence-Moon-Biedl syndrome—obesity, hypogonadism, polydactylism.
   g. Pseudohypoparathyroidism—hypocalcemia, obesity, bone abnormalities.
   h. Babinski-Fröhlich syndrome—hyperphagia and hypogonadism due to hypothalamic lesions.
   i. Abnormal thermogenesis (causal relationship not well established).

### Symptoms

Most obese patients are otherwise asymptomatic. When obesity is marked, easy fatigability, exertional dyspnea, depression, anxiety, and somnolence are likely to occur. Many of the symptoms attributed to obesity actually result from an underlying or associated disorder rather than from the obesity itself. The more common symptoms encountered in obese individuals are listed below.

1. Easy fatigability.
2. Depression with anxiety.
3. Malaise.
4. Weakness, hunger, fatigue, and dyspepsia—common in pregnancy.
5. Symptoms of reactive hypoglycemia—weakness, hunger, palpitation, and sweating—often seen in obese adult-onset diabetics about 3 to 5 hours after meals.
6. Excessive hunger—not uncommon in patients with adult-onset diabetes mellitus, islet cell tumors, the Babinski-Fröhlich syndrome, pregnant women, women taking oral contraceptives, and hypothalamic disorders.
7. Excessive weight gain in spite of a normal or reduced caloric intake, frequent in Cushing's disease or syndrome.
8. Weight gain not due to overeating, often in association with loss of libido, headaches, increased hair growth, and enlargement of the hands and feet—common in acromegaly.
9. Muscle cramps, numbness of the hands, feet, and face, seizures, and obesity—suggestive of pseudohypoparathyroidism.

---

## Signs

---

Some physical findings are produced by obesity per se, but most of the signs encountered in obese individuals are primarily related to the underlying disease.

1. Obesity that is generalized in distribution is typical of exogenous obesity. However, truncal accentuation (presumably genetic) is frequently observed.
2. Pink striae are commonly distributed over the axillae, breasts, abdomen, flanks, thighs, and buttocks, particularly in young women if the weight gain has been rapid. Usually, the pink color tends to fade and eventually disappear, leaving the striae shiny and white.
3. The blood pressure is usually normal, unless systemic hypertension due to another cause coexists or the blood pressure cuff is ill-fitting.
4. Intertrigo is quite common in the folds below the breasts and in the inguinal regions.
5. Ankle edema is occasionally noted.
6. Plethora involving the cheeks and neck is not unusual.
7. When obesity is massive, tachypnea may be evident.
8. The presence of a thyroidectomy scar, typical changes in the skin, and a delayed return of deep tendon reflexes suggest hypothyroidism.
9. Purpura, moon facies, truncal obesity, plethora, and weakness are common in Cushing's syndrome or disease.
10. Xanthomata, xanthelasma, and arcus senilis suggest hyperlipoproteinemic abnormalities.
11. Brachydactylia, a round facies, a stocky build, and tetany are found in patients with pseudohypoparathyroidism.
12. Excessive growth of the hands, feet, and jaw are typical of acromegaly.
13. Hypogonadism may occur in the hypothalamic obesity syndromes.
14. Hirsutism may occur in the polycystic ovary syndrome.

---

## Diagnostic Approach

---

### Initial Evaluation

1. CBC and platelet count.
2. Urinalysis.
3. Glucose tolerance testing.

    **a.** Several normal 2-hour postprandial glucose level tests may be adequate in most cases to exclude diabetes mellitus.

    **b.** A 5-hour glucose tolerance test may be indicated in patients with symptoms of reactive hypoglycemia to document the hypoglycemia.

**4.** Fasting triglycerides.

**5.** Thyroid function tests (TSH; free $T_4$; or $T_4$ and $T_3$ RIA).

**6.** BUN and serum electrolytes (biochemical profile).

**7.** Serum uric acid, primarily to obtain a baseline value, because hyperuricemia often occurs with restricted caloric intake and after weight loss.

**8.** Chest films.

**9.** Electrocardiogram.

**10.** Psychiatric consultation is especially valuable in planning treatment and estimating prognosis in patients with serious weight problems.

    As a rule, the aforementioned laboratory tests are normal in patients with exogenous obesity who have not been on diuretic therapy or on a dietary regimen. However, serum triglyceride levels frequently are elevated, particularly when obesity is marked.

## Subsequent Evaluation

In patients in whom the symptoms, signs, or initial laboratory studies suggest the possibility of an associated disorder or systemic disease, additional workup, as follows, is indicated.

**1.** Fasting total lipids and lipoprotein electrophoresis when the serum triglyceride or cholesterol levels are markedly elevated, or if the glucose tolerance test is abnormal.

**2.** Pulmonary function studies and arterial blood gases, if somnolence or exertional dyspnea is present. Sleep study may be necessary.

**3.** Thyroid antibodies, when thyroid dysfunction is suspected.

**4.** Growth hormone measured in association with a glucose tolerance test, if acromegaly is being considered. Growth hormone levels are measured while fasting, and at 1- and 2-hour intervals after glucose administration.

**5.** Skull films (and, if indicated, CT scanning, MRI, and arteriography), when acromegaly, Cushing's disease, or infiltrative pituitary-hypothalamic disease is suspected.

**6.** Fasting insulin and fasting blood sugar determinations. Both of these parameters should be measured serially during a 72-hour fast if hyperinsulinism is suspected. Insulin levels may also be helpful in the evaluation of patients who exhibit symptoms of reactive hypoglycemia during glucose tolerance tests.

**7.** If truncal adiposity, weakness, plethora, and other symptoms or signs suggest concomitant Cushing's disease or syndrome, an overnight dexamethasone suppression test should be performed in the following manner: A plasma cortisol level is obtained in a blood sample drawn at 8 A.M. on the day of the test. Dexamethasone (1.0 mg) is given at midnight. The plasma cortisol level is determined on a sample drawn at 8 A.M. the next morning. Normally, the administration of dexamethasone causes a reduction in the plasma cortisol level to 5 to 7 μg/100 ml or less. If the plasma cortisol level is not suppressed by this maneuver or if Cushing's disease or syndrome is suspected, further evaluation of adrenal function is necessary. The following procedure is recommended: Daily 24-hour urine specimens for 17-ketogenic steroids and creatinine are collected before and during the test period. After an adequate collection of baseline urine (two specimens) has been obtained, dexamethasone is given orally (0.5 mg every 6 hours for a 2- to 3-day period, followed by 2.0 mg every 6 hours for an additional 2- to 3-day period). Normally, steroid excretion is reduced to at least 50 percent of the control values by the second day of dexamethasone administration. In patients with adrenocortical hyperplasia, suppression of steroid excretion is ordinarily apparent by the fourth to sixth day of dexamethasone therapy. Steroid excretion is usually not suppressed in patients with neoplasms of the adrenal cortex. When the test results are equivocal, the study can be repeated. The metyrapone and ACTH stimulation tests are important adjuncts that are helpful in differentiating between adrenal hyperplasia, tumor, and carcinoma. ACTH assay should be carried out. The specimens may be collected before and after dexamethasone suppression and may give helpful adjunctive information. Urinary free cortisol measurements may be substituted for 17-ketogenic steroid determinations.

8. Measurement of plasma free testosterone, and plasma FSH and LH may be helpful in those cases in which the polycystic ovary syndrome is suspected. Pelvic ultrasound and CT scanning may be indicated.

## THYROID ENLARGEMENT
Janet E. Schemmel

### Definition

Enlargement of the thyroid gland is referred to as goiter. A goiter may be congenital or acquired, endemic or sporadic. Throughout the world, regions exist in which goiter is endemic. In such areas, the incidence of thyrotoxicosis, thyroiditis, and thyroid malignancy is increased. Malignancy of the thyroid gland occurs frequently in individuals who have received radiation therapy to the head, neck, or face during infancy and childhood.

### Etiology

Enlargement of the thyroid gland may be due to many causes. Various classifications of goiter, based on the palpatory findings, the histologic examination, the state of thyroid function, or the results of laboratory tests, have been proposed. The more common causes of goiter are as follows:

1. Diffuse goiter.
   a. Euthyroid.
      (1) Endemic or sporadic diffuse goiter; colloid goiter.
      (2) Drug-induced goiter.
      (3) Abnormality of hormone synthesis.
      (4) Thyroiditis.
         (a) Acute.
         (b) Subacute.
         (c) Chronic.
         (d) Hashimoto's struma.
         (e) Postpartum thyroiditis; silent thyroiditis.
   b. Hypothyroid.
      (1) Cretinism.
      (2) Juvenile hypothyroidism.
      (3) Thyroiditis and Hashimoto's struma.
      (4) Drug-induced goiter.
      (5) Abnormality of hormone synthesis.
   c. Hyperthyroid.
      (1) Graves' disease.
      (2) Subacute thyroiditis.
2. Multinodular goiter: endemic or sporadic.
   a. Nontoxic.
   b. Toxic.
3. Solitary nodular goiter.
   a. Nontoxic.
      (1) Benign.
      (2) Malignant.
   b. Toxic.

---

## Symptoms

1. Many patients with goiters are asymptomatic. The mass in the neck may be the presenting complaint, having been discovered by the patient or brought to his attention by a relative or friend. At other times, the goiter is found by a physician during the course of a routine physical examination.
2. Absence of symptoms is common in patients with endemic or sporadic goiter, drug-induced goiter, multinodular goiter, solitary nodular goiter, early thyrotoxicosis, and Hashimoto's struma.
3. The presence or absence of systemic symptoms may provide a clue to the state of thyroid function or the presence of coexisting disease.
4. Fatigue, lethargy, a 10- to 20-pound weight gain, intolerance to cold, dry skin, and arthralgia suggest hypothyroidism. This may be the result of inadequate or abnormal thyroid hormone synthesis, thyroiditis, multinodular goiter, or drug-induced goiter.
5. Weakness, weight loss, heat intolerance, palpitation, and exophthalmos suggest thyrotoxicosis.
6. Pain in the thyroid during deglutition, or radiation of pain to the ear or jaw, may be indicative of subacute thyroiditis, cancer, or hemorrhage or other degenerative changes in an adenoma or cyst.
7. Dyspnea may occur when large thyroids encroach on the trachea or bronchus.
8. Dysphagia suggests esophageal obstruction due to chronic thyroiditis or carcinoma but may occur whenever the gland is massively enlarged.
9. Symptoms of systemic illness, such as rheumatoid arthritis or nontuberculous Addison's disease, should raise the possibility of associated Hashimoto's struma.
10. Growth retardation in infants and children is common in hypothyroidism. Precocious puberty may also occur infrequently.
11. A history of x-ray therapy to the thymus, pharynx, or face during infancy or childhood should suggest the possibility of thyroid carcinoma or multiple nodularity.

---

## Signs

1. The findings on general examination depend largely on the status of thyroid function. Every patient with a goiter should be examined for clinical evidence of thyrotoxicosis or hypothyroidism. If the patient is euthyroid, the findings are usually limited to the neck area.
2. A diffusely and symmetrically enlarged thyroid that is smooth or lobulated is found in neonatal and childhood goiters, endemic or sporadic goiters, thyroiditis, and Graves' disease. The gland is usually soft in colloid goiter and firm in hyperthyroidism. In Hashimoto's thyroiditis, the gland tends to be firm and lumpy. Stony hard glands are usually indicative of malignancy or Riedel's struma. The presence of a vascular thrill or bruit over the thyroid gland suggests hyperthyroidism.
3. Multinodular enlargement of the thyroid gland may be observed in toxic or nontoxic endemic or sporadic goiters and, occasionally, in carcinoma or chronic thyroiditis.
4. The occurrence of a solitary nodular goiter suggests toxic or nontoxic adenoma, carcinoma, or a cyst.
5. The presence of cervical lymphadenopathy suggests carcinoma but may occur in Hashimoto's thyroiditis.
6. Evidence of tracheal or esophageal obstruction, or both, may occur in carcinoma, retrosternal goiter, or Hashimoto's struma, or whenever the gland is massively enlarged.
7. Fixation of the gland is typical of carcinoma but occurs occasionally in thyroiditis.
8. Hoarseness due to compression of the recurrent laryngeal nerve suggests a ma-

lignant neoplasm of the thyroid, although hoarseness may occur in Hashimoto's struma.

## Diagnostic Approach

### Clinical Features

1. The duration of a goiter, the age, sex, and geographic origin of the patient, the family history, evidence of previous irradiation to the pharynx, thymus, or face, or prior exposure to goitrogenic agents may provide important clues to the cause of thyroid enlargement.
2. The nodularity of the thyroid gland is of diagnostic significance. Multinodular goiters are most often nontoxic and are rarely malignant. Solitary nodular goiters occur much more frequently in women than in men, but the incidence of carcinoma is higher in men than in women and is greatest below the age of 40 years. Functioning nodules are more likely to be benign than are nonfunctioning nodules. Solitary nodules may be toxic or nontoxic. Nodularity of the thyroid gland in a patient of either sex with a history of head or neck irradiation is suggestive of carcinoma.
3. When signs of thyrotoxicosis are present, the thyroid gland is usually diffusely enlarged, although it is sometimes nodular or lobulated. Thyrotoxicosis rarely coexists with malignancy.

### Laboratory Studies

1. CBC and platelet count. Leukopenia and a relative lymphocytosis are common in thyrotoxicosis.
2. Thyroid function tests.
   a. Thyroid profile. In the past, the usual thyroid profile included $T_4$ and $T_3$ uptakes. Now, a reliable free $T_4$ coupled with a $T_3$ RIA may replace the profile of the past. These values are usually normal unless hyperthyroidism or hypothyroidism is present. Abnormal values may occur in thyroiditis, pregnancy, or absence of thyroid-binding globulin, and as a result of the effect of drugs (e.g., diphenylhydantoin, estrogen). The many factors that may affect the results of these tests are beyond the scope of this discussion.
   b. TSH (ultrasensitive). This test is now widely available. TSH can be used to diagnose thyrotoxicosis as well as hypothyroidism. In the former, the value is suppressed to $< 0.1$ mIU/ml. This determination is of value in distinguishing between primary and secondary hypothyroidism: TSH values are increased in the former condition but are low or immeasurable in the latter. In order to differentiate between pituitary and hypothalamic causes of secondary hypothyroidism, a TRH test can be performed. TRH is injected intravenously with measurement of TSH prior to, and 30 and 60 minutes after, the administration of the TRH. At least a threefold rise in TSH occurs at 30 minutes if pituitary function is intact. Should TSH fail to rise after the administration of TRH, pituitary disease should be suspected. TSH is suppressed in hyperthyroidism unless a TSH secreting pituitary tumor is present.
3. Thyroglobulin antibodies. Increased serum levels of antithyroglobulin antibodies and microsomal antibodies may occur in Hashimoto's thyroiditis, as well as in simple goiter, thyrotoxicosis, and malignancy. Usually, the incidence of positive tests and the antibody titer are higher in Hashimoto's struma than in the other conditions. Positive tests may be considered specific for Hashimoto's struma in the appropriate patient.
4. Ultrasonography is useful in differentiating between thyroid cysts and solid nodules and in delineating the thyroid gland.
5. Thyroxin-binding globulin determination may be indicated when thyroid function tests do not correlate with the clinical picture, when hepatitis or nephrosis is

present, when there is an uncertain history of previous drug therapy (e.g., diphenylhydantoin, estrogens), or if the diagnosis of primary thyroxin-binding globulin deficiency is suspected.

6. RAI uptake. This test is usually carried out at 6 and 24 hours after the administration of $^{123}$I or $^{131}$I. An abnormally low level may occur in hypothyroidism, iodine contamination, and acute and subacute thyroiditis. An elevated value may be seen in iodine deficiency, certain types of thyroid hormone synthesis abnormalities, thyrotoxicosis (both diffuse and nodular types), and Hashimoto's struma. It may be normal in thyroiditis, multinodular goiter, toxic nodular goiter, and $T_3$ thyrotoxicosis.

7. Thyroid scan with $^{123}$I is usually not necessary in the thyrotoxic patient with diffuse thyroid enlargement and exophthalmos. However, a scan may be helpful in differentiating between toxic and nontoxic nodular goiter. It is particularly valuable when the iodine uptake is within the normal range. Under such circumstances, the demonstration of a single area of intense uptake is significant. In the case of nontoxic solitary nodules, radioisotope scanning may be helpful in management of the patient. Thyroid scanning is recommended for all patients who have had x-ray therapy to the head and neck during infancy and childhood.

8. Needle aspiration of the thyroid gland with cytologic studies is indicated to differentiate between thyroiditis, carcinoma, and colloid goiter. Conventional surgical biopsy is also employed for diagnostic purposes in selected cases.

9. An elevated $T_3$ by RIA confirms the diagnosis of $T_3$ thyrotoxicosis in a patient with symptoms of hyperthyroidism and a normal $T_4$.


### Further Investigations

1. Serum calcium and phosphorus levels are occasionally abnormal in both hyperthyroidism and hypothyroidism. The serum alkaline phosphatase is frequently elevated in thyrotoxicosis.

2. TRH stimulation test. This test can be used to confirm the diagnosis of autonomous thyroid nodules. TSH may be suppressed before and after TRH administration even when $T_4$ and $T_3$ measurements are normal. This test replaces the Cytomel suppression test used previously.

3. Perchlorate study. This test is indicated if an organification defect is suspected. A tracer dose of RAI is given. After a suitable interval, 500 mg of potassium perchlorate is administered by mouth. Normally, because of the rapid organic binding of the iodide, no thyroid loss of $^{131}$I occurs. However, when organification is impaired, the potassium perchlorate causes a partial or complete discharge of $^{131}$I from the thyroid gland within a 30-minute period. This test is also useful in the occasional case of Hashimoto's struma in which the RAI uptake is elevated.

4. Thyroid stimulating immunoglobulins. Measurement of immunoglobulins may be helpful in confirming neonatal Graves' disease, in the differential diagnosis of exophthalmos, and sometimes in predicting spontaneous remission or cure of Graves' disease.

5. Indirect laryngoscopy is indicated in dysphonic patients to exclude intrinsic lesions of the larynx.

6. Investigation of other family members is indicated when familial disease is suspected.

7. Hearing and taste tests should be carried out in children with thyroid enlargement in whom either multinodular goiter or Pendred's syndrome (familial goiter with deafness) is suspected.

8. Other tests of thyroid function, the determination of iodinated products in serum, and chromatography of thyroid hormone precursors are either research procedures or as yet not readily available clinically.

9. Despite the number of available tests, the cause of a goiter is not always easily determined. In such cases, thyroid hormone suppression treatment over a 6-month period may be indicated. If at the end of this period no reduction in thyroid

size has occurred, surgical exploration may be advisable. Surgical exploration for both diagnostic and therapeutic purposes is indicated whenever malignancy is a reasonable possibility. Surgical exploration is also advisable in patients with previous x-ray therapy to the head or neck if the thyroid examination or a technetium thyroid scan is abnormal.

## HYPERCALCEMIA

Janet E. Schemmel

### Definition

Hypercalcemia is said to exist when the serum calcium is 10.5 mg/100 ml or greater, as determined by the autoanalyzer, using the Gitelman modification of the Kessler and Wolfman colorimetric method. This figure may vary slightly depending on the normal values of the method as established by the individual laboratory. Hypercalcemia is emerging as an even more complex diagnostic problem than it was in the past. With automation of laboratory procedures, biochemical screenings or profiles are often done routinely, both in the physician's office and in the hospital. The serum calcium is generally included in these screenings, and elevations are often seen in asymptomatic patients. Elevations of the serum calcium level are found in about 1 percent of routine biochemical screens.

### Etiology

Multiple causes for hypercalcemia have been elucidated, hence the diagnosis may be difficult. Sometimes the diagnosis can be established only by observation of the patient over a period of time. The various known causes of hypercalcemia include the following conditions:

1. Malignancy—probably most common in hospitalized patients.
   a. Carcinoma.
   b. Multiple myeloma.
   c. Leukemia; lymphoma.
   d. Nonendocrine, parathyroid hormone–secreting carcinoma (e.g., lung, kidney, ovary, colon, cervix, pancreas), ectopic hyperparathyroidism.
2. Primary hyperparathyroidism (0.1 percent).
   a. Tumor.
   b. Hyperplasia.
   c. Carcinoma.
3. Drug-induced hypercalcemia, including the thiazides and spironolactone—increasingly common.
4. Vitamin D intoxication.
5. Milk-alkali syndrome.
6. Multiple endocrine neoplasia, I and II; Zollinger-Ellison syndrome.
7. Benign familial hypercalcemia (familial hypocalciuric hypercalcemia).
8. Others.
   a. Hypothyroidism and hyperthyroidism.
   b. Adrenal insufficiency.
   c. Sarcoidosis and other granulomatous diseases.
   d. Acromegaly.
   e. Immobilization.
   f. Idiopathic hypercalcemia of infancy (William's syndrome).
   g. Vitamin A intoxication.
   h. Pheochromocytoma.

## Symptoms

It is obvious from the many possible causes of hypercalcemia that a variety of symptoms may occur. Frequently, an asymptomatic patient is found to have an elevated serum calcium on routine biochemical screening. As a general rule, patients with slightly elevated serum calciums usually have fewer symptoms than those with higher values. Usually, most patients with serum calciums below 11 mg/100 ml are relatively asymptomatic, whereas most patients with serum calciums above 12 mg/100 ml are symptomatic. The following symptoms may occur:

1. None—particularly common at this time.
2. Nocturia—perhaps the earliest symptom.
3. Polydipsia, polyuria—both early symptoms.
4. Easy fatigability.
5. Irritability, difficulty in concentrating, depression, confusion.
6. Constipation, obstipation.
7. Urinary tract stones and urinary tract infections—may antedate other modes of presentation by a number of years.
8. High blood pressure—may antedate other symptoms by a number of years.
9. Muscle weakness, generalized or involving the shoulders and hips.
10. Anorexia, nausea, vomiting, abdominal pain, peptic disease.
11. Weight loss.
12. Joint pain.
13. Deep pain (e.g., arms, legs, back).
14. Instability when walking.
15. Headache.
16. Difficulty in focusing the eyes.

## Signs

The physical examination may yield no abnormalities, particularly if hypercalcemia has been of short duration or if the serum calcium is 11 mg/100 ml or less. In patients with malignancy, marked weight loss may occur. Physical findings in hypercalcemia may include the following:

1. Elevated systolic blood pressure with or without elevated diastolic pressure. This is a common finding.
2. Rarely, a parathyroid tumor may be palpable and then usually is more than 4 g in weight. (Most palpable anterior neck masses are of thyroid origin.)
3. Bone or muscle tenderness on pressure.
4. Proximal or generalized muscle weakness.
5. Dysequilibration.
6. Emotional lability, mental confusion, depression.
7. Weight loss, varying from 10 to 30 pounds, although none may be noted.
8. Reflexes may be normal or reduced; hypotonia may be present.
9. Skin lesions, such as purpura, ecchymosis, and petechia may be present.
10. An enlarged liver or spleen may be palpable; lymphadenopathy may be present.
11. Recurring, intermittent urticaria.
12. Somnolence, coma.
13. Band keratopathy on slit lamp examination of the eyes. This is an uncommon finding.

## Diagnostic Approach

### Initial Workup

In view of the paucity of signs that may be present, the workup may be particularly difficult. The purpose of the initial study is to establish a diagnosis, or failing that, to reduce the number of diagnostic possibilities. Patients with marked hypercalcemia (serum calcium $\geq$ 13 mg/100 ml) should be treated immediately in order to reduce the serum calcium level. Once this has been accomplished, diagnostic studies may be performed at a later and more appropriate time. The following initial studies are recommended:

1. Serial determinations of serum calcium and phosphorus to establish that hypercalcemia is present. These should be obtained while the patient is not on excessive intake of phosphate because this ion may reduce the serum calcium levels.
2. A careful review of all of the patient's medications and diet. All drugs that are not essential or that are known to influence serum calcium levels (e.g., calcium, vitamin D, thiazides, and spironolactone) should be withheld.
3. Hemoglobin and hematocrit determinations.
4. WBC and differential counts.
5. Platelet count.
6. Serum electrolytes.
7. BUN and serum creatinine.
8. Serum alkaline phosphatase.
9. Serum protein electrophoresis.
10. Urine protein electrophoresis in selected cases.
11. Serum immunoglobulins in selected cases.
12. Sedimentation rate (Westergren).
13. 24-hour urine for calcium, phosphorus, and creatinine determinations.
14. X-rays—chest (PA and lateral), lumbar spine (AP and lateral), skull, and PA views of both hands.

If continuous hypercalcemia and associated hypophosphatemia are documented, the most likely diagnosis is primary or ectopic hyperparathyroidism, myeloma, or sarcoidosis. However, if normal phosphate levels are found, the diagnosis remains uncertain. If the drug history indicates the use of medications known to influence serum calcium, the drugs should be withdrawn and the patient reevaluated for hypercalcemia after approximately 4 to 6 weeks.

Patients with hypercalcemia may demonstrate slight anemia. Profound anemia is usually seen only in patients with leukemia, myeloma, malignancy, and secondary renal disease. The white blood cell, differential, and platelet counts may not be helpful except in leukemia and occasionally in myeloma. The erythrocyte sedimentation rate is frequently normal in primary hyperparathyroidism but may be elevated in malignancy, leukemia, and myeloma. It may also be elevated in patients with vitamin D intoxication and, presumably, in patients with parathyroid hormone–secreting nonendocrine tumors. The serum sodium and potassium levels may be normal or reduced in primary hyperparathyroidism. The serum chloride is frequently, but not always, elevated in this disease. In patients with adrenal crisis, the serum sodium and chloride may be normal or reduced in association with elevated calcium and phosphorus levels. Elevation of the BUN and serum creatinine can be expected if hypercalcemia has been present for a long period of time or if the serum calcium is over 12 mg/100 ml. Obtaining the BUN and creatinine is helpful in determining the duration of the disease, the selection of additional tests, the appropriate treatment, and the prognosis of the renal disease that may be present.

The serum alkaline phosphatase may be normal in the presence of hypercalcemia. Elevation of this enzyme suggests the bone disease of hyperparathyroidism. However, patients with malignancy of any type may have high alkaline phosphatase levels. Measurement of the serum enzyme gamma glutamyl transpeptidase (GGT), or fractionation of the alkaline phosphatase levels, or both, can usually clarify whether an elevated alkaline phosphatase is of bony or hepatic origin.

Routine protein electrophoresis is useful in excluding sarcoidosis and multiple myeloma. Urine protein electrophoresis should also be performed to identify the rare patient who may have an abnormal protein in the urine that is not detectable by serum protein electrophoresis. Immunoglobulins are determined for the same reason.

A 24-hour urine collection (with the patient on a normal phosphate intake) for calcium, phosphorus, and creatinine determinations may be useful. Hypercalciuria and hyperphosphaturia are commonly seen in primary or ectopic hyperparathyroidism. However, they may also occur in vitamin D overdose, myeloma, and sarcoidosis. The 24-hour urine calcium level is usually less than 150 mg in benign familial hypercalcemia.

X-ray studies may provide the following information:

1. Chest films may disclose the presence of a hilar or peripheral lung lesion. The distal portions of the clavicles should be examined for subperiosteal resorption.
2. Lumbar spine films may reveal osteoporosis or the lytic lesions of multiple myeloma, or both. In addition, nephrolithiasis and urinary tract stones may be visualized.
3. Hand films may be normal, may demonstrate subperiosteal resorption, or may reveal osteoporosis. Subperiosteal resorption of bone is pathognomonic of hyperparathyroidism. Its absence, however, is not helpful in clarifying the diagnosis. At present, osteoporosis is perhaps the most common radiologic finding in hyperparathyroidism.
4. Skull films may demonstrate osteoporosis or the presence of a pituitary tumor, or both. Occasionally, intracranial calcification suggestive of sarcoidosis can be identified.

### Subsequent Workup

1. Further evaluation of the patient with hypercalcemia is dependent on the results of the initial studies and their correlation with the symptoms and signs. If the patient has lost a considerable amount of weight, has anemia, has an elevated sedimentation rate, and has normal phosphorus levels, malignancy should be strongly suspected. If the chest x-rays are normal, further radiologic investigation should be done. A barium enema, an upper GI series, and an intravenous pyelogram may be indicated. The IVP should be delayed until the results of the protein electrophoresis and immunoglobulins are known and the diagnosis of multiple myeloma has been virtually excluded. The latter is important because acute renal failure may be precipitated by pyelography in myeloma patients. In addition, sigmoidoscopy should be performed. An abdominal CT scan may be substituted as a preliminary investigative technique. A bone marrow biopsy is indicated, especially in the presence of anemia or abnormal white cell, differential, or platelet counts; or if multiple myeloma, leukemia, or lymphoma is suspected.
2. Parathyroid hormone (PTH) measurements. A number of commercial assays are available; it is important to know which fragments of PTH are being measured in order to interpret assay results. Recently, an immunoradiometric (IRMA) PTH has been developed. This assay is extremely useful in differentiating the hypercalcemia of primary hyperparathyroidism from the hypercalcemia of malignancy. The level is elevated in the former and suppressed in the latter.
3. Other tests.
   a. Ionized calcium. Measurement of the serum level of ionized calcium, if available, may be helpful. Although this value is high in hyperparathyroidism, it may be elevated in other conditions associated with hypercalcemia.
   b. Urinary cyclic AMP measurements. Urinary cyclic AMP levels are elevated in primary hyperparathyroidism if renal function is normal. A decreased level virtually excludes primary hyperparathyroidism in the presence of normal renal function. Unfortunately, cyclic AMP measurements may be elevated in malignancy and other conditions associated with hypercalcemia.
   c. Serum magnesium is usually normal or decreased in primary hyperparathyroidism.
   d. Vitamin D. 1,25(OH) Vitamin D may be elevated in lymphomas, vitamin D intoxication, and granulomatous diseases (e.g., sarcoidosis).

4. Localization techniques.
   a. A number of tests have been utilized to localize parathyroid tumors. These include cervical CT scan, cervical ultrasonography, and a number of isotopic scans. Unfortunately, none of these radiologic tests have been particularly useful, probably because parathyroid tumors are usually small.
   b. A barium swallow may show extrinsic pressure at the site of the tumor.
   c. Measurement of the intact molecule of PTH in multiple venous samples from the neck obtained by venous catheterization is useful in localizing parathyroid tumors. This procedure is recommended for patients who have had previously negative surgical exploration of the neck.

#### Comments

At present, there is no practical or widely available method for differentiating hyperparathyroidism due to an adenoma from that caused by hyperplasia or parathyroid carcinoma. The latter condition, however, is rare.

If hyperparathyroidism is considered the most probable cause of hypercalcemia, other associated endocrine abnormalities should be considered. These include pituitary tumor, islet cell tumors, pheochromocytoma, and medullary carcinoma of the thyroid. Acromegaly is sometimes associated with hypercalcemia and may occur in the presence of multiple endocrine neoplasia. Even if other endocrine syndromes are not found in hypercalcemic patients with hyperparathyroidism, repeated examinations for this purpose over a period of years are advisable because of the frequency with which this association occurs. Also, since hyperparathyroidism may be familial, other members of the family should be evaluated.

Occasionally, a diagnosis cannot be made using any of the aforementioned procedures. Under such circumstances, the case should be followed and laboratory studies repeated at appropriate intervals.

## HYPOCALCEMIA
### Janet E. Schemmel

### Definition

Hypocalcemia exists when the serum calcium value is less than 8.5 mg/100 ml as determined by the autoanalyzer using the Gitelman modification of the Kessler and Wolfman colorimetric method. This value may vary depending on the normal values of the method as established by the individual laboratory.

### Etiology

The most common cause of hypocalcemia is surgically induced hypoparathyroidism. Hence, if a thyroidectomy scar is present, the diagnosis is usually obvious. A history of antecedent illness, past gastrointestinal surgery, or known underlying renal disease may elucidate the cause in other cases. The various causes of hypocalcemia include the following conditions:

1. Hypoparathyroidism.
   a. Surgically induced, partial or complete—most common.
   b. Idiopathic.
   c. Transient hypoparathyroidism of infancy (newborn)—usually partial.
   d. Bioinactive parathyroid hormone (PTH).
2. Reduction in serum albumin.
   a. Malabsorption states.
   b. Short bowel syndrome.

      **c.** Chronic liver disease and liver failure.
      **d.** Nephrotic syndrome.
      **e.** Malnutrition.
**3.** Pancreatitis.
**4.** Renal disease.
      **a.** Renal tubular dysfunction.
      **b.** Acute tubular necrosis.
      **c.** Chronic renal failure.
**5.** Rickets and osteomalacia.
**6.** Pseudohypoparathyroidism, types I and II.
**7.** Hypoparathyroidism in association with other disease states, which may be familial.
      **a.** Addison's disease.
      **b.** Pernicious anemia.
      **c.** Candidiasis.
**8.** Medullary carcinoma of the thyroid with or without associated endocrinopathies.
**9.** Hyperphosphatemia.

## Symptoms

Symptoms of hypocalcemia usually occur when the serum calcium value is below 7.5 mg/100 ml, but they sometimes occur at higher levels when there has been a rapid decrease in the serum calcium concentration. The symptoms are generally those of neuromuscular irritability. Patients with chronic renal disease have such symptoms infrequently because of coexisting metabolic acidosis. Patients with primary gastrointestinal disease may have remarkably few symptoms, complaining chiefly of weakness, weight loss, diarrhea, increased number of stools, and abdominal cramping. Children and adults with pseudohypoparathyroidism often complain of weight problems. Patients with rickets or osteomalacia may have bone pain or problems related to the growth of bone. Hypocalcemic individuals may be asymptomatic or exhibit one or more of the following symptoms:

**1.** Numbness and tingling of the face, hands, and feet.
**2.** Muscle cramps in the arms, hands, abdomen, legs, and feet.
**3.** Increased number of stools or diarrhea.
**4.** Headaches, usually frontal; irritability, anxiety.
**5.** Difficulty in breathing, particularly noisy breathing during exercise or sleep.
**6.** Seizures, which are common; in infants this may be the only complaint.
**7.** Decreased vision.
**8.** Nail growth abnormalities and infections; delay in "cutting" teeth.
**9.** Dry skin, often infected.
**10.** Weight problems.
      **a.** Weight loss in association with chronic systemic disease.
      **b.** Difficulty in losing weight in pseudohypoparathyroidism.
**11.** Bone growth abnormalities or pain (in rickets and osteomalacia).

## Signs

Physical signs may help to clarify the underlying disease. Signs of neuromuscular irritability occur most often. It should be remembered that even when a patient has previously undergone thyroidectomy, other signs may suggest a coexisting disease. The following findings may be noted on physical examination:

**1.** None.
**2.** Thyroidectomy scar.
**3.** Dry skin.
**4.** Abnormal or infected nails; delayed dentition.
**5.** Cataracts.

6. Chvostek's sign.
7. Trousseau's sign.
8. Crowing noises during sleep.
9. Seizure disorder—may be the only finding in infants.
10. Hypotension—infrequently seen.
11. Coma—rare, but does occur.
12. Bone pain or bone abnormalities, including abnormal growth, bowing, and brachydactylia—findings that suggest rickets, osteomalacia, or pseudohypoparathyroidism.
13. Goiter, if present, may suggest medullary carcinoma of the thyroid, thyroiditis, or Graves' disease.
14. Other findings suggestive of underlying chronic disease (e.g., hepatomegaly, edema, surgical abdominal scars).

## Diagnostic Approach

### Initial Investigation

As mentioned previously, the most common cause of hypocalcemia is surgically induced hypoparathyroidism. The demonstration of hypocalcemia, hyperphosphatemia, and normal serum alkaline phosphatase, BUN, and serum albumin in a patient with a thyroidectomy scar is virtually diagnostic of hypoparathyroidism. The initial workup should include the following tests:
1. Several determinations of serum calcium and phosphorus.
2. BUN, creatinine.
3. Serum albumin and globulin.
4. Hemoglobin and hematocrit determinations.
5. WBC and differential counts.
6. Platelet count.
7. Urinalysis.
8. Electrolytes, including magnesium.
9. Thyroid function tests, if the patient is not on replacement therapy.

### Subsequent Investigation

1. If hypoparathyroidism has been documented by the initial investigation, the following studies should be carried out:
   a. Slit lamp examination of the eye for cataracts.
   b. Skull films for evaluation of calcification.
   c. EEG to evaluate seizure activity.
   d. Routine chest x-rays.
   e. Routine ECG (may show Q-T interval increase).
   f. PTH determination. PTH is usually low. A high level suggests bioinactive PTH, pseudohypoparathyroidism, or rickets.
2. Because many patients with hypocalcemia due to hypoparathyroidism have an increased number of stools, it may be difficult to know whether primary gastrointestinal disease coexists. In these patients, the following tests may be helpful:
   a. Serum carotene—usually within normal limits.
   b. D-Xylose absorption test—usually within normal limits, but may be reduced.
   c. Seventy-two–hour stool fat—usually abnormal, with a high fat content, resembling that seen in steatorrhea of gastrointestinal origin.
      Following therapy and restitution of the serum calcium level to normal, a 72-hour stool fat determination can be repeated. It should be normal if the hypocalcemia is secondary to hypoparathyroidism.
3. Further investigation is indicated if the patient is thought to have another underlying disease or if no previous thyroid surgery has been performed. In addition to the aforementioned tests, the following tests may be warranted if symptoms and signs suggest other disease states:

   a. Liver function tests.
   b. Creatinine clearance, urine electrolyte excretion, urine amino acid chromatography, and ammonium chloride loading in patients with renal dysfunction from varying causes.
   c. Throat, urine, and blood fungus cultures in patients suspected of candidial infections.
   d. Long bone and hand films in patients with obesity, round facies, and brachydactylia, as may be seen in patients with pseudohypoparathyroidism.
   e. Glucose tolerance test—frequently abnormal in pseudohypoparathyroidism.
   f. Barium enema, upper GI series, small bowel study, serum iron, and vitamin $B_{12}$ and folic acid levels in patients with malabsorption or short bowel syndrome.
   g. Long bone, skull, and rib films in rickets (osteomalacia in adults).
   h. If idiopathic hypoparathyroidism is proved, the patient should be followed and studied, as indicated, for Addison's disease, pernicious anemia, diabetes mellitus, or polyglandular autoimmune syndromes.
   i. If a goiter is present, RAI uptake and scan and thyroid antibody measurement may be indicated. If medullary carcinoma is suspected, neck x-rays, urinary catecholamines and VMA, and thyrocalcitonin assay, before and after pentagastrin administration, should be determined.
   j. PTH measurement may be invaluable in determining the cause of hypocalcemia. The level is immeasurable or low in idiopathic and surgically induced hypoparathyroidism, and elevated in rickets, pseudohypoparathyroidism, and patients with bioinactive PTH.
   k. Vitamin D measurement is indicated to clarify the various forms of rickets and osteomalacia.
   l. Bone biopsy may be necessary particularly if several diseases coexist with osteomalacia.
   m. PTH infusion with measurement of urinary cyclic AMP and phosphorus is indicated if pseudohypoparathyroidism is present.

## HYPERLIPIDEMIA (HYPERLIPOPROTEINEMIA)
Fred H. Katz

### Definition

The central role of elevated cholesterol level in the cause of coronary artery disease has now been securely established. Hyperlipidemia is defined as an excess concentration of lipids in plasma or serum. Because fats are practically insoluble in plasma water, they must circulate in the bloodstream bound to soluble proteins known as lipoproteins. Therefore, the terms *hyperlipidemia* and *hyperlipoproteinemia* are used synonymously. However, clinical laboratories usually do not measure the lipoproteins but only the lipids, mainly cholesterol and triglyceride. Thus, hyperlipidemia is elevation of either serum cholesterol or triglyceride value, or both.

### Laboratory Diagnosis

1. Standing plasma test (refrigerator test). Prior to laboratory measurement of the two lipids, cholesterol and triglyceride, many hyperlipidemias can be at least partially diagnosed at or near the bedside by visual inspection of the serum. When serum triglyceride exceeds 300 mg/100 ml (normal range is up to 175 mg/100 ml), the serum has an opalescent or cloudy appearance. Furthermore, the large fat-containing globules, chylomicrons, form a characteristic layer of "cream" on top

of a clear or cloudy serum, especially when such a specimen is allowed to settle in a refrigerator overnight. Thus, the hyperlipidemias with elevated triglycerides and those with circulating chylomicrons, usually absent from the normal peripheral circulation in the postabsorptive (fasting) state, can be detected by the clinician without the aid of the laboratory. Elevation of serum cholesterol (normal range is 150 to 250 mg/100 ml) does not alter the gross appearance of serum. Most clinical laboratories measure serum cholesterol and triglyceride.

2. Lipoprotein electrophoresis. Because lipoproteins, like other serum proteins, have characteristic migration rates in an electrophoretic field, they can be separated in many clinical laboratories by standard electrophoresis methods. The electrophoretic strip is then stained for fat and the location of the fats (i.e., cholesterol and triglyceride) identified by comparison with a simultaneously run strip that has been stained for proteins. In such a system, chylomicrons (rich in triglycerides) remain at the origin and the nonchylomicron lipoproteins richest in triglyceride travel just in front of the beta globulins and are therefore known as the *pre-β–lipoproteins*. The lipoproteins richest in cholesterol travel with the beta globulins and are therefore known as β-lipoproteins. The lipoproteins richest in phospholipids travel with the alpha globulin and are known as α-lipoproteins. The α-lipoproteins also contain significant amounts of cholesterol.

3. Ultracentrifugation. Lipoproteins can be characterized not only by their electrophoretic mobility but also by their density on ultracentrifugation. The largest and least dense particles are the chylomicrons, with a density from 0.9 to 0.96 g/ml. Next come the pre-β–lipoproteins, which are called *very low-density lipoproteins* (VLDL) and have a density from 0.96 to 1.006 g/ml in the ultracentrifuge. The low-density lipoproteins (LDL) in the ultracentrifugal separation have a density of 1.006 to 1.063 g/ml and correspond to the β-lipoproteins on the electrophoretogram. Finally, the high-density (1.063 to 1.21 g/ml) lipoproteins (HDL) correspond to the α-lipoproteins. Although ultracentrifugal separation and identification of the lipoproteins are not routinely available to the clinician, the lipoprotein electrophoresis suffices for making a specific diagnosis of a hyperlipoproteinemia.

4. HDL-cholesterol is now routinely measured in the laboratory by simple differential solubility. The non-HDL lipoproteins are precipitated by the addition of phosphotungstic acid and magnesium sulfate. After centrifugation, the HDL-cholesterol in the supernatant solution is easily determined.

5. The concentration of VLDL-cholesterol can be estimated by dividing the triglyceride concentration in mg/100 ml by 5, if the triglyceride level is not over 400 mg/100 ml, and the patient does not have type III hyperlipoproteinemia. The LDL-cholesterol can then be estimated by subtracting the HDL-cholesterol and VLDL-cholesterol from the total serum cholesterol.

6. Immunologic measurements of a number of the specific apolipoproteins associated with the circulating lipid fractions can now be obtained. These include apolipoproteins B and AI. Apolipoprotein B is the sole protein of LDL and a major protein of VLDL. Apolipoprotein AI is the major structural protein of HDL. Although it has been claimed that these apolipoproteins may provide a better estimate of coronary risk than LDL- and HDL-cholesterol measurements, problems in the laboratory estimation of these apolipoproteins are frequent enough to make it wise to restrict their use to the research laboratory for the present.

7. The ratio of total to HDL cholesterol is used to assess the coronary risk. Table 9-2 summarizes this relationship for the two sexes. The National Cholesterol Education Program (NCEP), on the other hand, recommends that the absolute level of LDL-cholesterol be used to determine this risk. They advise that efforts be made to keep LDL-cholesterol below 160 mg/dl to minimize the risk in individuals without any evidence of coronary disease. The NCEP goes on to recommend that the level be kept below 130 mg/dl in individuals with known previous coronary events or with any two of the following risk factors: male gender, family history of premature coronary disease, cigarette smoking, hypertension, diabetes mellitus, HDL cholesterol under 35 mg/dl, severe obesity or proven cerebrovascular or peripheral vascular disease.

**Table 9-2.** Risk of coronary heart disease according to ratio of total cholesterol to HDL cholesterol

| | Ratio | |
|---|---|---|
| Risk of heart disease | Men | Women |
| Low risk | Under 4.2 | Under 3.8 |
| Average risk | 4.3–7.3 | 3.9–5.7 |
| Moderate risk | 7.4–11.5 | 5.8–9.1 |
| High risk | Over 11.5 | Over 9.2 |

**Table 9-3.** Laboratory diagnosis of hyperlipidemias

| | Plasma lipids | | Appearance of standing plasma test | Principal lipoprotein abnormality |
|---|---|---|---|---|
| Type | Cholesterol | Triglyceride | | |
| I | N or ↑ | ↑ | Creamy layer on top, clear below | Chylomicrons ↑ |
| IIa | ↑ | N | Clear | β-lipoprotein ↑ |
| IIb | ↑ | ↑ | Clear or slightly turbid | β-lipoprotein ↑ Some ↑ of pre-β |
| III | ↑ | ↑ | Turbid, creamy layer sometimes | Broad β band |
| IV | N or ↑ | ↑ | Clear or turbid | Pre-β ↑ |
| V | N or ↑ | ↑ | Creamy layer on top, turbid below | Chylomicrons ↑ Pre-β ↑ |

N = normal, ↑ = increased

## Clinical Features

Most cases of hyperlipidemia are diagnosed by laboratory screening or determinations; it is for this reason, and because the various types are defined by the results of the laboratory tests, that the laboratory findings have been discussed first.

Historically, an early system for classifying the hyperlipidemias was that of Frederickson, who divided them into Types I through V, with a further subdivision into two subgroups of Type II. The laboratory abnormalities of these six types of hyperlipidemias are described in Table 9-3. Each group has characteristic clinical features.

1. Type I is a very rare type of hyperlipidemia that can be seen in children or adults. The usual complaint is recurrent episodes of abdominal pain associated with ingestion of dietary fats. Hepatosplenomegaly is common, as are eruptive xanthomas of the papular type, principally over the extensor surfaces. Pancreatitis and lipemia retinalis are occasional features. Inheritance is recessive.

2. Type II is more common than Type I, and both subtypes are associated with an increased risk of atherosclerosis from deposition of β-lipoproteins and their cholesterol in plaques. Homozygous dominantly inherited Type II, or familial, hypercholesterolemia often progresses to fatal ischemic heart disease by early

adulthood or before. The heterozygous form is less malignant. Other common clinical features are xanthelasma (lipid deposits on the eyelids), extensor tendon xanthomas, and premature corneal arcus.

3. Type III hyperlipoproteinemia is relatively uncommon and inherited by an autosomal recessive mechanism. Premature arteriosclerosis, coronary and elsewhere, is seen in men in their thirties but in women a decade or two later. Orange-yellow, palmar crease xanthomas are said to be typical, but tuberoeruptive xanthomas of elbows, knees, and buttocks as well as tendinous xanthomas may occur. Impaired glucose tolerance or diabetes is common.

4. Type IV is the most common type of hyperlipidemia. It is probably inherited as a dominant trait, but there may be genetic heterogeneity with Types III, V, and possibly, II. Early atherosclerosis is commonly seen above age 30 but xanthomas are rare unless triglycerides are very high. When xanthomas are present, hepatosplenomegaly may be seen. Obesity, diabetes, and hyperuricemia are frequent.

5. Type V is rather similar to Type I in its clinical presentation. In addition, abnormal glucose tolerance, hyperuricemia, and obesity are common. Inheritance is probably dominant but may involve genetic heterogeneity with Type IV.

## Etiology

1. Type I appears to be due to an impaired ability to clear chylomicrons from the blood after absorption of exogenous fats (triglycerides) because of a severe congenital deficiency of the enzyme lipoprotein lipase, which can be determined by an assay of this enzyme activity. Poorly controlled diabetes can sometimes be causative, and high fat intake can be aggravating.

2. Type II hyperlipoproteinemia appears to be caused by a defect in clearance of cholesterol-rich β-lipoproteins from the plasma. In the familial syndrome, there is a defect in the configuration or function of the plasma membrane receptors for these low-density lipoproteins. This induces a marked increase in plasma LDL, and HDL is diminished. This hyperlipidemia can also be secondary to hypothyroidism, nephrotic syndrome, or various dysproteinemias. Thus, these conditions should be ruled out.

3. Type III, which is characterized by a "broad beta" band on electrophoresis, may be due to a block in normal conversion of triglyceride-laden pre-β–lipoprotein to triglyceride-poor β-lipoprotein. Glucocorticoid therapy or hypothyroidism can be the cause. High fat or carbohydrate intake can be aggravating. Recent cessation of estrogen therapy can induce the appearance of this syndrome, because estrogen has a paradoxical hypolipidemic effect in this condition.

4. Type IV hyperlipidemia is caused by either overproduction or decreased catabolism of pre-β–lipoproteins. In addition to the inherited abnormality, this syndrome can be caused by glucocorticoid therapy, diabetes, dysproteinemia, or estrogens (as in oral contraceptives). High-carbohydrate diets, alcohol, and obesity aggravate the condition.

5. Type V of the familial type is of uncertain origin because, unlike Type I, these patients do not have a significant lipase deficiency. This condition is aggravated by the same factors indicated for Type IV hyperlipidemia. Diabetes, nephrotic syndrome, and dysproteinemias can be etiologic.

## Genetic Classification

The hyperlipidemias may also be classified genetically as follows:

1. Familial hypercholesterolemia—Frederickson's Types IIa and occasionally IIb.
2. Polygenetic hypercholesterolemia—also Type IIa or IIb.
3. Familial combined hyperlipidemia—Types IIa, IIb, IV in similar numbers, and occasionally V.
4. Familial hypertriglyceridemia—Type IV or occasionally V.

5. Broad beta disease—Type III.
6. Familial lipoprotein lipase deficiency—Type I.

When families with early coronary disease are carefully studied, up to half have familial combined hyperlipidemia, and 15 percent have isolated low levels of HDL cholesterol. Considerable evidence has recently accumulated that the incidence of coronary disease is inversely related to the level of HDL, the cholesterol-rich α-lipoprotein. HDL cholesterol is sometimes called "good cholesterol" because it has been postulated that HDL transports cholesterol out of atheromatous deposits back to the liver for catabolic disposal or excretion.

## Conclusion

Hyperlipidemia can be determined clinically very readily by obtaining the family history and three measurements in the laboratory: cholesterol, triglyceride, and HDL cholesterol. Elevated values can then be checked off against the genetic and Frederickson classifications to determine the specific diagnosis.

# 10

## Neurologic Problems

### COMA

Sidney Duman
Stanley H. Ginsburg

### Definition

Coma, stupor, and lethargy are altered states of consciousness. *Coma* may be defined as "unarousable unresponsiveness" to stimulation. *Stupor,* like coma, represents a state of marked unresponsiveness, but arousal is possible by stimulation. *Lethargy,* which represents lesser impairment of consciousness, is characterized by dullness, decreased mental alertness, some mental confusion, and especially by excessive drowsiness. However, responsiveness to auditory or physical stimuli is retained. Altered states of consciousness should be distinguished from other mental disturbances such as delirium and dementia. *Delirium* is an acute confusional state characterized by clouding of the sensorium, decreased alertness, irritability, agitation, sensory misinterpretations, and often, hallucinations. Delirium is usually associated with metabolic or toxic encephalopathy as well as multifocal cerebral disease. *Dementia* is a state of mental deterioration characterized by failing memory and loss of intellectual and cognitive functions usually due to chronic and often progressive brain disease of multiple etiologies.

### Etiology

Metabolic abnormalities, alcoholism, drug overdose, and trauma are the most common causes of coma encountered in hospital emergency rooms.

The etiology of coma is listed in Table 10-1. It is important to bear in mind that more than one cause may be responsible for coma in any given patient.

Based on the anatomic location of the lesion and the mechanisms by which neurologic diseases produce coma, the causes of coma can be classified into four major groups:[1]

1. Supratentorial lesions (epidural hematoma, subdural hematoma, cerebral hemorrhage, cerebral infarction, tumor, and abscess).
2. Infratentorial lesions (brainstem or cerebellar infarction, hemorrhage, tumor, and abscess).
3. Metabolic and diffuse cerebral disorders (hypoxia, ischemia, hypoglycemia, endogenous and exogenous toxins, meningitis, concussion, postictal states, metabolic and electrolyte disorders).

[1]F. Plum and J. B. Posner, *The Diagnosis of Stupor and Coma,* 2nd ed. Philadelphia: Davis, 1972. P. 3.

**Table 10-1.** Etiology of coma

A. Craniocerebral trauma
  1. Subdural hematoma
  2. Epidural hematoma
  3. Concussion
  4. Contusion
B. Metabolic encephalopathy
  1. Exogenous
    a. Alcoholism
    b. Drug overdose
    c. Poisoning
  2. Endogenous
    a. Endocrine
      (1) Diabetes (ketoacidosis, lactic acidosis, nonketotic hyperosmolar hyperglycemic coma, hypoglycemia)
      (2) Hyperpituitarism and hypopituitarism
      (3) Hyperthyroidism and hypothyroidism
      (4) Hyperadrenocorticism and hypoadrenocorticism
      (5) Hyperparathyroidism and hypoparathyroidism
    b. Nonendocrine
      (1) Renal failure
      (2) Hepatic failure
      (3) Respiratory failure
      (4) Vitamin deficiency (e.g., thiamine, vitamin $B_{12}$)
      (5) Other systemic illnesses
    c. Fluid, acid-base, and electrolyte disorders
      (1) Hypernatremia and hyponatremia
      (2) Hyperkalemia and hypokalemia
      (3) Hypercalcemia and hypocalcemia
      (4) Hypermagnesemia and hypomagnesemia
      (5) Hyperosmolarity and hypoosmolarity
      (6) Acidosis (metabolic and respiratory)
      (7) Alkalosis (metabolic and respiratory)
      (8) Water intoxication
C. Cerebral vascular disease
  1. Intracerebral hemorrhage
  2. Subarachnoid hemorrhage
  3. Hypertensive encephalopathy
  4. Cerebrovascular ischemia from any cause
  5. Occlusion of a major cerebral artery
  6. Hyperviscosity encephalopathy
  7. Eclampsia
  8. Systemic vasculitis
D. Infection
  1. Meningitis
  2. Encephalitis
  3. Cerebritis or abscess
  4. Systemic infections and septicemia
E. Neoplasms and other space-occupying lesions
F. Miscellaneous
  1. Psychiatric (hysteria, depression, catatonia)
  2. Syncope
  3. Seizures and postictal states

4. Psychiatric disorders.

In Plum and Posner's series of "comas of unknown origin," approximately 45 percent were due to metabolic encephalopathy or diffuse cerebral disorders; 30 percent to supratentorial or infratentorial lesions; 25 percent to drug intoxication; and a few to psychiatric disorders.

## Clinical Features

1. *Supratentorial lesions* are characterized by the following:
   a. Premonitory symptoms such as headaches or seizures.
   b. Focal hemispheric symptoms or signs (e.g., sensory or motor disturbances, aphasia, visual field defects).
   c. Signs of bilateral hemispheric dysfunction (e.g., decorticate posturing).
   d. Absence of signs of infratentorial involvement, except terminally (see paragraph **2** below).
   e. When progressive, signs of transtentorial herniation.
      (1) Uncal herniation.
         (a) Ipsilateral dilated and eventually fixed pupil with oculomotor nerve paralysis.
         (b) Progressive impairment of the level of consciousness.
         (c) Hemiparesis, which may be ipsilateral.
      (2) Central herniation.
         (a) Progressive impairment of the level of consciousness.
         (b) Evidence of respiratory dysfunction: sighing, yawning, Cheyne-Stokes respiration.
         (c) Preservation of pupillary light responses and oculovestibular reflexes until increasing brainstem dysfunction occurs (see paragraph **2** below).
         (d) Bilateral rigidity and spasticity with extensor plantar reflexes.
2. The onset of coma in acute *infratentorial lesions* is usually more rapid than in supratentorial lesions. Premonitory symptoms frequently include occipital headache, nausea and vomiting, ataxia, dysarthria, and diplopia. The specific findings depend on the site of the lesion.
   a. Midbrain—upper pons.
      (1) Fixed, nonreactive pupils that are usually in midposition (about 5–6 mm in size).
      (2) Nuclear ophthalmoplegia.
      (3) Signs of long motor tract involvement, including decerebrate rigidity.
      (4) Central neurogenic hyperventilation (deep, rapid breathing).
   b. Pons.
      (1) Constricted, nonreactive pupils.
      (2) Altered or absent oculovestibular reflexes.
      (3) Signs of long motor tract involvement.
      (4) Apneustic breathing (prolonged inspiration followed by an expiratory pause) or sometimes Biot's respiration.
   c. Lower pons—medulla.
      (1) Miotic nonreactive pupils that dilate terminally.
      (2) Absence of oculovestibular reflexes.
      (3) Flaccid quadriplegia.
      (4) Ataxic (irregular) breathing culminating in respiratory arrest.
   d. Cerebellum.
      (1) Signs of cerebellar involvement may precede the onset of coma.
      (2) Signs of progressive brainstem dysfunction, as outlined in paragraph **c** above, ultimately occur.
3. Depending on the cause, the signs of *metabolic encephalopathy* are quite variable. The findings include
   a. Respiratory abnormalities such as hyperventilation or hypoventilation.

**b.** Preservation of pupillary light reflexes. However, certain drugs (e.g., atropine, glutethimide) may cause alterations in pupillary light reflexes.
**c.** Random eye movements, but not persistent ocular deviations.
**d.** Disorders of motor tone, strength, and reflexes.
**e.** Tremor, asterixis, multifocal myoclonic jerks, and seizures.
**4.** *Psychogenic coma* is rare. The condition is characterized by the following:
    **a.** Absence of signs of structural disease of the brain.
    **b.** A normal response to ice water caloric testing, which often has the added advantage of waking up the patient.

---

## Diagnostic Approach

---

**1.** Coma is a medical emergency. No time should be wasted. It is often necessary to perform the physical examination while obtaining the history.
**2.** Life-sustaining measures have precedence over diagnostic procedures. Quickly evaluate the status of the respiratory and cardiovascular systems. Check to see that the patient has an adequate airway, is not hypotensive or in shock, and is not bleeding. Institute appropriate therapy if any of these abnormalities is detected.
**3.** Insert a large-bore intravenous catheter or needle and immediately draw a blood sample for laboratory tests (outlined p. 384). Because hypoglycemia and thiamine deficiency can mimic many intoxications, all patients with stupor or coma of unknown etiology should be given 50 ml of 50 percent glucose and 50 mg of thiamine intravenously. Lethargic, stuporous, or comatose patients with pinpoint pupils and hypoventilation should also receive naloxone, 0.4 to 1.2 mg intravenously, because of the possibility of narcotic overdose.
**4.** The history is vital in the diagnosis of altered states of consciousness. It is usually necessary to obtain the requisite information from relatives, friends, or bystanders. Do not permit anyone with information about the patient to leave until the diagnosis is established, or until it becomes clear that additional information will no longer be helpful. Salient points to be checked in the history include the following:
    **a.** The presenting symptom or symptoms.
    **b.** The rapidity of onset, whether sudden or gradual.
    **c.** The evolution of the clinical picture.
    **d.** The state of the patient's health prior to the onset of coma.
    **e.** The patient's accessibility to drugs or poisons.
    **f.** Conditions that commonly cause coma.
        **(1)** Trauma.
        **(2)** Epilepsy.
        **(3)** Drug abuse.
        **(4)** Cardiovascular disease.
        **(5)** Pulmonary disease.
        **(6)** Cerebrovascular disease.
        **(7)** Metabolic disorders.
        **(8)** Infections.
        **(9)** Neoplasms.
**5.** The initial examination should be as thorough as the patient's condition permits. Examine the patient's personal effects for cards or medical identification tags that may reveal any other existing conditions. After a preliminary observation of the patient, systematically check the following:
    **a.** Vital signs (temperature, respiratory and heart rates, and blood pressure).
        **(1)** Temperature.
            **(a)** Fever may suggest infection.
            **(b)** Hyperthermia of any cause.
            **(c)** Hypothermia may be indicative of alcoholic or barbiturate intoxi-

cation, myxedema, hypopituitarism, peripheral circulatory collapse, or exposure.

**(2)** Heart rate.

    **(a)** A slow heart rate may suggest heart block. If combined with periodic breathing and hypertension, consider increased intracranial pressure.

    **(b)** Marked tachycardia (> 140/min) may suggest an ectopic paroxysmal tachyarrhythmia.

**(3)** Blood pressure.

    **(a)** Hypotension is commonly found in barbiturate or alcoholic intoxication, hemorrhage, shock, and other conditions.

    **(b)** Hypertension may be a manifestation of hypertensive encephalopathy as well as increased intracranial pressure of any etiology.

**(4)** Respiratory rate.

    **(a)** Slow breathing may indicate intoxication or myxedema.

    **(b)** Rapid breathing is common in a variety of conditions.

**(5)** Respiratory pattern.

    **(a)** Cheyne-Stokes respiration implies bilateral hemispheric dysfunction with the brainstem intact. It may be the first sign of transtentorial herniation. It may occur in metabolic disorders and congestive failure.

    **(b)** Central neurogenic hyperventilation (deep rapid breathing) usually indicates involvement of the brainstem between the midbrain and pons.

    **(c)** Apneustic respiration (prolonged inspiration followed by an expiratory pause) signifies a pontine lesion.

    **(d)** Ataxic (irregular) breathing is usually a terminal event and implicates a medullary lesion.

    **(e)** Coma with hyperventilation is frequently seen in metabolic encephalopathy associated with either metabolic acidosis or respiratory alkalosis.

**b.** Skin.

    **(1)** Look for cyanosis, rashes, bruises.

    **(2)** Check the skin turgor.

    **(3)** Note whether the skin is dry or moist.

**c.** Body orifices.

    **(1)** Bleeding from the ears or nose suggests cranial trauma.

    **(2)** Bleeding from other orifices suggests a bleeding disorder or hemorrhage as the cause of coma.

**d.** Odor of the breath.

    **(1)** The odor of alcohol is characteristic.

    **(2)** A fruity odor is observed in diabetes ketoacidosis.

    **(3)** A musty odor generally signifies hepatic coma.

    **(4)** A uriniferous odor is found in uremia.

**e.** Central nervous system.

    **(1)** Posture in bed.

        **(a)** Decorticate rigidity, characterized by flexion of the arms and extension of the legs, signifies bilateral hemispheric dysfunction with the brainstem intact.

        **(b)** Decerebrate rigidity, in which the arms, legs and head are in an extended position, implies bilateral involvement of the upper brainstem or lesions deep in the hemispheres.

    **(2)** Meningeal signs.

        **(a)** Resistance of the neck limited to active flexion or extension is a sign of meningeal irritation, which may be due to meningitis or subarachnoid hemorrhage.

        **(b)** Positive Kernig's or Brudzinski's signs.

        **(c)** Restriction of movement of the neck in all directions may occur in generalized rigidity or disease of the cervical spine.

    **(3)** Level of consciousness.
        **(a)** Reduced awareness, but with appropriate responses to auditory or physical stimulation, indicates lethargy.
        **(b)** Limited responsiveness to noxious stimulation is found in stupor.
        **(c)** Complete absence of responsiveness to stimulation is diagnostic of coma.
    **(4)** Cranial nerves. Localization of a lesion may be assisted by detecting involvement of specific cranial nerves.
    **(5)** Eye movements.
        **(a)** In comatose patients without involvement of the neural pathways influencing ocular movements, the eyes are usually directed straight ahead or display slow, roving movements.
        **(b)** Sustained involuntary conjugate deviation of the eyes toward the unaffected side of the body suggests a hemispheric lesion; toward the paralyzed side, a pontine lesion.
        **(c)** Absence of oculocephalic (doll's eye movements) and corneal reflexes indicates pontine dysfunction.
        **(d)** Oculovestibular reflexes, demonstrable by testing, may be lost in brainstem lesions.
    **(6)** Pupils.
        **(a)** Reactive pupils indicate that the midbrain is intact.
        **(b)** Reactive pupils in association with absent oculocephalic and corneal reflexes generally signify a metabolic encephalopathy or drug overdose.
        **(c)** Pinpoint pupils may be due to drugs such as opiates or pilocarpine, or to pontine dysfunction.
        **(d)** Dilated fixed pupils may occur with severe midbrain lesions or in response to such drugs as atropine or glutethimide.
        **(e)** A unilateral fixed, dilated pupil with oculomotor nerve paralysis occurs in uncal herniation.
    **(7)** Fundi.
        **(a)** Papilledema is a sign of increased intracranial pressure.
        **(b)** The presence of specific types of retinopathy may suggest an etiologic diagnosis.
    **(8)** Sensory system. Sensory loss may be suspected if the patient exhibits variations in responsiveness to noxious stimuli.
    **(9)** Motor system.
        **(a)** Hemiplegia, hyperreflexia, and an extensor plantar response implicate a structural lesion of the brain as the cause of coma.
        **(b)** Hyporeflexia without paralysis and with preservation of normal plantar responses suggests a metabolic cause or drug ingestion.
   **(10)** Movements.
        **(a)** Yawning, swallowing movements, and licking of the lips suggest preservation of brainstem function.
        **(b)** Multifocal myoclonic jerks are typical of metabolic or anoxic encephalopathy.
        **(c)** Multifocal seizures may occur in metabolic encephalopathies such as uremia.
        **(d)** Jacksonian seizures preceding the onset of coma suggest a cortical lesion.
        **(e)** Tremors and asterixis are prominent manifestations of metabolic brain disease.
        **(f)** Laboratory procedures. Unless the diagnosis is obvious from the history and physical examination, the following procedures should be obtained in *coma of unknown etiology:*
            **(i)** CBC and platelet count.
            **(ii)** Urinalysis.
            **(iii)** Prothrombin and partial thromboplastin times.
            **(iv)** Toxicology screen.

   **(v)** Arterial blood gases and pH.
  **(vi)** Serum electrolytes.
 **(vii)** Biochemical screening.
**(viii)** Chest films.
   **(ix)** Lumbar puncture (may be advisable provided there are no contraindications such as infection at the site of lumbar puncture, suspected mass lesion, and papilledema).
    **(x)** Cardiac rhythm monitoring.
   **(xi)** Computed tomography is indicated if a structural intracranial lesion is suspected. An MRI (magnetic resonance imaging) scan may add further information.
**(g)** Repeated observation and examination of the patient at frequent intervals are essential to ensure appropriate management.
**(h)** Supportive measures having been previously instituted, specific therapy is begun once the cause of the coma is determined.

## DELIRIUM

Sidney Duman
Stanley H. Ginsburg

### Definition

Delirium is an acute confusional state characterized by clouding of the sensorium, irritability, restlessness, agitation, and abnormal mental phenomena, such as illusions, delusions, and hallucinations. It is usually of relatively brief duration. Delirium and stupor may alternate in the same patient.

### Etiology

1. Delirium is most common in toxic and metabolic aberrations.
    a. Use and abuse of various cerebroactive drugs (e.g., acute atropine intoxication).
    b. Withdrawal from various cerebroactive drugs (e.g., alcohol, barbiturates).
    c. Metabolic disturbances, such as uremia, liver failure, hyponatremia, hypoxemia.
    d. Fever.
    e. Postictal states.
    f. Head trauma.
2. Delirium is unusual in primary cerebral disease but may occur in encephalitis and other multifocal brain disorders.
3. Underlying brain disease of various etiologies (e.g., senility, various structural brain lesions) often allows for the development of delirium with relatively minor metabolic disturbances.

### Clinical Features

Varying degrees of confusion, agitation, restlessness, and emotional lability are seen. Attention is poor and perception is altered. Delusions, illusions, and hallucinations (usually visual) are common. These symptoms may fluctuate considerably, with swings from intense agitation to stupor, depending on environmental stimuli, use of sedative agents, or the advent of exhaustion. During periods of stupor, especially when drug-induced, hypotension and its attendant complications may occur. Cerebral hypoxia may result and further complicate the picture.
   *Delirium tremens* is a striking example of an acute delirium. It is characterized

by profound confusion, agitation, sleeplessness with delusions, and vivid hallucinations. Increased autonomic activity prevails (e.g., fever, tachycardia). Delirium tremens occurs in the chronic alcoholic in whom, for whatever reason, alcohol is withdrawn. Symptoms, initially consisting of irritability, restlessness, tremulousness, poor appetite, and insomnia, typically begin 2 to 3 days after withdrawal. Frightening dreams may occur. These symptoms then lead to the full-blown picture outlined above. The patient also becomes increasingly tremulous, and autonomic hyperfunction occurs. Convulsive seizures may occur. Improvement may be rapid, with the entire illness lasting only several days. However, death may occur in as many as 15 to 20 percent of cases.

## Differential Diagnosis

1. The distinction between acute delirium and psychiatric disorders such as manic or catatonic excitement can be difficult. Table 10-2 lists the diagnostic criteria for delirium.
   a. The behavior may be identical, although in psychiatric disorders lethargy and confusion are less prominent.
   b. Absence of localizing neurologic signs is not unusual in either.
   c. Longitudinal observation usually helps to resolve the question.
   d. The EEG may be helpful in distinguishing acute delirium from behavioral disorders. It tends to be abnormally slow in hepatic failure, encephalitis, and other organic conditions, and abnormally fast in drug withdrawal states. A normal EEG, however, does not rule out organic delirium.
2. Delirium must also be distinguished from dementia. Delirium is characterized by an acute onset. It is not caused by central nervous system disease, but it is associated with prominent autonomic nervous system symptoms, fragmented

**Table 10-2.** Diagnostic criteria for delirium

A. Reduced ability to maintain attention to external stimuli (e.g., questions must be repeated because attention wanders) and to appropriately shift attention to new external stimuli (e.g., perseverates in answering a previous question).
B. Disorganized thinking, as indicated by rambling, irrelevant, or incoherent speech.
C. At least two of the following:
   1. Reduced level of consciousness (e.g., difficulty keeping awake during examination).
   2. Perceptual disturbances: misinterpretations, illusions, or hallucinations.
   3. Disturbance of sleep-wake cycle with insomnia or daytime sleepiness.
   4. Increased or decreased psychomotor activity.
   5. Disorientation in time, place, or person.
   6. Memory impairment (e.g., inability to learn new material, such as the names of several unrelated objects after five minutes, or to remember past events, such as history of current episode of illness).
D. Clinical features develop over a short period of time (usually hours to days) and tend to fluctuate over the course of a day.
E. Either 1 or 2:
   1. Evidence from the history, physical examination, or laboratory tests of a specific organic factor (or factors) judged to be etiologically related to the disturbance.
   2. In the absence of such evidence, an etiologic organic factor can be presumed if the disturbance cannot be accounted for by any nonorganic mental disorder (e.g., manic episode accounting for agitation and sleep disturbance).

Reprinted with permission from the American Psychiatric Association. *Diagnostic and Statistical Manual of Mental Disorders, 3rd ed. rev.,* 1987.

thoughts, and a labile course. On the other hand, in dementia the onset is insidious. The etiology is of central nervous system origin. Autonomic nervous system symptoms are absent. Impoverished thoughts and a relatively stable course are characteristic features.

## Diagnostic Approach

1. Careful history and physical examination are indicated, with special reference to drug (and alcohol) habits, withdrawal from medications, head trauma, and evidence of neurologic disease.
2. An EEG is often helpful (see above).
3. A detailed search for metabolic derangements (including anemia, biochemical disturbances such as uremia, hepatic dysfunction, and impairment of oxygenation) and toxins should be instituted.
4. A CT or MRI scan of the head is usually worthwhile.

## DEMENTIA
### H. Harold Friedman

## Definition

Dementia is a state of mental deterioration characterized by failing memory and loss of intellectual and cognitive functions.

## Etiology

Dementia may be associated with clinical and laboratory evidence of medical disease. It may also occur in neurologic diseases, either as the only evidence of a neurologic disorder or accompanied by other neurologic signs related to the primary neurologic illness.

Presenile and senile dementia are most commonly caused by Alzheimer's disease. It is now generally accepted that Alzheimer's disease (formerly considered presenile dementia) and senile dementia are the same disease. It is estimated that it is the cause of 65 percent of cases of presenile and senile dementia. Vascular disease is probably the cause in only about 10 to 15 percent of such cases.

The various causes of dementia are listed in Table 10-3.

## Characteristics of Dementia

1. Lack of orientation to time, place, and person.
2. Poor memory for past and recent events. Immediate recall also defective.
3. Inability to perform simple calculations.
4. Difficulty or inability to think in abstract fashion.
5. Difficulty with language.
   a. Impaired fluency of speech and writing.
   b. Difficulty in following simple oral or written commands.
   c. Impaired ability to read and understand written or printed material.
   d. Difficulty in writing or copying.
6. Visual agnosia (the ability to see but not recognize objects).
7. Apraxia (the loss of purposive movement without paralysis).
   Figure 10-1 lists diagnostic criteria for dementia.

**Table 10-3.** Classification of dementing diseases of the brain

Dementia associated with medical disease
 Hypothyroidism
 Cushing's syndrome
 Nutritional deficiency states (pellagra, vitamin $B_{12}$ deficiency, Wernicke-Korsakoff's syndrome)
 Hepatolenticular degeneration (familial and acquired)
 Chronic meningoencephalitis (general paresis, meningovascular syphilis)
 Drug intoxication (brominism and chronic barbiturism)
Dementia associated with neurologic disease
 Other neurologic signs invariably present
  Huntington's chorea
  Schilder's disease
  Lipid storage disease (e.g., amaurotic familial idiocy)
  Jakob-Creutzfeldt disease
  Myoclonic epilepsy
  Spastic paraplegia
 Other neurologic signs commonly present
  Vascular disease (thrombotic and embolic)
  Brain tumor
  Brain abscess
  Cerebral trauma
  Communicating (low-pressure) or obstructive hydrocephalus
Dementia as the sole evidence of neurologic disease
 Alzheimer's disease
 Pick's disease

Source: Modified from R. D. Adams and M. Victor, *Principles of Neurology.* New York: McGraw-Hill, 1977. P. 275.

## Clinical Features of Dementing Disorders

Dementia is sometimes misdiagnosed as a primary psychologic disturbance (especially, reactive depression). Usually the conditions can be differentiated without too much difficulty. Psychogenic disorders are almost invariably associated with a positive psychiatric history; not so with dementing diseases. In psychological disorders, the onset is usually acute with rapid evolution of the symptomatology. The loss of cognitive functions is generally not severe and tends to remain static. Vegetative signs occur commonly, and there is usually improvement with appropriate therapy. On the other hand, the onset of dementia tends to be insidious and the course subacute but progressive. Cognitive functions tend to decline steadily, vegetative signs are often absent, and there is little or no response to medications.

It is impossible to describe the clinical features of all the many possible causes of dementia in a text of this size. Listed below are the findings in some of the more common and important causes of dementia.

### Medical Disorders

It is usually possible to exclude medical causes such as *hypothyroidism* and *Cushing's syndrome* on clinical grounds and with simple laboratory tests. *Pellagra* is characterized by dermatitis, pigmentation of the skin, glossitis, stomatitis, and diarrhea, all correctable by the administration of niacin. Patients with *Wernicke-Korsakoff psychosis* classically exhibit retrograde and antegrade amnesia with

A. Demonstrable evidence of impairment in short- and long-term memory. Impairment in short-term memory (inability to learn new information) may be indicated by inability to remember three objects after 5 minutes. Long-term memory impairment (inability to remember information that was known in the past) may be indicated by inability to remember past personal information (e.g., what happened yesterday, birthplace, occupation) or facts of common knowledge (e.g., past presidents, well-known dates).

B. At least one of the following:
   1. Impairment in abstract thinking, as indicated by inability to find similarities and differences between related words, difficulty in defining words and concepts, and other similar tasks.
   2. Impaired judgment, as indicated by inability to make reasonable plans to deal with interpersonal, family, and job-related problems and issues.
   3. Other disturbances of higher cortical function, such as aphasia (disorder of language), apraxia (inability to carry out motor activities despite intact comprehension and motor function), agnosia (failure to recognize or identify objects despite intact sensory function), and "constructional difficulty" (e.g., inability to copy three-dimensional figures, assemble blocks, or arrange sticks in specific designs).
   4. Personality change, such as alteration or accentuation of premorbid traits.

C. The disturbance in **A** and **B** significantly interferes with work or usual social activities or relationships with others.

D. Not occurring exclusively during the course of delirium.

E. Either 1 or 2:
   1. There is evidence from the history, physical examination, or laboratory tests of a specific organic factor (or factors) judged to be etiologically related to the disturbance.
   2. In the absence of such evidence, an etiologic organic factor can be presumed if the disturbance cannot be accounted for by any nonorganic mental disorder (e.,g., major depression accounting for cognitive impairment).

Criteria for severity of dementia:

Mild: Although work or social activities are significantly impaired, the capacity for independent living remains, with adequate personal hygiene and relatively intact judgment.

Moderate: Independent living is hazardous, and some degree of supervision is necessary.

Severe: Activities of daily living are so impaired that continual supervision is required (e.g., unable to maintain minimal personal hygiene; largely incoherent or mute).

**Fig. 10-1.** Diagnostic criteria for dementia. (From the American Psychiatric Association. *Diagnostic and Statistical Manual of Mental Disorders,* 3rd ed. rev., 1987. With permission.)

lesser impairment of cognitive functions. Confabulation may be present. *Vitamin B$_{12}$ deficiency* is almost invariably associated with megaloblastic anemia and not infrequently with subacute combined degeneration of the cord. *Liver disorders* are usually recognized by clinical examination and laboratory tests.

## Neurologic Disorders

### VASCULAR DISEASE OF THE BRAIN

Arteriosclerotic dementia is the result of multiple cerebral infarctions. There is often a history of hypertension, diabetes, and vascular disease involving other organs. The course is often episodic. Focal neurologic signs such as bilateral py-ramidal tract signs, pseudobulbar palsy, cerebellar signs, and hemiparesis may be present. CT scans of the head typically reveal areas of infarction.

BRAIN TUMOR

Frontal lobe tumors may occur without localizing signs, but there may be abnormal frontal lobe reflexes (snout, suck, grasp). In other areas, there are usually focal neurologic abnormalities. If obstructive hydrocephalus occurs, dementia may appear. Headaches are a common feature of metastatic tumors to the brain. Seizures, hemiplegia, and visual and psychic disturbances may also occur. Subtle changes in mental status may be clues to metastatic disease.

SUBDURAL HEMATOMA

There may or may not be a history of trauma. The course is variable; it may be acute or prolonged over a period of weeks or months. Headache is generally present. A CT scan usually leads to diagnosis.

NORMAL PRESSURE HYDROCEPHALUS

This condition is usually idiopathic, but it may follow trauma, meningitis, or subarachnoid hemorrhage. The disease may be rapidly progressive. Psychomotor slowing, ataxia, and urinary incontinence are characteristic features. The CT cranial scan shows enlargement of the ventricles without cerebral atrophy.

JAKOB-CREUTZFELDT DISEASE

This disease has a rapid course usually terminating in death in a matter of months. Upper motor neuron signs, myoclonus, basal ganglia signs, and EEG changes are features of this disorder.

ALZHEIMER'S DISEASE

The onset is usually insidious and the course is usually progressive over a period of years. It may be familial. Its only manifestation is presenile or senile dementia. There are no associated neurologic signs. A cranial CT scan reveals ventricular enlargement and diffuse cortical atrophy.

PICK'S DISEASE

The clinical picture is exactly like that of Alzheimer's disease. However, the temporal and frontal lobes are affected to a greater degree than the remainder of the brain.

## Diagnostic Approach

### History and Physical Examination

1. Obtain a careful history from both the patient and the patient's family. Observations by family members are particularly important because abnormalities unknown to the patient may have been noted.
2. Check the family history; Alzheimer's disease is often familial.
3. Make inquiries about symptoms or illnesses that might establish a medical cause for the dementia.
4. Careful physical and neurologic examinations are indicated in all cases.
5. Differentiate between dementia and delirium (see page 386).

### Mental Status Examination

Evaluation of the mental status is mandatory. The mental status can often be defined by using simple tests at the bedside or in the physician's office. The patient's educational level and prior intellectual capabilities must be considered in evaluating the results.

1. Orientation.
   a. Determine if the patient is aware of the time, date, month, and year.
   b. Check whether the patient is cognizant of where he is and of his surroundings.
2. Memory.
   a. Can the patient recall remote events (e.g., dates of graduation from school, date of marriage, names of the last two presidents)?
   b. Can the patient recall recent events (e.g., newspaper stories, items eaten at his last meal, activities within the past day or so)?
   c. What is the patient's capacity for immediate recall? Name three common objects (e.g., hat, car, pencil). Can the patient name them 5 minutes later?
3. General information. Can the patient discuss current events, weather conditions, common geography (e.g., names of major cities, states, rivers), important dates in history?
4. Calculation.
   a. Ask the patient to count backward by seven starting with 100.
   b. Give the patient a simple problem. For example, if he purchases four apples at 9 cents each, how much change should he receive from $1.00?
5. Abstraction. Can the patient think in abstract terms?
   a. Ask him to describe how a ball and an orange are alike.
   b. Ask him to tell the difference between a child and a dwarf.
6. Naming. Ask the patient to name such objects as a pencil, book, knife, table, and coin.
7. Apraxia. Ask the patient to lock an imaginary door with an imaginary key or to use an imaginary pair of scissors.
8. Language.
   a. Ask the patient to read a paragraph in a newspaper. Is it read accurately? Is it comprehended?
   b. Ask the patient to write a sentence of his choosing. Dictate one for him to write.
   c. Ask the patient to follow a simple command or commands (e.g., "Take a pencil and place it on a desk").
   d. Ask the patient to draw or copy a simple object, such as a cube.
   e. Ask the patient to repeat, "No ifs, ands, or buts."
   f. Ask the patient to complete and interpret a proverb (e.g., "A new broom sweeps . . .," or "A rolling stone gathers no . . .").

## Additional Studies

If the mental status evaluation is indicative of dementia, further workup is indicated. It is not necessary to perform a sophisticated battery of psychological tests to evaluate the mental status, except under unusual conditions.

Depending on the circumstances and clinical information, some or all of the following procedures should be performed.

1. CBC.
2. Urinalysis.
3. Biochemical screening (including liver function tests).
4. Serum vitamin $B_{12}$ level.
5. Serum electrolytes.
6. Arterial blood gases.
7. Thyroid function tests ($T_4$; $T_3$ resin uptake or $T_3$ RIA, or both; TSH).
8. Drug levels (when appropriate).
9. Serologic tests for syphilis.
10. Chest films.
11. Electroencephalogram.
12. Lumbar puncture.

**13.** Cranial CT or MRI scan.
**14.** HIV antibodies if AIDS is suspected.

---

## HEADACHES AND FACIAL PAIN
Sidney Duman
Stanley H. Ginsburg

---

### Headache

---

Headache is a symptom, not a disease.

### Diagnostic Approach

HISTORY

1. Age, sex, occupation.
   a. Migraine headaches are more frequent in teenagers and young adults, with a slightly higher occurrence in females. Migraine may occur in later years coincident with the development of systemic hypertension.
   b. Cluster headaches occur almost exclusively in males.
   c. Cranial arteritis occurs more frequently in late middle age and in the elderly.
   d. Exposure to occupational toxins (e.g., carbon monoxide, lead, nitrates) may predispose to headache.
2. Duration.
   a. Tension headaches often have symptoms of long duration.
   b. Headaches due to expanding intracranial disease are usually of short duration. It should be mentioned that patients with chronic subdural hematoma may give no history of head trauma (often the injury is forgotten).
   c. Headaches due to meningeal causes (e.g., spontaneous subarachnoid hemorrhage, acute meningitis) are usually acute in onset.
   d. Posttrauma headache, although of variable duration, tends to be self-limiting. Undue prolongation of symptoms suggests nonorganic factors.
   e. Vascular and migraine headaches are usually recurrent over a long period of time with symptom-free intervals between attacks.
3. Location of headache.
   a. As a general rule, localized headache is of greater significance than diffuse headache.
   b. Tension headaches are typically generalized, bandlike, or bioccipital.
   c. Classic migraine is often unilateral and frequently more prominent anteriorly. Although the side of involvement may alternate, one side tends to be affected more frequently.
   d. Common or simple migraine is frequently bilateral.
   e. The cluster variety of migraine is invariably limited to the same side of the head in any given attack. It is usually periorbital.
   f. Headache early in the course of expanding intracranial lesions is often appreciated at the site of the expanding mass. When there is a progressive increase in intracranial pressure, the headache may become generalized.
   g. The headache of acute subarachnoid hemorrhage is not only sudden in onset but usually is generalized, with predominant occipital localization.
   h. Headache due to meningitis is often predominantly occipital.
   i. Cranial arteritis is initially manifested by localized temporal headache.
4. Quality of the pain.
   a. Tension headaches are pressing, squeezing, tight, or heavy.
   b. Vascular or migraine headaches are usually throbbing or pounding.
   c. The headache associated with an expanding intracranial lesion is usually relatively mild.

    **d.** In acute subarachnoid hemorrhage, the pain tends to be explosive and intense. Unruptured intracranial aneurysms are usually not associated with pain. Cerebral infarction is commonly painless.

**5.** Prodromal symptoms.

    **a.** Migraine headaches are commonly preceded by such systemic complaints as euphoria, anorexia, or nausea.

    **b.** Migraine headaches are often preceded by such neurologic symptoms as scintillating scotomata, transient hemianopias, hemimotor or hemisensory disturbances, and dysphasia.

**6.** Associated symptoms.

    **a.** Tension headaches are usually associated with other psychophysiologic disturbances.

    **b.** Migraine headaches may be accompanied by all of the prodromal symptoms listed above. On occasion, transitory blindness or paresis of eye movements may occur.

    **c.** Cluster headaches are typically associated with ipsilateral lacrimation, conjunctival injection, rhinorrhea, and facial flushing. Focal cerebral symptoms or signs are absent.

    **d.** In the case of intracranial mass lesions, the associated symptomatology is often more prominent than the headache. The symptoms that occur depend on the anatomic location of the lesion. Some intracerebral lesions (e.g., tumors, arteriovenous malformations) may exhibit seizures, whereas extracerebral masses (e.g., chronic subdural hematoma) are less likely to be accompanied by seizures.

    **e.** Cranial arteritis is often associated with systemic symptoms, including fever, anorexia, and rheumatic symptoms (polymyalgia rheumatica). Focal cerebral symptoms may be related to intracranial arterial occlusion. Ocular involvement is frequent.

**7.** Precipitating and aggravating factors.

    **a.** Tension headaches and vascular headaches are commonly induced or aggravated by emotional factors.

    **b.** Factors such as alcohol, hypoxia, systemic hypertension, and hormonal changes (e.g., menses, oral contraceptives, pregnancy) may affect the frequency of vascular headaches.

    **c.** The headache of intraventricular and posterior fossa tumors may be accentuated by changes in head position, coughing, and the Valsalva maneuver.

**8.** Frequency, duration, and diurnal variation of headaches.

    **a.** Tension headaches are often persistent and may worsen as the day progresses.

    **b.** The frequency of migraine headaches is variable and unpredictable. Although the usual duration is from 6 to 36 hours, they may persist for days. Migraine headaches frequently begin in sleep but may occur at any time of the day.

    **c.** Cluster headaches usually occur repetitively over a period of weeks or months. Often there are one or two attacks daily. The headaches are typically nocturnal and of brief duration (30 minutes to a few hours). The peak incidence is in the spring and fall.

    **d.** Expanding intracranial lesions exhibit no specific pattern.

    **e.** The headache of acute spontaneous subarachnoid hemorrhage is persistent.

**9.** Family history.

    **a.** There is usually a strong family history of migraine in patients with this type of headache. Cluster headaches are not familial.

    **b.** Some brain tumors, especially the phakomatoses, may be reported in the family history.

PHYSICAL EXAMINATION

**1.** General physical examination.

    **a.** A flushed face, lacrimation, and unilateral rhinorrhea may be noted in cluster headaches.

  **b.** Facial hemangiomas and neurofibromatosis may be observed in the phako-
    matoses.
  **c.** Systemic signs of disease, such as fever, weight loss, and anemia, may be seen
    in the following conditions:
     **(1)** Infectious disease.
     **(2)** Specific infections of the central nervous system.
     **(3)** Metastatic disease to the brain or meninges, or both.
     **(4)** Cranial arteritis.
**2.** Neurologic examination.
  **a.** No neurologic abnormalities are noted in patients with tension headaches.
  **b.** A small percentage of patients with migraine may exhibit permanent residual
    neurologic evidence of cerebral ischemia. Most patients, however, show no
    neurologic abnormalities.
  **c.** Horner's syndrome is sometimes seen during a migraine headache, but it is
    rarely permanent.
  **d.** With any expanding intracranial lesion, localizing signs are the rule. The
    findings depend on the location of the lesion.
     **(1)** Chronic subdural hematomas may not have localizing or lateralizing
       physical signs.
     **(2)** Midline neoplasms may have no localizing neurologic signs.
     **(3)** Confusion and obtundation may be the only positive findings in chronic
       subdural hematomas and in midline intracranial lesions.
  **e.** Papilledema is observed in intracranial lesions producing increased intracra-
    nial pressure, but it may also be seen in benign intracranial hypertension
    (pseudotumor cerebri).
  **f.** Bruits may be audible over the eyes or cranium in vascular malformations of
    the brain.
  **g.** Signs of meningeal irritation are noted in lesions affecting the meninges.

DIAGNOSTIC STUDIES

**1.** If the history does not suggest significant neurologic disease and the clinical examination reveals nothing remarkable, no further investigation is warranted.
**2.** If either the history or the examination suggests organic disease, additional studies are indicated. These should include an electroencephalogram, CT or MRI scan,
  and mapping of the visual fields. Angiography may be needed.
**3.** Lumbar puncture is indicated in suspected subarachnoid hemorrhage, encephalitis, or meningitis. It may also be of value in the investigation of other neurologic
  diseases producing headache. A spinal tap is contraindicated in the presence of
  increased intracranial pressure, with an occasional specific exception (e.g., bacterial meningitis with associated papilledema).
**4.** The need for other studies is ordinarily suggested by the history and physical
  examination (e.g., sedimentation rate and biopsy in suspected cranial arteritis,
  various diagnostic x-ray studies to rule out primary neoplasm metastatic to the
  brain).

---

## Facial Pain

---

### Neuralgia

Neuralgia may be defined as recurrent, usually brief, paroxysmal, intense, lancinating pain of unknown cause, localized to the distribution of a specific nerve,
and not associated with objective evidence of nerve dysfunction.
**1.** Trigeminal neuralgia (tic douloureux).
  **a.** Trigeminal neuralgia may involve one or more of the sensory divisions of the
    trigeminal nerve.
  **b.** The condition usually occurs in older people. Its occurrence in patients under
    35 years of age is rare and should suggest the possibility of multiple sclerosis.

    **c.** The frequency of episodes of pain is variable. Pain may occur many times each day or may occur infrequently. Various stimuli, such as talking, eating, exposure to cold, and local pressure, may trigger paroxysms of pain.

    **d.** The presence of signs of dysfunction of the fifth cranial nerve in association with neuralgia should suggest the possibility of such entities as multiple sclerosis or tumors of the nerve.

    **e.** The diagnosis is based entirely on the history and the absence of neurologic, radiologic, and laboratory abnormalities.

**2.** Glossopharyngeal neuralgia.

    **a.** This condition is found much less frequently than trigeminal neuralgia.

    **b.** The pain is generally referred to the throat or ear.

    **c.** The frequency of attacks is variable.

    **d.** The pain is often triggered by swallowing, talking, or contact with pharyngeal structures.

    **e.** Occasionally, glossopharyngeal neuralgia is accompanied by syncope due to associated vagal stimulation.

**3.** Postherpetic facial pain (postherpetic neuralgia).

    **a.** Postherpetic neuralgia involving any of the divisions of the trigeminal nerve may follow herpes zoster.

    **b.** The pain differs from typical neuralgic pain in its tendency to be more constant, its nonparoxysmal quality, and its failure to be triggered by stimuli that ordinarily aggravate conventional neuralgic pain.

    **c.** Objective sensory loss is usually present, and the skin of the affected area is sensitive to touch.

### Atypical Facial Pain

**1.** The term *atypical facial pain* refers to pain that does not conform to the anatomic distribution of a nerve.

**2.** The pain is quite variable in character, frequency, and duration.

**3.** Some authorities think that it may represent a form of migraine.

**4.** No abnormalities are noted on physical examination. Laboratory and x-ray findings are also negative.

### Other Facial Pains

Many facial pains are related to local disease affecting the teeth, nose, paranasal sinuses, mouth, eyes, ears, temporomandibular joints, and other structures. Careful examination supplemented by appropriate x-ray studies usually establishes the diagnosis in these disorders.

## SYNCOPE
### H. Harold Friedman

### Definition

Syncope, or fainting, is a brief period of unconsciousness caused by reversible disturbances in cerebral function. The most common mechanism is a decrease in cerebral blood flow due to diminished cardiac output, arterial hypotension, or cerebral arterial obstruction. Altered patterns of central nervous system activity or impairment of cerebral metabolism by systemic disorders may be contributory mechanisms in some instances.

---

## Etiology

---

1. Vasovagal or vasodepressor syncope (simple faint).
   a. This is the most common form of syncope, accounting for more than 50 percent of cases. Its primary mechanism is a fall in blood pressure. The symptoms and signs of the faint result from vasodepressor and vagal responses usually initiated by pain, fear, or anxiety. Contributory factors include excessive intake of food or alcohol, close quarters, and excessive heat.
   b. Fainting occurs *only* when the patient is sitting or standing.
   c. Vasodepressor syncope occurs typically in young people. Fainting that begins in middle age or later in life is usually due to other causes.
   d. The clinical picture is well known. The faint is almost always preceded by prodromal symptoms such as a feeling of warmth, nausea, abdominal stress, yawning, or belching. The premonitory symptoms are followed by weakness, lightheadedness or faintness, pallor, sweatiness, coldness of the hands and feet, and eventually, loss of consciousness. During the premonitory phase, the heart rate is rapid, but when the systolic pressure falls to a critical level of 55 or 60 mm Hg, the heart rate slows (instead of accelerating) and the radial pulse usually becomes weak. Consciousness is rapidly regained with recumbency. However, symptoms may recur for a brief period after the faint if the patient tries to sit up or stand.
2. Cardiac syncope.
   a. Syncope may result from lesions or structural abnormalities of the heart and from cardiac arrhythmias. A decreased cardiac output is the fundamental mechanism of this type of syncope.
   b. On the left side of the heart, the most common causes of cardiac syncope are aortic stenosis, idiopathic hypertrophic subaortic stenosis, malfunction or thrombosis of a prosthetic mitral or aortic valve, left atrial myxoma, and a ball-valve thrombus.
   c. Right-sided lesions that may be responsible for syncope include Eisenmenger's syndrome, the tetralogy of Fallot, primary pulmonary hypertension, pulmonary embolism, and pulmonary stenosis.
   d. Certain congenital or familial syndromes characterized by prolongation of the Q-T interval may be associated with syncope due to ventricular dysrhythmias.
   e. Fainting is a common occurrence in organic heart disease. The relationship to exertion may have diagnostic significance.
      (1) Severe aortic stenosis, *on exertion* (effort syncope).
      (2) Primary pulmonary hypertension, *on exertion.*
      (3) Idiopathic hypertrophic subaortic stenosis, *after exertion.*
   f. Syncope may occur when the heart is beating too fast or too slow, or, obviously, when it is not beating at all. Heart block and cardiac arrhythmias are the most common causes.
   g. *Heart block,* whether complete or incomplete, may be permanent or intermittent. Unconsciousness usually occurs when the block is complete and the idioventricular pacemaker fails to initiate impulses. However, syncope is not uncommon in second-degree atrioventricular block when the ventricular response is slow. The term *Adams-Stokes attack* refers to syncope occurring in association with heart block. The mechanism is ventricular tachyarrhythmia or asystole.
   h. Fainting may occur at the onset and during paroxysmal tachycardias because of the sudden fall in cardiac output. The arrhythmias that may produce syncope are supraventricular tachycardia, ventricular tachycardias, and torsades de pointes. It may also occur at the termination of a paroxysm with asystole from overdrive suppression.
   i. Syncope may be the result of *sinus arrest* or *sinoatrial block* and is common in the *sick sinus syndrome.* Marked sinus bradycardia, especially in the elderly, may sometimes produce syncope.

    **j.** *Pacemaker malfunction* may sometimes produce syncope.

    **k.** Common underlying causes of cardiac arrhythmias associated with syncope include: sinus node dysfunction, the WPW syndrome, the LGL syndrome, cardiomyopathy, mitral valve prolapse, long Q-T interval syndromes, drugs, and metabolic disturbances.

**3.** Vascular syncope.

    **a.** Vascular syncope may be divided into three categories: orthostatic, cerebrovascular, and miscellaneous.

    **b.** Orthostatic hypotensive syncope.

        **(1)** Orthostatic syncope occurs *only* in the upright position (sitting or standing). The faint occurs *without* warning; its mechanism is a precipitous drop in blood pressure.

        **(2)** Orthostatic syncope may occur *physiologically* in some individuals after prolonged standing or upon assumption of an upright position after a long period of recumbency.

        **(3)** Orthostatic syncope may occur after *venous pooling or volume depletion* as a result of factors such as hemorrhage and sodium depletion. It may also occur following the use of drugs such as diuretics, guanethidine, L-dopa, carbidopa, phenothiazines, tricyclic antidepressants, MAO inhibitors, and prazosin.

        **(4)** Orthostatic syncope may be due to *neurologic disease or disease with neurologic complications,* such as diabetic neuropathy, and tabes dorsalis. The mechanism appears to be a loss of normal sympathetic compensatory mechanisms.

        **(5)** *Idiopathic orthostatic hypotension* and the Shy-Drager syndrome may be associated with syncope. The causes of these syndromes are unknown. They are often associated with impotence, anhidrosis, and parkinsonian-like symptoms.

    **c.** Cerebrovascular syncope.

        **(1)** Cerebrovascular disease is one of the less common causes of syncope. It is usually the result of a reduction in cerebral blood flow due to atherosclerotic narrowing of vessels, thrombosis, or embolism.

        **(2)** Cerebrovascular syncope is a common feature of vertebrobasilar arterial insufficiency. It may occur in the subclavian steal syndrome and the aortic arch syndrome. Unilateral carotid artery insufficiency usually does not cause fainting unless the contralateral artery is compressed. Cerebral arterial obstructive disease may make a patient more susceptible to syncope from other causes.

**4.** Miscellaneous causes of syncope.

    **a.** The *carotid sinus syndrome* is an uncommon cause of syncope. The vasodepressor type is characterized by a drop in blood pressure without a change in heart rate; the cardioinhibitory type, by cardiac standstill; and the cerebral type, by a loss of consciousness without a change in either pulse rate or blood pressure. The diagnosis should be suspected when fainting is induced by turning the head, looking upward, or wearing tight collars.

    **b.** *Glossopharyngeal neuralgia* is characterized by paroxysmal pain in the throat, bradycardia, hypotension, and syncope.

    **c.** *Micturition syncope* is not unusual in elderly men. It is usually nocturnal. Syncope occurs during or immediately after urination.

    **d.** *Cough syncope* is a faint preceded by a violent coughing spell. It usually occurs in overweight men with chronic obstructive pulmonary disease.

    **e.** *Hysterical fainting* occurs in neurotic young people, more often in women. The faint characteristically takes place in the presence of other people. Usually there are no premonitory symptoms. The vital signs are unchanged at the time of the syncope episode. Although the fainting is usually involuntary, some individuals can produce a faint at will. Beyond early adult life the diagnosis of hysterical fainting is unlikely, and other causes of the fainting should be sought.

    **f.** Syncope may occur during *hypoglycemic episodes.* The diagnosis is established by the clinical picture and low blood sugar values. Injection of glucose intravenously usually leads to a prompt return of consciousness. Although hypoglycemia may be spontaneous, the vast majority of cases occur in diabetics who are receiving insulin or oral hypoglycemic medications.

g. *Hyperventilation* may cause syncope. Paresthesias, numbness, lightheadedness, coldness, and at times, tetany are the associated telltale signs of hyperventilation.

h. Rarely, syncope may occur in the absence of heart disease as a result of reflex cardiac asystole *(vasovagal syncope)*.

5. Combined causes of syncope.
    a. In many cases, particularly in the elderly, several factors may be responsible for syncope.
    b. Such conditions as arrhythmias, volume depletion, decreased cardiac output, decreased peripheral resistance, in combination may result in syncopal episodes.
    c. In some cases, especially in the elderly, in spite of thorough investigation no apparent cause for syncope can be found.

---

## Diagnostic Approach

---

As a first step, conditions such as coma, dizziness and vertigo, seizures, and other neurologic symptoms should be excluded.

### History

1. Check for systemic conditions that predispose to volume depletion and venous pooling, or for drugs that have these effects (e.g., nitrates, beta blockers, nifedipine, prazosin, quinidine, methyldopa, and verapamil).
2. The age of the patient may be significant. Vasodepressor syncope and hysterical fainting are rare beyond early adult life. Syncope that begins during or after middle age is usually due to other causes.
3. Inquire into the circumstances of the attack.
    a. Symptoms.
        (1) Fainting preceded by pain, fear, or anxiety suggests a vasovagal origin.
        (2) Premonitory symptoms (e.g., weakness, sweating, pallor) are commonly present in vasodepressor and hypoglycemic syncope.
        (3) Associated symptoms of numbness, paresthesias, and coldness of the extremities suggest the diagnosis of hyperventilation.
        (4) Syncope preceded by prolonged standing is probably orthostatic.
        (5) Absence of warning symptoms is typical of cardiac or orthostatic syncope.
    b. Effect of posture.
        (1) In vasovagal syncope, the patient is always upright at the time of the faint.
        (2) In orthostatic hypotensive syncope, fainting occurs after prolonged standing or upon a shift from recumbency to the erect position; it never occurs in recumbency.
        (3) Fainting in the upright position with little or no warning is indicative of cardiac or orthostatic syncope.
        (4) Syncope in recumbency is almost always cardiac.
    c. Sleep. Syncope while the patient is asleep (manifested by inability to arouse the patient) suggests the cause may be cardiac, hypoglycemic, or epileptic.
    d. Meals. Syncope in the fasting state or long after a meal requires investigation for hypoglycemia.
    e. Relationship to exercise. Effort syncope is often due to aortic stenosis or primary pulmonary hypertension; posteffort syncope, to idiopathic hypertrophic subaortic stenosis.

   **f.** Duration of syncope. Syncope lasts but a few seconds, except in aortic stenosis, hypoglycemia, and hysteria, when it may be of longer duration.
   **g.** Other factors.
   **(1)** Nocturnal fainting in men in relationship to the act of urination suggests micturition syncope.
   **(2)** Fainting following a coughing episode is characteristic of cough syncope.
   **(3)** Fainting that occurs in relationship to head and neck movements or the wearing of tight collars may be indicative of carotid sinus syncope.
   **(4)** Fainting in diabetics receiving insulin or hypoglycemic medications suggests hypoglycemia.
   **(5)** Syncope associated with palpitation suggests a cardiac arrhythmia.
**4.** Obtain a record, if available, of the blood pressure, heart rate, and associated findings during the attack. Hypotension with a slow rate suggests vasodepressor syncope. Marked bradycardia with normal or elevated pressure implicates atrioventricular block or sinoatrial node dysfunction. Marked hypotension with a normal or rapid heart rate suggests orthostatic syncope. The presence of bifascicular, trifascicular, or bilateral bundle branch block in the electrocardiogram suggests AV block as a possible cause of syncope. Electrocardiographic monitoring may be useful in the diagnosis of syncope due to cardiac arrhythmias.
**5.** Check for a history of organic heart disease, neurologic disease, diabetes, anemia, or cerebrovascular disease, all of which may predispose to syncope.

## Physical Examination and Special Studies

**1.** Look for diseases or disorders (listed in the preceding paragraph) that predispose to syncope.
**2.** Listen for carotid bruits, and examine the patient for other evidence of cerebrovascular disease.
**3.** Search for signs of organic heart disease, particularly for such conditions as aortic and mitral valve disease, primary pulmonary hypertension, and the tetralogy of Fallot.
**4.** When cardiac arrhythmia is suspected, record an electrocardiogram, and, if necessary, monitor the patient continuously.
**5.** Determine the heart rate and blood pressure with the patient recumbent and after he has been standing still for at least 1 minute. Because there is normally little change in these parameters on change of position, a significant fall in blood pressure implicates postural hypotension. Orthostatic hypotension is also demonstrable on a tilt table.
**6.** Have the patient hyperventilate for a 2-minute period while seated, to see if the symptoms of hyperventilation are similar to those of spontaneous attacks.
**7.** When carotid sinus syncope is suspected, massage first the right and then the left carotid bulb with the patient seated. Observe the patient for changes in clinical status, heart rate, and blood pressure. Carotid massage should be employed with great caution in the elderly and is contraindicated in cerebrovascular and some cardiac disorders.
**8.** When spontaneous hypoglycemia is suspected, blood sugar determinations and 5-hour glucose tolerance tests may be indicated.
**9.** Specialized procedures may be necessary for the diagnosis of cardiovascular lesions: ambulatory monitoring (preferably with loop recorders), determination of systolic time intervals, exercise testing, signal-averaged electrocardiography, echocardiography, angiography, cardiac catheterization, radioisotopic studies, upright tilt testing, and electrophysiologic studies.
   Signal-averaged electrocardiography may be useful in identifying patients at risk for ventricular tachycardia as a cause of syncope. It is most valuable in patients with coronary artery disease.
   Upright tilt testing may provide a means for substantiating a basis for syncope in some patients with autonomic dysfunction or a neurally mediated hypotension-bradycardia syndrome. The prognosis in such patients is relatively benign.

**Table 10-4.** Differential diagnosis of syncope and seizures

| Parameter | Syncope | Seizures |
|---|---|---|
| Onset | Gradual in vasodepressor type; often sudden in other types | Sudden |
| Warning symptoms | Usual in vasodepressor; absent in other types | Aura common |
| Duration of unconsciousness | Brief | Prolonged except in absence seizures |
| Position at onset | Usually erect or on change to erect; rarely recumbent | Any |
| Convulsions | Rare | Common |
| Incoherence, tongue biting | Rare | Common |
| Postictal symptoms (headache, drowsiness, confusion) | Usually absent | Usually present |

Electrophysiologic studies are an important part of the workup in some patients with syncope of unexplained cause. The best candidates for electrophysiologic studies are patients with organic heart disease and unexplained syncope. Electrophysiologic testing may have significant limitations, however, both in diagnosis and in the interpretation of the results.

10. Diagnostic evaluation of cerebrovascular syncope may require ophthalmodynamometry, Doppler flow studies, skull films, and angiography.

### Differential Diagnosis

1. *Coma* is differentiated from syncope by the prolonged duration of the state of unconsciousness.
2. *Dizziness and vertigo* are not associated with unconsciousness and are characterized by a subjective sensation of motion.
3. The differential diagnosis of *seizures* and *syncope* is summarized in Table 10-4.

## EPILEPSY (SEIZURES)
Sidney Duman
Stanley H. Ginsburg

### Definition

Epilepsy is a paroxysmal disorder of the central nervous system, sudden in onset, usually recurrent, and characterized by one or more of the following manifestations:

1. Unconsciousness.
2. Localized or generalized tonic spasms or clonic muscle contractions, or both.
3. Sensory disturbances.
4. Psychic disturbances.

The disorder may be classified into two major categories: (1) idiopathic (*generalized seizures without focal onset* as termed by the International Classification of Seizures) and (2) symptomatic (*partial seizures,* according to the International Classification).

## Idiopathic Epilepsy

Idiopathic epilepsy refers to seizures not directly attributable to demonstrable organic brain disease. The condition usually begins in the first two decades of life and may last well into adult life. A hereditary factor may be present. Idiopathic epilepsy may be manifested as grand mal or petit mal seizures.

### Clinical Features

MAJOR MOTOR SEIZURES (GRAND MAL)

Grand mal seizures are characterized by sudden loss of consciousness, often preceded by a cry, following which the patient falls. Various injuries may occur. Usually a tonic phase, consisting of generalized muscle rigidity, precedes a clonic phase of generalized muscle activity. During this period, the patient may be incontinent of either urine or feces, and he may lacerate his tongue or buccal mucous membranes. Frothing at the mouth may occur. During the tonic phase, respirations often cease and cyanosis may occur. After cessation of the convulsive activity, flaccidity supervenes, but unresponsiveness may persist for a variable period of time. Upon awakening, the patient often is sleepy and confused. He may complain of headache or sore muscles. The postictal symptoms may persist for several hours to several days. The duration of an individual convulsion is variable, lasting from less than a minute to 30 minutes or longer. The frequency of seizures is also extremely variable. They may happen at any time of the night or day. Convulsions may occur only during sleep in some patients.

MINOR MOTOR SEIZURES (PETIT MAL)

1. The petit mal triad consists of the following:
   **a.** Myoclonic jerks, which are brief, sudden, involuntary muscle contractions.
   **b.** Akinetic seizures, in which there is a transitory loss of motor tone sufficient to cause falling without associated clonic muscle activity. Consciousness may be lost briefly.
   **c.** Brief absences or loss of contact with the environment without a loss of muscle tone.
2. Classic petit mal is characterized by a blank or vacant expression and momentary cessation of motor activity without loss of muscle tone.
3. Petit mal seizures are not followed by a postictal state. Consciousness returns promptly. Voluntary motor activity may resume immediately. Petit mal episodes often occur with great frequency. As many as 50 or more attacks in a day may occur. The onset of true petit mal epilepsy is invariably in childhood.
4. Patients with idiopathic epilepsy often have both major and minor seizures. Although petit mal seizures usually cease spontaneously before the age of 20 years, they occasionally persist into adult life. Idiopathic grand mal seizures, however, frequently continue in adult life.

### Physical Examination

Examination of the patient with idiopathic epilepsy demonstrates no localizing neurologic abnormalities. Following a grand mal seizure, bilateral extensor plantar reflexes are often present.

## Symptomatic Epilepsy

The term *symptomatic epilepsy* refers to seizures attributable to demonstrable organic brain disease. The anatomic localization of the lesion determines the clinical features of the seizure. Symptomatic epilepsy may begin at any age. The various manifestations of symptomatic epilepsy are described below.

## Clinical Features

GENERALIZED CONVULSIONS

The generalized convulsions encountered in symptomatic epilepsy do not differ from the grand mal seizures of idiopathic epilepsy. Unlike the latter, they may be preceded by an aura. The nature of the aura depends on the focus of origin of the seizures. For example, the aura may be a sensation such as unpleasant odor or paresthesia in a limb. The aura should be regarded as the initial manifestation of the seizure, although it sometimes represents the entire seizure. In some instances, seizures are manifested by unconsciousness without associated involuntary motor activity. It is worth noting that a generalized convulsion may follow any variety of symptomatic epilepsy.

TEMPORAL LOBE EPILEPSY (PARTIAL SEIZURES
WITH COMPLEX SYMPTOMATOLOGY)

1. *Absences* found in symptomatic epilepsy are of themselves clinically indistinguishable from those of petit mal epilepsy. However, associated temporal lobe phenomena (e.g., lip smacking) assist in identifying their origin.
2. *Automatisms* ("psychomotor epilepsy") may be defined as repetitive automatic behavior patterns.
3. *Dreamy states,* or feelings of familiarity *(déjà vu)* or unfamiliarity *(jamais vu)* and forced or compulsive thinking.
4. *Auditory, vertiginous, olfactory, or gustatory hallucinations.*
5. *Abdominal sensations,* usually unpleasant or peculiar epigastric feelings that not uncommonly seem to radiate to the head.
6. *Visual hallucinations* are well formed in temporal lobe disturbances but tend to be ill-defined in more posteriorly situated (occipital lobe) lesions.

FOCAL MOTOR AND SENSORY EPILEPSY (PARTIAL SEIZURES
WITH ELEMENTARY SYMPTOMATOLOGY)

Focal motor seizures originate in the precentral cortex and are characterized by tonic or clonic muscle activity limited to one extremity, one side of the body, or one side of the face. Focal sensory seizures are similarly localized sensory phenomena that have their origin in the postcentral cortex.

1. Jacksonian seizures are motor or sensory phenomena that spread peripherally in accordance with the anatomic cortical location of the lesion.
2. Epilepsia partialis continua are continuous focal motor seizures of exceptionally prolonged duration, sometimes lasting for months.

ADVERSIVE SEIZURES

Adversive seizures are of frontal lobe origin. They result in deviation of the head and eyes, and occasionally the body, to the side opposite the lesion. These are a form of partial seizures with elementary symptomatology.

UNCLASSIFIED SEIZURES

1. Reflex epilepsy. Reflex epilepsy refers to seizures precipitated by some form of external stimulation. Examples are photic stimulation, reading (reading epilepsy), and music (musicogenic epilepsy).
2. Tonic postural seizures. This type of epilepsy refers to the paroxysmal occurrence of generalized muscle rigidity, often with opisthotonos. The limb posture may resemble that observed in decerebrate rigidity. Such seizures are presumed to originate in the brainstem.
3. Infantile massive spasms. This uncommonly occurring syndrome of varied causes is characterized by frequent, abrupt, myoclonic, and akinetic seizures. It is often

accompanied by mental retardation and a typical electroencephalographic pattern (hypsarrhythmia).
4. Myoclonus epilepsy (Unverricht's syndrome). This is a rare familial disorder, beginning in childhood, that is manifested by generalized convulsive and myoclonic seizures and progressive intellectual deterioration. So-called Lafora's bodies are a characteristic pathologic finding in the brain.

## Postictal Symptoms

In addition to the general postictal symptoms just noted, patients with symptomatic epilepsy may experience focal neurologic symptoms representing dysfunction of that portion of the brain responsible for the seizure. Dysphasia following a generalized convulsion is an example of this type of symptom. The occurrence of such a localized symptom makes it possible to deduce that the seizure is focal in origin, arising from the dominant hemisphere.

## Physical Examination

Examination may demonstrate localizing neurologic abnormalities that may be transient (e.g., Todd's postictal paralysis) or permanent. The presence of localizing signs implies a focal lesion and thus rules out the diagnosis of idiopathic epilepsy.

## Etiology

The occurrence of symptomatic epilepsy implies a focal lesion in the brain but does not specify its cause. Search for a lesion amenable to specific therapy is imperative. The types of lesions responsible for symptomatic epilepsy are listed below.
1. Localized structural lesions.
   **a.** Static—local brain atrophy.
   **b.** Progressive—neoplasms, abscesses, vascular malformations.
   **c.** Vascular.
      **(1)** Thrombotic cerebral infarction—seizures uncommon.
      **(2)** Embolic cerebral infarction and intracerebral hemorrhage—seizures somewhat more common.
      **(3)** Cortical vein thrombosis—seizures frequent.
   **d.** Various other encephalopathic disorders, such as HIV encephalopathy.
2. Diffuse structural lesions.
   **a.** Infections (e.g., encephalitis).
   **b.** Metabolic (e.g., uremia, hypoxia, hyponatremia, hypothyroidism).
   **c.** Degenerative (e.g., Tay-Sachs disease).
3. Cerebral trauma. Seizures may occur in cerebral trauma, especially in penetrating brain injuries.
4. Febrile seizures. Seizures may be caused by fever alone in children from 6 months to 3 years of age. Seizures due to focal brain lesions may sometimes be triggered by fever.

# Diagnostic Approach to Epilepsy

1. All patients with epilepsy should have an EEG and usually a CT or MRI scan of the head, as well as determinations of the fasting blood sugar, serum calcium, electrolytes, and BUN or creatinine. An isotope brain scan may also be helpful.
2. All patients with the onset of seizures in adult life should have a CT scan. Children with seizures in whom structural brain disease is suspected should also have a CT scan.

## Status Epilepticus

Status epilepticus refers to the failure of a patient to recover from one seizure before the next attack occurs. Vigorous attempts to terminate the seizures are mandatory, since death may occur. Petit mal status epilepticus and focal status epilepticus occur occasionally.

## DIZZINESS AND VERTIGO
### Sidney Duman
### Stanley H. Ginsburg

## Definitions

*Vertigo* is a subjective sensation of movement. The patient may feel either that he is revolving in space or that objects in his environment are moving around him. *Dizziness* is the term most commonly used by patients to describe vertigo. However, since this term may have a different meaning to different individuals, the patient should be asked to describe his symptoms in detail. It will then become apparent whether the patient is suffering from vertigo or other symptoms such as giddiness, lightheadedness, faintness or a sensation of "passing out," a feeling of fullness in the head, swaying or swimming sensations, or visual disturbances (e.g., diplopia).

## Clinical Features of Nonvertiginous Dizziness

1. The etiology is varied. Psychogenic, cerebrovascular, neurologic, arthritic, otologic, or visual disturbances may play a role, separately, or in various combinations.
2. Nonvertiginous dizziness is easily distinguished from true vertigo by the absence of the sensation of rotary movement of either the patient or his environment.

### Evaluation of Dizziness

1. Clues to the causes of dizziness may be obtained from the history. Specific inquiry should be made concerning the following:
   a. Symptoms of anxiety, hyperventilation, or both.
   b. Cerebrovascular disease, especially vertebrobasilar insufficiency.
   c. Cardiovascular disease, with special reference to disorders of the heartbeat, the sick sinus syndrome, and orthostatic hypotension.
   d. Neurologic disease, particularly with reference to the neuropathies.
   e. Cervical osteoarthritis and spondylosis.
   f. Visual disturbances, especially cataracts.
   g. Medications.
   h. Precipitating factors—change of position, effort, cough, anemia.
2. In the general physical examination, special attention should be paid to the following:
   a. The blood pressure in both arms during recumbency and standing.
   b. Disorders of cardiac rhythm.
   c. Auscultation of the neck for bruits.
   d. The effect of carotid sinus massage.
   e. Relationship of symptoms to neck movements.
   f. Attempted reproduction of the symptoms by hyperventilation.

  **g.** Visual disturbances.
  **h.** Neurologic examination, including, if indicated, the procedures elaborated be-
     low in the workup for vertigo.
**3.** Routine laboratory studies such as CBC, urinalysis, biochemical screening, serologic study, and an electrocardiogram are probably indicated in most patients.
**4.** Dizziness due to postural change is especially common in middle-aged and elderly
   patients. It is probably related to unstable vasomotor reflexes, cerebrovascular
   disease, cervical spondylosis, or any combination of these. The occurrence of transient giddiness accompanied by dimming of vision and spots before the eyes following an abrupt change from a recumbent or sitting position to an erect one is
   typical.
**5.** Psychogenic dizziness is more frequently encountered in younger, tense, and anxious individuals who often exhibit symptoms of hyperventilation.
**6.** Disturbances in cardiac rhythm as a cause of dizziness may not be apparent from
   the history, examination, or electrocardiogram. Electrocardiographic monitoring
   may be necessary to establish the diagnosis.
**7.** Miscellaneous but less common causes of dizziness are the sensory neuropathies,
   autonomic nervous system dysfunction, orthostatic hypotension, poor vision, and
   vestibular disturbances.
**8.** Any of the conditions that can cause syncope may also be responsible for dizziness.

---

## Clinical Features of Vertigo

---

Vertigo may result from lesions of the labyrinth, the eighth cranial nerve, the
brainstem, or the cerebral cortex.

### Labyrinthine Vertigo

Labyrinthine vertigo is generally sudden in onset and of variable duration (several days to several weeks). The vertigo is often aggravated by changes in position. Recurrence is frequent.

ACUTE LABYRINTHINE VERTIGO

Attacks of acute labyrinthitis are usually self-limiting. The vertigo is not associated with hearing loss, tinnitus, or symptoms of brainstem dysfunction. However,
nausea and vomiting occur frequently. Aside from nystagmus and dysequilibrium
of gait, no abnormalities are detectable on neurologic examination. It is worth
noting, however, that vertical nystagmus is indicative of brainstem rather than
labyrinthine disease.

CHRONIC LABYRINTHINE VERTIGO (MÉNIÈRE'S SYNDROME)

Chronic labyrinthitis is characterized by recurrent, acute, usually brief episodes
of vertigo associated with tinnitus, hearing loss, nausea, and vomiting. The tinnitus and hearing loss may persist between attacks. No signs of brainstem dysfunction are noted on examination.

TOXIC LABYRINTHINE VERTIGO

Many drugs, such as streptomycin, kanamycin, aspirin, and ethacrynic acid, may
affect labyrinthine and cochlear function and thereby produce vertigo.

TRAUMATIC LABYRINTHINE VERTIGO

Vertigo may result from relatively mild to severe cranial trauma (e.g., temporal
bone fracture). Resolution of the vertigo usually occurs spontaneously.

LABYRINTHINE ISCHEMIA

The acute vertigo sometimes found in the elderly or in patients with cerebrovascular disease may be the result of interruption of the blood supply to the labyrinth (via the auditory artery). The clinical picture may be similar to or indistinguishable from that which occurs in acute labyrinthitis or brainstem ischemia, but usually there are differences (see Brainstem Lesions, below).

BENIGN POSITIONAL VERTIGO

Benign positional vertigo of the peripheral type is characterized by brief (10 seconds or less) vertigo and nystagmus that appear within seconds of a change in head position, using Bárány's test, and are fatigable. There is no hearing loss, and caloric testing is normal. Positional vertigo and nystagmus of central origin, on the other hand, begin immediately, may last longer, and are not fatigable. Lesions of central origin are likely to be associated with physical signs of central nervous system dysfunction.

## Acoustic Nerve Lesions

Patients with eighth nerve or cerebellopontine angle tumors often complain of dizziness, when in fact they mean imbalance or unsteadiness of gait. True vertigo is rare. Involvement of adjacent structures, such as the trigeminal and facial nerves, in association with unilateral ataxia, are clues to the diagnosis of such lesions.

## Brainstem Lesions

Vertigo is a common symptom of acute or chronic brainstem dysfunction due, most commonly, to ischemic disease. It may also result from demyelinating diseases, inflammatory and toxic disorders, or, unusually, from destructive intramedullary lesions (e.g., neoplasms, vascular malformations, syringobulbia). The presence or absence of physical signs of brainstem dysfunction permits the differentiation between vertigo due to lesions of the brainstem and labyrinthine disturbances, respectively.

## Cerebral Cortex Lesions

Vertigo may in rare instances be the manifestation of a temporal lobe cortical discharge (temporal lobe seizure).

---
## Diagnostic Approach
---

### History and Physical Examination

It is usually possible to determine the anatomic location of the lesion causing vertigo from the history and examination.

1. Labyrinthine vertigo, which is most common, is characterized by nystagmus and dysequilibrium of gait and the absence of other neurologic abnormalities.
2. Acoustic nerve lesions are characterized by evidence of both auditory dysfunction (deafness and tinnitus) and vestibular abnormality (nystagmus and ataxia), as well as by the presence of "neighborhood" neurologic signs.
3. Brainstem lesions are characterized by (1) horizontal or vertical nystagmus, or both, (2) evidence of eye muscle dysfunction or involvement of other cranial nerve nuclei, and (3) abnormalities of long tract motor, sensory, or cerebellar pathways.
4. Cerebral cortical lesions (temporal lobe seizures) are rare causes of vertigo.
5. Ischemic labyrinthine disease can usually be differentiated from ischemic brainstem disease by the absence of the neurologic abnormalities described in paragraph 3 above.

## Caloric and Audiometric Testing

These procedures are valuable in suggesting labyrinthine rather than cerebral cortex or brainstem lesions as the cause of vertigo. Electronystagmography, a more sophisticated type of caloric investigation, is employed in some medical centers in place of conventional caloric testing. Brainstem evoked potentials may confirm a CNS origin of vertigo.

## Imaging Procedures

1. CT or MRI scans of the internal auditory canals are helpful.
2. Cervical spine x-rays may be useful in demonstrating vertebral foraminal encroachment, which sometimes causes obstruction of the arterial blood flow to the brainstem and the peripheral auditory apparatus.

## Electroencephalogram (EEG)

The EEG may be of help in the identification of irritable cortical foci producing temporal lobe seizures.

## Lumbar Puncture

Examination of the spinal fluid is occasionally helpful diagnostically. For example, the protein concentration is typically elevated in acoustic neurinomas, abnormal protein electrophoretic patterns, and oligoclonal bands may be observed in the demyelinating diseases.

## Computerized Tomography (CT) and Magnetic Resonance Imaging (MRI) Scans

These procedures are of great assistance in the diagnosis of mass intracranial lesions. The outline of the internal auditory canals may also be visualized.

## Contrast Angiography, Pneumoencephalography, or Contrast Cisternography

Contrast studies may be necessary for the demonstration of specific intracranial lesions.

# WEAKNESS OF NEUROMUSCULAR ORIGIN

Sidney Duman
Stanley H. Ginsburg

Weakness is one of the most common complaints presented to the physician. This section deals only with weakness produced by neuroanatomic or neurophysiologic lesions. Other causes of weakness are considered elsewhere in the book. Since weakness of neuromuscular origin is manifested by objective evidence of reduced muscle strength, manual testing of muscle function is an important early step in the evaluation of weakness.

## Etiology

The various neuromuscular causes of weakness and paralysis can be divided into five major groups:

**Table 10-5.** Common causes of neuromuscular weakness and paralysis

| Anatomic site of involvement | Location | Disease state |
|---|---|---|
| Upper motor neurons (long motor pathways) | Brain | Infarction<br>Hemorrhage<br>Neoplasm<br>Infection |
| | Brainstem | Infarction<br>Motor neuron disease (progressive pseudobulbar palsy)<br>Neoplasm |
| | Spinal cord | Demyelinating diseases<br>Neoplasm<br>Primary lateral sclerosis |
| Lower motor neurons | Brainstem | Progressive bulbar palsy<br>Syringobulbia<br>Poliomyelitis |
| | Spinal cord | Progressive primary muscular atrophy<br>Syringomyelia<br>Poliomyelitis |
| Nerve roots and peripheral nerves | Nerve roots | Intervertebral disk herniation<br>Metabolic radiculopathies (e.g., diabetic neuropathy) |
| | Peripheral nerves | Metabolic disorders<br>Inflammatory disorders<br>Trauma |
| Myoneural junction | | Myasthenia gravis<br>Botulism |
| Muscle | | Polymyositis<br>Muscular dystrophies |

1. Disease of the upper motor neurons (the long motor pathways of the brain and spinal cord, consisting of the corticobulbar and corticospinal pathways).
2. Disease of the lower motor neurons (the anterior horn cells of the spinal cord and the motor nuclei of the brainstem).
3. Disease of the nerve roots and the peripheral nerves.
4. Disease of the myoneural junction.
5. Disease of skeletal muscle.
   Table 10-5 lists the more common causes of these anatomic lesions.

## Clinical Features

### Upper Motor Neuron Disease

CHRONIC LESIONS

1. The weakness is located below the anatomic level of the lesion.
2. Unilateral lesions situated above the pyramidal decussation in the medulla produce weakness on the contralateral side, whereas those situated below this level produce ipsilateral weakness.

3. The weakness is in "elective distribution"; that is, in patients who are not completely paralyzed, the pattern of involvement is selective.
   a. In the upper extremity, the muscles that produce abduction, external rotation, and extension of the joints are primarily affected. The antagonistic muscle groups are usually less severely involved.
   b. In the lower extremity, the muscles responsible for flexion and internal rotation of the articulations are the ones that are primarily involved. However, with respect to the ankle, it is the dorsiflexors that are weakened and the plantar flexors that are relatively spared.
   c. The demonstration of weakness in elective distribution is virtually diagnostic of disease of the long motor tracts.
4. Spasticity of the involved extremities is seen commonly.
5. The deep tendon reflexes are increased and the superficial reflexes are lost on the affected side.
6. Pathologic reflexes, such as the Babinski sign, are noted frequently.

ACUTE LESIONS

1. The onset of weakness is sudden.
2. An elective pattern of weakness is observed, as with chronic lesions.
3. Flaccidity or hypotonia is commonly present during the acute phase.
4. The deep tendon reflexes may be depressed or absent.

COMMENTS

1. Weakness with any of the aforementioned characteristics indicates disease of the central nervous system but does not imply a specific cause. All disease processes involving the long motor pathway produce similar findings.
2. Lesions of the extrapyramidal tracts (e.g., parkinsonism) or cerebellar pathways may also present as weakness but without objective evidence of decreased muscle strength.

PSEUDOBULBAR PALSY

Bilaterally situated corticobulbar lesions, regardless of cause, may produce the syndrome referred to as pseudobulbar palsy. It is characterized by dysphagia, dysarthria associated with clumsy movements of a spastic tongue, loss of emotional control with frequent outbursts of crying or laughter, exaggerated jaw and pharyngeal reflexes, and the appearance of sucking and snout reflexes.

## Lower Motor Neuron Disease

1. The motor involvement is segmental in distribution.
2. The affected musculature is flaccid and ultimately becomes atrophic.
3. Fasciculations of the involved muscles are typically observed.
4. Depression or loss of tendon reflexes occurs in the involved segments.
5. Sensory abnormalities do not occur.
6. Lesions of the motor nuclei of the brainstem produce the syndrome of bulbar palsy. The clinical picture is similar to that of pseudobulbar palsy. However, as with other lower motor neuron lesions, the muscles innervated by the motor nuclei of the brainstem (e.g., the tongue) become weak, flaccid, and atrophic, and usually show fasciculations. The jaw jerk and gag reflex are diminished or absent. Loss of emotional control is not a feature of bulbar palsy.

## Disease of the Nerve Roots and Peripheral Nerves

MONORADICULOPATHIES AND MONONEUROPATHIES

1. Weakness is limited to those muscles innervated by the affected nerve roots or nerves.

2. The weakness produced by these lesions is similar to that found in disease of the lower motor neurons.
   a. Hypotonia is commonly present, and the deep tendon reflexes are depressed or absent.
   b. Although atrophy often occurs, it is less prominent than that noted with involvement of the anterior horn cells.
   c. Fasciculations are a rare occurrence in lesions of the nerve roots or peripheral nerves.

POLYNEUROPATHIES

1. The quality of the muscle weakness and the associated phenomena, such as hypotonia and depressed reflexes, is similar to that seen with anterior horn cell disease or lesions of the nerve roots or peripheral nerves.
2. The distinguishing feature of the polyneuropathies is the more widespread distribution of the weakness. It tends to be bilateral, symmetric, and more prominent in the distal than in the proximal portions of the affected extremities. The legs are more likely to be involved than the arms.
3. Sensory changes may or may not accompany the weakness caused by peripheral nerve lesions.

## Disease of the Myoneural Junction

Diseases of the myoneural junction resemble the myopathies more than the neuropathies. As a general rule, muscle weakness is more prominent proximally than distally, sensory changes do not occur, and there are no significant early reflex changes.

*Myasthenia gravis* is a disease of the myoneural junction with very specific clinical characteristics, as listed below.

1. There is undue fatigability of the musculature. The weakness of the muscles is greatest after physical exercise and at the end of the day. Following rest, there is improvement in the muscle strength.
2. Although weakness may be generalized, there is a predilection for involvement of the muscles supplied by the nuclei of the brainstem as well as the proximal limb musculature. Involvement of the ocular muscles is especially frequent.
3. Improvement of muscle strength following the administration of anticholinesterase drugs (neostigmine or edrophonium) is typical and virtually diagnostic.
4. In advanced cases, the muscle weakness may be permanent and may fail to respond either to rest or to drugs.
5. A progressive diminution in the muscle response to repetitive electric nerve stimulation is typical and often diagnostic.
6. Myasthenic features may occur in patients with myopathy due to various malignancies (Eaton-Lambert syndrome). Electrodiagnostic studies may help in differentiating this condition from myasthenia gravis. In the Eaton-Lambert syndrome, repetitive electric nerve stimulation at slow frequencies produces decreased response, but at higher frequencies there is an augmentation of muscle potentials.

## Disease of Skeletal Muscle (Myopathies)

1. Muscle weakness is usually symmetrically distributed but tends to affect the proximal musculature more than the distal musculatures.
2. Sensation is unimpaired.
3. The deep tendon reflexes are preserved.
4. Muscle atrophy is not an early feature.

## Diagnostic Approach

1. In the patient with bona fide muscular weakness, it is usually possible to determine clinically whether the lesion is located in the upper motor neurons, the lower motor neurons, the nerve roots or peripheral nerves, the myoneural junction, or the muscles.
2. In the case of suspected central nervous system lesions, it may be advisable to obtain CT or MRI scan and an electroencephalogram. When spinal cord involvement is suspected, appropriate x-ray studies of the spine (cervical, dorsal, or lumbar) are indicated. Myelography may be necessary. Systemic laboratory studies that may assist in establishing the cause are also warranted.
3. In the case of peripheral lesions, the following routine studies are advisable: CBC, sedimentation rate, muscle enzyme levels, serum protein electrophoresis, immunoglobulins, ANA, $B_{12}$, thyroid function studies, and serologic test for syphilis. Under some circumstances, investigation for porphyria or heavy-metal poisoning may be indicated.
4. The edrophonium and neostigmine tests and electrodiagnostic tests are the procedures of choice for the diagnosis of myasthenia gravis.
5. Electromyography is useful in evaluating suspected lesions affecting the anterior horn cells, muscle, and peripheral nerves.
6. In myopathies, muscle biopsy (with examination of the tissue under both light and electron microscopy) and histochemical studies may be helpful.
7. Evoked potentials (visual brainstem and somatosensory) are of diagnostic value, especially in multiple sclerosis.

## SELECTED NEUROGENIC PAIN SYNDROMES

Sidney Duman
Stanley H. Ginsburg

### Central Nervous System Pain

Pain arising from disease of the central nervous system is an infrequently diagnosed occurrence clinically. The anatomic structures from which such pain most commonly originates are the thalamus and spinal cord. The causes of painful central lesions are varied.

Pain of central origin is typically constant, intractable, burning in quality, and agonizing. Exacerbations of more severe pain often occur spontaneously or in response to minimal cutaneous stimulation. The associated neurologic findings depend on the anatomic site of the lesion.

The thalamic syndrome is a classic example of central pain that is cerebral in origin. It is characterized by severe, intractable pain as well as by contralateral hemiparesis and hemihypesthesia, both of which may become permanent. Any lesion of the thalamic structures (e.g., infarction, neoplasm) may produce the thalamic syndrome.

Central pain originating in the spinal cord results from trauma or disease affecting the spinothalamic pathways (e.g., cord injuries, multiple sclerosis). The precise nature of the associated neurologic abnormalities depends on the anatomic site of the lesion.

In the case of cerebral disease, CT scan of the head and an electroencephalogram should be obtained. When the spinal cord appears to be involved, appropriate x-rays of the spine should be done. Lumbar puncture and myelography may also be indicated.

## Painful Upper Extremity

### Cervical Radiculopathies

HISTORY

The patient usually complains of neck pain that radiates in dermatomal distri
bution. Suprascapular pain on the affected side is also common. Dysesthesias in
the distribution of the involved nerve root may be noted. Both the pain and the
dysesthesias are frequently aggravated by neck movements and by the Valsalva
maneuver. The nerve roots most commonly involved are C7 and C6. Involvement
of C5 and C8 occurs less frequently.

PHYSICAL FINDINGS

Tenderness in the cervical and paracervical regions is common. Motor and sen
sory changes, as well as decreased or absent reflexes, are usually noted. The type
of abnormalities that occur are listed in Table 10-6.

ETIOLOGY

Of the variety of causes, the most common causes are nerve root compression from
foraminal encroachment by bony spurs or intervertebral disk herniation. Less
frequent causes are inflammatory masses or neoplasms.

DIAGNOSTIC APPROACH

The level of the lesion can usually be determined clinically. Cervical spine films
including AP, lateral, and oblique views, should be obtained. Other diagnostic
studies that may be helpful are electromyography and myelography. In some in
stances, the correct diagnosis can be established only at the time of surgery.

### Brachial Plexus Neuropathy

1. Brachial plexus neuropathy may be idiopathic, or it may follow infectious dis
   eases or inoculations.
2. An acute onset with severe pain, usually located about the shoulder and upper
   arm, is typical.
3. Muscle weakness usually develops eventually. It has a predilection for the prox

**Table 10-6.** Neurologic signs in the cervical radiculopathies

| Type of abnormality | Nerve root affected | | | | |
| --- | --- | --- | --- | --- | --- |
| | C5 | C6 | C7 | C8 | T1 |
| Major sensory abnormality (hypalgesia) | Lateral arm | Lateral forearm and thumb | Middle finger | Little finger | Medial forearm |
| Major motor abnormality (weakness) | Biceps, supraspinatus, infraspinatus, deltoid | Brachio-radialis | Triceps | Wrist and finger flexors | Intrinsic hand muscle |
| Reflex changes (decreased or absent reflexes) | Biceps | Brachio-radialis | Triceps | None | Finger flexors |

imal musculature of the arm, but any of the muscles of the upper extremity may be involved. The deltoid, infraspinatus, and supraspinatus muscles are most commonly affected; the trapezius and serratus anterior muscles, somewhat less often.
4. Involvement of the phrenic nerve may cause diaphragmatic paralysis.
5. Physical examination (see above) reveals weakness and often atrophy of the affected musculature. Sensory changes may occur but are less prominent than the motor abnormalities.
6. Spontaneous recovery, which is often complete, generally takes place over a period of several months or years. The recovery time tends to be longer when the distal portion of the limbs is the major site of involvement.

### Other Brachial Plexus Lesions

Direct (penetrating injuries) and indirect (torsion, pressure) trauma accounts for about 50 percent of brachial plexus lesions. Pain is usually caused by the musculoskeletal injury rather than by damage to the plexus. Tumors involving the brachial plexus are usually quite painful. Most often these are metastatic (e.g., Pancoast's tumor). In addition to the motor and sensory deficits, Horner's syndrome is a not uncommon finding.

### The Thoracic Outlet Syndrome

1. The thoracic outlet syndrome comprises a number of conditions in which the neurovascular bundle is subjected to pressure at the thoracic outlet. The subclavian and axillary vessels as well as the brachial plexus may be compressed.
2. Pain and paresthesias, usually in C8 and T1 distribution, are the most common symptoms. However, sensory disturbances may affect other parts of the extremity. Numbness and clumsiness are also frequent complaints. Ischemic symptoms are present in some cases, but muscle weakness is less common. Positional and postural changes may initiate or aggravate the symptoms.
3. Objective signs of neurologic dysfunction are absent in most cases, but motor weakness and sensory disturbances in C8 and T1 distribution are observed occasionally.
4. The reproduction of the pain and paresthesias and the diminution or obliteration of the pulse by various maneuvers are considered to have diagnostic significance. The reader is referred to the sections Chest Pain, Chapter 3, and Painful Shoulder, Chapter 8, for additional information.
5. Plethysmography, nerve conduction studies, and angiography may be helpful diagnostically.

### Peripheral Nerve Lesions

ULNAR NEUROPATHY

Paresthesias involving the little finger and the ulnar side of the ring finger are the major manifestation of ulnar neuropathy. Objective sensory changes occur in similar distribution. Pain is relatively slight. Weakness and atrophy of the intrinsic muscles of the hand, such as the interossei and the two lateral lumbricals, may be noted.

MEDIAN NEUROPATHY (CARPAL TUNNEL SYNDROME)

1. Pain and paresthesias are the most prominent symptoms of the carpal tunnel syndrome. Although these sensations are generally referred to the area of distribution of the median nerve, many patients also complain of discomfort of the forearm. The symptoms are frequently aggravated by inactivity. Nocturnal pain is often quite severe and may awaken the patient.
2. The syndrome may occur unilaterally or bilaterally. It tends to occur most frequently in individuals whose occupations require repeated wrist movements (e.g.,

typists). Median neuropathies are also prevalent in such diseases as rheumatoid arthritis, myxedema, and acromegaly.

3. Examination usually discloses tenderness over the transverse carpal ligament. Percussion at this site may reproduce the discomfort (Tinel's sign). Wrist movements may act in a similar fashion. Sensory loss may occur over the palmar surface of the first three fingers, the radial half of the ring finger, and the medial portion of the hand. Weakness, with or without atrophy, of the short abductor of the thumb and the opponens pollicis is commonly observed.

4. Electrodiagnostic studies may be helpful.

## Painful Lower Extremity

### Lumbosacral Radiculopathies

HISTORY

The patient typically complains of low back and gluteal pain that radiates to the lower extremity. The distribution of the pain in the lower extremity depends on the nerve root affected. Involvement of the lower nerve roots (L5 and S1) is generally manifested by pain that radiates along the posterior and lateral aspects of the thigh and leg. Lesions of the upper lumbar nerve roots usually produce pain that radiates more anteriorly, especially to the thigh. The pain is characteristically aggravated by back movements and the Valsalva maneuver.

PHYSICAL FINDINGS

Motor and sensory changes as well as decreased or absent reflexes are usually noted. The types of abnormalities encountered are summarized in Table 10-7.

ETIOLOGY

1. Intervertebral disk herniation is the most common cause. The S1 and L5 nerve roots are most frequently affected, although L4 involvement also occurs. Additional information about herniated intervertebral disks may be found in the section Low Back Pain, Chapter 8.

2. Diabetic radiculopathy is also a common cause. The L4 root is most frequently involved in this condition.

3. Primary and metastatic neoplasms may also cause radiculopathies.

**Table 10-7.** Neurologic signs in the lumbosacral radiculopathies

| Type of abnormality | Nerve root affected | | |
| --- | --- | --- | --- |
| | L4 | L5 | S1 |
| Major sensory abnormality (hypalgesia) | Medial calf | Lateral calf, dorsomedial aspect of foot and great toe | Posterior calf; sometimes, lateral aspect of the foot |
| Major motor abnormality (weakness) | Quadriceps and iliopsoas; sometimes, adductors of the thigh | Extensors of the toes and ankle | May have weakness of the hamstrings and gastrocnemiu |
| Reflex changes (decreased or absent) | Knee jerk | None | Ankle jerk |

DIAGNOSTIC APPROACH

Usually, a fairly accurate diagnosis can be established from the history and physical examination. Lumbosacral spine films should be obtained. Electromyography and myelography may also be helpful diagnostically.

## Meralgia Paresthetica (Lateral Femoral Cutaneous Neuropathy)

*Meralgia paresthetica* is the term applied to the syndrome of entrapment of the lateral femoral cutaneous nerve at the lateral aspect of the inguinal ligament. The primary symptom is a burning, superficial type of discomfort located in the anterior and lateral aspects of the thigh. Complaints of itching and "numbness" may also be noted. Examination usually reveals hypalgesia of the involved area of the thigh. There are no motor or reflex changes.

## SPINAL FLUID FINDINGS IN DISEASE
Sidney Duman
Stanley H. Ginsburg

The spinal fluid findings in the more common neurologic abnormalities are shown in Table 10-8 (pp. 416–418).

**Table 10-8.** Spinal fluid findings in disease

| Disease | Initial pressure (mm CSF) | Appearance | Cells (per cubic mm) | Protein (mg/100 ml) | Culture | Sugar (mg/100 ml) | Chlorides | Comments |
|---|---|---|---|---|---|---|---|---|
| Normal | 70 to 150 | Clear, colorless | 0 to 5; monos | 15 to 45 | | 40 to 80 | | |
| | | | | Infections of the central nervous system | | | | |
| Tuberculous meningitis | Often ↑ | Opalescent, faintly yellow; fibrin clot | 50 to 300; monos | 60 to 700 | Positive for acid-fast bacilli | < 20 | Diminished | Polys in acute phase |
| Fungal and yeast meningitis | Often ↑ | Opalescent | 30 to 500; monos | 100 to 700 | Positive (smear may demonstrate fungi) | < 30 | Diminished | Positive India ink prep in cryptococcosis |
| Acute purulent meningitis | Often ↑ | Turbid | Few to 20,000; chiefly polys | 100 to 1000 | Positive (smear often positive) | < 20 | Often N | Early, or in partially treated forms, cell count may be low |
| Acute anterior poliomyelitis | N | Clear, colorless | 50 to 250; chiefly monos | 40 to 200 | Negative | N | N | In preparalytic stage, polys may exceed 80% |
| Viral meningitis and encephalitis | N (rarely elevated) | Clear, colorless | Few to 350; chiefly monos | 40 to 100 | Negative | N | N | Polymorphonuclear reaction early; virus cultures may be positive |
| Brain abscess | May be ↑ | Clear, colorless; may be xanthochromic | Few to 100; monos predominate | 40 to 140 | Negative | N | N | |
| Landry-Guillain-Barré disease | N | Clear, colorless | N | 50 to 1000 | Negative | N | N | Similar changes in various other polyneuropathies (e.g., diabetes) |

| | | | | | | | | |
|---|---|---|---|---|---|---|---|---|
| Acute syphilitic meningitis | N to slightly ↑ | Clear to slightly opalescent | 300 to 2000; monos | 50 to 400 | Negative | N | N | Serologic tests nearly always positive |
| Meningo-vascular syphilis | N | Clear, colorless | 10 to 50; monos | 50 to 100 | Negative | N | N | Serologic tests positive in 60% |
| Parenchymatous syphilis | N | Clear, colorless | 10 to 40; monos | 50 to 100 | Negative | N | N | Serologic tests positive in practically all untreated paretics; usually negative in tabes |
| **Miscellaneous conditions** | | | | | | | | |
| "Bloody tap" | N | Blood-tinged; *supernatant fluid colorless* | RBC; WBC ratio similar to peripheral blood | Slightly ↑ (depends on amount of blood introduced) | Negative | N | N | Progressively less bloody in consecutive tubes |
| Early subarachnoid hemorrhage | Elevated | Bloody; faintly yellow supernatant | Many RBCs | 50 to 400 | Negative | N | N | |
| Late subarachnoid hemorrhage | Elevated | Slightly bloody; supernatant deep yellow | Fewer RBCs; WBCs ↑ due to aseptic meningitis | 100 to 800 | Negative | May be depressed | N | RBCs disappear in about 2 weeks; xanthochromia may persist for several weeks |
| Spinal cord tumor (with "block") | Low | Deep yellow; may coagulate | 5 to 50; monos | Up to 6000 | Negative | N | N | No rise of pressure on jugular compression |

**Table 10-8** (continued)

| Disease | Initial pressure (mm CSF) | Appearance | Cells (per cubic mm) | Protein (mg/100 ml) | Culture | Sugar (mg/100 ml) | Chlorides | Comments |
|---|---|---|---|---|---|---|---|---|
| Brain tumor | May be ↑ | Clear or yellow | Usually normal; may have few monos | N to 150 | Negative | N | N | Occasionally cytologic examination reveals tumor cells |
| Meningeal carcinomatosis (carcinomatous meningitis) | May be ↑ | Clear to turbid | 20 to 300 (may be mixture of malignant and inflammatory cells) | 60 to 200 | Negative | Often depressed | N | Cytologic examination often reveals tumor cells |
| Multiple sclerosis | N | Clear, colorless | 5 to 50 monos | N to 80 | Negative | N | N | Gamma globulin fraction may be ↑; oligoclonal bands may be present; myelin basic protein is elevated |
| Cerebral infarction | N (occasionally elevated) | Clear | Usually normal; occasionally a few monos (RBCs frequent in embolic infarction) | N to 80 | Negative | N | N | Pleocytosis when infarct is in proximity to ventricle or subarachnoid space |
| Cerebral hemorrhage | Often ↑ | Blood-tinged (sometimes grossly bloody) | RBCs; varying number WBCs, especially late | 50 to 200 | Negative | N | N | |

N = normal, ↑ = increased, monos = mononuclear leukocytes, polys = polymorphonuclear leukocytes.
Source: Modified from R. R. Grinker, P. C. Bucy, and A. L. Sahs, *Neurology*, 6th ed. Springfield, Ill.: Thomas, 1966.

# Appendix: Normal Values of Standard Laboratory and Function Tests

## Alimentary Tract Function Tests

Gastric secretion

  Volume
    Fasting                            20–100 ml/h
    Nocturnal                    < 800 ml/10 h

Acid output (mean ± standard deviation)

  Basal (BAO)
    Male                            3.7 ± 2.1 meq/h
    Female                        2.2 ± 1.7 meq/h
  Stimulated after betazole (Histalog), 0.5
    mg/kg or pentagastrin 6 µg/kg
    subcutaneously (PAO)
    Male                            23 ± 7 meq/h
    Female                        18 ± 5 meq/h
  BAO/PAO ratio                  < 0.5

Gastrin, serum                   < 150 pg/ml

Gastrin, serum following stimulation with intravenous secretin 2 units/kg      Increases of 110 pg/ml or 100% of basal level 1, 2, 5, 7, 10, 15, or 30 min after secretin indicate Z-E syndrome (gastrinoma)

Intestinal absorption

  Stool fat on diet containing 80–100 g fat/ day (72- to 96-h collection)      < 8 g/24 h
  D-Xylose absorption (25 g D-xylose administered orally after overnight fast)
    5-h urine collection after D-xylose      > 5 g
    1- or 2-h serum level after D-xylose      > 25 mg/dl
  Triolein breath test (5 µCi $^{14}$C-triolein administered in 30 ml Lipomul; breath collected hourly for 6 h for measurement of breath $^{14}CO_2$)      > 3.5% of dose/h

Source: Reprinted from J. H. Stein (Editor-in-Chief), *Internal Medicine*, (3rd ed.). Boston: Little, Brown. 1990. Used by permission.

Lactose absorption (50 g lactose administered after overnight fast; baseline and 1-, 2-, and 3-h serum samples obtained; alternatively, breath hydrogen can be measured in expired air 90–120 min after lactose administered)

> 25 mg/dl increase in serum glucose
> 20 PPM $H_2$ in expired air

Schilling test (see Hematologic Normal Values)

Pancreatic secretion
  Secretin test (2 units secretin/kg body weight, intravenously; duodenal fluid collected for 4 periods of 20 min thereafter)
    Volume
    Bicarbonate output
    Bicarbonate concentration

> 1.5 ml/kg/80 min
> 16 meq/80 min
> 80 meq/L

  Bentiromide (N-benzoyl-L-tyrosyl-p-aminobenzoic acid) test (500 mg administered after overnight fast followed by oral hydration and collection of a 6-h urine sample)

> 50% urinary recovery of ingested PABA/6 h

## Cardiovascular Function Tests

Cardiac index

$$L/min/m^2 = \frac{C.O.}{body\ surface\ area\ (BSA)}$$
$$Normal = 2.8\text{--}4.2$$

Cardiac output

$$C.O. = heart\ rate \times stroke\ volume$$

Cardiac output (Fick principle)

$$C.O.\ (L/min) = \frac{O_2\ consumption\ (ml\ O_2/min)}{AV\ O_2\ difference\ (ml\ O_2/L)}$$

where

$O_2$ consumption (basal state estimate) $= 3$ ml $O_2$/min/kg body weight

AV $O_2$ difference $=$ arterial $O_2$ content $-$ venous $O_2$ content (ml $O_2$/L)

$O_2$ content (vol %) $=$ Hb (g/dl) $\times 1.39$ (ml $O_2$/g Hb) $\times$ % saturation

$O_2$ content (ml $O_2$/L) $=$ vol % $\times 10$

Therefore

$$C.O.\ (L/min) = \frac{3\ (ml/min) \times weight\ (kg)}{(SaO_2 - S\bar{v}O_2)\ (1.39) \times Hb\ (g/dl) \times 10}$$

Mean arterial pressure

Mean arterial pressure

$\qquad = $ diastolic pressure $+$ ⅓ (systolic pressure $-$ diastolic pressure)

Resistance—can be expressed in absolute resistance units (ARU) of dyne-sec-cm$^{-5}$ or hybrid resistance units (HRU) of mm Hg/L/min; ARU $= 80 \times$ HRU

## Cardiovascular Normal Values

**Table A-1.** Normal pressures in the heart and great vessels*

| Pressures | Average (mm Hg) | Range (mm Hg) |
|---|---|---|
| Right atrium | | |
|    Mean | 2.8 | 1–5 |
|    a wave | 5.6 | 2.5–7.0 |
|    z point | 2.9 | 1.5–5.0 |
|    c wave | 3.8 | 1.5–6.0 |
|    x wave | 1.7 | 0–5 |
|    v wave | 4.6 | 2.0–7.5 |
|    y wave | 2.4 | 0–6 |
| Right ventricle | | |
|    Peak systolic | 25 | 17–32 |
|    End diastolic | 4 | 1–7 |
| Pulmonary artery | | |
|    Mean | 15 | 9–19 |
|    Peak systolic | 25 | 17–32 |
|    End diastolic | 9 | 4–13 |
| Pulmonary artery wedge | | |
|    Mean | 9 | 4.5–13.0 |
| Left atrium | | |
|    Mean | 7.9 | 2–12 |
|    a wave | 10.4 | 4–16 |
|    z point | 7.6 | 1–13 |
|    v wave | 12.8 | 6–21 |
| Left ventricle | | |
|    Peak systolic | 130 | 90–140 |
|    End diastolic | 8.7 | 5–12 |
| Brachial artery | | |
|    Mean | 85 | 70–105 |
|    Peak systolic | 130 | 90–140 |
|    End diastolic | 70 | 60–90 |

*Reference elevation = 10 cm above the spine of the recumbent subject.

Systemic vascular resistance (SVR)

$$SVR = \frac{\overline{SA} - \overline{RA}}{C.O.} \text{ (Normal = 1130 dyne-sec-cm}^{-5} \pm 178)$$

Pulmonary arteriolar resistance (PAR)

$$PAR = \frac{\overline{PA} - \overline{LA}}{C.O.} \text{ (Normal = 67 dyne-sec-cm}^{-5} \pm 23)$$

Total pulmonary resistance (TPR)

$$TPR = \frac{\overline{PA}}{C.O.} \text{ (Normal = 205 dyne-sec-cm}^{-5} \pm 51)$$

Total systemic resistance (TSR)

$$TSR = \frac{\overline{SA}}{C.O.}$$

where

$\overline{RA}$ = mean right atrial pressure
$\overline{PA}$ = mean pulmonary artery pressure
$\overline{LA}$ = mean left atrial pressure
$\overline{SA}$ = mean systemic arterial pressure
C.O. = cardiac output

## Cerebrospinal Fluid Normal Values

| | |
|---|---|
| Bilirubin | 0 |
| Cells | 0–5/mm³, all lymphocytes |
| Chloride | 110–129 meq/L |
| Glucose | 48–86 mg/dl or $\geq$ 60% of serum glucose |
| pH | 7.34–7.43 |
| Pressure | 7–20 cm water |
| Protein, lumbar | 15–45 mg/dl |
|   Albumin | 58% |
|   $\alpha_1$-globulins | 9% |
|   $\alpha_2$-globulins | 8% |
|   $\beta$-globulins | 10% |
|   $\gamma$-globulins | 10 (5–12)% |
| Protein, cisternal | 15–25 mg/dl |
| Protein, ventricular | 5–15 mg/dl |

## Endocrinologic Normal Values

### Hormone and Metabolite Normal Values

| | |
|---|---|
| Adrenocorticotropin (ACTH), serum | 15–70 pg/ml |
| Aldosterone (mean $\pm$ standard deviation) | |
|   Serum | |
|     210 meq/day sodium diet | |
|       Supine | 48 $\pm$ 29 pg/ml |
|       Upright (2h) | 65 $\pm$ 23 pg/ml |
|     110 meq/day sodium diet | |
|       Supine | 107 $\pm$ 45 pg/ml |
|       Upright (2h) | 532 $\pm$ 228 pg/ml |
|   Urine | 5–19 µg/24 h |
| Calcitonin, serum | None detectable |
| Catecholamines, free urinary | < 110 µg/24 h |
| Chorionic gonadotropin, serum | |
|   Pregnancy | |
|     First month | 10–10,000 mIU/ml |
|     Second and third months | 10,000–100,000 mIU/ml |
|     Second trimester | 10,000–30,000 mIU/ml |
|     Third trimester | 5,000–15,000 mIU/ml |
|   Nonpregnant | 0 |

Cortisol
  Serum
    8 A.M. — 5–25 µg/dl
    8 P.M. — < 10 µg/dl
    Cosyntropin stimulation (30–90 min after 0.25 mg cosyntropin intramuscularly or intravenously) — > 10 µg/dl rise over baseline
    Overnight suppression (8 A.M. serum cortisol after 1 mg dexamethasone orally at 11 P.M.) — ≤ 5 µg/dl
  Urine — 20–70 µg/24 h

C-peptide, serum — 0.28–0.63 pmol/ml

11-Deoxycortisol, serum
  Basal — 0–1.4 µg/dl
  Metyrapone stimulation (30 mg/kg orally 8 h prior to level) — > 7.5 µg/dl

Estrogens, urine (increased during pregnancy; decreased after menopause)

| | Male | Female |
|---|---|---|
| Total | 4–25 µg/24 h | 5–100 µg/24 h |
| Estriol | 1–11 µg/24 h | 0–65 µg/24 h |
| Estradiol | 0–6 µg/24 h | 0–14 µg/24 h |
| Estrone | 3–8 µg/24 h | 4–31 µg/24 h |

Etiocholanolone, serum — < 1.2 µg/dl

Follicle-stimulating hormone, serum
  Male — 6–18 mIU/ml
  Female
    Follicular phase — 5–20 mIU/ml
    Peak midcycle — 12–30 mIU/ml
    Luteal phase — 5–15 mIU/ml
    Postmenopausal — > 50 mIU/ml

Free thyroxine index, serum — 1–4 ng/dl

Gastrin, serum (fasting) — 60–200 pg/ml

Growth hormone, serum
  Adult, fasting — < 5 ng/ml
  Glucose load (100 g orally) — < 5 ng/ml
  Levodopa stimulation (500 mg orally in a fasting state) — > 5 ng/ml rise over baseline within 2 h

17-Hydroxycorticosteroids, urine
  Male — 2–12 mg/24 h
  Female — 2–8 mg/24 h

5'-Hydroxyindoleacetic acid (5'-HIAA), urine — 2–9 mg/24 h

Insulin, plasma
  Fasting — 6–26 µU/ml
  Hypoglycemia (serum glucose < 50 mg/dl) — < 5 µU/ml

17-Ketosteroids, urine

| | |
|---|---|
| Under 8 years old | 0–2 mg/24 h |
| Adolescent | 0–18 mg/24 h |
| Adult | |
|   Male | 8–18 mg/24 h |
|   Female | 5–15 mg/24 h |

Luteinizing hormone, serum

| | |
|---|---|
| Male | 6–18 mIU/ml |
| Female | |
|   Basal | 5–22 mIU/ml |
|   Ovulation | 30–250 mIU/ml |

Metanephrines, urine      < 1.3 mg/24 h
  plasma      150–450 pg/ml

Norepinephrine, urine      < 100 μg/24 h

Parathyroid hormone, serum      150–300 pg/ml
  C-terminal      150–350 pg/ml
  N-terminal      230–650 pg/ml

Pregnanediol, urine

| | |
|---|---|
| Female | |
|   Follicular phase | < 1.5 mg/24 h |
|   Luteal phase | 2.0–4.2 mg/24 h |
|   Postmenopausal | 0.2–1.0 mg/24 h |
| Male | < 1.5 mg/24 h |

Progesterone, plasma

| | |
|---|---|
| Female | |
|   Follicular phase | 0–5.3 ng/ml |
|   Luteal phase | 0–21 ng/ml |
|   Postmenopausal | < 2 ng/ml |
| Male | < 2 ng/ml |

Prolactin, serum

| | |
|---|---|
| Nonpregnant | |
|   Day | 5–10 ng/ml |
|   Night | 20–40 ng/ml |
| Pregnant | 150–200 ng/ml |

Radioactive iodine ($^{131}$I) uptake (RAIU)      5–25% at 24 h (varies with iodine intake)

Renin activity, plasma (mean ± standard deviation)

| | |
|---|---|
| Normal diet | |
|   Supine | 1.1 ± 0.8 ng/ml/h |
|   Upright | 1.9 ± 1.7 ng/ml/h |
| Low sodium diet | |
|   Supine | 2.7 ± 1.8 ng/ml/h |
|   Upright | 6.6 ± 2.5 ng/ml/h |
| Diuretics and low sodium diet | 10.0 ± 3.7 ng/ml/h |

Testosterone, total plasma

| | |
|---|---|
| Bound | |
|   Adolescent male | > 100 ng/dl |

| Adult male | 300–1100 ng/dl |
| Female | 25–90 ng/dl |
| Unbound | |
| Adult male | 3–24 ng/dl |
| Female | 0.09–1.30 ng/dl |

Thyroid-stimulating hormone, serum  $< 10 \ \mu U/ml$

Thyroxine ($T_4$), serum
    Total                           4.5–11.5 $\mu$g/dl
    Free                            0.8–2.4 ng/dl

Thyroxine-binding globulin capacity, serum   15–25 $\mu$g $T_4$/dl

Thyroxine index, free               1–4 ng/dl

Tri-iodothyronine ($T_3$), serum    70–190 ng/dl

$T_3$ resin uptake                  25–45%

Vanillylmandelic acid (VMA), urine  1–8 mg/24 h

## Endocrine Function Tests

Adrenal gland
    Glucocorticoid suppression: overnight      $\leq 5 \ \mu$g/dl
        dexamethasone suppression test (8
        A.M. serum cortisol after 1 mg
        dexamethasone orally at 11 P.M.)
    Glucocorticoid stimulation: cosyntropin    $> 10 \ \mu$g/ml more than baseline
        stimulation test (serum cortisol 30–        serum cortisol
        90 min after 0.25 mg cosyntropin
        intramuscularly or intravenously)
    Metyrapone test, single dose (8 A.M.       $> 7.5 \ \mu$g/dl
        serum deoxycortisol after 30 mg/kg
        metyrapone orally at midnight)
    Aldosterone suppression: sodium            $< 20 \ \mu$g/24h
        depletion test (urine aldosterone
        collected on day 3 of 200 meq/day
        sodium diet)

Pancreas
    Glucose tolerance test* (serum glucose
        after 100 g glucose orally)
        60 min after ingestion                 $< 180$ mg/dl
        90 min after ingestion                 $< 160$ mg/dl
        120 min after ingestion                $< 125$ mg/dl

Pituitary gland
    Adrenocorticotropic hormone (ACTH)
        stimulation. See Adrenal gland,
        Metyrapone test
    Growth hormone stimulation: insulin        $> 5$ ng/ml rise over baseline
        tolerance test (serum growth
        hormone after 0.1 U/kg regular
        insulin intravenously after an

*Add 10 mg/dl for each decade over 50 years of age.

overnight fast to induce a 50% fall
in serum glucose concentration or
symptomatic hypoglycemia)

Levodopa test (serum growth hormone
after 0.5 g levodopa orally while
fasting)

$> 5$ ng/ml rise over baseline
within 2 h

Growth hormone suppression: glucose
tolerance test (serum growth
hormone after 100 g glucose orally
after 8 h fast)

$< 5$ ng/ml within 2 h

Luteinizing hormone (LH) stimulation:
gonadotropin-releasing hormone
(GnRH) test (serum LH after 100 μg
GnRH intravenously or
intramuscularly)

4- to 6-fold rise over baseline

Thyroid-stimulating hormone (TSH)
stimulation: thyrotropin-releasing
hormone (TRH) stimulation test
(serum TSH after 400 μg TRH
intravenously)

$> 2$-fold rise over baseline within
2 h

Thyroid gland

Radioactive iodine uptake (RAIU)
suppression test (RAIU on day 7
after 25 μg tri-iodothyronine orally
4 times daily)

$< 10\%$ to $< 50\%$ baseline

Thyrotropin-releasing hormone (TRH)
stimulation test. See Pituitary
gland, TSH stimulation

| | **Hematologic Normal Values** |
|---|---|
| Acid hemolysis test (Ham) | No hemolysis |
| Carboxyhemoglobin | |
|   Nonsmoker | $< 1\%$ |
|   Smoker | 2.1–4.2% |
| Cold hemolysis test (Donath-Landsteiner) | No hemolysis |
| Complete blood count (see Table A-3) | |
| Erythrocyte life span | |
|   Normal | 120 days |
|   $^{51}$Cr-labeled half-life | 28 days |
| Erythropoietin by radioimmunoassay | 9–33 mU/dl |
| Ferritin, serum | |
|   Male | 15–200 μg/L |
|   Female | 12–150 μg/L |
| Folate, RBC | 120–670 ng/ml |
| Fragility, osmotic | |
|   Hemolysis begins 0.45–0.38% | |
|   Hemolysis completed 0.33–0.30% | |

**Table A-2.** Differential cell count of bone marrow

| | |
|---|---|
| Myeloid cells | |
| Neutrophilic series | |
| Myeloblasts | 0.3–5.0% |
| Promyelocytes | 1–8% |
| Myelocytes | 5–19% |
| Metamyelocytes | 9–24% |
| Bands | 9–15% |
| Segmented cells | 7–30% |
| Eosinophil precursors | 0.5–3.0% |
| Eosinophils | 0.5–4.0% |
| Basophilic series | 0.2–0.7% |
| Erythroid cells | |
| Pronormoblasts | 1–8% |
| Basophilic normoblasts | |
| Polychromatophilic normoblasts | 7–32% |
| Orthochromatic normoblasts | |
| Megakaryocytes | 0.1% |
| Lymphoreticular cells | |
| Lymphocytes | 3–17% |
| Plasma cells | 0–2% |
| Reticulum cells | 0.1–2.0% |
| Monocytes | 0.5–5.0% |
| Myeloid/erythroid ratio | 0.6–2.7 |

| | |
|---|---|
| Haptoglobin, serum | 100–300 mg/dl |
| Hemoglobin | |
| Hemoglobin $A_{1C}$ | 0–5% of total |
| Hemoglobin $A_2$ by column | 2–3% of total |
| Hemoglobin, fetal | < 1% of total |
| Hemoglobin, plasma | 0–5% of total |
| Hemoglobin, serum | 2–3 mg/ml |
| Iron, serum | |
| Male | 75–175 µg/dl |
| Female | 65–165 µg/dl |
| Iron-binding capacity, total serum (TIBC) | 250–450 µg/dl |
| Iron turnover rate (plasma) | 20–42 mg/24 h |
| Leukocyte alkaline phosphatase (LAP) score | 30–150 |
| Methemoglobin | < 1.8% |
| Osmotic fragility | |
| Hemolysis begins 0.45–0.38 NaCl | |
| Hemolysis completed 0.33–0.30 NaCl | |

Reticulocytes
    Male                                  4.6–6.2
    Female                              4.2–5.4

Schilling test (urinary excretion of radiolabeled vitamin $B_{12}$ after "flushing" intramuscular injection of $B_{12}$)    6–30% of oral dose within 24 h

| | Male | Female |
|---|---|---|
| Sedimentation rate | | |
|   Wintrobe | 0–5 mm/h | 0–15 mm/h |
|   Westergren | 0–15 mm/h | 0–20 mm/h |
| Transferrin saturation, serum | 20–50% | |
| Volume | Male | Female |
|   Blood | 52–83 ml/kg | 50–75 ml/kg |
|   Plasma | 25–43 ml/kg | 28–45 ml/kg |
|   Red cell | 20–36 ml/kg | 19–31 ml/kg |

**Table A-3.** Complete blood count

| Parameter | Male | Female |
|---|---|---|
| Hematocrit (%) | 40–52 | 38–48 |
| Hemoglobin (g/dl) | 13.5–18.0 | 12–16 |
| Erythrocyte count ($\times 10^{12}$ cells/L) | 4.6–6.2 | 4.2–5.4 |
| Reticulocyte count (%) | 0.6–2.6 | 0.4–2.4 |
| MCV (fL) | 82–98 | 82–98 |
| MCH (pg) | 27–32 | 27–32 |
| MCHC (g/dl) | 32–36 | 32–36 |
| WBC ($\times 10^9$ cells/L) | 4.5–11.0 | 4.5–11.0 |
| Segmented neutrophils | 1.8–7.7 | 1.8–7.7 |
|   Average (%) | 40–60 | 40–60 |
| Bands (cells) | 0–0.3 | 0–0.3 |
|   Average (%) | 0–3 | 0–3 |
| Eosinophils (cells $\times 10^9$/L) | 0–0.5 | 0–0.5 |
|   Average (%) | 0–5 | 0–5 |
| Basophils (cells $\times 10^9$/L) | 0–0.2 | 0–0.2 |
|   Average (%) | 0–1 | 0–1 |
| Lymphocytes (cells $\times 10^9$/L) | 1.0–4.8 | 1.0–4.8 |
|   Average (%) | 20–45 | 20–45 |
| Monocytes (cells $\times 10^9$/L) | 0–0.8 | 0–0.8 |
|   Average (%) | 2–6 | 2–6 |
| Platelet count (cells $\times 10^9$/L) | 150–350 | 150–350 |

## Coagulation Normal Values

| | |
|---|---|
| Template bleeding time | 3.5–7.5 min |
| Clot retraction, qualitative | Apparent in 30–60 min; complete in 24 h, usually in 6 h |

Coagulation time (Lee-White)

| | |
|---|---|
|   Glass tubes | 5–15 min |
|   Siliconized tubes | 20–60 min |
| Euglobulin lysis time | 120–240 min |
| Factors II, V, VII, VIII, IX, X, XI, or XII | 100% or 1.0 unit/ml |
| Fibrin degradation products | $< 10$ µg/ml or titer $\leqslant 1.4$ |
| Fibrinogen | 200–400 mg/ml |
| Partial thromboplastin time, activated | 20–40 s |
| Prothrombin time (PT) | 11–14 s |
| Thrombin time | 10–15 s |
| Whole blood clot lysis time | $> 24$ h |

---

## Pulmonary Function Tests

---

Abbreviations

    $P_B$ = barometric pressure (mm Hg)

  $F_{I}O_2$ = inspired oxygen fraction (0.21 = room air)

$PaCO_2$ = partial pressure of carbon dioxide in arterial blood (mm Hg)

$P_ACO_2$ = partial pressure of carbon dioxide in alveolar gas (mm Hg)

  $PaO_2$ = partial pressure of oxygen in arterial blood (mm Hg)

  $P_AO_2$ = partial pressure of oxygen in alveolar gas (mm Hg)

Alveolar-arterial oxygen gradient ($F_{I}O_2$ = 0.21)

  $P_{(A-a)}$ in adolescents = $< 10$ mm Hg

    adults $< 40$ years = 10 mm Hg

        $> 40$ years = 10–15 mm Hg

Alveolar oxygen partial pressure (sea level, $F_{I}O_2$, = 0.21)

  $P_AO_2 = 150 - (1.2 \times PaCO_2)$

Blood gases ($F_{I}O_2$ = 0.21)

| | *Arterial* | *Alveolar* |
|---|---|---|
| $PO_2$ | 80–105 mm Hg | 90–115 mm Hg |
| $PCO_2$ | 38–44 mm Hg | 38–44 mm Hg |
| pH | 7.35–7.45 | |

Spirometric volumes and lung volumes are size-dependent.
Typical normal values for adults are provided.

| *Lung volumes* | *Male* | *Female* |
|---|---|---|
| Total lung capacity (TLC) | 6–7 L | 5–6 L |
| Functional residual capacity (FRC) | 2–3 L | 2–3 L |
| Residual values (RV) | 1–2 L | 1–2 L |

| *Measures of air flow* | | |
|---|---|---|
| Forced vital capacity (FVC) | 4.0 L | 3.0 L |
| One second forced vital capacity ($FEV_1$) | > 3.0 L | > 2.0 L |
| Pulmonary resistance (RL) | < 3.0 cm $H_2O$/sec/L | |
| Airway resistance (Raw) | < 2.5 cm $H_2O$/sec/L | |

| *Other* | |
|---|---|
| Pulmonary compliance (CL) | 0.2 L/cm $H_2O$ |
| Diffusing capacity (DLCO) | 25 ml CO/min/mm Hg |

## Renal Function Tests

Anion gap

$$Na^+ - HCO_3^- + Cl^- = 10 \pm 2 \text{ meq/L}$$

Osmolality

$$\text{Osmolality (serum)} = 2\,Na\,(meq/L) + \frac{BUN\,(mg/dl)}{2.8} + \frac{glucose\,(mg/dl)}{18}$$

Bicarbonate deficit

$$HCO_3^- \text{ deficit} = \text{body weight (kg)} \times 0.4\,(\text{desired } HCO_3^- - \text{observed } HCO_3^-)$$

Glomerular filtration rate

$$\begin{aligned}
GFR &= \frac{Ucr \times V}{Pcr} \\
&= 130 \pm 20 \text{ ml/min in males} \\
&= 120 \pm 15 \text{ ml/min in females} \\
&\cong \frac{Ucr}{Pcr} \times 70
\end{aligned}$$

where

Ucr = urine creatinine (mg/dl)
Pcr = plasma creatinine (mg/dl)
V = urine volume/24 h (ml/min)

Renal plasma flow

$$\begin{aligned}
RPF &= \frac{Upah \times V}{Ppah} \\
&= 700 \pm 130 \text{ ml/min in males} \\
&= 600 \pm 100 \text{ ml/min in females}
\end{aligned}$$

where

Upah = urine para-aminohippuric acid (mg/dl)
V = urine volume/24 h (ml/min)
Ppah = plasma para-aminohippuric acid (mg/dl)

| | Serum Normal Values |
|---|---|
| Acetoacetate | 0.3–2.0 mg/dl |
| Acid phosphatase | 0–0.8 U/ml |
| Acid phosphatase, prostatic | 2.5–12.0 IU/L |
| Albumin | 3.0–5.5 g/dl |
| Aldolase | 1–6 IU/L |
| Alkaline phosphatase<br>  15–20 years<br>  20–101 years | <br>40–200 IU/L<br>35–125 IU/L |
| Alpha-1 antitrypsin | 200–500 mg/dl |
| Ammonia | 11–35 μmol/L |
| Amylase, serum | 2–20 U/L |
| Anion gap | 8–12 meq/L (mmol/L) |
| Ascorbic acid | 0.4–1.5 mg/dl |
| Bilirubin<br>  Total<br>  Direct | <br>0.2–1.2 mg/dl<br>0–0.4 mg/dl |
| Bromosulphalein (BSP) | Normal retention: 0–5% at 45 min |
| Calcium, serum | 8.7–10.6 mg/dl |
| Carbon dioxide, total | 18–30 meq/L (mmol/L) |
| Carcinoembryonic antigen, serum | < 2.5 μg/L |
| Carotene (carotenoids) | 50–300 μg/dl |
| C3 complement | 55–120 mg/dl |
| C4 complement | 14–51 mg/dl |
| Ceruloplasmin | 15–60 mg/dl |
| Chloride, serum | 95–105 meq/L (mmol/L) |
| Cholesterol, total<br>  12–19 years<br>  20–29 years<br>  30–39 years<br>  40–49 years<br>  50–59 years | <br>120–230 mg/dl<br>120–240 mg/dl<br>140–270 mg/dl<br>150–310 mg/dl<br>160–330 mg/dl |
| Copper | 100–200 μg/dl |
| Creatine phosphokinase, total | 20–200 IU/L |
| Creatine phosphokinase, isoenzymes<br>  MM fraction | <br>94–95% |

| | |
|---|---|
| MB fraction | 0–5% |
| BB fraction | 0–2% |
| Normal values in | |
| Heart | 80% MM, 20% MB |
| Brain | 100% BB |
| Skeletal muscle | 95% MM, 2% MB |
| Creatinine, serum | |
| Female adult | 0.5–1.3 mg/dl |
| Male adult | 0.7–1.5 mg/dl |
| Delta-aminolevulinic acid (ALA) | < 200 μg/dl |
| α-Fetoprotein, serum | < 40 μg/L |
| Folate, serum | 1.9–14.0 ng/ml |
| Gamma glutamyl transpeptidase | |
| Male | 12–38 IU/L |
| Female | 9–31 IU/L |
| Gastrin | 60–200 pg/ml |
| Glucose, serum | 70–120 mg/dl |
| Glucose 6-phosphate dehydrogenase | 5–10 IU/g Hb |
| G6PD screen, qualitative | Negative |
| Haptoglobin | 100–300 mg/dl |
| Hemoglobin $A_2$ | 0–4% of total Hb |
| Hemoglobin F | 0–2% of total Hb |
| Immunoglobulin, quantitation | |
| IgG | 700–1500 mg/dl |
| IgA | 70–400 mg/dl |
| IgM | |
| Male | 30–250 mg/dl |
| Female | 30–300 mg/dl |
| IgD | 0–40 mg/dl |
| Insulin, fasting | 6–26 μU/ml |
| Iron binding capacity | 250–400 μg/dl |
| Iron, total, serum | 40–150 μg/dl |
| Lactic acid | 0.6–1.8 meq/L |
| LDH, serum | 20–220 IU/L |
| LDH isoenzymes | |
| $LDH_1$ | 20–34% |
| $LDH_2$ | 28–41% |
| $LDH_3$ | 15–25% |
| $LDH_4$ | 3–12% |
| $LDH_5$ | 6–15% |
| Leucine aminopeptidase (LAP) | 30–55 IU/L |

| | |
|---|---|
| Lipase | 4–24 IU/dl |
| Magnesium, serum | 1.5–2.5 meq/L |
| 5′-Nucleotidase | 0.3–3.2 Bodansky units |
| Osmolality, serum | 278–305 mOsm/kg serum water |
| Phenolsulfonphthalein (PSP) | > 25% excreted within 15 min after injection of 1 ml dye |
| Phenylalanine | 3 mg/dl |
| Phosphorus, inorganic, serum | 2.0–4.3 mg/dl |
| Potassium, plasma | 3.1–4.3 meq/L |
| Potassium, serum | 3.5–5.2 meq/L |

Protein, total, serum
| 2–55 years | 5.0–8.0 g/dl |
|---|---|
| 55–101 years | 6.0–8.3 g/dl |

Protein electrophoresis, serum
| Albumin | 3.5–5.2 g/dl |
|---|---|
| Alpha-1 | 0.6–1.0 g/dl |
| Alpha-2 | 0.6–1.0 g/dl |
| Beta | 0.6–1.2 g/dl |
| Gamma | 0.7–1.5 g/dl |

| | |
|---|---|
| SGOT | 5–40 IU/L |
| Sodium, serum | 135–145 meq/L |
| Sulfate | 0.5–1.5 mg/dl |
| $T_3$ uptake | 25–45% |
| $T_4$ | 4.5–11.5 µg/dl |

Triglycerides
| 2–29 years | 10–140 mg/dl |
|---|---|
| 30–39 years | 20–150 mg/dl |
| 40–49 years | 20–160 mg/dl |
| 50–59 years | 20–190 mg/dl |
| 60–101 years | 20–200 mg/dl |

Urea nitrogen, serum
| 2–65 years | 5–22 mg/dl |
|---|---|
| 65–101 years | |
| Male | 10–38 mg/dl |
| Female | 8–26 mg/dl |

Uric acid
| 10–59 years | |
|---|---|
| Male | 2.5–9.0 mg/dl |
| Female | 2.0–8.0 mg/dl |
| 60–101 years | |
| Male | 2.5–9.0 mg/dl |
| Female | 2.5–9.0 mg/dl |

| | |
|---|---|
| Viscosity | 1.4–1.8 (serum compared to $H_2O$) |
| Vitamin A | 0.15–0.60 µg/ml |
| Vitamin $B_{12}$ | 200–850 pg/ml |

## Stool Normal Values

| | |
|---|---|
| Bulk | |
| Wet weight | < 197 g/24 h |
| Dry weight | < 66.4 g/24 h |
| Coproporphyrin | 12–832 mg/24 h |
| Fat (on a diet containing 30 g fat/day) | < 7.2 g/24 h or < 30% of dry weight |
| Nitrogen | < 2.2 g/24 h |
| Urobilinogen | 40–280 mg/24 h |
| Water | Approximately 65% |

## Synovial Fluid Normal Values

| | |
|---|---|
| Cells | < 200 cells/mm³ |
| Polymorphonuclear cells | < 25% |
| Crystals | None |
| Fibrin clot | None |
| Glucose | Same as serum |
| Hyaluronic acid | 2.45–3.97 g/L |
| pH | 7.31–7.64 |
| Protein | < 2.5 g/dl |
| Albumin | 63% |
| $\alpha_1$-Globulins | 7% |
| $\alpha_2$-Globulins | 7% |
| β-Globulins | 9% |
| γ-Globulins | 14% |
| Relative viscosity | > 300 |
| Uric acid | Same as serum |

## Toxicology

**Table A-4.** Serum values for drugs and toxic substances

| Substance | Therapeutic range | Toxic range |
|---|---|---|
| Acetaminophen | 10–20 mg/L | > 150 mg/L 4 h after ingestion |
| Alcohol | 0 | 150–300 mg/dl: confusion<br>300–450 mg/dl: stupor<br>> 400 mg/dl: coma → death |
| Amphetamine | 0 | |
| Amobarbital | 7–15 µg/ml | |
| Bromide | 20–120 mg/dl | > 150 mg/dl |
| Carbamazepine | 6–10 µg/ml | |
| Clonazepam | 0.02–0.10 µg/ml | |
| Digitoxin | 5–40 ng/ml | |
| Digoxin | 0.5–2.0 ng/ml | > 2.0 ng/ml |
| Diphenylhydantoin | 10–20 µg/ml | |
| Ethosuximide | 40–100 µg/ml | |
| Glutethimide | 1–7 µg/ml | |
| Lead | < 40 µg/dl; occupational < 80 µg/dl | |
| Lithium | 0.5–1.5 meq/L | 2.0 meq/L |
| Meprobamate | 10–20 µg/ml | 30–70 µg/ml: coma |
| Methanol | 0 | |
| Pentobarbital | 4–6 µg/ml | |
| Phenobarbital | 5–30 µg/ml | > 40 µg/ml |
| Primidone | 4–12 µg/ml | |
| Procainamide | 4–6 µg/ml | |
| Propranolol | 100–300 ng/ml | |
| Quinidine | 3–5 µg/ml | > 8 µg/ml |
| Salicylate | 20–25 mg/dl | 30 mg/dl |
| Secobarbital | 3–5 µg/ml | |
| Theophylline | 10–20 µg/ml | |
| Valproic acid | < 100 µg/ml | |

| | **Urine Normal Values** |
|---|---|
| Acidity, titratable | 20–40 meq/24 h |
| Ammonia | 30–50 meq/24 h |
| Amylase | 35–260 Somogyi units/h |
| Bence Jones protein | None detected |
| Bilirubin | None detected |
| Calcium | |
|   Unrestricted diet | < 300 mg/24 h (men)<br>< 250 mg/24 h (women) |
|   Low calcium diet (200 mg/day for 3 days) | < 150 mg/24 h |
| Chloride | 120–240 meq/24 h (varies with dietary intake) |
| Copper | 0–32 μg/24 h |
| Creatine | |
|   Male | 0–40 mg/24 h |
|   Female | 0–100 mg/24 h |
| Creatinine | 1.0–1.6 g/24 h or 15–25 mg/kg body weight/24 h |
| Cysteine, qualitative | Negative |
| Delta-aminolevulinic acid | 1.3–7.0 mg/24 h |
| Glucose | |
|   Qualitative | None detected |
|   Quantitative | 16–300 mg/24 h |
| Hemoglobin | None detected |
| Homogentisic acid | None detected |
| Iron | 40–140 μg/24 h |
| Lead | 0–120 μg/24 h |
| Myoglobin | None detected |
| Osmolality | 50–1200 mOsm/L |
| pH | 4.6–8.0 |
| Phenylpyruvic acid, qualitative | None detected |
| Phosphorus | 0.8–2.0 g/24 h |
| Porphobilinogen | |
|   Qualitative | None detected |
|   Quantitative | 0–2.4 mg/24 h |
| Porphyrins | |
|   Coproporphyrin | 50–250 μg/24 h |
|   Uroporphyrin | 10–30 μg/24 h |

| | |
|---|---|
| Potassium | 25–100 meq/24 h |
| Protein | |
|   Qualitative | None detected |
|   Quantitative | 10–150 mg/24 h |
| Sodium | 130–260 meq/24 h (varies with dietary sodium intake) |
| Specific gravity | 1.003–1.030 |
| Uric acid | 80–976 mg/24 h |
| Urobilinogen | 0.05–3.5 mg/24 h; < 1.0 Ehrlich units/2 h |

# Index